# Also Available

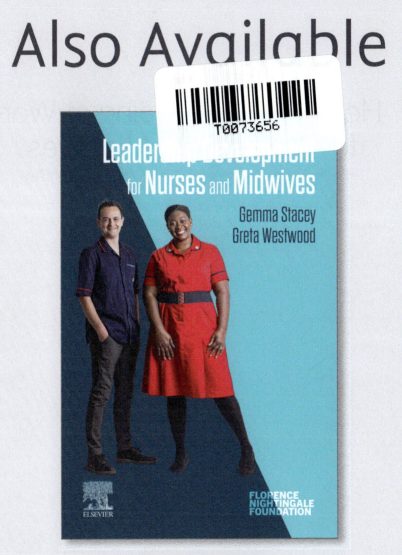

ISBN: 9780323870498

ELSEVIER

# Health and Wellbeing at Work for Nurses and Midwives

# Health and Wellbeing at Work for Nurses and Midwives

**HOLLY BLAKE, PhD, CPsychol, PGCHE, BA (Hons), SFHEA**

Professor of Behavioural Medicine
School of Health Sciences, University of Nottingham
Nottingham, UK

**GEMMA STACEY, PhD, MN, RN (MENTAL HEALTH), PGCHE, PFHEA**

Director of Academy
Florence Nightingale Foundation
London, UK

ELSEVIER

ISBN: 9780323880534

Content Strategist: Poppy Garraway
Content Project Manager: Kritika Kaushik
Design: Ryan Cook
Marketing Manager: Belinda Tudin

Last digit is the print number: 9  8  7  6  5  4  3  2  1

Working together
to grow libraries in
developing countries

www.elsevier.com • www.bookaid.org

# CONTENTS

Health and wellbeing amongst the nursing and midwifery workforce has long been a consideration but not always a priority. With concerns about the retention of early career and established health care professionals rising, we are seeing an increased commitment to systematically address the factors that influence and undermine health and wellbeing in the full range of health and social care environments.

In this book, we aim to explore these factors in an accessible and practical way. The purpose is to highlight issues that impact on health and wellbeing and offer examples of strategies that have been implemented to support and enhance the wellbeing of the workforce. Authors with expertise in nursing, midwifery, workplace health, and psychology will offer their insights informed by theory, research, and policy. The book will be helpful to individuals looking to enrich their own wellbeing and experiences at work and those of their colleagues, team leaders committed to creating team cultures and working environments that foster wellbeing, and senior leaders influencing the policies and practices of the organisation that have the potential to embed wellbeing into the fabric of the clinical environment.

## Section 1: The Case for Health and WellBeing at Work

The first section outlines the cost of ill health to employers and provides the business case for organisations to invest in wellbeing by outlining the costs to employers of ill health in the workforce. We offer perspectives on the way in which health and wellbeing can be impacted by the health and social care environment and the nature of the work nurses and midwives engage in on a day-to-day basis. This section demonstrates why health and wellbeing should be a primary consideration for employers in terms of the impact of health and ill health on individuals, the workforce, and the organisation, and how it impacts on the quality of care that nurses and midwives can provide. This section includes the following chapters:

1. Why Health Care Employers Should Promote Health: The Costs of Ill Health at Work
2. Caring for Yourself, To Care for Others: Prioritising Self-Care
3. How Staff WellBeing Relates to Patient Experiences of Care
4. How Stress and Anxiety Affect the Body
5. Understanding Compassion Fatigue and Burnout

## Section 2: Managing Emotions in Difficult Times

The second section advances to explore the ways in which ongoing concerns that diminish wellbeing can progress into more significant challenges associated with mental health issues. This section is intended to highlight the early warning signs of deterioration in mental health and offer strategies that destigmatise and encourage an open dialogue amongst nurses and midwives in relation to their emotional wellbeing. Chapters focus on how to manage emotions in challenging times:

6. Untangling Difficult Emotions on the Job
7. Starting Conversations About Your Mental Health
8. Dealing With Anxiety and Low Mood

## Section 3: WellBeing Needs at Different Times

The third section is a discussion of the varying wellbeing needs that impact at various stages of our careers or because of different job-related or lifestyle factors. It is an acknowledgement of the transient and fluctuating variables that can impact on wellbeing and emphasises the importance of wellbeing strategies that are purposefully targeted to meet the unique needs of our diverse workforce. Chapters include:

9. Shiftwork, Sleep, and Managing Fatigue
10. WellBeing Needs During Periods of Fasting
11. WellBeing and Late Career Nurses and Midwives
12. Mental WellBeing in Nursing and Midwifery Students

## Section 4: Enhancing WellBeing at Work

The final section offers examples of factors that enhance wellbeing in the workplace. Underpinning this is the creation of psychologically safe working environments where nurses and midwives feel encouraged to share their challenges and raise their concerns. It is argued that this is the foundation for wellbeing interventions, strategies, and innovations to be received by the nursing and midwifery workforce as a valued investment in them and their holistic health. This section also includes a focus on strategies for self-care and healthy lifestyles and concludes with the learning that has arisen from the psychological impact of responding to the Covid-19 pandemic. Chapters include:

13. Psychologically Safe Working Environments
14. Clinical Supervision and WellBeing
15. Developing Teamwork and Social Support Across Occupational Boundaries
16. Enhancing Health and WellBeing Through Shared Governance
17. Acknowledging the Emotional and Social Challenges of Nursing and Midwifery Through Schwartz Rounds
18. Supporting Distressed Colleagues Using Psychological First Aid
19. Being Physically Active
20. Healthy Eating, Diet, and Obesity
21. The Impacts of Dehydration and Staying Hydrated at Work
22. The Challenge of Health and WellBeing in a Crisis

We end the book with our final chapter:

23. The Future of Health and WellBeing at Work

The Covid-19 pandemic is a contemporary crisis that has caused an unprecedented disruption and pressure on the nursing and midwifery workforce. This has reinforced the importance of protecting the workforce wellbeing across healthcare services. However, we must acknowledge that the emotional implications of healthcare practice have *always* been significant. The occurrence of moral injury, working with limited resources, and lack of access to appropriate reflective learning spaces have been a longstanding experience of nurses and midwives. Sustained and embedded wellbeing strategies must therefore be an organisational priority and not simply a reactive remedial response to a crisis.

*Holly Blake and Gemma Stacey*

Supporting patients and clients 24 hours a day, 7 days a week, nurses and midwives have the highest levels of occupational stress and resulting distress compared with other groups. Working in an environment where the human needs of others are often an urgent priority, it easy for nurses and midwives to put their own needs last.

The health and wellbeing of the nursing and midwifery workforce have been considered important but not always absolute essential priorities. The Covid-19 pandemic changed this by shining a light on the critical significance of the psychological wellbeing of healthcare staff, particularly nurses working on the frontline. At the beginning of the pandemic in 2020, we wrote:

> *As researchers who have studied nurse wellbeing for decades, it is gratifying to see the increased focus on health care staff wellbeing, yet sad that it takes a pandemic to recognise its critical importance.*

The immense challenges and trauma that nurses experienced during their working lives were finally being recognised and acknowledged, and we hoped that this was an opportunity to:

> *fully recognise the inherent stresses and emotional strain that nurses bear on behalf of society and ensure support, not only through this crisis but after it is all over. When healthcare is back to "normal," ongoing support for nurses' wellbeing will remain critically important.*

From research undertaken with nurses and midwives during the pandemic, which highlights the stress, trauma, and distress experienced by nurses (see Chapter 22), we know how important this ongoing support is and will continue to be for some time to come. This book is therefore both timely and important.

Significantly, this text recognises that the responsibility for nurses' and midwives' psychological health is a collective national and organisational responsibility, not just an individual one. Placing responsibility for good mental health on individuals and exhorting them to improve their resilience neglects the wider structural and organisational constraints that negatively affect staff psychological wellbeing and lets organisations off the hook, so to speak. Remaining resilient in, for example, the face of staff shortages is an impossible expectation. Yet, staff need to keep going and manage work challenges.

This book therefore provides critical information on the ways to manage emotions in difficult times and start conversations about mental health at work. It also has some important insights into the links between psychological and physical health and identifies wellbeing needs at different times and career stages. It provides practical and accessible guidance to nurses and midwives on managing their psychological wellbeing at work and includes a wealth of helpful case studies to inspire innovation and change.

Our national study evaluating Schwartz Rounds identified the importance of interprofessional support and psychological safety at work. Chapters in this book pick up these important points, showing how to create psychologically safe work environments and social support across occupational boundaries within teams. This book provides tangible action to support the promotion of a culture of psychological safety where wellbeing can be openly discussed—an important step in reducing stigma and recognising the impact of providing emotional support for people accessing health and care services, and colleagues, in the face of challenging work situations and trauma.

Finally, and importantly, the authors in this book show that there is a link between staff psychological wellbeing at work and patient experiences and outcomes of care. Over a decade ago, my colleagues and I demonstrated that the experience of healthcare staff shapes people's experiences of care, whether good or bad.

We now know there are significant costs to nurses themselves (stress, burnout, and ill health), to health and care organisations (high rates of sickness absence and poor retention rates), and to the delivery of high-quality care for people accessing health and care services, when nurses' and midwives' health and wellbeing is not prioritised.

Health and care professionals come to work to support people at some of the most difficult times of their lives, support their colleagues, and ultimately make a difference by providing high-quality care and support. To do this they should be able to gain help with their psychological health, not as an add-on but as an expected and central part of work.

Changing the work environment to promote positive staff wellbeing at work starts here. I hope this book provides new ideas, inspiration, and support to nurses in the vital work that they do and enables them to do what they came into the profession to do: care well for people and have a rich and satisfying career, thriving at work within an organisational culture that support this at its core.

Professors Holly Blake and Gemma Stacey have brought together an important range of topics, insights, and case studies providing varied and novel perspectives not included in other nursing- and midwifery-focused texts on workplace wellbeing.

Happy reading, keep well, and I hope it inspires and supports you in the important work that you do.

*Professor Jill Maben, OBE*

The editors would like to acknowledge and offer grateful thanks for the input of all contributors, without whom this edition would not have been possible.

**Maria Armaou, PhD Education, MSc Occupational Psychology, BSc Psychology**
Postgraduate Research Assistant
Psychology, Health and Professional
  Development
Oxford Brookes University
Oxford, UK

**Aimee Aubeeluck, PhD, MSc, PGCHE, BA (Hons)**
Professor of Health Psychology Education
School of Health Sciences
University of Nottingham
Nottingham, UK

**Kiran K. Bains**
Health Psychologist
University of London
London, UK
Honorary Research Fellow
School of Health Sciences
University of London
London, UK

**Holly Blake, PhD, CPsychol, PGCHE, CPsychol, BA (Hons), SFHEA**
Professor of Behavioural Medicine
School of Health Sciences, University
  of Nottingham
Nottingham, UK

**Louise Bramley, PhD, MA (Research Methods), BSc**
Head of Nursing and Midwifery Research
Institute of Care Excellence
Nottingham University Hospitals NHS Trust,
  Nottingham, UK

**Charles Anthony (Tony) Butterworth, CBE, FRCN, FMed, Sci, PhD, MSc, RNT, RMN, RGN.**
Professor Emeritus of Healthcare Workforce
  Innovation
University of Lincoln
Lincoln, UK

**Liz Charalambous, PhD, MSc, PGCHE, BSc (Hons), RN**
Assistant Professor
School of Health Sciences
The University of Nottingham
Nottingham, UK

**Aquiline Chivinge, MSc, BN, Diploma in OH, Diploma in Midwifery, and Diploma in Nursing**
Assistant Director of Nursing
Corporate Nursing
Nottingham University Hospital NHS Trust
Nottingham, UK

**Joanne Cooper, PhD, RN**
Assistant Director of Nursing
Nottingham University Hospitals NHS Trust
Nottingham, UK

**Dr Emma Coyne, ClinPsyD, BSc**
Consultant Clinical Psychologist
Nottingham University Hospitals NHS Trust
Nottingham, UK

**Jo Daniels, DClinPsy**
Academic Director, Doctorate in Clinical
  Psychology
Senior Lecturer FHEA, Department of
  Psychology
University of Bath, Bath, UK
Specialist Clinical Psychologist
North Bristol NHS Trust, Bristol, UK

**Joy Darch**
Health and Social Care
University of Gloucestershire
Cheltenham, UK

**Anne Felton, PhD, MN, PGCHE, BA (Hons), RN (Mental Health), RNT SFHEA**
Head of Department
Institute of Health and Allied Professions
School of Social Sciences, Nottingham Trent
  University
Nottingham, UK

**Sue Haines, DHSci, MA, BSc (Hons), RGN**
Assistant Director of Nursing (Education,
    Professional Development and Leadership)
Institute of Care Excellence
Nottingham University Hospitals
    NHS Trust
Nottingham, UK

**Katharine Halford, OBE, RN, RSCN**
Chief Nurse
Barking, Havering and Redbridge University
    Hospitals
NHS Trust, UK

**Charlotte Halls**
Community Mental Health Nurse, Perinatal
    Service
Nottinghamshire Healthcare Trust
Nottingham, UK

**Juliet Hassard, BA (Hons) MSc PhD PGCHE**
Associate Professor of Occupational Health
    Psychology
Mental Health and Clinical Neuroscience,
School of Medicine
Nottingham, UK

**Valerie James**
Independent Consultant
Corporate Psychologist
Visiting Senior Fellow, Kingston University
    and St George's
University of London
London, UK

**Samantha Kelly, PhD, MSc, PGCAP, BA (Hons)**
Consultant Nurse
Crisis Resolution Home Treatment
Derbyshire Healthcare NHS Foundation
    Trust
Derby, UK

**Richard Kyle, PhD, MA (Hons)**
Professor of Interprofessional Education
Academy of Nursing
University of Exeter
Exeter, UK

**Olga Lainidi**
University of Macedonia
Thessaloniki, Greece

**Paul Maloret, RN (LD) DipHE, BSc, PG Cert,
MSc, DHres**
Interim Head of School
Associate Head of School
School of Nursing, Midwifery and Allied
    Health
Buckinghamshire New University
Uxbridge, UK

**Maria Moirasgenti, PhD, MSc, RN**
Nurse Manager
Coronary Care Unit
AHEPA University Hospital of Thessaloniki
Thessaloniki, Greece

**Anthony Montgomery, PhD**
Professor of Occupational and Organisational
    Psychology
Psychology
Northumbria University
Newcastle, UK

**Rachel Paskell, DClinPsy, MSc, BSc Hons**
Clinical Psychologist and Lecturer
Department of Psychology
University of Bath
Bath, Somerset, UK

**Sally Pezaro, PhD, MSc, FRCM, SFHEA, BA
(Hons), RM, DipMid**
Adjunct Associate Professor, The University
    of Notre Dame, Australia
Assistant Professor
Centre for Healthcare Research
Coventry University
Conventry, UK

**Aggie Rice, MSc, BA (Hons)**
Schwartz Rounds Community Lead
Staff Experience Team
The Point of Care Foundation
London, UK

**Rohit Sagoo, MRes, BSc, Dip HE**
PhD Student
Institute for Health Research
University of Bedfordshire
Luton, UK

**Jessica Sainsbury, RN, Bachelor of Nursing (Adult and Mental Health)**
Research and Policy Associate
Florence Nightingale Foundation
London, UK

**Stefan Schilling, PhD, MSc, MA, FHEA**
UKRI/ESRC Research Fellow
Department of Psychology, Health & Professional Development
Oxford Brookes University
Oxford, UK
Associate Fellow
School of Security Studies
King's College
London, UK

**Kerry Sheldon, DClinPsy, PhD, MSc, BA (Hons), PGCert**
Principal Clinical Psychologist
Windermere Lodge/Older Adult Mental Health Unit
Rotherham, Doncaster & South Humberside NHS Trust (RDASH)
Doncaster, UK

**Gemma Stacey, PhD, MN, RN (Mental Health), PGCHE, PFHEA**
Director of Academy
Florence Nightingale Foundation
London, UK

**Hollie Starbuck, BSc Mental Health Nursing, BA (Hons) Drama and Theatre**
Senior Mental Health Practitioner
Oxford Children and Adolescent Eating Disorder Service
Oxford Health Foundation Trust
Oxford, UK

**Kevin Teoh, PhD, MSc, BSc**
Senior Lecturer in Organizational Psychology
Department of Organizational Psychology
Birkbeck, University of London
London, UK

**Rebecca Thomas, MSc, BSc, HNDip, PgCEd**
Senior Nurse Improvement
Improvement and Innovation
Cwm Taf Morgannwg University Health Board
Merthyr Tydfil, South Wales, UK

**Jane Wills, MSc, PGCE, BA**
Professor Health promotion
Institute of Health and Social Care
London South Bank University
London, UK

This book is dedicated to nurses and midwives across the
world who have courageously and selflessly provided care
during the pandemic. Through their commitment, tenacity
and determination, many lives have been saved. Now we
must wait patiently as colleagues slowly repair and recover
from the frenetic work of the last two years. We owe them
our wholehearted gratitude.

We remember the nurses, midwives, nursing associates
and health care support workers who sadly lost their lives
during the pandemic. "Fallen in the cause of saving lives,
a glory that shines upon our tears." We thank them for
their leadership, courage and compassion. They surely give
their today for our tomorrow.

Professor Greta Westwoon CBE – Chief Executive Officer,
Florence Nightingale Foundation

# The Case for Health and WellBeing at Work

Kevin Rui-Han Teoh ■ Juliet Hassard ■ Holly Blake

## SECTION OUTLINE

1 Why health care employers should promote health: the costs of ill health at work

2 Caring for yourself, to care for others: prioritising self-care

3 How staff wellbeing relates to patient experiences of care

4 How stress and anxiety affect the body

5 Understanding compassion fatigue and burnout

# Why Health Care Employers Should Promote Health: The Costs of Ill Health at Work

Kevin Rui-Han Teoh ■ Juliet Hassard ■ Holly Blake

## KEY POINTS

1. Work-related ill health comes at a cost to the individual, to patients, and to the organisation. These exist as workforce issues, poor patient care, and financial costs.
2. The financial costs can be separated into direct costs (that which incurs a monetary exchange such as medication costs), indirect costs (loss of productivity), and intangible costs (the pain and suffering experienced).
3. Not all costs are immediately visible as some nurses and midwives will still go to work when ill (i.e., presenteeism) and costs manifest over a longer period (such as the development of moral injury and compassion fatigue or leaving the workforce).
4. The different costs of ill health are inherently interlinked, with one type of cost having a knock-on effect on other costs. This means that over time there can be a perpetuating downward cycle, where the scale and impact of workplace ill health get cumulatively worse overtime.
5. There is considerable data available within organisations that can be harnessed to understand the costs within a specific context and to create a rationale for intervention.

## Introduction

We know that ill health is becoming more common among nurses and midwives. A review written for the Royal College of Nursing Foundation (Kinman et al., 2020) shows that nurses and midwives are at considerable risk of work-related stress, burnout, and mental health problems (such as depression and anxiety). This risk is greater than that of the general working population and appears to be increasing in response to rising demands on health and care services, staffing shortages, and concerns about limited funds and resources available to the health and care sector.

Action is needed to promote and support the health and wellbeing of nurses and midwives as there is a moral and ethical responsibility to do so. However, understanding the economic costs of ill health can help make a stronger case for action to employers and decision makers. In this chapter, we introduce three arguments as to why health care employers should aim to promote employee health: (i) to address staffing issues such as sickness absence, turnover (employees that leave and need to be replaced), and presenteeism (being present at work in ill health); (ii) to improve the standards of care provided; and (iii) to reduce the financial cost to organisations associated with employee ill health. We then offer some guidance on using data and estimating costs of ill health within a more specific individual or organisational context.

# The Cost of Ill Health

## COST IN RELATION TO WORKFORCE ISSUES

There are rising workforce challenges in the health and care services, with high rates of sickness absence, high turnover, and many vacancies. As rates of ill health increase, sickness absence rates also rise, as workers need time away from work to rest and recuperate. This in turns exacerbates staff shortages, placing additional pressure on colleagues who are working and increasing their risk of ill health.

To avoid the feeling of letting colleagues or patients down, nurses and midwives might engage in presenteeism. This refers to carrying on working while feeling unwell. While the exact reasons for doing this may vary, some do so to protect their income. Presenteeism is common among health care professionals. In 2020, 49.7% of the 157,000 nurses and midwives who took part in the National Health Service (NHS) Staff Survey (NHS Staff Survey Coordination Centre, 2020) reported engaging in presenteeism in the previous 3 months. While individuals might perceive this as a noble act, presenteeism not only jeopardises individual health but can reduce patient safety. People who work when they are sick may not perform at optimal level, and in health and care settings this might increase the risk of errors or reduce care quality. Coming to work with a viral infection also risks spreading it among colleagues and vulnerable patients. When employees do eventually go on sick leave they are often off work for a longer period. Longer sickness absence is problematic as it results in a longer gap on the rota, and in some cases it can reduce the likelihood of the individual successfully returning to the workplace again.

Research shows that between 40% and 60% of nurses and midwives are considering leaving their jobs (Kinman et al., 2020). The reasons for this are complex, but ill health is one of the primary factors for wanting to leave. For example, one study found that nurses experiencing burnout were more than twice as likely to consider leaving than those who were not burnt out (Heinen et al., 2013). While poor working conditions (e.g., long working hours, bullying, staff shortages) are key factors in nurses' and midwives' decisions to leave, many describe leaving to protect their wellbeing. While the focus here has been on ill health, where nurses and midwives report better wellbeing, they report higher levels of commitment to their organization (Kinman et al., 2020).

## COST TO PATIENT CARE

There is growing evidence that ill health among nurses and midwives has a negative impact on the care that they provide (Kinman et al., 2020). This happens in several different ways. For example, when a worker struggles with poor mental health, this person is more likely to make errors or to not follow established protocols, all of which can have serious repercussions for patients. It can also change the way in which the worker interacts with patients and colleagues, including being more rushed and perceived as less compassionate or empathetic. Not being able to provide the level of care that workers would like is linked with higher rates of compassion fatigue and moral injury among nurses and midwives, perpetuating the cycle between ill health and its costs. Compassion fatigue refers to when emotional and physical exhaustion diminishes one's ability to empathise or feel compassion for others. Moral injury occurs when an individual takes part in, sees, or fails to prevent events that clash with moral values and beliefs.

It is not only the individual nurse or midwife who is affected. Research shows that nurses who experience burnout also rate the care that their unit provides as being poor or being more unsafe (Kinman et al., 2020). While we do not have specific information for nurses and midwives, we do know that ill health among health care workers can be associated with poorer clinical care outcomes, more patient deaths, and higher rates of infections (Teoh et al., 2020). However, research findings are inconsistent since other studies have found no relationship between ill health of health care workers and patient care (Teoh et al., 2020). This is often attributed to health care workers working harder (e.g., taking no breaks, working longer hours, increasing concentration) to ensure that patients are not harmed. The danger, however, is that over an extended period this will take a toll on the individual nurse and midwife, leading to increased rates of ill health, sickness absence, and high turnover. All this has a disastrous effect on the long-term sustainability of the nursing and midwifery workforce.

## FINANCIAL COSTS

The previous sections begin to illustrate how ill health can carry a financial cost to organisations. To quantify this, we first need to recognise the different types of costs that economists will typically consider: direct costs, indirect costs, and intangible costs (Hassard et al., 2018).

Direct costs involve everything that has an exchange of money, such as the cost of medication, insurance fees, agency fees, or travel expenses. Indirect costs refer to costs that do not have a fixed price and includes, for example, loss of productivity, presenteeism, and sickness absence. These might be estimated by using the daily rate of a worker and multiplying that by the number of days that the worker is off (sickness absence) or the level in which a worker believes to be working at (presenteeism). Finally, intangible costs are about trying to cost the pain and suffering that someone might experience due to ill health. This not only includes a person's own suffering from ill health but also potentially related experiences (such as damaged personal relationships). Intangible costs are difficult to estimate, but they are typically estimated by asking individuals how much they would be willing to pay to avoid the issue they face.

To date, we are not aware of any attempt to quantify the cost of ill health to health care workers, not least nurses and midwives. However, analysis of the general UK workforce shows that the cost of mental ill health is between £41 and £102 per worker (Hassard et al., 2018). Focusing on workplace bullying alone, which is strongly associated with mental ill health, one estimate costed this at £2.281 billion to the NHS (Kline & Lewis, 2019), which is approximately £1885 for each NHS worker. This total was comprised of the summed costs of sickness absence (£302.2 million), presenteeism (£604.4 million), turnover (£231.9 million), and productivity (£575.7 million), as well as industrial relations, compensation, and litigation costs (£83.5 million). This shows not only the great expense but also the many ways in which costs are incurred for a single factor that influences health. Importantly, the complexity that goes into these calculations means that most of these figures are believed to be underestimates, with the genuine cost being substantially higher.

## Identifying Costs to a Specific Context

Having discussed the three forms of costs, we now consider how individuals and organisations can best identify how these costs might manifest in their local contexts.

Data relating to costs exists everywhere, and we can start by recognising what is available to us that can help us understand the scale of the issue. Most organisations routinely collect data on workforce issues, including sickness absence and turnover rates. Similarly, health care organisations also collect data around quality of care, including patient satisfaction, care outcomes, and safety reports. Information about the work experiences and health of workers is often collected as part of annual staff surveys, research studies, and occupational health data. This can provide a wealth of information about an organisation (or sections of it). For example, the UK NHS Staff Survey (NHS Staff Survey Coordination Centre, 2020) publicly releases its findings, which not only provides a local picture on measures such as work-related stress, presenteeism, and patient safety but also allows data on specific organisations to be compared against other organisations, professional groups, or the NHS more generally.

From these data sources it might be possible to compare teams with elevated levels of ill health or sickness absence to see how they are different on quality-of-care measures when compared with teams with low levels of ill health. Even on their own, issues of concern (e.g., high turnover rates, poor satisfaction scores) provide a starting point in which to explore why they occur and a plausible reason for interventions to be implemented.

In terms of estimating the financial costs (Hassard et al., 2018), some organisations have systems in place that allow for this to be calculated. Others may have data on costs such as agency spend on sickness absence or occupational health costs. It is also possible to provide a rough estimate of the cost of a single day's sickness absence by taking the total cost of an employee to the organisation (salary with overheads) and dividing it by 220 (the number of working days in a year). If this figure is not available, then the annual salary or the average salary for an employee would provide a basic picture.

This daily cost provides the basis to estimate the cost of sickness absence of a team or organisation by multiplying it by the number of sick days taken. It can also be used to estimate the cost of presenteeism or productivity. Here, employees would be asked at what capacity they were working, and this estimate would be applied to their daily cost. For example, an employee who was only able to work at 70% would cost the employer the daily cost multiplied by 30%.

Having a more specific picture of how ill health is affecting an organisation is vital to understanding the scale of the issue. Understanding all the different types of costs and impacts allows us to utilise a wider set of data and resources. In turn, this allows us to create a more accurate, and hopefully stronger, argument for taking action.

## Conclusion

Rates of ill health are high among the nursing and midwifery workforce. It is imperative that we recognise the associated costs that this has not only to individuals but to health and care employers as well. Costs to individuals, the broader workforce, organisations, and patient care are not separate from each other but are inherently interlinked. High levels of sickness absence, turnover, presenteeism, and poor standards of care come with higher financial costs to health and care organisations. In contrast, better wellbeing is associated with better care quality, greater productivity at work, and financial savings (Kinman et al., 2020). This provides a sound justification for urgent action to support the health of individual nurses and midwives and the collective health and care workforce.

### ACTIVITY

- Think about the last time you were ill. Did you go to work or not? What *type* of costs might this have incurred?

  _____

  _____

  _____

  _____

  _____

- Using the formula from this chapter, what might the financial cost of you (or another member) be for a day of sickness absence? What might the cost be of the last day you were not able to work at your usual level?

  _____

  _____

  _____

  _____

  _____

- Who are the stakeholders in your organisation who need to be convinced to take ill health more seriously? What data and information can you use to strengthen your case?

  _____

  _____

  _____

  _____

  _____

| CASE STUDY 1.1 | **Creating a Business Case to Support Staff Mental Health** |
|---|---|

Creating a business case for more support to improve staff wellbeing can be difficult when resources are limited. However, this is possible with a strong rationale. We share in this case study how we obtained more funding for staff posts over several years to better support staff wellbeing at Mid-Yorkshire NHS Hospitals Trust in the United Kingdom.

Our Head of Service commenced employment in 2016 and began an audit of departmental functions at clinical and nonclinical levels. An important finding was the difference between the level of mental health support needed versus what was offered. Discussions with the Head of Clinical Psychology highlighted the need for the Occupational Health & Wellbeing Service (OH&WbS) to have a more robust approach to supporting staff wellbeing. This was imperative given increasing local, national, and international evidence that health care workers were not coping as well with the pressures of work as they had in previous decades. It was clear that we needed additional longer-term input and proactive work to offset the reactive case management provision already in place. Subsequently, in 2017, it was agreed that the Clinical Psychology Service would be funded by the OH&WbS to provide an additional post to support it. This was for a Clinical Psychologist to provide proactive support for staff in services that were deemed to be struggling.

Over the next 18 months the demand for mental health support grew. By 2019, the subsequent increase in wait times for staff to receive support was acknowledged as an organisational risk. Discussions were held with agreements to fund an additional post. We then had to make more changes to acknowledge the impact of the COVID-19 pandemic on staff. Drawing on internal rostering data and international evidence for the numbers of staff that would require psychological treatment postpandemic, we predicted that 10% of staff (excluding medics) working in settings with the highest risk patients (known as red areas) will require psychological intervention following their experiences. This necessitated an additional 2.8 full-time equivalent clinicians, not including additional capacity for debriefing (learning conversations that occur soon after clinical events), group work, risk management, and more. Furthermore, these calculations do not include staff whose mental health has been impacted by the pandemic but who have not worked in red areas.

Additional investment would better allow us to support our staff across four levels by developing a (1) positive psychological wellbeing culture focus, (2) proactive psychological wellbeing focus, (3) responsive team focus, and (4) responsive individual focus. The anticipated benefits of this investment should translate to better outcomes on a range of existing organisational measures, including the NHS Staff Survey, sickness absence, staff retention, and Freedom to Speak Up data (relating to raising concerns whistleblowing policy for the NHS). Not investing in the proposed staff wellbeing services could also lead to distressed staff, poorer patient experience, and increased risk of errors or complaints. Crucially, NHS England estimates sickness absence costs more than £3 million annually for a midsized hospital trust and that even small improvements can equate to serious savings. For example, a 1% reduction in sickness absence equates to £1 million savings—a substantial savings compared to the approximate £300,000 required to fund the additional requested posts. This proposal led to the Executive sanctioning the additional posts to better support our staff's mental wellbeing.

**ELIZABETH A. WOOD**
Specialist Nurse Practitioner, Occupational Health & Wellbeing Centre,
The Mid-Yorkshire Hospitals NHS Trust

## References

Hassard, J., Teoh, K. R. H., Visockaite, G., Dewe, P., & Cox, T. (2018). The cost of work-related stress to society: A systematic review. *Journal of Occupational Health Psychology, 23*(1), 1–17. https://doi.org/10.1037/ocp0000069.

Heinen, M. M., van Achterberg, T., Schwendimann, R., et al. (2013). Nurses' intention to leave their profession: A cross sectional observational study in 10 European countries. *International Journal of Nursing Studies, 50*(2), 174–184. https://doi.org/10.1016/j.ijnurstu.2012.09.019.

Kinman, G., Teoh, K. R. -H., & Harriss, A. (2020). The mental health and wellbeing of nurses and midwives in the United Kingdom. *Society of Occupational Medicine.* https://www.som.org.uk/sites/som.org.uk/files/The_Mental_Health_and_Wellbeing_of_Nurses_and_Midwives_in_the_United_Kingdom.pdf.

Kline, R., & Lewis, D. (2019). The price of fear: Estimating the financial cost of bullying and harassment to the NHS in England. *Public Money & Management*, *39*(3), 166–174. https://doi.org/10.1080/09540962.2 018.1535044.

National Health Service Staff Survey Coordination Centre. (2020). *NHS Staff survey results—key findings by occupational groups.* https://www.nhsstaffsurveyresults.com/homepage/national-results-2020/breakdowns-questions-2020/.

Teoh, K. R. -H., Kinman, G., & Hassard, J. (2020). The relationship between healthcare staff wellbeing and patient care: It's not that simple. In A. H. de Lange, & L. Lovseth (Eds.), *Integrating the organization of health services, worker wellbeing and quality of care* (pp. 221–244). Springer International Publishing. https://doi.org/10.1007/978-3-030-59467-1_10.

# Caring for Yourself, To Care for Others: Prioritising Self-Care

Joy Darch

## KEY POINTS

1. Self-care for nurses and midwives is essential rather than desirable.
2. Individuals can consider and improve personal resilience, but this does not replace the responsibility of organisations to support staff health and wellbeing.
3. Learning to care for yourself to care for others should be a priority in nursing and midwifery education.
4. Key priorities to support the health and wellbeing of nurses are physical and psychological safety, access to water and food, breaks, and shifts.
5. Considering your personal strategies, strengths, resources, and insights can be helpful in developing a self-care toolkit.

## Introduction

Have you ever wondered why some nurses and midwives do not prioritise self-care when they are so good at caring for others? It is an occupational strength that the nature of those attracted to the nursing and midwifery profession have a desire to meet the needs of others, which attracts those who are often givers in nature. This chapter considers the dilemma for such caregivers to balance care for others with care for themselves when the lives of others are the focus of everyday on the job. Working in an environment when the human needs of others are a priority and often urgent, it is quite easy to lose sight of your own needs. Have you ever missed a break, become dehydrated during a busy day, left work hungry and grabbed an easy but high-calorie snack before falling into bed exhausted? Sound familiar? Those that support others in times of intense need mostly have a nurturing quality that is often evident in both work and home life, which can also manifest itself in never putting themselves first with family and friends. Ever felt exhausted when still agreeing to do a favour for someone? Felt guilty when saying no? Listened to a friend's problems for an entire evening without sharing your own worries? As one experienced nurse explained to me, for many giving in does not come as naturally as giving out.

My own research and experience within nurse education have often led me to consider the phenomenon of nurse as a wounded healer (Conti-O'Hare, 2002). Many people are attracted to caring professions because they have experienced suffering in life, either their own or those close to them, which has provided personal insight. Often prospective students reveal at interview that their reason or catalyst for entering the profession is that they have lost a family member, a relative has a life-threatening illness, or they have experienced care or ill health themselves. Some also appear to have unresolved trauma about such experiences they bring with them to the start of their educational journey. Self-healing and self-care are therefore essential components of nurse and midwifery education for self-preservation, to ensure that person-centred care is delivered without self-sacrifice.

## Considering Resilience

Resilience has recently become a buzzword as the health and wellbeing of the nursing profession has risen up the agenda. Definitions of resilience include 'the capacity to recover quickly from difficult situations' and 'the ability to spring or bounce back'. Resilience training is offered at many organisations, and nurses and midwives are often praised for being resilient when coping with stressful situations. Is resilience therefore a personal requirement of the role? Or should those who are caring for others be supported sufficiently that such resilience is desirable rather than essential? With more support in place would such a level of resilience be required?

Consider for a moment a female staff nurse on a hospital ward who has worked in an understaffed ward all day due to unforeseen sickness, trying to teach and support learners whilst delivering the best care possible. Feeling frustrated that she must prioritise care during the shift, she is aware that many basic needs of those she is caring for have not been met to the standard that she would wish. This does not sit comfortably with her, she misses a meal break to try to compensate, hardly stops for a drink of water, and leaves the ward thirsty, hungry, desperate for a visit to the bathroom, and feeling that she has not done the best for the patients in her care that day. Getting into bed she feels exhausted and suspects that her experience will be the same the next day so does not sleep well. Such experience is well recognised by many and sadly the reason for burnout in some individuals. Becoming disillusioned or disappointed when not being able to deliver the highest quality care does not maintain professional vitality and creates stress. To be successful in the caring professions, depleted caring must be avoided and for some the challenge is just too great and too much giving of self (Skovholt & Trotter-Mathison, 2016). Many good nurses leave the profession because they feel stressed that they are not able to deliver the standard of care the way they would wish in an organisation where they do not always feel valued. Consider for a moment if these individuals lack resilience. Is it not the organisational culture that should be resilient in supporting those who care for others to care for themselves? If we expect personal resilience to be an essential requirement for nurses and midwives, are we not buying into a blame culture by focusing on the individual rather than insisting that organisations take further responsibility to meet the needs of individuals? Resilience should therefore not be the flavour of the month, where individuals are sent on a training day or a workshop as a tickbox exercise, but integral to organisational culture by supporting strategies for self-care and ensuring that the health and wellbeing of employees is on every agenda. Facilities for rest and relaxation, clinical supervision, healthy reasonably priced food available at all times, hydration stations, and mandatory breaks as part of organisational culture encourage self-care.

Having just challenged the idea that there should be organisational responsibility for supporting self-care strategies, it is still important to recognise that individuals can of course take steps to consider their own personal resilience. We are all familiar with the relevant expression 'you can't pour from an empty jug', a metaphor to remind us to take care of ourselves. However, the advice given to us each time we take a flight is also worthy of application to all nurses and midwives every day: **'Please place the mask over your own mouth and nose before assisting others.'** This might seem counterintuitive to many, but the message is clear: You simply are of more help to others if you take care of yourself and survive.

## Considering Your Own Strengths, Strategies, Resources, and Insights

So how do we begin considering personal resilience? Some years ago, I had the privilege to learn from and work with one of the United Kingdom's leading resilience trainers, a medical doctor and psychologist who experienced burnout and depression as a junior doctor. Since then, his approach has been adopted and adapted to support those who care for others to care for themselves by considering personal resilience in a semistructured workshop, resulting in the development of a personal self-help toolkit (Johnstone, 2019). The goal of the session is to identify four types of tools available to each of us, strengthen skilfulness in using each tool, and explore potential new tools by listening to others. This session has now been used with many groups of nurses, midwives, and student nurses in the United Kingdom and integrated into the curriculum for students to provide time for self-reflection as they begin their educational journey. Such teaching strategies can also support self-healing and personal resilience whilst preparing students for the challenges that lie ahead in practice (Darch et al., 2019). Self-healing may be required for some students, and therefore such teaching strategies as considering personal resilience in the curriculum will facilitate this, thus supporting those who care for others to care for themselves. Those taking part in the workshop firstly work individually, then, if comfortable, in pairs, and finally in a group discussion led by an experienced facilitator.

The self-help toolkit consists of four types of tools categorised as strengths, strategies, resources, and insights (SSRI). Johnstone (2019) refers to this as the SSRI toolkit for its relevance to the potential impact on depression and the common group of drugs called selective serotonin reuptake inhibitors.

Strategies: These are practical things we do that make us feel better, lift our mood, or offer us comfort (e.g., taking a walk in the country, spending time with friends, playing certain music, gardening, baking a cake).

Strengths: Our personal qualities that help us through tough times are often our strengths (e.g., determination, persistence (holding the line), sense of humour).

Resources: What we look to for guidance, support, or inspiration are resources (e.g., places we feel safe and good (countryside, garden, beach), things or people that help us (friends, family, pets)).

Insights: Personal perspective or wisdom as a result of our own experiences in life can often provide powerful messages that carry us through challenging situations. Examples of this are often experiences that have been difficult but have provided some personal insight (e.g., the death of a family member or friend at a young age making us realise that life is for living so we give everything a go, try new things, and be grateful for being alive).

Taking the time to consider our own personal SSRIs is helpful because often when we are feeling down, stressed, or anxious, it is not always possible to take action to do something to help yourself. That is not the moment when you can consider what might make you feel better. However, if you have already gained self-awareness of the tools that work for you, it is much easier to take the time for yourself and shift your mood in a direction that you want: 'Ok, so it's been a bad day but if I take the dogs for a walk/phone a friend/put reggae music on when I get home, it might help.'

These are all healthy coping mechanisms to help us get through everyday challenges. However, some of us develop strategies that are not so healthy: smoking, alcohol/other drugs, or even regular comfort eating. There is evidence that some nurses and midwives do have unhealthy coping mechanisms, and there is some debate whether this is appropriate if they are supposed to be healthy role models (Darch et al., 2017). Many of us will reach for a glass of wine or a bar of chocolate at the end of a bad day, but these are not useful tools to have in your self-help toolbox if used to excess and without any healthy strategies to support you. If this sounds familiar, is it time to give it some careful thought?

## Key Priority Areas to Facilitate Self-Care in the Working Environment

In the United Kingdom, in 2019, the Chief Nursing Officer (CNO) Health and Wellbeing Reference Group was formed to share and lead initiatives nationally and to inform policy. The group identified key priority areas to support the health and wellbeing of nurses:

1. Physical and psychological safety
2. Access to water and food
3. Breaks
4. Shift patterns

Despite the rise of health and wellbeing of nurses on the agenda, initiatives were found to be localized, and quality of support for self-care offered by organisations varies across the United Kingdom. The recent global pandemic has accentuated the need to improve the working environment for many nurses and midwives. Nurses still report that in some areas they are discouraged from drinking water as it appears unprofessional. You will find more on the importance of staying hydrated elsewhere in this book. Reports of a lack of hot, healthy food available for all shifts remain in certain areas, and the culture of some organisations still accepts work breaks being missed. On a positive note, some health and care environments have introduced designated health and wellbeing spaces and have a culture that values their staff by fully embracing the requirements for self-care, hydration stations, healthy food, mandatory breaks, and more flexible shift patterns. Psychological safety and wellbeing are increased when individuals feel valued by their organisations, which is a win-win for both the organisation and those trying to care for themselves while caring for others.

This chapter has considered some key points surrounding self-care for nurses and midwives. To ensure that person-centred care is delivered without self-sacrifice, we as individuals have 'an obligation in attitude that involves a constant allegiance to one's own wellbeing as necessary for competent other-care' (Skovholt & Trotter-Mathison, 2016). Employing organisations and educational institutions have a responsibility to support those who care for others to care for themselves.

## ACTIVITY

Complete this Activity in 30 minutes.
- Reflect on the things that you are aware of that lift your mood (strategies) at the end of a challenging day and write a list.

_____
_____
_____
_____
_____

- Consider your own personal qualities that will help you through challenging times.

_____
_____
_____
_____

- List your existing resources that support or inspire you.

_____
_____
_____
_____
_____

- Reflect on previous life experience and consider what insight it has given you.

_____
_____
_____
_____

If you feel comfortable to do so, consider completing this exercise with someone you trust, share your list, and discuss it. This person may suggest something to add to your toolkit!

| CASE STUDY 2.1 | **Self-Care and Nurse Education—University of Gloucestershire** |
|---|---|

Prioritising your own self-care is a fundamental lesson to learn. At our university, we have acted on the seminal work undertaken by Darch and colleagues to embed self-care within the nursing programme curriculum. Time has been allocated within the taught curriculum, specifically to provide nursing students with opportunity to focus on the importance of their own self-care. Students are encouraged and taught to develop self-care strategies through trying a range of different activities to promote their own health and wellbeing.

Evaluation of sessions has confirmed the importance of self-care education in laying the foundations for practice following graduation and registration with the UK Nursing and Midwifery Council (NMC). It has enabled students to recognise the need to take steps to keep well and proactively take some 'me time.' The development of triggers to recognise their own self-care needs has also provided opportunity to support others through sharing of strategies and make recommendations to colleagues from a position of understanding. Of value was the opportunity to try out different approaches to promoting self-care, including reflective practice (the process of making sense of events, situations, and actions through reflection on practice), hand massages, Pilates, and meditation. One student reported the positive impact of learning to use mindfulness and reflection, particularly taking time to stop on a Sunday to reflect on what was achieved over the previous week, set plans for the coming week, and taking time for yoga to enhance wellbeing. We believe it is important to encourage student nurses to develop and practice self-care during training, encouraging them to balance care for others with care for themselves.

Self-care is not only the responsibility of the individual but also the employing organisation. It is easy to wait for graduates to filter through the system to influence future practice, raising the importance of self-care as they move into influential roles. However, if we wait, we run the risk of self-care education becoming diluted by the many demands on practitioners in our current health and care system. Our approach to designing our current portfolio of nurse education has centred around coproduction and development of a systems approach, with partners, academics, experts by experience (service users), and students to meet the future workforce need. We are currently working collaboratively with practice partners to develop postqualifying education to further empower practitioners and the wider community with self-care tools to expand the support provided around health and wellbeing of nurses to midwives and other health and care professions. Additionally, we are working across disciplines within the university and with our practice partners to develop a Centre for Arts, Health and Wellbeing that embraces the importance of self-care not only for nursing students but as an important philosophy for our community, and to build an evidence base through research that helps to rebalance the delivery of health and care to recognise the importance of self-care and all its benefits.

**LORRAINE DIXON**

Head of School for Health and Social Care, University of Gloucestershire, United Kingdom to the end of the Case Study box as in Chapter 1.]

## *References*

Conti-O'Hare, M. (2002). *The nurse as the wounded healer: From trauma to transcendence.* Sudbury, MA: Jones and Bartlett Publishers.

Darch, J., Baillie, L., & Gillison, F. (2017). Nurses as role models in health promotion: A concept analysis. *British Journal of Nursing, 26*(17), 982–988. https://doi.org/10.12968/bjon.2017.26.17.982.

Darch, J., Baillie, L., & Gillison, F. (2019). Preparing student nurses to be healthy role models: A qualitative study. *Nurse Education in Practice.* (40):102630. https://doi.org/10.1016/j.nepr.2019.102630.

Johnstone, C. (2019). *Seven ways to build resilience: Strengthening your ability to deal with difficult times.* Robinson.

Skovholt, T. M., & Trotter-Mathison, M. (2016). The resilient practitioner. *Burnout and compassion fatigue prevention and self-care strategies for the helping profession* (3rd ed.). Routledge/Taylor & Francis Group.

## CHAPTER 3

# How Staff WellBeing Relates to Patient Experiences of Care

Anthony Montgomery ■ Maria Moirasgenti

## KEY POINTS

1. Burnout needs to be publicly recognised as a professional risk for all nurses and midwives, and thus needs to be described and discussed within the education and training programs for these professions.
2. Burnout will become less of a major problem if nurses/midwives-in-training have learned what it is, what are effective coping and recovery strategies, how to work effectively with colleagues and patients, and how to build a positive social culture of appreciation.
3. Organisational interventions and system change is needed to improve factors that cause burnout and changes to established ways of behaving.
4. Hospital managers should aim to give nurses and midwives space at the beginning and end of their shifts, to implement the coping strategies they need to mentally prepare.
5. To improve outcomes for patients, nurses/midwives and their organisations must be supported to name and discuss openly care that was not completed at the end of a shift.

## Introduction

Nurses and midwives are faced with serious responsibilities, acutely ill patients, high caseloads, and limited resources over long periods of time. Health care takes place around the clock, and many employees need to work various shifts, including night work. The high levels of burnout that we see reported in the nursing and midwifery profession are rooted in the fact that (1) the relationship between nurses and patients is central to the work, and (2) the provision of service and care can be a highly emotional experience. Within occupations such as nursing and midwifery the norms are clear, if not always stated explicitly: to be selfless and put others' needs first, to work long hours and do whatever it takes to help the patient, to go the extra mile, and to give one's all—in other words, the work is considered a calling rather than simply a job (Montgomery & Maslach, 2019). Unfortunately, the picture of the ideal nurse and midwife who goes the extra mile for our care is also one that puts the health and wellbeing of nurses and midwives at risk. Health care culture is one that had strong attendance demands, meaning that nurses and midwives come to work even when they feel ill, from a sense of duty. For nurses (compared to doctors), working in health care organisations is even more demanding as they have less work autonomy, fewer career development opportunities, fewer alternatives for career change (Aiken et al., 2001), and less social recognition. Indeed, nurses report that they can feel invisible to society under the shadow of doctors. Following from this, the interesting question to assess is to what degree the wellbeing of nurses and midwives impacts upon patient care.

There is a symbiotic relationship between nurse/midwife wellbeing and patient outcomes. Take burnout, for example. Job burnout is a special type of work-related stress—a state of physical or emotional exhaustion that also involves a sense of reduced accomplishment and loss of personal identity. Burnout is driven by small, burdensome, chronic events that erode the spirit of frontline nurses. Burnout, which is common and likely to increase, is a threat to the ability of nurses and midwives to provide appropriate care, and a threat to their own wellbeing. Burnout is becoming more common among nurses and midwives. Those who experience burnout may be more likely to engage in risky behaviours, such as heavy drinking, smoking, and being physically inactive. Some of these behaviours (such as alcohol misuse) might lead to mistakes at work and compromise patient safety. A high level of burnout in nurses and midwives is associated with high rates of health care-associated infections, suboptimal care, and compromised patient safety. The problem of burnout is compounded by the fact that it can lead to feelings of depression and affect cognitive skills (e.g., memory and concentration issues), which increases the risk of involvement in patient safety problems for nurses and midwives.

## What About the Organisation?

When discussing the relationship between nurse/midwife wellbeing and patient care, it is important not to ignore the role that the organisation plays in this equation. The support and resources provided by the organisation in which nurses and midwives work has both direct and indirect effects on patient care. For example, there is good evidence that safe nurse-to-patient ratios (e.g., 1:2 in intensive care units (ICUs) or 1:6 in postnatal wards) are associated with shorter hospital stays for patients, lower failure-to-rescue rates (i.e., death within 30 days among patients who experienced complications), and lower death rates (Lang et al., 2004). Moreover, evidence suggests that when patients rate their hospital as excellent or would recommend their hospital to other patients, this is associated significantly with nurses' satisfaction with their hospital work environment (Aiken et al., 2012). However, burnout plays a mediating role between organisational factors and patient care, meaning that increasing the number of nurses/midwives and improving working environments are less impactful if nurses and midwives are still suffering from burnout. Therefore for nurses and midwives it would appear that hiring more staff, having better facilities, and ensuring that management helps solve problems in patient care is desirable and has the potential to impact positively on patients, but the effectives of such measures will be less effective if we do not also improve the wellbeing of nurses and midwives at the same time. This is an excellent example of how satisfying different needs of employees leads to different outcomes. The general literature on motivation in organisational psychology suggests that addressing work needs (e.g., fair pay, reasonable work shifts) can make employees more satisfied but will not necessarily lead to more increased feelings of job engagement (i.e., the opposite of burnout). Put practically, we should not expect that only providing more resources (e.g., more staff, better facilities) will directly result in better wellbeing, when the factors that are driving burnout have not been addressed. The most common organisational factors driving burnout are workload, control, reward, community, fairness, and values (Montgomery & Maslach, 2019). For example, it should be obvious that increasing the number of nurses available to patients will have a limited impact if nurses and midwives feel that they are not treated like other professionals, especially doctors (i.e., fairness) or that they do not feel appreciated by senior members of the health care team (i.e., being valued by our employer). Thus, the message is clear: Improving the working conditions of nurses and midwives is essential to improving patient care, but such measures must also improve these workers' individual wellbeing.

# Impact of the Handover Period on Staff WellBeing and Patient Care

We can all bring problems from our personal/family life into our work and equally bring problems from our work back home with us. This is what psychologists call spillover, and it can occur from both domains. Conversely, it is also possible to experience positive spillover, meaning that we bring helpful energy from either our work or nonwork life into the other domain. The handover period for nurses/midwives is critical and worthy of special mention given that it represents the transition point for both their exit and entry from work.

We know little about the strategies nurses and midwives use immediately before and immediately after their shift. This crossover period, from one shift to another, has a critical impact for patient outcomes. The need to mentally prepare (switch on) for the stressful hospital environment is a necessity for nurses and midwives working shifts. In addition, nurses often miss opportunities for breaks during work to deal with patient needs, and midwives skip breaks to care for newborns in need. Even when there is time for a break, it is often too brief and ineffective and cannot offer sufficient recovery time. Moreover, after the end of a shift, nurses and midwives frequently must deal with family and household duties. We should not underestimate how nonwork demands can be experienced as a second shift, with most of the international research showing that women still carry much of the burden when it comes to family and household chores.

The beginning or end of a shift can involve important rituals that help nurses cope with the challenges of their work. For example, some nurses say that they drink coffee and smoke before and after work to prepare or disengage themselves mentally (Manomenidis et al., 2016). This can be explained by the fact that both coffee and cigarettes are considered simultaneously as tools that can both stimulate and decompress. Nurses prefer to drink coffee at the workplace while chatting with colleagues instead of drinking it at home. Such rituals function as a prework transitional stage that might indeed be helpful for the transition to the work atmosphere. Humour is an important way for nurses and midwives to emotionally decompress from difficult days at work. The second author of this chapter, who worked in an ICU with COVID-19 dying patients in 2021, found that daily humour was lifesaving for nurses, helping them cope with the stressors of working life.

The handover period is a time to share information about what has happened and what needs to be done. However, nurses and midwives are aware that they cannot always provide full care, so they are forced to make decisions daily to ration care and/or leave it undone. The problem is that this could be become a pattern or habit over an extended period. The question is whether they admit to missing certain elements of patient care or inform the incoming staff at the handover. Missed care is a significant problem in modern health care (Kirwan & Matthews, 2020) and one that is likely to happen more often when nurses and midwives are exhausted, fatigued, and burnt out. The rationing of care is unavoidable and common, but it is likely to go under the radar with regard to nursing and midwifery. This is an opportunity for nurse and midwife managers to play a constructive role in acknowledging that sometimes care is missed and rationed, and thus make it part of the conversation.

## Focusing on What's Going Right

Today there is enough evidence to suggest that expecting health professionals to deliver safe, efficient, and patient-centred care while they are getting increasingly burnt out is not only ineffective but also costly and dangerous. For health care systems to be truly patient centred, safe, and efficient, they need primarily to protect the health and wellbeing of their workers. Positive psychology is a relatively new field in psychology that prompts us to look at optimal functioning rather than identifying what is going wrong. In short, we should not ignore the many problems that are common at work, but we should find out what is going well and see how we can use this as a lever to change other elements of our work.

In general, health care is an environment in which we are prompted to focus on what is going wrong (a pathogenic approach) rather than what is going right (a salutogenic approach). We need a mental shift in the way we think about our work. It can be easier to focus on what is going wrong, as health care training has reinforced us to diagnose the disease and prescribe the correct medicine. This medical model is not effective when it comes to our wellbeing. Getting out of bed every day and coming to work can be reduced to two elements: how motivated we feel to be good at our job and whether we feel in control/competent at work. So the challenge is to help nurses and midwives feel more motivated to come to work and have a feeling of being in charge of their work day. Health care is all about being able to adapt to changing circumstances. West et al. (2020) have identified the three core work needs for nurses and midwives that must be met to ensure wellbeing and motivation at work and to minimise workplace stress: (1) autonomy, the need to have control over their work lives; (2) belonging, the need to be connected to, cared for by, and caring of others around them at work; and (3) contribution, the need to experience effectiveness in what they do and deliver valued outcomes. This ABC of needs is a practical way for us to assess the impact of interventions and policies. Finally, we need to be clear on what is the bigger picture of supporting staff wellbeing. The profile of a resilient nurse/midwife is an individual who has invested in their own education, experiences low levels of anxiety, and utilizes mental preparation strategies effectively. If you are reading this as a nurse manager or clinical leader, ask yourself how well you are supporting these goals among your staff.

## The Bigger Picture

We run the risk of underestimating the crucial role that nurses and midwives play as gatekeepers of health care. As noted by Kirwan and Matthews (2020), understanding the work of nurses involves appreciating the following: (1) nurses and midwives are key players in the delivery of patient care and make up the largest number of workers across all health care systems; (2) they are frequently seen as coordinators of care in both acute and nonacute settings, promoting interprofessional collaboration and helping other health care professionals provide comprehensive patient care; (3) nurses therefore, due to their proximity to the patient, are somewhat uniquely placed to influence the quality and safety of care provision and are often the last link in the chain of delivery of care. All the aforementioned create bullet-proof arguments as to why nurse and midwife wellbeing must be addressed and why, until we do, patient care will suffer.

---

**ACTIVITY**

We often think about stress as an individual phenomenon that reflects an inherent weakness in the person who is suffering from stress. Additionally, we tend to look for solutions that focus on the person. A good exercise for you as a nurse/midwife is to evaluate the degree to which your work environment can provide you with help at the primary, secondary, and tertiary levels of health prevention as described here.

Try these three questions:

*Questions to Appreciate The Three Levels of Prevention*

| Level | Example |
|---|---|
| Primary | Do I have adequate opportunities for rest and relaxation at work? |
| Secondary | Does my workplace have procedures that allow for identifying people at risk of burnout? |
| Tertiary | Does my workplace have policies to help people who suffer from stress and burnout? |

## CASE STUDY 3.1     The DNA of Care: Patient Voices Programme

*"No one's looking after us, but we're expected to provide the service that is looking after other people. How are we going to do that if we feel this bad?"*

The Patient Voices Programme (www.patientvoices.org.uk) is a social enterprise dedicated to the sharing of the voices in health and social care that 'wait patiently to be heard'—whether patients, relatives, staff, or managers—through the medium of digital storytelling. Digital stories are short multimedia films created by the storyteller through a facilitated, inclusive, and coproductive process. By developing their own script and curating images and music, the storytellers produce an artifact (i.e., digital) story that communicates their lived experiences to wider audiences and so initiates change.

In 2016, NHS England commissioned the Patient Voices Programme to facilitate workshops with the National Health Service staff to cocreate digital stories around five key themes: compassion, staff as carers, staff in distress (wounded healers), learning from serious incidents, and leading change. The project title, 'The DNA of Care', reflected how its premise likened the intertwined relationship between patient care and staff wellbeing to the characteristic double helix of DNA. It was hoped the stories would powerfully articulate this inextricable connection and motivate employers to address workplace culture and invest in and prioritise staff wellbeing.

In five 3-day reflective digital storytelling workshops, 34 digital stories were created by a diverse group of staff, including midwives, nurses, anaesthetists, paediatricians, general practitioners, speech-language therapists, psychologists, health care assistants, and a mortuary and bereavement service lead. The workshops required a fine balance between vulnerability and courage, which is necessary to create and share important personal stories that have an emotional impact on the audience. Storytellers described the process as beneficial—even therapeutic. They attributed new insights and greater courage in their personal and professional lives to the storytelling process and began using their stories to stimulate improvements to workplace culture.

The stories from the workshops offer tangible examples of the relationship between staff wellbeing and their ability to care for patients. Themes centred on the significant and enduring emotional impact of engaging in clinical practice, secondary trauma from exposure to distressing events, conflicts between personal values and dehumanising models of care, and how compassion fatigue affected their ability to remain emotionally connected to their work. Throughout the stories it was clear that the emotional demands of their roles were not attended to, and there was little meaningful support to respond to these challenges. For some, this resulted in an armoured approach to practice focused on self-protection. Others doubted if they could remain in their profession.

NHS England recognised that the existing statistics and data that demonstrated the relationship between wellbeing and patient experience had failed to initiate this impetus for change. The stories were used to influence culture and emphasise the importance of staff wellbeing to individuals, the organization, and patient care by integrating them into a national learning and development programme (http://www.patientvoices.org.uk/what-we-do/workbooks.htm). Stakeholders and storytellers reported important themes in reactions to the stories: maintaining authenticity by bringing their whole selves to their practice and fidelity to the personal values that motivated them to pursue a career in caring for others.

The DNA of Care digital stories can be seen at www.patientvoices.org.uk/dnaoc.htm

**PIP HARDY**  ■  **TONY SUMNER**

## References

Aiken, L. H., Clarke, S. P., Sloane, D. M., Sochalski, J. A., Busse, R., Clarke, H., Giovannetti, P., Hunt, J., Rafferty, A. M., & Shamian, J. (2001). Nurses' reports on hospital care in five countries. *Health Affairs, 20,* 43–53.

Aiken, L. H., Sermeus, W., Van den Heede, K., Sloane, D. M., Busse, R., McKee, M., Bruyneel, L., Rafferty, A. M., Griffiths, P., Moreno-Casbas, M. T., Tishelman, C., Scott, A., Brzostek, T., Kinnunen, J., Schwendimann, R., Heinen, M., Zikos, D., Sjetne, I. S., Smith, H. L., & Kutney-Lee, A. (2012). Patient safety, satisfaction, and quality of hospital care: Cross sectional surveys of nurses and patients in 12 countries in Europe and the United States. *BMJ (Clinical Research Ed.), 344,* e1717. https://doi.org/10.1136/bmj.e1717.

Kirwan, M., & Matthews, A. (2020). Missed nursing care: The impact on patients, nurses, and organizations. In A. Montgomery, M. Van der Doef, E. Panagopoulou, & M. Leiter (Eds.), *Connecting health care worker wellbeing, patient safety and organisational change: The triple challenge* (pp. 25–40). Springer.

Lang, T. A., Hodge, M., Olson, V., Romano, P. S., & Kravitz, R. L. (2004). Nurse-patient ratios: A systematic review on the effects of nurse staffing on patient, nurse employee, and hospital outcomes. *The Journal of Nursing Administration, 34*(7–8), 326–337. https://doi.org/10.1097/00005110-200407000-00005.

Manomenidis, G., Panagopoulou, E., & Montgomery, A. (2016). The 'switch on–switch off model': Strategies used by nurses to mentally prepare and disengage from work. *International Journal of Nursing Practice, 22*(4), 356–363. https://doi.org/10.1111/ijn.12443.

Montgomery, A., & Maslach, C. (2019). Health care professionals' wellbeing. *Cambridge handbook of psychology, health and medicine.* Cambridge University Press, 353–370.

West, M., Bailey, S., & Williams, E. (2020). *The courage of compassion supporting nurses and midwives to deliver high-quality care.* The Kings Fund. https://www.kingsfund.org.uk/publications/courage-compassion-supporting-nurses-midwives.

## CHAPTER 4

# How Stress and Anxiety Affect the Body

Aimee Aubeeluck ■ Kiran K. Bains ■ Samantha Kelly

## KEY POINTS

1. Workplace stress and anxiety can have a negative impact on our physical health.
2. Unhealthy organisational culture can increase stress and anxiety in the workplace.
3. Individual cultural differences may influence how stress and anxiety are interpreted and experienced.
4. How we react and respond to stress and anxiety differs from person to person.
5. We can actively manage our stress response to improve wellbeing at work.

## Introduction

Workplace stress and anxiety can be described as how we feel when the demands placed on us at work are more than we feel we can cope with. But what do we mean by stress and anxiety in this context, and how can we better understand what is happening in our bodies to manage how we feel? This chapter will discuss the impact of stress and anxiety on the body. It will begin by operationalising stress and anxiety as both emotional and physiological constructs, considering the mind-body connection and how stressors are interpreted. We will discuss the active management of workplace stressors and how emotional regulation and cognitive reappraisal may reduce negative emotions in the workplace. The influence of individual cultural differences on how we express our thoughts, behaviours, and emotions will be explored. Consideration will be given to the impact of organisational culture on the health and wellbeing of individuals.

## Stress and Anxiety

What do we mean by stress? There are many operational definitions of stress that can be drawn from different disciplines; for example, the definition proposed by Hans Selye (1936) simply states that stress is 'the non-specific response of the body to any demand'. This generic definition suggests that stress is part of the human experience as just existing creates a demand for a life-maintaining response. Within the contexts of health care and psychology, we have come to consider stress as the 'perception of threat, with resulting anxiety discomfort, emotional tension, and difficulty in adjustment' (Fink, 2009); when we are experiencing stress, this is probably the definition that will most resonate with us. Another element to add to our understanding and experience of stress is that the situations and circumstances that individuals find stressful will differ from person to person. Therefore the way we appraise a situation as stressful (or not) will have an impact on our experiences of that situation (Katana et al., 2019). This is great news for any of us experiencing stress as it offers the potential to reappraise the situations we are in and see them in a different light with a view to reducing those negative feelings.

If we have experienced stress in the workplace, it is likely that this has led to feelings of anxiety as well. Anxiety can be defined as 'state of worry over a future unwanted event, or fear of an actual situation' (Franklin et al., 2017) and is like stress in that both are emotional responses. However, stress is generally triggered by external pressures, and anxiety is triggered by internal and excessive worries that do not go away even after a stressful situation has passed.

One important aspect of our understanding of stress and anxiety is that they are not just feelings of being overwhelmed, or worrying over a future unwelcome event, or actual situations. There can also be a physiologic impact of experiencing stress and stressors in the workplace. Therefore stress and anxiety in the workplace can impact upon both our physical and mental wellbeing. If we think about our brain as the command centre that speaks to the rest of the body, we can begin to understand how our thoughts and feelings can present physiologically with our mind and body being intertwined. If we reflect on a situation that we found stressful or anxiety provoking, we may recall an increased heart rate, loss of appetite, or insomnia, for example.

So, what is happening when we experience stress and anxiety? When we are stressed and anxious, our body releases a surge of hormones, including adrenaline and cortisol. These hormones are meant to provide us with a short burst of energy so we can flee a dangerous situation. However, in the modern world, we are not often running from life-threatening situations. It may be more likely that we are experiencing an excessive workload, difficult relationships with colleagues, or a lack of control over how we do our jobs. Sometimes there is no single cause of work-related stress but a buildup of smaller things that begin to overwhelm us. Even in these situations where there is no real danger to escape, our bodies can release these hormones leading to long-term negative effects on the body such as chronic disease or a weakened immune response.

We also experience additional physiologic changes in response to stress and anxiety, particularly with relation to critical organs in the cardiovascular system such as the heart and the lungs, where in stressful situations the release of adrenaline increases heart rate and expands air passages to aid oxygen uptake. For a healthy person, this short-term stress response is likely to lead to nothing more than hyperventilation, heart palpitations, and sometimes dizziness or chest pain that passes within a few moments. However, when an individual has a chronic health condition such as chronic obstructive pulmonary disease, this can cause a flare-up leading to longer-term health implications. Stress responses can also trigger the release of histamine and leukotrienes in the body that create a narrowing of airways causing breathing difficulties such as asthma.

Stress and anxiety can further impact on the musculoskeletal, endocrine, and digestive systems, and many people are unaware that the physical symptoms they are experiencing are in fact caused by external (environmental) stressors or internal negative thought processes. Individuals may experience fatigue from being in a state of high alertness or headaches, migraines, muscle aches, and pains caused by tension. Ongoing stress and anxiety can stop the immune system from working effectively leading to inflammation within the body that can present as tingling sensations, joint pain, and stiffness. People can also experience digestive discomfort such as heartburn, constipation, and diarrhoea. Chronic digestive problems (e.g., irritable bowel syndrome alongside food intolerance and sensitivities) can also be a symptom of ongoing stress and anxiety.

## Managing Stress and Anxiety

We are learning that stress and anxiety are an expected part of life. When we can see stress as a positive challenge and an opportunity for growth and change, it may motivate us to success and we may see our anxiety levels reduce (Kiecolt-Glaser et al., 2020). However, when stressors are viewed as a negative challenge or a threat, they can overwhelm us and lead to long-term health concerns. Certainly within the health care profession there is evidence that the workforce is experiencing high levels of stress, burnout, anxiety, and depression as part of their working lives (Hunter et al., 2019). So how can we take control of some of the stressful workplace situations in which we find ourselves? Cognitive reappraisal is one way of nudging our emotions back toward a baseline level or status quo. This technique requires us to recognise negative thought patterns and change them into something more positive. For example, imagine you cannot park when you arrive at work, and this makes you significantly late. Your first response may be to get frustrated, appraising the situation by thinking, 'There is never anywhere to park! My workplace needs to sort this out if they want people to arrive on time!' This appraisal may make you feel irritated and stressed causing you to be flustered and on the back foot on arrival to your shift. However, just take a moment to reappraise and look at this from a different perspective. What if instead of feeling frustrated you can think, 'I'm late but, life happens, the parking situation is well known, and it is not my fault.' These two different perspectives both exist, but if you can teach yourself to notice when you are experiencing negative thoughts and consider your emotions from a few different angles, for example: 'What's really the worst that could happen?' or 'If I were in a better mood, would I still think about this in the same way?' then you can potentially begin to reduce some of the stressors around you.

## Cultural Differences

As individuals, we all react to stress in different ways so the physical impact of stress may present very differently from one person to another. Moreover, there may be cultural differences or differences that relate to protected characteristics that also influence how we express our thoughts, behaviours, and emotions when experiencing stress and anxiety. When considering cultural differences in stress and anxiety it can help to break down how these may manifest themselves. People may experience differences in attribution (what they believe to have triggered stress and anxiety), expression (how we might observe them behaving in response to these emotions), and the coping strategies they may find acceptable to use when they are struggling. It has been previously thought that some ethnic minorities may somatise their distress through repression of emotion; that is, they would report physical manifestations of stress, distress, and anxiety but not necessarily understand its underlying cause. However, Kawanishi (1992) questioned the assumptions underlying this and pointed to research that (1) suggested that those who somatise their distress can label their affective symptoms if asked and (2) argued that somatisation of distress was widespread in primary care and not unique to minoritised ethnic communities. Stress and anxiety can often lead to physical symptoms such as nonspecific pain and fatigue, as outlined earlier. Chronic stress can lead to increased allostatic load (wear and tear on the body), inflammation, and cellular ageing. Additionally, people from minoritised ethnic communities carry a higher burden of chronic illness, including diabetes and cardiovascular disease. For example, increased allostatic load among minoritised communities (including racial minorities) is associated with experiences of disadvantage and discrimination in Westernised contexts and implicated in chronic illnesses and poorer health outcomes, including psychological distress and lowered self-esteem. Those experiencing multiple indices of marginalisation appear to be at greater risk. However, social support, good interpersonal relationships, and greater education (high school or beyond, including having qualifications in nursing and midwifery) appear to be protective factors, reducing allostatic load and its deleterious effects on mental and physical health.

Effective communication and understanding that distress can be an embodied experience are key, and more recent research has begun to explore the idioms of distress that people use in different cultural contexts. These include physical, cognitive, and emotional symptoms, as well as naming relational and social elements in the process (such as relating thinking too much to stressors ranging from the spiritual to relational and economic stressors) in various cultural contexts across sub-Saharan Africa (Backe et al., 2021). In contrast, use of the terms *depression* and *anxiety* can often be loaded with shame and stigma, as such terms may be conflated with serious mental illness. Whilst experiencing distress in relation to everyday stressors is accepted in sub-Saharan Africa, seeking mental health or integrative support to manage mental and physical health concerns may not be as broadly acceptable or normalised as undertaking a medical consultation for physical illness. There may be greater pressure to be able to cope with stressors and temptations (e.g., alcohol use) and shame associated with seeking help with these concerns due to a link between help-seeking and perceived failure, though, as with the wider Western population, beliefs may change over time.

In Western cultures we can often feel under pressure to be enthusiastic, joyful, and positive. Unhappiness, stress, and anxiety can be perceived to be negative states to fix; however, there are efforts to break down stigma in seeking psychological support where a person may be overwhelmed and struggling with mental health difficulties via therapy, expressive writing, support groups, and self-help literature. An overview of what emotions may be acceptable to express by the people of the global majority would be far beyond the scope of this chapter and deserving of significant exploration in its own right. However, as an example, in some East Asian cultures it is important to be emotionally restrained and harmonious, thus showing excessive emotional distress may be considered disruptive. Nevertheless, in many contexts it is acceptable to seek out pastoral and spiritual guidance or sometimes informal conflict mediation.

It can be common for professionals in nursing and midwifery to experience stress and anxiety for many reasons, including job stress, interpersonal conflict, grief, and loss. The same stressors would also likely impact ethnic minorities in the profession, particularly where ethnic minorities are at disproportionate risk of morbidity and mortality from certain illnesses (e.g., COVID-19, HIV, diabetes) and community grief may also present itself. However, a person-centred approach can be key to help us and our colleagues to cope with stress and anxiety rather than making generalised assumptions. It is important to remember that cultural diversity in emotional expression (the degree and what type of emotion) exists. Generational differences may also exist between migrants regarding language, communication, models of health and wellbeing, and acceptability of various coping mechanisms and avenues for receiving support. Using everyday language (such as *stress, worry, low mood*) rather than *anxiety* or *depression* can be helpful to address stigma when a person is struggling, so that the person is willing to seek support. Identifying sources of positive support in a person's life can also be helpful.

Whilst some people desire to have support from within their own communities, others will prefer to be supported by people outside of their social or community groups. For the former, there may be a comfort in shared rituals or practice in providing support or sense of identification with the person. However, with the latter, there may be some concerns about being judged or ostracised within the community (especially in close-knit protective social groups or where a person experiences multiple marginalisation (e.g., chronic illness/disability, domestic violence, LGBT+ identity) or seeks out others they perceive to have a different perspective). It is important that assumptions are not made, and appropriate signposting resources are created for ethnic minority community support providers in the local area and for people experiencing multiple marginalisation (as available) and services that are more generic for nurses and midwives to access.

## Organisational Culture

Working in health care can be high pressured and low staffed, with an underlying culture and expectation that individuals should do more and an overreliance on goodwill. However, research from the field of positive psychology demonstrates that this kind of culture can be harmful to both productivity and to the individual over time. The stress of belonging to a hierarchical organisation (such as a health care organisation) has been linked to disease and death with a strong link between leadership behaviours and heart disease in employees. In these types of environments, staff can disengage from their work feeling high levels of stress and anxiety, which may be accompanied by feeling a lack of support, value, and respect. However, a positive working culture that provides support, avoids blame, and demonstrates gratitude can improve the workplace at all levels and the experience of those within it. Positive workplaces are more successful and tend to increase positive emotions and wellbeing of all employees. Organisations that develop positive cultures are likely to achieve greater levels of overall effectiveness such as patient satisfaction, productivity, and employee engagement. These positive environments buffer against the negative experiences of stress and anxiety, allowing staff to be more resilient in the face of challenges and difficulties and reducing the likelihood of negative impacts on physical health.

## ACTIVITY

### Managing Emotions Through a Reflective Positive Stress Diary

Mild stress and anxiety respond well to a variety of coping mechanisms (e.g., physical activity, a nutritious diet, good sleep hygiene, use of a stress diary). This activity will take you through the process of how to log anxious moments in a stress diary to pinpoint the causes of stress in your life. A stress diary can also be used to give you an insight into how you react to stress. Stress diaries are used to regularly record information about the stressors you are experiencing so that you can reflect upon them, consider them, and manage them. Stress diaries can help you to understand the following:
- Causes of stress in more detail
- Levels of stress at which you operate most effectively
- Ways to improve how you manage stress

### Step 1: Diary Entries

Try to make regular entries in your diary after every shift, recording the following:
- Date and time
- Stressful situation(s)
- Fundamental cause of the stress (Is it the workplace or is something else also going on?)
- How you managed the situation (Could you have done anything differently?)
- Level of happiness on a scale of 0 (not happy at all) to 10 (I couldn't be happier); note the mood you are feeling and any physical changes (e.g., increased heart rate).
- How effectively you are working now—a subjective assessment, on a scale of 0 (ineffective) to 10 (highly effective)

### Step 2: Reflection and Analysis

After about 1 week of diary entries, you can reflect on your experiences, analyse them, and consider different ways to reduce your experiences of stress:
1. Explore the different stressors you experienced during the past week. Highlight the most frequent and most difficult stressors.
2. Look at your evaluation of their fundamental causes, how you manged the situation and whether you thought you could have done things differently. Are there issues that need to be resolved? If so, list these issues.
3. Take this list of issues and reflect on how you might be able to change the situations these occurred in for the better.
4. Think about how you felt when you were feeling stressed and consider how this affected your happiness and effectiveness. Was there a middle level of pressure at which you were happiest and performed best?

### Step 3: Consolidation

When you've reflected on your diary, you should have a better understanding of your stressors, what you are able to change, and the level of pressure where you work best. You should be able to identify the types of situations that cause you the most stress, allowing you to begin to feel in more control of these situations and to manage them in the best way for you.

CASE STUDY 4.1          **Managing Stress to Reduce Sickness Absence**

As part of the leadership team of a busy, inner-city community mental health team, we noticed an increase in staff sickness and felt a general sense of unease in the work environment, and so the team manager asked people how they were feeling in their supervision. Some of the short-stay staff (rotational doctors, students, and bank nurses) told her that they often felt isolated and undervalued by their colleagues. They said that they didn't fully understand some of the working practices or systems, and they described feeling left out by the core staff team, with many of them not using their names, so referring to them as 'the bank nurse' or 'the student.' Consequently, they described feeling stressed and unsafe in the workplace and said they often experienced worry and anxiety about coming to work. They also felt unable to perform their jobs either safely or effectively. They had tried to cope in various ways, but some had started to isolate themselves, avoid the main team office whenever possible, and at times some staff said they had not felt able to come into work at all.

Collectively, the leadership team decided to revisit the team's core values of compassion, respecting each other, and working together and to think about what changes could be made in the work environment to better promote these values. They led a series of focus groups with the team to explore how people were feeling and how they felt these values were reflected in their day-to-day practice. Together they were able to recognise that they felt overwhelmed by the amount of work and so just focused on getting everything done in the day. This meant they had no time to take a break, to talk to each other, or notice what was going on around them. They also didn't feel they had time to engage in more formal professional activities, such as clinical supervision or case discussions, and so felt ill-equipped to do their jobs safely.

Together they agreed some actions that they thought would provide them with the structure and support they needed to work more effectively and compassionately together. They set up a peer supervision group, which, together with individual clinical supervision, was allocated protected time. One of the rotational doctors also started a reflective practice group to provide staff with the opportunity to share how they were feeling and support each other when working with complex clinical situations. They also changed the physical layout of the work environment to reduce the risk of isolation and to create more opportunities for interaction. An induction programme was developed so that new staff would enjoy a period of supernumerary status to participate in shadowing before being expected to work independently. This allowed them the time and space to become familiar with the working practices of the team, ask questions, get to know their colleagues, and understand how the various disciplines in the team work individually and collectively in the provision of care.

Whilst initially these changes meant that staff had less time to tackle the clinical workload, in time, as staff felt safer, more connected, better supported, and happier, efficiency improved and sickness absence reduced.

**SAMANTHA KELLY**

### References

Backe, E. L., Bosire, E. N., Kim, A. W., & Mendenhall, E. (2021). 'Thinking too much': A systematic review of the idiom of distress in sub-Saharan Africa. *Culture Medicine and Psychiatry*, 1–28. https://doi.org/10.1007/s11013-020-09697-z.

Fink, G. (2009). Stress: Definition and history. In L. R. Squire (Ed.), *Encyclopaedia of neuroscience* (pp. 549–555). Elsevier.

Franklin, E., McLean, M., McNally, C., et al. (2017). Defining anxiety disorders. In *Treating and preventing adolescent mental health disorders: What we know and what we don't know*. Oxford University Press. https://www.oxfordclinicalpsych.com/view/10.1093/med-psych/9780199928163.001.0001/med-9780199928163-chapter-9.

Hunter, B., Fenwick, J., Sidebotham, M., & Henley, J. (2019). Midwives in the United Kingdom: Levels of burnout, depression, anxiety and stress and associated predictors. *Midwifery*. https://doi.org/10.1016/j.midw.2019.08.008.

Katana, M., Röcke, C., Spain, S. M., & Allemand, M. (2019). Emotion regulation, subjective wellbeing, and perceived stress in daily life of geriatric nurses. *Frontiers in Psychology*. https://doi.org/10.3389/fpsyg.2019.01097.

Kawanishi, Y. (1992). Somatization of Asians: An artifact of Western medicalization? *Transcultural Psychiatric Research Review, 29*(1), 5–36.

Kiecolt-Glaser, J. K., Renna, M. E., Shrout, M. R., & Madison, A. A. (2020). Stress reactivity: What pushes us higher, faster, and longer—and why it matters. *Current Directions in Psychological Science.* https://doi.org/10.1177/0963721420949521.

Selye, H. (1936). A syndrome produced by diverse nocuous agents. *Nature, 138,* 32.

## CHAPTER 5

# Understanding Compassion Fatigue and Burnout

Sally Pezaro

## KEY POINTS

1. Compassion toward both patients and colleagues is essential for excellence in health care.
2. The effects of both compassion fatigue and burnout can negatively impact upon the safety and quality of health care.
3. Compassionate rather than punitive approaches are required in pursuit of recovery.
4. The assessment of workplace imbalances between staff and organisations can be useful in identifying areas in need of address.
5. Settings that enable midwives and nurses to practise in line with their values may be most useful in the mitigation of burnout and compassion fatigue overall.

## Introduction

Midwives and nurses join their respective professions to deliver excellence in care. This requires compassion toward service users, defined as 'the combination of underpinning emotions (such as sympathy and empathy), with altruistic values (particularly a desire to help others), which together motivate an individual to take action, which would ultimately be experienced as "care" by the recipient' (Kneafsey et al., 2016). In this context, empathy (the ability to imagine and share the feelings of another person) is also fundamental, as it facilitates one's ability to feel and act with compassion (i.e., to feel concern and wishing to relieve a person of suffering) (Klimecki & Singer, 2012). Yet it is also important for midwives and nurses to foster and maintain workplace compassion toward colleagues.

Many may ponder as to what shows workplace compassion in health care. In our research, we asked a variety of health care professionals via Twitter what '#ShowsWorkplaceCompassion' means from their perspective (Clyne et al., 2018). Statements included: '[n]urturing good people by valuing, respecting, rewarding them' and '[a] moment to make a cup of tea, to share a difficult time.'

Small acts of kindness, an embedded organisational culture of caring for one another, and recognition of the emotional and physical impact of health care work were the most frequently cited characteristics considered to show workplace compassion in health care. But what happens when compassion fatigue sets in?

## Compassion Fatigue

Building on earlier theories, Coetzee and Klopper (2010) defined compassion fatigue in the caring professions as 'the final result of a progressive and cumulative process that evolves from compassion stress after a period of unrelieved compassion discomfort, which is caused by prolonged, continuous and intense contact with patients, the use of self, and exposure to stress' (p. 237). A lack of resources, inadequate positive feedback, and individual reactions to distress have also been noted causes of compassion fatigue (Coetzee & Laschinger, 2018).

## Burnout

There is a significant relationship between compassion fatigue and burnout. We hear about burnout quite frequently, both from our colleagues and ourselves. But what are we really talking about and what does this mean? Earlier in my career I had the pleasure of meeting the inspirational Christina Maslach, who first introduced the classic definition of burnout as 'a syndrome of emotional exhaustion, depersonalisation, and reduced personal accomplishment that can occur among individuals who do 'people work' of some kind' (Maslach et al., 1986). It consists of the following three dimensions:

**Personal (Exhaustion):** Exhaustion is more than a feeling of tiredness easily resolved by sleep. It can be both physical and emotional, where one feels depleted, overstretched, and/or empty to the point of being potentially dysfunctional.

**Interpersonal (Cynicism):** Those experiencing cynicism in their burnt-out state may lose feeling toward colleagues and those in their care. This does not necessarily mean that they are not caring people, yet it may mean that they may feel unable to provide caring responses during this time. They may also become negative, snappy, and/or disengaged in the workplace.

**Self-Evaluation (Reduced Professional Efficacy):** It is important for midwives and nurses to experience feelings of competence and achievement in their work. Burnout can develop when these people do not feel that they are doing what they are meant to do, that their skills are being wasted, and/or that they have little ability to manage environmental demands and/or exercise control.

## What Might Compassion Fatigue and Burnout Look Like in Practice?

The physical effects of compassion fatigue may be similar to those of burnout. They may be displayed as lethargy, apathy, and/or poor performance in the workplace. There are also emotional effects to consider. These may be displayed as inurement (toughening up), irritability, detachment, callousness toward service users and colleagues, a reduced ability to self-evaluate, disengagement with self-care, poor judgement, and ultimately professional impairment. Take a moment here to reflect on how these effects may impact upon quality of care, professionalism, relationships, and the reputation of the professions in this context.

There is also a risk that such symptoms of compassion fatigue and burnout may be misinterpreted. For example, think of a midwife or nurse who seems uncaring, rude, and unkind to students, staff, and patients. This person may even say things to shock you, such as 'I don't care' or 'Screw them.' This behaviour may not define the person as uncaring, and whilst the behaviour may be construed as unprofessional and even uncivil or bullying in nature, the person may actually be showing symptoms of compassion fatigue and burnout. This does not mean that such behaviours are acceptable, but they may require a compassionate and practical, rather than punitive, response in promoting recovery.

# What Can Be Done?

Given that both compassion fatigue and burnout can have such negative personal and professional effects, we now need to look at how these may be mitigated. In this task, Maslach et al. (1986) suggest it is important to decipher where mismatches lie between the professional and the organisation. It is then important to instigate resolutions that rebalance such mismatches within each of the following six interconnected areas:

**Workload:** Job demands that are too high can increase work stress. It is important therefore to take both mental/physical breaks and reduce unmanageable workloads. Task changes at work can also be useful in rebalancing workloads.

**Control:** Increased autonomy is important and is linked to increased job satisfaction. Strong leadership and participation in decisions that affect one's work may promote balance in this area.

**Reward:** The rewards one receives for doing a job are significant in the promotion of wellbeing. Increased praise in teams may redress negative imbalances in this area.

**Community:** Communities that offer us a sense of purpose and belonging are psychologically good for us. Ongoing dialogues, civility, and a consistent information flow can bolster the quality of collegial relationships in this area.

**Fairness:** Inequity and injustices can cause disgruntlement. Do you and your colleagues have consistent and equitable rules to follow? Robust antidiscrimination interventions may reduce injustices in this regard.

**Values:** In pursuit of professional wellbeing, it is important that our values match those of our team/organisation. Due to the nature of our professional motivations, settings that support midwifery/nursing models of care may be most effective in enabling us to work in line with our values.

Following a brief exploration of compassion in health care organisations, this chapter has outlined the interrelations between compassion fatigue and burnout and suggested some of the ways in which their negative effects might be mitigated. Overall, despite the negative behavioural symptoms associated with these conditions, it remains important to foster compassionate collegial and managerial responses to foster recovery. Ultimately, staff and patient wellbeing are two sides of the same coin. In understanding context-specific issues, organisations may be better enabled to tailor workplace changes designed to mitigate the effects of any causes for concern identified.

| CASE STUDY 5.1 | Boats on an Ocean (with Activity) |
| --- | --- |

Following is the script of an audio artwork entitled 'Boats on an Ocean.' This piece was inspired by the narratives of health care professionals working during the COVID-19 pandemic as they reflected on their experiences and our workplace compassion research (Clyne et al., 2018). It was written and directed by Nick Walker following an innovative arts-based research workshop hosted with China Plate Theatre as part of the Humans Not Heroes project (which I am proud to be a part of) and the Coventry Creates initiative funded by Coventry University and the University of Warwick for Coventry City of Culture 2021. You can access the audio here:

For the activity, as you read the scripts consider how these experiences may relate to the themes discussed in this chapter.

### 1. Ext. Layby - Morning 1

It's morning and we're in a stationary car with its window open.

VOICE

This is a layby on a busy trunk road in the early morning. This is where I stop. In the rear-view mirror, I can see the hills and trees near my home. Ahead of me I can see the spires of the city, an orange glow of streetlights hovering above them. This is my coffee in a cup holder, its steam makes a tiny circle of fog on the windscreen. This is a delivery lorry rushing past, rocking my car like a boat on choppy seas, its horn blaring like an ocean liner. This is my breath, coming quickly. This is my heart, beating strongly so it makes my shirt quiver. This is the moment when everyone else will just see sunshine today, but for me, I know this is the beginning of it.

### 2. Int. Hospital - Morning 2

We're in the corridor outside the ICU.

VOICE

And there's another moment. The one when we put on our boots; the one when we close the door to our home, or the hotel room which has become our home; the one when we get off the bus; or when we smell the burnt bacon in the hospital cafe. Or even the night before, in front of the mirror, when you decide whether you need a shave or not. It's a different moment for all of us, but mine is when I put my lanyard over my head and turn my photo towards the world. It's when I feel a change both small and huge, and one that flows from my feet to the top of my head. It's the moment when 'me' becomes 'work me.' And for some, when 'her' becomes 'hero.'

We hear a bleep as she enters.

### 3. Int. Icu - Day 3

We're in a hospital room.

VOICE

The team is different again today. A paramedic has swapped a shift with someone who has a poorly dog. A receptionist has swapped a shift with someone who was coughed on in the street. A nurse has swapped a shift with a student who abandoned her lectures and her holiday to come and stand by our side. And me, I've swapped a shift with someone who hasn't seen her daughter for 8 weeks. And we do it because our lives are interlaced. Our feelings are interlaced, too. And I know there are lots of poems about love in the world, about roses and sunsets and mixtapes, but this is what love is here, and what it is now. We can't hug to show it, and so we show it by swapping shifts.

### 4. Int. Bedside - Day 4

We're at a bedside.

VOICE

There is no script for this, so this is what I will do. I will be at his bedside for you. I will whisper your words into his ear. I will whisper them softly and with love. I will whisper them as his wife. I will whisper them as his daughter. I will whisper them as his mother. I will make your words the sea breeze for him. I will make your words a sigh as you sit in the sun on a holiday from long ago. I will make your words feel like a kiss before bedtime. And when I've whispered them, I will remove the medical devices, I will wrap him in a blanket. And I will hear his last breath for you.

### 5. Ext. Hospital - Evening 5

We're outside in the hospital grounds. It's raining.

VOICE

None of us know what the weather does all day. Stepping outside, the sun has given way to rain, and it looks like it's been coming down for hours. And because today we sometimes said words to each other that we didn't mean; and we snapped at each other when we shouldn't have snapped; and some patients died in the company of strangers, compassionate strangers, but strangers all the same; because of all that I look up and feel the rain on my face and it brings me back to myself. Clear drops down my cheeks, not tears. I think how the goslings I've seen grow up in Swanswell Park will be splashing about in puddles. How my hay fever won't be so bad. How the weather will keep people inside and safe. And also, I thank this rain that's falling, because I won't need to water my plants tonight.

## 6. Ext. Street - Night 6

We're on a residential street.
> VOICE
> I drove off in the dark and I arrive home in the dark. Uniform gone. Lanyard hidden. I take my coffee cup out of the car to make room for tomorrow's. And although I haven't launched a ship today, and I haven't given a speech, and I haven't done a magic trick; I haven't scored a goal and I didn't win a gold medal, and I haven't been in a play and taken a bow; I haven't kissed the bride or graduated from college or arrived home as a war hero; although all I've done is my job today, just that, nevertheless, I can hear clapping. And I smile a thank you. And I mean it. And I also don't mean it. And I think of the comfort it brings. And I think of the babies it wakes up.

## 7. Int. Bedroom - Night 7

It's midnight.
> VOICE
> To help me sleep I say the word 'compassion.' If you say it softly it sounds like the sea breaking over the shore. Compassion. Compassion. Compassion. Swish swish swish. And I'm on a boat. It's not the same boat that everyone is in. Other boats are in calmer waters. Other boats are drifting. Other boats are fishing happily. Other boats are already lost beneath the waves. My boat is far out, in the swell of the storm, sails flapping, wood creaking, looking for land. And I will find it. Tomorrow I'll find it. Or the day after. It's the same ocean, though. Different boats, yes, but all of us are in the same ocean.
> The sea fades out.
> End.

## References

Clyne, W., Pezaro, S., Deeny, K., & Kneafsey, R. (2018). Using social media to generate and collect primary data: The #ShowsWorkplaceCompassion Twitter research campaign. *JMIR Public Health and Surveillance, 4*(2), e41.

Coetzee, S. K., & Laschinger, H. K. (2018). Toward a comprehensive, theoretical model of compassion fatigue: An integrative literature review. *Nursing & Health Sciences, 20*(1), 4–15.

Coetzee, S. K., & Klopper, H. C. (2010). Compassion fatigue within nursing practice: A concept analysis. *Nursing & Health Sciences, 12*(2), 235–243.

Klimecki, O., & Singer, T. (2012). Empathic distress fatigue rather than compassion fatigue? Integrating findings from empathy research in psychology and social neuroscience. *Pathological Altruism*, 368–383.

Kneafsey, R., Brown, S., Sein, K., Chamley, C., & Parsons, J. (2016). A qualitative study of key stakeholders' perspectives on compassion in healthcare and the development of a framework for compassionate interpersonal relations. *Journal of Clinical Nursing, 25*(1-2), 70–79.

Maslach, C., Jackson, S. E., & Leiter, M. P. (1986). *Maslach burnout inventory*. stylefix: Scarecrow Press.

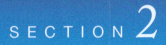

SECTION 2

# Managing Emotions in Difficult Times

**SECTION OUTLINE**

## CHAPTER 6

# Untangling Difficult Emotions on the Job

Olga Lainidi ■ Anthony Montgomery

## KEY POINTS

1. Being a nurse or midwife involves significant emotional demands that can increase during difficult times (e.g., a pandemic).
2. People experience very different emotions after the same events, despite choosing the same course of action.
3. The need to always be 'on the job' can significantly increase stress for nurses and midwives, which is known as emotional labour.
4. Nurses and midwives are sometimes forced to make undesirable decisions to achieve the best care possible based on the available resources for their patients, which can result in moral injury.
5. Employee silence in health care challenges the role of nurses and midwives as patient advocates.

## Introduction

Nurses and midwives are faced with emotionally demanding situations daily. These demands include dealing with patients and their relatives, communicating with colleagues effectively in pressured situations, coping with limited resources, increased workloads, and rationing care as a result of multiple demands on time and effort. Moreover, all these demands occur daily where nurses and midwives are expected to maintain standards and quality of care. The focus of this chapter will be on the challenge of managing emotions through difficult times (e.g., such as a pandemic). There is no doubt that empathy and compassionate care are beneficial for patients, but these core elements of the nursing profession can take a huge toll on nurses' and midwives' wellbeing. We will first provide a brief introduction to the science of emotions and then discuss the impact of moral injury and employee silence.

## From Emotion Physiology to the Subjective Emotional Experience

The ability to experience emotion is one of the most powerful and universal characteristics of humankind. Happiness and sadness convey the same meaning across cultures, continents, and even centuries, and humans have been investing energy and resources in communicating emotions for a very long time. For example, we are all familiar with the way that music and art can portray, communicate, and invoke emotional reactions in us and people around us. We all accept that we experience a broad range of emotions, but psychology is a discipline that tries to help us understand how emotions are experienced and how they affect our everyday lives. The psychological theories about emotions are almost as many as the number of emotions known to psychologists. According to the American Psychological Association, emotions are defined as complex reaction patterns experienced on three levels: a physiological response, a behavioural response, and a subjective experience. We should be careful here to avoid any confusion between emotions, feelings, and mood; feelings are related to the emotional experience and can be classified in the same taxonomy as pain; mood is any short-lived emotional state, usually of low intensity and, compared with emotions, lacks an apparent starting point. For example, a nurse might feel exhausted (feeling) at work, angry (emotion) after not being heard by the medical director, and spend the rest of the day in frustration at home (mood).

The element of physiological responses is a subject of the biology of emotions. The physiological activity of the nervous system is central to our understanding of emotions: the autonomic nervous system controls all those involuntarily physical reactions that arise when we have an emotional experience. For example, when someone experiences fear, they might have symptoms such as numb hands and/or legs, increased heartbeat, and shortness of breath/difficulty breathing. Those physiological symptoms indicate the body is in a situation that requires a stress-response mechanism to take over: fight, flight, or freeze.

The second element is the behavioural response. For example, when we are angry our expressions of anger can include shouting, keeping it to ourselves, talking about it to someone, or using alcohol to drown our sorrows. So, the behaviour refers to the action we take to express an emotion, and this action can be either positive or negative. From facial expressions to rituals and coping strategies, how we act in response to the way we feel varies within the same individual across different emotions and different situations and of course varies across different people. We will return to the behavioural aspect of the emotional experience later in the chapter when we discuss the issue of employee silence.

Last but not least is the element of the subjective experience of the emotion, and this is of critical importance when we think about managing emotions at work. Even when different people have identical physiological experiences (what happens in the body) followed by very similar behavioural responses (how we act in response to the way we feel), the purely emotional experience is still extremely subjective. For example, two nurses are the recipients of patient care concerns by a family member for not having dedicated enough time to a patient (same situation); both experience elevated heart rate and shortness of breath (physiological response), and both choose to apologise and proceed to the next patient (behavioural response). However, if we were to ask Nurse A, their subjective experience could be identified as anger, while for Nurse B it could be fear. This shows how people experience quite different emotions after the same events despite their own body responding in a similar way and despite choosing a similar or the same course of action.

From the perspective of nursing, our understanding of how we manage emotions in difficult times can be traced back to the ground-breaking work of sociologist Arlie Hochschild (1983), in her study of what she termed emotional labour, which is based on the idea that employees are often forced to display emotions at odds with what they truly feel. The basic argument is that professions such as nursing, where you are called upon to control and regulate your emotional expression continuously, contribute to burnout and fatigue. Daily in the workplace, nurses and midwives encounter different situations that can involve tremendous emotional effort. For example, nurses and midwives can be expected to express appropriate emotions, whereby they are expected to be empathetic, caring, compassionate, and considerate. Congruently, nurses and midwives frequently encounter challenging situations but are expected to modify or control unpleasant emotions such as anger, distress, sadness, and frustration.

Since the identification of emotional labour as a phenomenon, researchers have also realised that emotional states can be shared in work teams by the process of emotional contagion, which refers to a process where members of a group come to be infected by others' emotional states (insofar as they begin to mimic other members' facial expressions, body language, and vocal tone). Thus how nurse leaders and colleagues regulate their emotions at work can have a ripple effect on the members in their departments and units (as well as their patients). This leads us to the phenomena of moral injury and employee silence.

## Moral Injury

Moral injury is the psychological distress that results from either taking or not taking action in a way that violates our ethical or moral code. Missed nursing care is an example where nurses and midwives must make decisions—most of them in the moment—about what type of patient care should be urgently provided and which can be postponed or left undone due to lack of resources, lack of time, or insufficient support provided in the organisation. With between 55% and 98% of nurses reporting that necessary patient care work remains undone at the end of their shift due to lack of time and resources (Jones et al., 2015), it becomes clear that during a typical workday nursing staff might often experience psychological distress due to implicitly rationed nursing care. The need to make a forced, involuntarily decision to achieve the best care possible based on the available resources and/or time in a situation requires (most of the time) for the nurses and midwives to decide against their ethical or moral code, which in turn results in moral injury.

Nursing care as a profession entails emotional labour, but in difficult times (e.g., during a pandemic) it can become even more challenging. For example, at times, a shift from patient-centred ethics to public health ethics might be required, and whereas public health ethics is focused on equity, common good, and the risk and benefit to society, patient-centred ethics focuses on the duty to care for a particular patient (Hossain & Clatty, 2021). When dealing with scarcity of resources nurses and midwives might be called upon to make tough decisions regarding allocating resources and their time. There might be many instances where nurses and midwives must ignore a patient who wants more emotional support to attend to a patient who is more vulnerable, whereas in situations of intensive care or terminal diseases, nurses might be called upon to provide end-of-life care to patients and be a surrogate family for them. Finally, in situations where strict protocols that prevent family members from visiting dying patients might need to be enforced, considerable strain on the moral and ethical values of nurses and midwives can be placed.

The experience of moral injury carries a chain of negative emotions: guilt, shame, anger, disgust, and negative thoughts about ourselves, our job, the organisation we belong to, and the world in general. We use the word *chain* because even in situations where we can identify a very particular event that affected us intensely, the aforementioned reactions usually appear as a sequence of events—like links of a chain—while the emotional and moral burden is holding us back—like chains would do. The description of the emotional and cognitive burden of moral injury can be more easily understood if we think about depression or grief. Depression incorporates a persistent pattern of negative emotions and thoughts about the self, the people around us, and the world, and in that sense the experience of moral injury is characterised by negative thoughts and emotions experienced by the nurses and midwives about the self, the organisation, and the health care system in total. The first stages of grief, on the other hand, include states of disbelief and numbed feelings, moral pain and guilt, anger, and bargaining before we are ready to start moving toward acceptance. Moral injury can be viewed as the subjective experience of emotions, and, combined with feelings of emotional labour and/or burnout, will inform how we act. The British Psychological Society (2020) has produced a useful guide on the psychological needs of health care staff, which recommends allowing space for taking stock, organising active learning events, focusing on acknowledgment and reward, needs assessment of staff, and providing spaces for peer support. This brings us appropriately to our next section on employee silence.

## Employee Silence

In difficult times such as a pandemic, nurses and midwives must cope with an extra burden beyond providing care. On some occasions they have been instructed to keep silent about the lack of personal and professional equipment (PPE) (Campbell, 2020; Dyer, 2020). The pressure put on health care workers to keep quiet about the shortage of equipment raises the larger issue of how big a problem is moral injury and employee silence in nursing and midwifery. We have known for a long time that it takes a huge psychological toll to actively inhibit the expression of one's thoughts, emotions, and behaviours, and that efforts to inhibit or suppress responses can accumulate over time, resulting in physiological and psychological symptoms. Keeping quiet about what we think is important for our work is referred to as employee silence.

Employee silence is the act of withholding any genuine expression about opinions or concerns that relate to something in our work from persons who are perceived to be capable of effecting change or redress. Silence in health care can take several forms, which include being silent about a patient safety concern, ethical issues, discrimination issues, inappropriate supervisor behaviour, neglected care, lack of resources etc. There is growing evidence in health care that employee silence is common and likely to go unnoticed (i.e., because we are silent). Silence in health care has been associated with concealing errors, reduced patient safety, and covering up errors made by others. Conversely, there is evidence that in organisations where employees are encouraged to speak up about concerns, and where concerns are responded to appropriately, better patient outcomes occur, such as improved patient safety and patient experience. Interventions to promote speaking up in health care (e.g., hotlines or training) have not been successful and are rooted in a professional culture that does not promote speaking out.

Nursing and midwifery play a key role in patient advocacy, which makes the issue of employee silence even more sensitive. The UK Nursing and Midwifery Code of Ethics states that nurses and midwives must act as an advocate for those in their care, helping them to access relevant health and social care, information, and support (i.e., speaking up on behalf of the patient). However, there are good reasons why not speaking up is the inevitable choice in different situations. For example, if nursing staff believe that certain forms of silence based on loyalty or not breaking ranks is expected of them, they run the risk of underestimating the impact of silence on their own wellbeing. Moreover, nurses and midwives can carry this rumination home—about speaking up or staying silent—which makes recovery from work less effective. Furthermore, we should not underestimate the positive forms of silence in health care, such as when we are requested to overlook a procedural issue to fast-forward patient care.

Remaining silent or speaking up are not by definition positive or negative behaviours; not all forms of silence will make us feel worse and not every form of speaking up will make us feel better. There is evidence that defensive voice—speaking up because of fear aiming to protect the self—is the behavioural element of experiencing moral injury and burnout. In the same way, involuntary silence can be linked to feelings of burnout and moral injury as well. These relationships can be pull and push, meaning that silence or defensive voice can both precede and follow moral injury and burnout.

Traditionally, moral injury is a term that has been applied to military settings. However, health care has transformed the way that we think about moral injury. The complexities of the nursing profession and health care mean that we need more than policies to effectively address all potential sources of burnout and moral injury for nurses and midwives. It is likely that a certain level of moral injury and burnout is inevitable since delivering health care involves daily exposure to human suffering and pain. We need to avoid moral injury and burnout becoming unmanageable, which requires a more specific focus on prevention, starting from nursing education. The same applies to employee silence as a culture of not speaking up develops during educational experiences.

## What Can We Do About Employee Silence and Moral Injury?

We recommend the following for nurses and midwives:

- Emotional writing has been linked to improved wellbeing as it can untangle the range of feelings and emotions we experience at work.

- Providing a forum for nurses and midwives to discuss experiences of moral injury can function as a supportive network.
- Promote speaking up about concerns even if the speaking-up is conducted in a nonwork environment.
- Create support groups for nurses and midwives who want to work through the emotional burden of care.
- Design policies that will better protect the nurses' and midwives' rights to raise concerns about patient care.

## ACTIVITY

Think about a day at work that felt like a good day and a day at work that felt like a really bad day. Try to identify what made the good day run well and the bad day hard to get through. You will probably find it easier to understand what makes a day at work bad rather than good. Reflect on what contributed to you having a good day at work, and think about ways that potentially could make your workday easier for you and your colleagues. This activity will highlight that typically good days rely on what we can do at work, and bad days result from things that happen to us that we feel little control over.

## CASE STUDY 6.1    Achieving Solace Through Outside Space

The intensive care unit (ICU) is known to be a highly stressful environment for the staff who provide care to critically ill patients and their families. During the COVID-19 pandemic, especially during the early stages in 2020, the stressors facing nurses and other clinicians increased significantly. The stressors faced by nurses caring for COVID-19-positive critically ill patients in ICU were immense, and for many the stressors manifested in physical and psychological symptoms. In more normal times, ICU nurses report high rates of burnout and depression, as well as posttraumatic stress disorder symptoms. The UK Impact of Covid on Nurses (ICON) study (Couper et al., 2022) found that these rates had increased among nurses during the first waves of the pandemic.

In one of the largest acute hospitals, the University Hospitals Plymouth (UHP) National Health Service Trust, the picture of Covid infections was different from that in the larger cities such as London and Manchester. Even so, the sight of a 27-bed ICU filling up with COVID-19-positive patients, many of whom were extremely ill and stayed for several weeks in the ICU receiving physical and emotional care, was one that no one had ever seen before. Like many health care organisations, strategies were put in place to assist and support staff, from access to online mental health support to the provision of one-to-one sessions with a clinical psychologist. Prior to the pandemic, UHP had created a secret garden (i.e., a space where critically ill patients could be taken outside and experience the benefits of the outdoors whilst still receiving all the necessary organ supporting interventions). This served to be a lifesaver for staff and patients during these stressful pandemic waves.

This unique and visionary garden is located in the depths of the hospital and was made possible through raising funds internally and externally. The cancellation of a major garden show resulted in one of the main exhibitors donating its show garden plants to the ICU to enable patients and staff to enjoy the sights in the secret garden. Whilst early on it was thought the patients benefited most from time in this space, it became clear just how beneficial time outside the stressful ICU was to the staff. Once the PPE had been safely doffed, staff were then able to sit in a calm and peaceful oasis in the centre of a busy hospital and recharge their personal batteries, helping them to face another period wearing full PPE.

When patients were not outside, nurses found that the time spent in the garden gave them recovery time, doing what helped them at the time. This might be sitting and eating food outside, enjoying the sunshine, chatting to colleagues, whilst in scrubs, and without fear of contaminating any other colleagues within the hospital, given that we were still learning a lot about how this virus spread.

The secret ICU garden truly helped many patients to turn the corner and begin to recover from their illness. The same could be said for many nurses and other health professionals as they found a place where they could spend a short amount of time in their recovery from moral injury. This special rehabilitation garden is something that should be, and is being, replicated in other hospitals worldwide.

**BRIDIE KENT**   ■   **KATE TANTAM**

## References

British Psychological Society. (2020). *The psychological needs of healthcare staff as a result of the coronavirus outbreak.* https://www.bps.org.uk/sites/www.bps.org.uk/files/News/News%20-%20Files/Psychological%20 needs%20of%20healthcare%20staff.pdf.

Campbell, D. (2020). *NHS staff 'gagged' over coronavirus shortages.* The Guardian UK. https://www.theguardian.com/society/2020/mar/31/nhs-staff-gagged-over-coronavirus-protective-equipment-shortages.

Couper, K., Murrells, T., Sanders, J., Anderson, J. E., Blake, H., Kelly, D., & Harris, R. (2022). The impact of COVID-19 on the wellbeing of the UK nursing and midwifery workforce during the first pandemic wave: *A longitudinal survey study. International journal of nursing studies, 127,* 104155.

Dyer, C. (2020). Covid-19: Doctors are warned not to go public about PPE shortages. *BMJ, 369.* https://doi.org/10.1136/bmj.m1592.

Hochschild, A. R. (1983). *The managed heart: Commercialization of human feeling.* University of California Press.

Hossain, F., & Clatty, A. (2021). Self-care strategies in response to nurses' moral injury during COVID-19 pandemic (2021). *Nursing Ethics, 28*(1), 23–32. https://doi.org/10.1177/0969733020961825.

Jones, T. L., Hamilton, P., & Murry, N. (2015). Unfinished nursing care, missed care, and implicitly rationed care: State of the science review. *The International Journal of Nursing Studies, 52*(6), 1121–1137.

## CHAPTER 7

# Starting Conversations About Your Mental Health

Hollie Starbuck  ■  Paul Maloret  ■  Holly Blake

## KEY POINTS

1. Nurses and midwives are at risk of mental ill health, but they often find it challenging to speak openly about their own mental health concerns.
2. The existence of stigma around mental health is a reality but is unhelpful and hinders disclosure and help-seeking behaviour.
3. Individuals can take small actions to benefit their own mental wellbeing that align with their values as health professionals: reflect on emotions, practice self-compassion, and start conversations about mental health.
4. Training courses on supporting conversations about mental health are beneficial to employees and line managers.
5. The responsibility for mental health is not that of the individual alone; line managers and the wider organisation play a critical role in tackling stigma, reviewing organisational structures, advocating psychologically safe work environments, and providing mental health support.

## Introduction

Have you ever found it difficult to speak about your mental wellbeing at work? Or support others to open up? In this chapter, we explore the benefits and associated challenges of speaking about your mental wellbeing within the working environment. People who have mental health conditions or poor mental wellbeing often find it difficult to talk about it in the workplace. They worry about facing stigma and discrimination. These worries are usually set in the context of responding to the daily demands and pressures of work: busy jobs, long hours, and trying to demonstrate a certain level of motivation and commitment to the job while experiencing poor health. This can feel like an untenable situation. One of the most important things we can do to foster positive mental health is to encourage open conversations about it. In this chapter, we therefore consider how you can start conversations about mental health and reflect on the positive actions that can be taken by line managers and the wider organisation to support this.

## Mental Ill Health in the Workforce

In the general workforce, one in five employees are affected by a mental health condition at any one time, leading to an estimated cost of between £33 billion - £42 billion a year (Farmer & Stevenson, 2017). You can read more about the costs of mental ill health and how they are estimated elsewhere in this book. In Great Britain, the Health and Safety Executive (HSE) published data gathered up to March 2021 on the prevalence of work-related stress, anxiety, or depression across occupations (HSE, 2021). This report shows that these conditions are more prevalent in public service industries such as health and social care. In fact, health care workers have higher levels of stress compared to all other jobs. A report published in July 2020, 'The Mental Health and Wellbeing of Nurses and Midwives in the United Kingdom (UK),' showed that nurses and midwives are at particular risk of mental ill health, with high rates of work-related stress, burnout, and mental health problems such as depression and anxiety (Kinman et al., 2020). Findings from the UK National Health Service (NHS) Staff Survey 2018 reflect the picture of mental ill health in nurses and midwives. Prior to the global COVID-19 pandemic:

- 43.5% of nurses and midwives were unwell due to work-related stress
- 34% showed symptoms of 'at least moderate' anxiety
- 37% showed symptoms of depression
- 5% of midwives fit the diagnostic criteria for posttraumatic stress disorder
- 20% to 39% of midwives were showing signs of posttraumatic stress
- Suicide rate in nurses was 23% higher than the occupational average for nurses between 2011 and 2015

These figures may escalate further due to the impacts of the pandemic on nurses and midwives across the world. Globally, there are approximately 28 million practicing nurses and midwives across various capacities. It is hard to estimate the true cost of mental illness in different countries and regions, but the average prevalence of burnout has been estimated at 11.23% in the world's nurses, and it has been suggested that the numbers are likely to be quite similar across nations (Woo et al., 2020). Mental health is therefore a global priority.

# What Stops Conversations About Mental Ill Health?

## FEAR OF STIGMA

Stigma around mental health is one of the biggest barriers to speaking openly about the way we feel. There are many definitions of stigma, but in brief it involves negative attitudes or discrimination against someone based on a distinguishing characteristic such as a mental health condition. In the workplace, stigma is an ongoing concern and has been increasingly challenged by antidiscrimination legislation as well as mental health promotion and antistigma campaigns (Stevenson & Farmer, 2017). However, the reaction to sharing mental health information remains difficult, and there are concerns that employees are defined by, or judged for, the information they have bravely offered.

Worldwide, mental health organisations advocate for people to speak up about mental ill health and seek help when it is needed. For example, Mind (a UK-based mental health charity) advocates speaking up as a mechanism for ending stigma, and Mental Health America provides tips on starting conversations about mental health. The reality is, however, that talking about mental distress for most people does not feel in parity with disclosing a physical health condition.

There are also strong cultural differences in the way in which mental health is perceived and discussed that may engender stigma or further prevent people from talking openly about their mental health. In many cultures, where there is the widely accepted notion that a person undergoing treatment for cancer or a broken leg cannot be blamed or responsible for the course of the illness, the same understanding or patience is not always attributed to the journey of a mental health condition. Asking ourselves whether we would be viewing the situation the same way as if we or the person affected was diagnosed with a physical health condition can be a good first step to noticing stigma in play within ourselves and our teams.

# Internalised/Self-Stigma

Stigma is a societal phenomenon, but when we are sharing society's air it is often impossible to not breathe it in, too. Self-stigma is the process of absorbing the views of those in our communities and turning them in on ourselves. For example, people who experience depression may hear from those around them that they are not trying hard enough to change their mindset and subsequently judge themselves in a similar fashion. What we do know about stigma is that it adds another layer of shame to our distress, which can have a paralysing effect. Those affected by societal and self-stigma are very unlikely to feel that opening up conversations about their mental health is going to be of benefit.

## STIGMA SPECIFIC TO HEALTH CARE

While nurses and midwives are at considerable risk for mental ill health, they are often reticent to talk about it due to worry about being perceived to be failing to cope (Kinman et al., 2020). This chapter and the reports we refer to bring hope of raising visibility to the overall picture. Consider this: if almost half of the nursing and midwifery workforce are losing days of work due to mental ill health, the likelihood is that half the members of our current team could be struggling; yet for most, this feels shrouded in secrecy. So why might this be happening?

From the perspective of the individual nurse or midwife, the most common fear is the possible ramifications of seeking help. What will my colleagues think? Will I be seen as incapable or incompetent? Will my registration be revoked? We tend not to ask these questions with relation to our physical heath. The oncologist who develops cancer is unlikely to be judged for not knowing how to have prevented the condition, but a nurse (especially one that works in the mental health field) can hold beliefs of somehow being able to foresee or control the course of a mental illness. This stigma, coupled with a desire to prioritise patients' health over their own, can result in nurses and midwives working through mental ill health, yet paradoxically this has a negative impact on care quality.

In recent times there has been a comparison of health and care workers to superheroes (i.e., working through challenging times of crisis and adversity). While this is well meaning, the comparison to superheroes could perpetuate the notion that nurses and midwives should be able to cope with superhuman levels of stress and illness, which oils the wheels of stigma surrounding discussions about health—in particular mental ill health. Trying to see oneself as human with the same basic physiological and psychological needs as those we care for is imperative.

The increasing global focus on mental health advocacy is slowly reducing the stigma around mental ill health and encouraging more open conversations. The rate at which this is happening, however, varies across regions and cultures, and we must remain realistic about the challenges that remain.

# What Will Talking Do to Help?

Outside of the other worries about what opening up may mean for us, a common thought is that simply discussing our struggles cannot change anything. Yet there is evidence to show that the process of supervision, debriefing, reflection, and expressing our emotions has a multitude of (often unexpected) positive outcomes.

Talking about the way you feel is not a sign of weakness. It is part of taking charge of your wellbeing and doing what you can to stay healthy. Discussing your issues can be a way of coping with the problem. Just being listened to can help you feel supported and less alone with your thoughts and your understanding of them. It can allow us to put our worries into perspective, which often means the worries themselves lose power and the individual feels able to have more control over such thoughts and feelings. It can also provide a signpost to support you in awareness and reassurance that you might need to take these avenues.

Aside from the individual benefits, us opening up and talking about our mental health helps our wider team and can act as a catalyst for positive change in the workforce. Breaking new ground and talking about our mental health can pave the way for others to follow suit.

## THE POWER OF BEING HEARD

The simple act of being heard can give individuals the time, space, and acknowledgment they need to process difficult thoughts and feelings. As mentioned previously, the self and external stigma are often the compounding issues that keep us in a cycle of isolation and despair. Being listened to and having our worries acknowledged and validated by another can be enough to break the shame and stigma and create a wider culture of acceptance. Feeling properly heard feeds a loop of mutual openness and helps individuals become less self-critical, more reflective, and therefore more open to changes of thought and behaviour (Rogers & Farson, 1957).

# What Can We Do to Help Ourselves?

Before we talk about the actions we can take as individuals, it is important to set these in the wider context of change. Kinman et al. (2020) differentiate between primary, secondary, and tertiary level interventions. Primary interventions are at the level of the individual employee and are all about personal actions and taking personal control. There is a place for personal control, but individual (primary) interventions can be seen as tokenistic and short term. At worst they can be detrimental when not backed up with higher level managerial (secondary) or systemic, organisational (tertiary) improvements. It is not our intention here to place the ultimate responsibility for opening conversations about mental health on the shoulders of individuals; this comes from the combined actions of individuals, line managers, organisations, and society. Yet, there are small, evidence-based changes that are within the individual's control that, when taken alongside wider considerations, can make a big difference.

## HAVING A CONVERSATION WITH OURSELVES

Before we start a conversation with managers or colleagues about our mental health, we first need to talk with ourselves. Before a discussion with others can take place, we should reflect on our awareness of this need and be kind to ourselves for identifying it. In a fast-paced world it is common to struggle with mental health and not even consciously recognise it. So, if we have recognised the need, we have achieved something already. So how do we identify what we are feeling?

Sometimes identifying our feelings can be difficult, and this is okay; in fact, researchers claim that there are tens of thousands of different emotions! It is very normal to feel many different emotions over a short period of time, or even at the very same time.

One way to identify them is to use an emotions wheel. There are many examples freely available online, and they help to bring clarity to emotions. As an example, Plutchik's wheel of emotions is a circular graphic divided into sections and subsections to help users better identify and understand their emotional experience at any given time, under any circumstance (Plutchik & Kellerman, 1980) (Fig. 7.1). It was developed by American psychologist Dr. Robert Plutchik, who proposed that there are eight primary emotions that serve as the foundation for all others: joy, sadness, acceptance, disgust, fear, anger, surprise, and anticipation.

## DEALING WITH THE INNER CRITIC

For several reasons, the outcome of this internal conversation may be the barrier to expressing ourselves more widely. Some of us talk to ourselves with a critical voice, one which we would never use to speak to anyone else. It is common to not be aware of this internal discussion and yet it certainly can deeply affect how we feel about ourselves and our ability to talk openly about our struggles. If you are finding it difficult to discuss your feelings and wellbeing with others, it's a good idea to think first about whether your own self-critical thoughts and self-stigma are potential barriers.

## SELF-COMPASSION

Interestingly, not everyone experiencing distress falls foul of the effects of stigma or self-criticism. When exploring the reasons why, Gilbert (2013) explains it comes down to self-acceptance. Our society is not yet where it needs to be to promote positive wellbeing, and it may be unrealistic to think we can change things dramatically overnight even though things are changing for the better. However, accepting yourself and practicing self-compassion has been shown to make an enormous difference in the way we feel about ourselves, our job, and the world (Gilbert, 2013).

Along with everything else in life, we can only control the controllable, and the only controllable factor is often how we view the challenges rather than the challenge themselves. Taking active steps to be more self-compassionate as a daily practice is likely to help improve your individual wellbeing.

> *'Caring for myself is not self-indulgence, it is self-preservation.'*
> —AUDRE LORDE

# Positive Line Manager or Team Responses

Line managers often have a good knowledge of what help is out there for their employees, but they can feel prohibited by time (Kinman et al., 2020). Making time to talk with the team preventatively about mental wellbeing, and the causes and impacts of stigma, is advised. Often these conversations happen too late when symptoms have already progressed. Incorporating signposting to available support into group supervision or team meetings will normalise the need for support and potentially spark supportive, stigma-busting conversations between colleagues.

Many line managers have themselves expressed feeling less confident in these discussions. Using active listening techniques as outlined later will be helpful, but prioritising enrolling in training courses in supporting conversations about mental health has been found to be hugely beneficial (Kinman et al., 2020).

Being aware of our own perceptions and assumptions about mental health and wellbeing is a priority and can act as a catalyst for positive change in your wider team. Finding time and resources to facilitate group and individual interventions should be a priority (Kinman et al., 2020).

## USING ACTIVE LISTENING

| *Do* | *Don't* |
|---|---|
| Pay attention and set aside any distractions. | Rush to solutions: 'Well, if you are depressed, it's best to exercise.' |
| Ask open questions (who/what/when/why/how): 'How did that feel for you?' 'What do you think would be most helpful?' Be curious about the person's reality. | Assume based on what you think you know: 'I have studied anxiety so you must be feeling this way.' Let your ideas and solutions stop you from listening. |

| *Do* | *Don't* |
|------|---------|
| Allow time for silence, which is when the individual can be free to think, process, and make links. | Place your judgments or values on the individual. |
| Paraphrase to ensure understanding: 'So, what I heard you are most upset about is ___. Does that sound right?' | Equate your experience with them. Everyone experiences everything differently. |
| Acknowledge and validate what the individual is saying: | Make the conversation about you. |
| 'I really can see why you feel overwhelmed with your caseload now that you've explained this to me.' | |
| 'It is understandable that you are feeling anxious about this.' | |

*True listening requires a setting aside of oneself.'*
—M. SCOTT PECK

*'If your mouth is open, you are not learning.'*
—BUDDHA

## RECOMMENDATIONS

| *Who* | *What* |
|-------|--------|
| Line Managers | • Advocating and providing protected time for group and individual interventions and approaches are priorities.<br>• Goal is to create an open environment in a nontokenistic way.<br>• Role model from above.<br>• Prioritise training and courses in open dialogue and mental health, not just clinical training.<br>• Prioritise group supervision/time for debrief.<br>• Ask about mental health more preventatively, not waiting for return to work or yearly appraisal although these are helpful, too.<br>• Monitor burnout (e.g., using a standardized measure).<br>• Use Health and Safety Executive framework to support staff with their mental health.<br>• Utilise referrals to Occupational Health Services. |
| Wider Trust | • Review staffing levels to allow reflective practice/self-care to be easier.<br>• Mental health treated with parity to physical health; take seriously the health and safety risks affecting mental health in line with regulations.<br>• All trusts should have a policy on work-related stress and managing mental health and wellbeing as a priority.<br>• Individuals can make some change themselves by engaging in self-care interventions, but the bigger focus needs to be on the organisational structures and tackling stigma at a wider level. |
| Individuals | • Monitor own mental health and start becoming aware of it.<br>• Role model openness even when it is difficult.<br>• Make small changes in your department: supervision groups/let's talk time/service improvement.<br>• Use the support systems in place.<br>• Be aware of the role of stigma and how internal and external stigma can keep us quiet.<br>• Participate in supportive services (e.g., psychoeducation initiatives, self-compassion training, reflective group practices, mindfulness-based stress reduction strategies, online discussion forums to improve coping skills). |

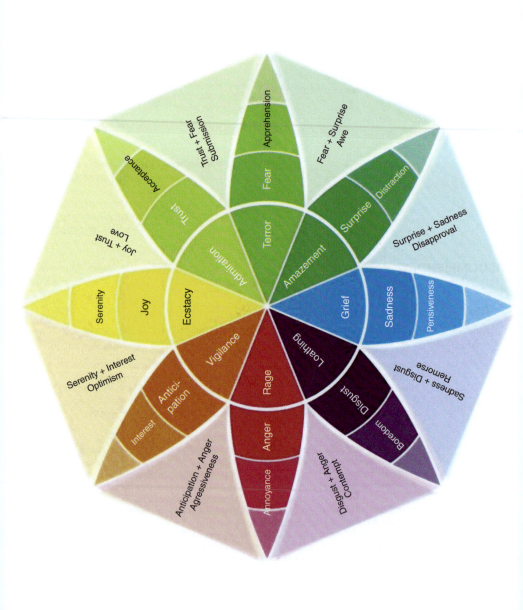

**ACTIVITY**

1. Set an alarm throughout the day. Each time the alarm goes off ask yourself how you are feeling. Write down which emotions are coming to mind. If it is helpful, use Plutchik's wheel of emotions to identify them.
2. When your alarm goes off, add to your notes what thoughts you have just been having about yourself. Try to identify what words your mind uses in your internal monologue. This will get easier the more you practice, and it will likely highlight some surprising findings. Common words to look out for:

   Never/always: 'I always let everyone down, I can't tell anyone I'm struggling.'

   Should/shouldn't: 'I shouldn't be feeling this way, others cope with a higher caseload' or 'I shouldn't be struggling myself, I am meant to be a nurse.'

   Next, reply to yourself as you would a friend.

---

**CASE STUDY 7.1**      **Creating Wellness Action Plans to Support Open Dialogue About Mental Health**

Starting a conversation around mental health can seem difficult. Research carried out through a workplace health initiative called the Mental Health and Productivity Pilot has revealed that employers want to do more to support mental health in the workplace. Why? Because we know that open conversations help to create healthy, happy workplaces where all staff can thrive. This case study provides two examples of how the workplace can reduce stigma and discrimination around mental health in the workplace and encourage staff to talk openly about mental health between themselves and with their line manager.

Every Mind Matters is Public Health England's first national mental health campaign. It aims to support all adults to feel more confident in understanding mental health and to take actions to improve and manage how they are feeling. Every Mind Matters offers a range of useful resources, including information on signs of common mental health issues, practical self-care tips, and where to seek further support. It has a free online tool (approved by the UK National Health Service), which will help you build a self-care action plan to deal with stress and anxiety, boost your mood, improve your sleep, and help you feel more in control.

Wellness action plans (WAPs) are an easy, practical way of helping you to support your own mental health at work and helping your line manager to support your mental health. A WAP is a personalised, practical tool we can all use—whether we have a mental health problem or not—to help us identify what keeps us well at work, what causes us to become unwell, and how to address a mental health problem at work should you be experiencing one. It can also be used to open up a dialogue with your manager or supervisor for them to better understand your needs and experiences and better support your mental health. This can lead to greater productivity, better performance, and increased job satisfaction.

How to get started with a WAP:
- Plan some time on your own to fill in your WAP.
- Schedule some confidential time with your manager to discuss it.
- Consider what it would be helpful for your manager to know before the meeting.

**Andy's Story (Nurse in a Busy NHS Trust)**

*'I don't have a mental health problem, but I think wellbeing and mental health shouldn't be something we only talk about when we get ill. My team and I have been under an immense amount of pressure during the pandemic, so when my manager suggested we all complete a WAP, I thought it would be a good opportunity to think about what makes me stressed at work and what helps me to perform well and be productive. As part of my WAP, I identified that a few things cause me stress—for example, not being kept informed of developments in the organisation that could affect me, a chaotic environment, and people not being supportive or approachable. Having set these out, I then considered ways they could be alleviated. I now feel more in control of my own mental health and feel listened to.'*

To learn more about how to look after your mental health and create your own action plan, visit Every Mind Matters (www.nhs.uk) and Wellness Action Plan (download: Mind, the mental health charity—help for mental health problems).

**KATE WOOD**

## References

Farmer, P., & Stevenson, D. (2017). *Thriving at work: the independent review of mental health and employers*. https://assets.publishing.service.gov.uk/government/uploads/system/uploads/attachment_data/file/658145/thriving-at-work-stevenson-farmer-review.pdf.

Gilbert, P. (2013). *The compassionate mind: a new approach to life's challenges*. London, Constable.

Health and Safety Executive. (2021). *Work-related stress, depression or anxiety statistics in Great Britain*. https://www.hse.gov.uk/statistics/causdis/stress.pdf.

Kinman, G., Teoh, K., & Harriss, A. (2020). *The mental health and wellbeing in nurses and midwives in the United Kingdom*. London: The Society of Occupational Medicine. https://www.som.org.uk/sites/som.org.uk/files/The_Mental_Health_and_Wellbeing_of_Nurses_and_Midwives_in_the_United_Kingdom.pdf.

Plutchik, R., & Kellerman, H. (1980). *Emotion: theory, research and experience*. Vol. 1, Theories of emotion. New York, Academic Press.

National Health Service. (2018). *Workforce health and wellbeing framework*. https://www.nhsemployers.org/sites/default/files/media/NHS-Workforce-HWB%20Framework-updated-July-18_0.pdf.

Rogers, C. R., & Farson, R. E. (1957). *Active listening*. Chicago, Industrial Relations Center, The University of Chicago.

Woo, T., Ho, R., Tang, A., & Tam, W. (2020). Global prevalence of burnout symptoms among nurses: A systematic review and meta-analysis. *J Psychiatr Res. 123*, 9–20.

## CHAPTER 8

# Dealing With Anxiety and Low Mood

Rachel Paskell  ▪  Jo Daniels

## KEY POINTS

1. Understand survival mechanisms and their role in normal mental health.
2. Use daily activity scheduling to keep the cogs turning.
3. Use daily activity scheduling to keep on top of mental health and wellbeing.
4. Recognise and challenge unhelpful thinking habits and behavioural responses.
5. Identify early warning signs and take simple steps to help improve mental health.

## Introduction

Mental health encompasses emotional, psychological, and social wellbeing. Mental health influences, and is influenced by, how we think, feel, behave, and relate to others. Our mental health naturally fluctuates over our lifetime and even over the course of a day; it is shaped by our preexisting and ever-changing biology, our life events and stressors, social support, and family histories. Around one in four people struggle with mental health on a day-to-day basis, and it is likely that we know someone close to us who is facing these difficulties. However, effective interventions are available, and many people go on to lead high-functioning lives that are not adversely affected by their mental health difficulties.

When we experience 'good' mental health we are likely to be feeling, generally on top of life's challenges and operating within what we might term our emotional and psychological window of tolerance (Siegel, 1999). Within this window we feel able to regulate our emotions, think clearly, and perform our best. The window of tolerance includes fluctuations around what is usually normal for us (i.e., our personal baseline) and can range from intense emotional states to intense calm; this is the emotional bandwidth that is optimal for us functioning effectively. For example, when hearing an alarm going off on the ward, operating within this window allows us to respond quickly and effectively, using skills and training to provide the necessary health care intervention. Or, conversely, we can deliver the calm, empathic warmth needed when giving news to a worried patient. We will each have a different window and range of emotions that we can tolerate before we begin to feel unsettled.

Over the course of our lives we all develop our own tools and techniques designed to help us stay cool, calm, collected, and connected at times of extreme stress, worry, or challenge (i.e., strategies that keep us within our window and not too far from our usual baseline). However, most of us will also experience episodes of stress that move beyond what is tolerable and manageable. In these times our emotions can become overly intense and difficult to manage (which is sometimes termed as 'dysregulated'), leaving us prone to experiencing overwhelm. This presents differently for different people and can be broadly separated into two types of responses: hyperarousal and hypoarousal. In hyperarousal, we can feel emotionally flooded, in a state of heightened alertness (hypervigilant), on edge, fearful, angry, experience racing thoughts and physical symptoms. This pattern of symptoms is often associated with an anxiety response. In hypoarousal, more commonly seen in low mood, we can feel  emotionally flat, lethargic, experience brain fog and thinking problems, and feel generally disconnected from the world. Over time, if experienced too regularly, these symptoms and patterns of symptoms can influence our ability to function effectively at home, at work, and in areas of self-care, which is why it is important to recognise the signs and develop strategies to address them.

## Anxiety and Low Mood

### ANXIETY

Fear and anxiety are normal evolutionary responses to feeling under threat. When we feel under threat, whether socially (e.g., judged by our peers), physically (e.g., exposure to a virus), or emotionally (e.g., difficult issues that feel personal and make you feel vulnerable), our brain triggers a self-protective survival mechanism that can result in a hormone-fueled fight-or-flight response designed to equip us to tackle or escape the pending threat. Our breathing increases to get more oxygen, blood vessels fill with oxygen-carrying red blood cells, our heart beats faster to distribute the oxygen and energy to the muscles we might need, our muscles tense and ready for action, and our thinking becomes more focused on the job at hand and less on things such as language. To gain an increased sense of safety, we then act to protect ourselves and/or others by avoiding or attempting to eliminate the threat. This response is triggered when the threat is real or merely perceived. Once we feel the threat has passed, the fear and anxiety resolve.

Anxiety can take many forms, however there are common patterns of thinking which allow anxiety to be better understood as specific subtypes, which include social anxiety disorder, obsessive-compulsive disorder, health anxiety, agoraphobia, panic disorder, and most commonly generalised anxiety disorder. All are maintained by the complex interaction between our thoughts, feelings, and behaviour (more on that later). Although these subtypes focus on particular concerns (e.g., health anxiety is associated with fears around having or contracting an illness), they share core characteristics when presenting in a way that is not just a passing concern but something more debilitating. Here are the key signs that normal anxiety and worry have transitioned into something that might need tackling:

- Worrying or feeling more anxious more often than you are not
- Anxiety that gets in the way of your usual hobbies, your relationships or you doing your job properly
- Regularly experiencing physical symptoms common in anxiety (e.g., palpitations, muscle tension, nausea, panic, irritability, sleep disturbance)
- Having thoughts that relate to fear of being unable to cope or wanting to escape a situation
- Anxiety that has persisted for months rather than days or weeks

While we might all experience some of these signs and symptoms from time to time, if they are consistent and affecting our daily lives, it is time to take steps to address difficulties in a more concerted way. It is easy to avoid dealing with mental health difficulties, hoping they will spontaneously improve, but we know that avoidance is key to maintaining these problems.

### LOW MOOD

Feeling low in mood is a normal response to difficult situations such as a relationship breakdown, loss of a loved one, feelings of disappointment, or reflections on difficult past events. This usually resolves naturally over time. However, if the symptoms of low mood become a more regular feature of daily life, this also warrants our attention. Like anxiety, there are key signs to indicate the transition from feeling low due to circumstances, to a spiral of low mood that feels difficult to shift:

- Having persistent negative views of self, the world, and the future (Beck, 1979)
- Low mood most of the day, on most days
- Loss of interest or pleasure in doing things you normally enjoy
- Low mood that gets in the way of your usual hobbies, relationships, or you being able to do your job properly
- Feeling foggy in your thinking, such as struggling with word finding or memory
- Physical symptoms such as losing or gaining weight, low energy, fatigue, loss of libido, and sleep problems

This inevitably leads to us doing less, disconnecting from others, and taking less care of ourselves, others, and our things. However, these shifts in behaviour are known to perpetuate the cycle of low mood, risking a downward spiral.

For some, negative thinking may lead to thoughts of suicide or self-harm. Very often this is the result of feeling like we do not have the resources to cope with a certain situation. Thoughts of suicide and self-harm are signs that we want the difficult problem to stop or end, and we might feel like the only way to achieve this is through suicide. These thoughts need to be addressed early on and should be taken very seriously-asking for help is the first step.

## Traumatic Experiences

Health care professionals are often at the frontline when it comes to some of life's most difficult events. Working in exceptional circumstances such as exposure to or threat of death, serious injury, or violence increases the likelihood of experiencing trauma-related distress. Health care workers are also at greater risk of moral distress, which arises when we witness or experience events that do not fit with our moral code of what is right/just. This might include being asked to do something you do not feel comfortable or trained to do, an unexpected loss of a patient, or making complex decisions that negatively impact others.

The initial fight-or-flight response often experienced in these difficult situations is an important and powerful natural coping mechanism for staying safe and responding quickly. However, in very emotionally charged situations, such as trauma or moral distress, the brain finds it difficult to process and make sense of what is happening. This can be very upsetting and can negatively impact our sense of self, perception of others, and the world in which we live and work.

In the immediate aftermath of difficult events, thoughts and images related to what happened may pop into our minds unexpectedly; we might dream about them or ponder them repeatedly during the day. This is a normal and essential stage of processing to make sense of the experience, though it can be quite distressing and worrying at the time. During this early phase you may notice you are more on edge, irritable, angry, distracted, low, or emotionally bruised. You may be more tearful or emotionally numb and may experience guilt or shame. For most people, these symptoms start to naturally improve as time passes.

During these early stages it is important to stay connected with people and do things that are healthy and important to us. Talking through the experiences with people we trust and feel supported by can be particularly helpful. This can be through informal connections or more formal structures provided by your organisation, such as staff wellbeing support (Daniels et al., 2021). However, if these difficult experiences persist for more than one month and impact significantly on your ability to function, it is important to seek specialist mental health support. Doing this early can help reduce the ripple effect of difficulties growing and impacting more broadly.

# Managing Mental Health

Managing our own mental health is a lifelong commitment. Therefore, a proactive approach to mental health, rather than waiting for difficulties to arise, is likely to reap long-term benefits. Taking inventory of early warning signs, triggers, and coping strategies is an important first step before tackling difficulties head on. The following paragraphs contain tips on how to start the ball rolling; an end-of-chapter activity will help to practice these skills.

## UNDERSTANDING THE MAINTENANCE OF ANXIETY AND LOW MOOD: WHAT KEEPS IT GOING?

The perceived threat responses that trigger our survival mechanisms are usually associated with thoughts about something bad happening in the future or having happened in the past. As we raised earlier, these commonly relate to our social selves, physical health, or the emotional side of things. These thoughts not only trigger the physiological (fight-or-flight) and emotional responses (e.g., fear/anxiety) but also lead us to take action to protect ourselves. How we respond to these thoughts can make us feel better about the situation, or in some circumstances, perpetuate a cycle of anxiety or low mood.

This cycle, involving our thoughts, feelings, behaviour, and physiology, is commonly conceptualised within a cognitive behaviour framework (Beck, 1979). A simplified version of this is the five-part model (Greenberger & Padesky, 2016) (Fig. 8.1), which includes the external environment; this is particularly important if you are working or living in a stressful setting. This model highlights the two-way relationship between each of these five dimensions and the strong role they play in the persistence of anxiety and low mood. The underpinning theory of this model forms the basis of cognitive-behavioural therapy (CBT), a prominent evidence-based psychological approach to treating anxiety, depression, and a range of other difficulties.

The premise of this model is that how we respond to our thoughts (e.g., 'I might embarrass myself') informs our choice of behavioural response (e.g., avoid social situations), which then directly affects how we feel both emotionally (e.g., fed up, anxious) and physically (e.g., on edge), feeding back into the cycle as belief in our negative thought is reinforced.

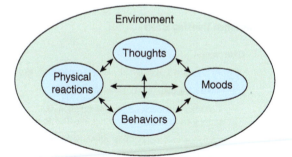

**Fig. 8.1** Five-part model to understand life experiences. (From Padesky, C.A. & Mooney, K.A. (1990). Clinical tip: Presenting the cognitive model to clients. *International Cognitive Therapy Newsletter, 6,* 13–14.)

## BREAKING THE CYCLE ONCE IT GETS GOING

There are simple steps that we can take if we are able to notice our 'early warning signs.' When we start to struggle with our mental health, many of us display subtle changes, such as loss of sense of humour, withdrawing from others, or doing less activity. These are our early warning signs and indications that now is a good time to step in and think about what steps we need to take to safe guard our mental health. See end of chapter activity for help to identify what you might need to look out for. These specifically relate to the physiological, cognitive, behavioural, and emotional aspects.

## Breathing and Moving

At times of stress and anxiety, hyperventilation and shallow breathing is common. Purposeful, regular breathing can therefore work to reset the fight-or-flight response, help us get a sense of control, and prevent the onset of panic and the unpleasant physical symptoms associated with anxiety. This is also true for exercise, which can help burn off the excess adrenaline associated with a stress response. It can also give much needed perspective.

## Identify and Challenge Negative Thinking

Our thoughts are central to triggering an episode of anxiety and low mood. Spotting common thinking patterns that can keep us in a negative loop (Table 8.1) and defining those hot (i.e., highly emotionally charged and powerful) thoughts are key to tackling it further. Ask yourself: 'Is there any evidence for this thought? Would someone else interpret the situation this way?' and then 'How can I counterbalance this thought to make it more accurate? What is another way of seeing this?' It is important to acknowledge that there is genuine worry and fear underpinning this thought, but there is also room to focus on developing an alternative way of thinking that is proportionate and believable. For example: 'I did a rubbish job today' is reviewed for evidence and results in a more balanced 'I made a mistake today, people make mistakes, and it has made me feel really uncomfortable. However, I did my best in those circumstances.' Sometimes this is quite tricky to do if you are already stuck in a negative loop. Imagining what a compassionate friend or colleague would say, or what you would say to a colleague or friend in this situation, can sometimes help. It is often easier to be kinder to others, so taking this outsider view can support us when doing that for ourselves. Once you have established your believable alternative thought, it is time to move on and shift your attention elsewhere.

## REFLECT ON RESPONSES

As we have explored, some of the ways we cope and respond can be useful, and other times they can be counterproductive despite intending to be helpful. This includes strategies such as

TABLE 8.1 **Examples of Common Thinking Errors**

| Thinking Error | Example(s) |
| --- | --- |
| All-or-nothing | 'I must be perfect at all times, with everyone in my life, especially my boss.' |
| Catastrophising | 'If I make a mistake, my boss will fire me.' |
| Discounting the postive | 'I got positive feedback on my presentation, but I know I made a mistake so they can't have been paying attention to me.' |
| Emotional reasoning | 'I am anxious and feel horrible, so something must be wrong.' |
| Mind-reading | 'My friend tensed up when I said I missed her, so she must be mad at me or not want to hang out anymore.' |
| Should statements | 'I should be working, not taking the night off! I have things that I should have done by now.' |
| Comparisons | 'Everyone else at work seems to be doing fine, what's wrong with me?' |
| False expectations | 'If my mum really loves me, she'll call this week—and I really want her to call because I am feeling low and sad right now.' |

avoidance, hypervigilance, reassurance seeking, or leaving a situation when you feel unable to cope. These ways of responding invariably perpetuate difficulties by reinforcing our fears and worries (i.e., 'I couldn't cope, I had to leave').

Instead, try and do something healthy and proactive. This may involve focusing on another task, allowing space to gain perspective and reevaluate, connecting and processing with a friend or colleague, or a taking a few moments of 'down-time'. It is important to accept that anxious or negative thinking is a common part of life, and accepting this can go a long way to minimise the ripple effect.

While these simple steps are likely to be useful to many, those struggling with anxiety or low mood daily may require more formal support that goes beyond what we have described here. If in doubt, always share concerns.

# Mental Health in the Workplace

## FOUNDATIONS OF WELLBEING: BEING HUMAN

It is important to adopt proactive and protective coping strategies at home and at work as much as we are able to. Without the correct fuel and maintenance, the brain and body will not have what they need to sustain us, especially when things get difficult. Aim to ensure you have a strategy for meeting the following basic human needs before, during, and after work. This might include planning the following into your day:

- Take physical space and psychological rest to decompress.
- Staying well hydrated with water, not being reliant on caffeinated or highly sugary drinks.
- Eat sufficient, nutritious, nourishing food.
- Engage in regular physical activity; this could be regular short walks or stretching, as a minimum.
- Schedule time for things you enjoy and get pleasure from (e.g., meeting a friend for a coffee; before your shift, reading a couple of pages of a book; making part of your journey to/from work a walk or cycle).
- Be aware of positive social support and connectivity. Seeking out, or letting in, people you feel supported by and can spend enjoyable time with will be important in helping reduce any sense of isolation and loneliness. Sharing difficult experiences with peers and work colleagues can help you see you are not alone and can also normalise your experiences and responses.

You have a role in creating a psychologically safe and supportive working environment. What ways could you help make changes to benefit you and your colleagues? Is there a staff suggestions forum/box? Could you make time in a team meeting, line management or supervision to explore together how positive change could be brought about? These suggestions may be a helpful starting point.

# Summary

Everyone has 'mental health', and we all see fluctuations in our mood, stress, and anxiety levels dependent on our life stressors and daily demands. This is particularly important when you work in high-stress or emotive environments such as nursing and midwifery. Early recognition of compromised mental health is important; simple evidence-based strategies can be helpful in kicking issues in to touch and maintaining good mental health on a day-to-day basis. Healthy working practices can play a key role in this. However, it is vital to identify when further support is needed, and to exercise compassion in the recognition that everyone struggles with their mental health from time to time, for varied reasons.

## ACTIVITY

Create your own mental health first aid plan:
1. What are the common things that trigger me feeling vulnerable or stressed at work?
    *Tip: Think back to the last time you had a particularly bad day, when you felt strong emotions.*
2. What are the early warning signs that I am starting to become overwhelmed?
    *Tip: Ask those closest to you, at work and home.*
3. What has helped before when you have felt anxious/stressed/upset?
    *Tip: This might be best figured out in a conversation with someone who has seen you in action!*
4. What are your top tips for mental health, for your future self?
    *Tip: Start with basic needs first, and don't be afraid to add in 'hug' from a friend!*
Once you have completed this, consider sharing it with those closest to you and use it as a conversation starter for what they could do if they noticed these signs, too.

---

### CASE STUDY 8.1 — Intensive Care Unit (ICU) WellBeing Team, The Royal United Hospitals Bath NHS Foundation Trust

A multidisciplinary team from ICU, anaesthetics, and operating theatres established a wellbeing team to provide immediate and ongoing support for all staff. They embedded and reinforced a strong work-based culture of well and happy health care staff providing safer patient care. They actively acknowledged and promoted that staff wellbeing (thus patient safety) is due to safe and well-designed working environments and working practices, including adequate bed numbers, staff levels and skill mix, ability to cope with surges in clinical demand, adequate and appropriate personal protective equipment, and provision of changing rooms/lockers/showers/bike racks/car parking/uniforms. They worked hard with the leadership team, including the ICU Matron, and managers to prioritise these. Key to their work was highlighting and facilitating the strategies that staff could implement to help themselves. They met regularly and put the following strategies in place:

- New wellbeing boards with useful resources, website links, and information about local and national initiatives and advice about how to contact the organisation's staff Employees Assistance Programme (EAP)
- Expanded the Trauma Risk Management (TRiM) system (Kelly et al., 2020), training 16 additional TRiM practitioners to support staff after a traumatic event
- Introduced a Team Immediate Meet tool for use by staff following a critical event
- Created/repurposed and decorated a staff quiet room on ICU
- Put care boxes in staff showers and rest rooms
- Introduced reclining chairs and blackout blinds in ICU handover rooms and anaesthetic department offices for staff breaks
- Facilitated 'Wellbeing Wednesday' dog walks, virtual coffees, and yoga sessions
- Optimised the existing doctor educational supervisor system and nursing development systems and introduced 'Corona-Comrade' buddies
- Added confidential boxes in coffee rooms to remove barriers for staff and make it easier to contact EAP for psychological support

The ICU wellbeing team have data showing that they had better than the UK national average staff recruitment/retention, helping maintain recommended staff-to-patient ratios, thus reducing a potential source of further stress. Staff have reported improved knowledge of how to access support for their wellbeing and reported that the wellbeing initiatives have been valuable/extremely valuable in maintaining their wellbeing and mental health. The team won the Intensive Care Society's 2021 Welfare and Wellbeing Award for prioritising staff welfare and wellbeing in the workplace.

The work undertaken by the Royal United Hospitals' ICU wellbeing team draws on recommendations from Blake and colleagues (Blake & Bermingham, 2020; Blake et al., 2020) in their *Psychological Wellbeing for Health and Care Workers* e-package on mitigating risk to staff wellbeing and the team being essential in this:

- Build team resilience and create a psychologically safe and supportive environment.
- Consider how the workplace impacts on wellbeing and how teams work under pressure.
- Set up good lines of communication.
- Maintain social connections (within and outside the workplace).
- Practice and model self-care.
- Practice and model positive coping strategies to manage stress (Blake et al., 2020).

## References

Beck, A. T. (Ed.). (1979). *Cognitive therapy of depression.* Guilford Press.

Blake, H., & Bermingham, F. (2020). *Psychological wellbeing for healthcare workers: mitigating the impact of covid-19.* The University of Nottingham. https://www.nottingham.ac.uk/toolkits/play_22794.

Blake, H., Bermingham, F., Johnson, G., & Tabner, A. (2020). Mitigating the psychological impact of CO-VID-19 on healthcare workers: A digital learning package. *International Journal of Environmental Research and Public Health, 17,* 2997. https://doi.org/10.3390/ijerph17092997.

Daniels, J., Ingram, J., Pease, A., Wainwright, E., Beckett, K., Iyadurai, L., & Carlton, E. (2021). The COVID-19 clinician cohort (CoCCo) study: empirically grounded Recommendations for forward-facing psychological care of frontline doctors. *International Journal of Environmental Research and Public Health,* 18(18), 9675.

Greenberger, D., & Padesky, C. A. (2016). *Mind over mood: Change how you feel by changing the way you think.* Guilford Publications.

Kelly, F. E., Osborn, M., & Stacey, M. S. (2020). Improving resilience in anaesthesia and intensive care medicine—learning lessons from the military. *Anaesthesia,* 75(6), 720–723.

Siegel, D. J. (1999). *The developing mind: How relationships and the brain interact to shape who we are.* New York. Guilford Publications.

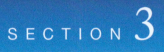

# Wellbeing Needs at Different Times

## CHAPTER 9

# Shiftwork, Sleep, and Managing Fatigue

Liz Charalambous

## KEY POINTS

1. Shift workers are mostly women. To reduce the negative impact of shift work on health, recommendations include employers being aware of the individual needs of staff and providing support for the challenges of each life stage (including the needs of breastfeeding mothers and those experiencing menopause).
2. A considerable proportion of shift workers are from lower socioeconomic groups. Recommendations include governments and policymakers taking this into consideration when formulating local and national policy to reduce the burden of social inequality and the subsequent impacts on health.
3. Shift work impacts physical and mental health. Recommendations to positively impact on the health of shift workers include employers supporting flexible working patterns tailored to the needs of the individual. This will facilitate their access to health care services, as well as healthy food and rest during breaks. With support, there are strategies that can be adopted by shift workers to support health.
4. Shift work can negatively impact social relationships, particularly aspects of family life and parenting. Recommendations include employers supporting flexible working to support those with caring responsibilities.
5. The impacts on health from working shifts can be tackled using several approaches. There is a responsibility for governments, organisations, and individuals to adopt healthy workplace practices.

## Introduction

Traditionally, work in hospitals has involved dividing the 24-hour period into two shifts of either 2 long days (7 a.m.–7.30 p.m. and 7 p.m.–7.30 a.m.) or early shift (7 a.m.–3 p.m.), late shift (1 p.m.–9:20 p.m.), and night shift (9 p.m.–8 a.m.) with nurses and midwives working internal rotation of nights and days over a 4-week rota. Many nurses and midwives find shift work challenging, however, and it can have consequences for health, particularly if it is not well managed. This chapter will explore the effect of shift work on health and set out the associated challenges, with suggestions for how shift workers' needs might be met.

Shift work is defined as 'a method of organisation of working time in which workers succeed one another at the workplace so that the establishment can operate longer than the hours of work of individual workers' (International Labour Organization, 1990). In practice, this could mean employees work outside the standard hours of 7 a.m. to 7 p.m., split shifts, overtime, on call, extended work periods of 12 hours or more, or rotating work hours (Health and Safety Executive (HSE), 2006).

## Numbers and Types of Shift Workers

Over the last 25 years the number of shift workers has increased in the United Kingdom, as 14% (or 3.6 million people) in the working population reported working shifts (HSE, 2006). Approximately one-third of these shift workers are men and one-fifth are women, with shift work being most common in the 16- to 24-year age group and least common among those aged over 55. Those from lower income households are more likely to work shifts and have less flexible work patterns (Dahlgren & Whitehead, 2006). This is an important consideration for maintaining health as health inequalities are associated with social inequalities and lower socioeconomic status (Marmot, 2010)

## The Importance of Sleep

Altered sleep patterns can disrupt our natural circadian rhythm (internal body clock) and have a negative effect on health. Sleep deprivation has many harmful effects. It can cause a lack of concentration, difficulty with decision making, increased risk of accidental injury, and mood alteration (National Health Service (NHS), 2021). Most people need about 8 hours of sleep in a 24-hour period, and this can give benefits that include boosted immunity, lower risk of weight gain and diabetes, increased sense of mental wellbeing, increased sex drive and fertility, and protection against heart disease (NHS, 2021).

## Impact of Shift Work on Health

A research study conducted in the United Kingdom showed that compared to those working regular hours, shift workers are more likely to report poor health and have one or more limiting longstanding illnesses; they are also more likely to be obese or develop diabetes (Weston, 2013). In this study, the number of smokers was found to be higher in shift workers, particularly in women. Fruit and vegetable consumption was lower among shift workers than nonshift workers, with shift workers being less likely than nonshift workers to eat five or more portions of fruit and vegetables per day. However, alcohol consumption was found to be less among shift workers when compared to nonshift workers, and no significant differences were found in levels of hypertension, cholesterol, or subjective self-reported wellbeing scores.

The needs of individual shift workers may vary during their life stages; for example, those undergoing menopause would have different needs than those who are breastfeeding or are pregnant.

As well as the physical impact of shift work on health, there are social challenges to consider. Factors affecting family and social relationships might include parents eating meals at separate times to the rest of the family or limited time spent with children, thereby impacting on parenting styles and relationships. Despite these challenges, having children may be a factor that influences parents to undertake shift work on the basis that they might save on child care costs by being available to provide care when off duty.

The following strategies can support shift workers from a national, local, and personal level.

### WHAT CAN BE DONE NATIONALLY?

Recommendations at the national level include adopting a strategy through effective social policy to address socioeconomic inequalities and their subsequent impact on health (Dahlgren & Whitehead, 2006). Efforts taken at the national level to reduce health inequalities will benefit the economy as a whole and reap greater societal benefits by reducing ill health associated with health inequalities, which result in loss of productivity, reduced tax revenue, increased welfare payments, and increased cost of health interventions (Marmot, 2010). Also, widening access to primary health care and out-of-hours services would facilitate the attendance of shift workers who may normally struggle to access services to support their own health and wellbeing during office hours.

Other helpful approaches include government attempts to rebalance gender inequality, which disproportionately impacts negatively on mothers who work shifts, and free early years support provided by the state to support child care costs. This includes a review of taxation to include tax incentives to subsidise the cost of child care for all workers, including shift workers. This could factor in child care payments as part of personal tax allowance rather than paying for child care out of the net salary. Governments could consider offering more generous child care benefits and longer paid parental leave for both parents, as well as child care costs or paid in proportion to their salary.

## WHAT CAN EMPLOYERS DO TO HELP?

Employers need to recognise the impact of hours and shift patterns on health. They should provide inclusive and equitable access to equal opportunities for career progression and access to support networks to reduce social isolation in those working less sociable hours (Strauss & Patel-Campbell, 2021). This is of particular importance for female shift workers from ethnic minority backgrounds who may be disproportionally affected by the impact of work on health. In the United Kingdom, legislation states that employers have a duty of care to safeguard the health of employees with the rights of employees protected by legislation (HSE, 2006). Practical examples of this could include an organisational infrastructure that focuses on meeting the needs of individual workers or engaging staff with child care responsibilities in conversations around flexible working to support school pick-up and drop-off times. In addition to this, some shift workers might also appreciate term-time only contracts.

Time could be factored in for employees to undertake voluntary work with the aim of improving their social capital, reduce social isolation (Marmot, 2010), and promote a sense of inclusion and value to maximise their sense of wellbeing.

Organisations should provide access to fresh and healthy food choices. This is important when considering the limited exposure to daylight and subsequent lack of vitamin D for those regularly working night shifts. Those from ethnic minority groups are at particular risk of vitamin D deficiency. Shift workers can be encouraged to maintain hydration by providing access to cold drinking water during shift times. While important for everyone, this is particularly important for menopausal women or lactating mothers. Staff need facilities for storing food; lactating mothers need a place to store expressed breast milk. Adequate rest facilities could also be provided to ensure employees can take rest or sleep during their breaktimes. This would be invaluable for those with child care responsibilities who choose shift work to save on the cost of child care and who may not have the opportunity to sleep after night shifts. Ensuring workspaces are clean will minimise the risk of infection to shift workers who are at greater risk of infection due to lowered immunity from shift work. It is important that shift workers have access to washing facilities, especially when traveling long distances. When uniforms are worn, these could be made of light, natural fabric to support menopausal shift workers who experience hot flashes and prolonged sweating.

All these suggestions are likely to be heavily dependent on workplace cultures and leadership styles adopted by organisations as well as the cost of business pressures driving service needs.

Line managers, human resources, and occupational health departments have a role to play in advocating employee wellbeing and promoting regular health checks, at times suitable for shift workers. This might include a focus on managing stress, with the aim of preventing mental as well as physical ill health (Marmot, 2010). Strategies to maximise a sense of social inclusion in the workplace could include efforts to support staff engagement, such as organising charitable fundraising efforts that have the potential to boost staff morale. However, it is important to recognise that employees from lower socioeconomic groups working shifts may not have the capacity, motivation, or resources to participate in such activities and could result in feeling further exclusion as a result.

## WHAT CAN NURSES AND MIDWIVES DO FOR THEMSELVES?

Along with the rights of shift workers to be supported by employers comes the individual responsibility for workers to stay as healthy as possible. General health advice includes maintaining a healthy weight; doing some type of physical exercise every day; eating a balanced diet (including at least 30 g of fibre, at least five portions of fruit and vegetables, and at least six to eight glasses of water a day); limiting consumption of saturated fat, sugar, and salt; smoking cessation; and managing alcohol consumption (NHS, 2021). Where shift workers are concerned, health strategies would also have a heavy focus on sleep hygiene. Aside from advice to take regular exercise and manage alcohol and caffeine consumption, shift workers could manage a sleep routine, including daytime naps (NHS, 2021).

Nurses and midwives can also safeguard their own health by accepting regular and recommended health checks and health screening by their health care provider if they are experiencing health concerns. Those shift workers concerned about ongoing fatigue can be screened for diseases such as coeliac disease, underactive thyroid, diabetes, vitamin D and vitamin B12 deficiency, folate deficiency anaemia, sleep apnoea, myalgic encephalomyelitis (sometimes called chronic fatigue syndrome), glandular fever, and restless legs syndrome, as well as anxiety, depression, and recent bereavement (NHS, 2021). Shift workers who experience ongoing fatigue could also consult their pharmacist to review medication as fatigue may be a side effect.

Other self-care strategies could include adapting one's lifestyle to establish a bedtime routine to factor in shift work, particularly rotational and night shift work schedules and subsequent disruption to routines (NHS, 2021). By this we mean ensuring the sleeping environment is dark, comfortable, and well ventilated at a temperature between 18°C (64°F) and 24°C (75°F). Thick curtains, eye masks, and ear plugs may be useful to block out extraneous light and noise. The bedroom should only be used for sleep or sex and digital devices avoided for about an hour before sleep as the light emitted from the screen can adversely affect sleep. Shift workers could also support their sleeping partner to seek help with snoring if this is a hindrance to sleep. A warm bath, relaxation strategies (e.g., meditation, yoga, mindfulness, massage), and listening to relaxing music or reading a book may help with winding down (NHS, 2021). A warm, milky drink might be helpful, as is keeping well hydrated, but large volumes of fluid at bedtime should be avoided to minimise the likelihood of toilet visits disturbing sleep. Stimulants such as alcohol and caffeine should also be avoided, as well as heavy meals just before sleep.

However, those from lower socioeconomic groups may experience extra challenges when striving to maintain a healthy lifestyle, particularly if they have issues with transport, housing, and access to shops selling fresh food (Dahlgren & Whitehead, 2006). Some may have caring responsibilities that may prevent them from adopting recommended healthy behaviours. This is of particular importance for women who may choose to work night shifts to reduce child care costs as they have the option to stay up during the day to provide care and so may be at increased risk of ill health as a result. Furthermore, living in poor housing in noisy urban environments may affect the quality of sleep should shift workers sleep during the day.

It appears that offering employees the option to choose flexible working is one solution to supporting healthy lifestyles, but this needs to be balanced against problems associated with shift workers from lower income families who may feel pressured to work as well as provide child care in their free time. This could be addressed by adopting democratic leadership practices to facilitate a constructive dialogue between employees, employers, and unions (Dahlgren & Whitehead, 2006)

## Conclusion

This chapter has explored the effect of shift work on sleep and the associated challenges to maintaining a healthy lifestyle. Suggestions are made to offer workable solutions to alleviate the burden of shift work on health. There appears to be scope for supporting shift workers at national and organisational levels, as employers can provide substantial support to shift workers with little effort or cost to organisations. Employees can ensure they take steps to safeguard their own health by using a range of self-care strategies to support health. Measures include meeting the needs of individual employees and providing access to healthy lifestyle choices while at work, which is of particular importance when considering the impact of shift work on those from lower socioeconomic groups who may be disproportionately affected due to inequalities in housing, transport, income, and education.

### ACTIVITY

Have you ever worked shifts? How did it make you feel?

Consider the challenges of the impact of shift work on health from a range of perspectives. What challenges might be experienced by governments when introducing new social policies? What might prevent organisations and managers from offering flexible working patterns? What difficulties might individuals experience when striving to achieve a healthy work-life balance while working shifts?

### CASE STUDY 9.1 — Newcastle Hospitals NHS Trust, a Whole-Team Approach to Co-production of a Fatigue Risk Management Strategy in Maternity Services

Fatigue—a sense of exhaustion, tiredness, or lack of energy—is detrimental to staff wellbeing and patient safety but is often overlooked. Fatigue increases risk-taking, risks of significant health conditions, and burnout. Doctors and nurses have died driving home, and driver fatigue from prolonged work and lack of sleep is considered a major contributor. Although the impacts of fatigue are well described, little attention has been given by health and care organisations to team- or unit-level comprehensive fatigue risk management strategies or systems, which remain rare despite potential risks.

However, top-down approaches are problematic, as standardised strategies imposed on clinical areas disregard the complexities of specialty/unit contexts and cultures, reduce ownership, and may constrain the flexibility needed to maintain safety.

In the United Kingdom, a multidisciplinary maternity services project team was established at Newcastle Hospitals NHS Trust in partnership with academics from Northumbria University Newcastle, with the aim of raising awareness, developing fatigue risk mitigation from the bottom up, and beginning a culture change. The project was funded by The Health Foundation (an independent charity committed to bringing about better health and health care for people in the UK).

The process, facilitated by academic researchers, involved:
- Delivering education and information about sleep, fatigue, and associated risk. A sleep specialist was a member of the group and developed a short information video for staff.

*Continued*

| CASE STUDY 9.1 | **Newcastle Hospitals NHS Trust, a Whole-Team Approach to Co-production of a Fatigue Risk Management Strategy in Maternity Services—cont'd** |

- Holding focus groups and drop-in meetings to gather information, experiences, and ideas for how to support staff
- Ranking and choosing suggested interventions
- Convening a fatigue risk management group comprised of a wide range of staff across all grades and levels, which met regularly, took ownership of the strategy development, and drove the implementation of the chosen interventions
- Implementing and monitoring interventions
- Assessing acceptability and perceived impact and monitoring physical activity using accelerometer data
- Drafting fatigue risk management strategy documents

The project resulted in raised awareness and an improved approach to identifying and managing staff fatigue. Over time, the culture changed to one where the team talked about tiredness, and staff expected to have power naps during their breaks. Lack of empathy and lapses in judgement were recognised as signs of fatigue. The project team made a presentation to the hospital-wide clinical risk management group, who are keen to develop the work further; they can see its potential in improving staff wellbeing. However, it has been quite challenging to have fatigue included on the risk register (a tool used for risk management) partly because the issue is so widespread, and some changes inevitably cost money. But the seeds are sown; staff fatigue is now seen as a hospital-wide safety issue and not just an occupational hazard.

Specific improvements from this initiative include:

- Education about fatigue and its impact on performance for midwifery, nursing, and medical staff; raising awareness of the value of a 20-minute power nap during the night shift
- Purchase of sofa beds for staff to sleep on during breaks
- Minimising routine tasks and managing the overall nighttime workload
- Managing timing of induction of labour to try and minimise the number of caesarean sections needed between midnight and 8 a.m.
- Establishing self-rostering for midwives so staff could choose a night shift pattern that better suited their own circadian physiology (meaning the 24-hour internal clock in our brain that regulates cycles of alertness and sleepiness)
- Having one extra trainee on call overnight in anaesthesia who can ensure other trainees are able to take a power nap

**ALISON STEVEN      NANCY REDFERN**

## References

Dahlgren, G., & Whitehead, M. (2007). *European strategies for tackling social inequalities in health: Levelling up part 2*. Studies on social and economic determinants of population health, no. 3. Copenhagen: World Health Organization Regional Office for Europe. https://www.euro.who.int/__data/assets/pdf_file/0018/103824/E89384.pdf.

Health and Safety Executive. (2006). Managing shift work. *Health and safety guidance*. https://www.hse.gov.uk/pUbns/priced/hsg256.pdf.

International Labour Organization. (1990). *Night work convention*. (No. 171). https://www.ilo.org/dyn/normlex/en/f?p=NORMLEXPUB:12100:0::NO::P12100_INSTRUMENT_ID:312316.

Marmot, M. (2010). *Fair society, healthy lives: The Marmot review. Strategic review of health inequalities in England post-2010*. Institute of Health Equity. https://www.gov.uk/research-for-development-outputs/fair-society-healthy-lives-the-marmot-review-strategic-review-of-health-inequalities-in-england-post-2010.

National Health Service. (2021). *Live well*. https://www.nhs.uk/live-well/.

Strauss, C., & Patel-Campbell, C. (2021). *Covid-19 and the female health and care workforce survey update. survey of health and care staff for the Health and Care Women Leaders Network*. February–March 2021. NHS Confederation. https://www.nhsconfed.org/-/media/Confederation/Files/Networks/Health-and-Care-Women-Leaders-Network/COVID19-and-the-female-health-and-care-workforce-survey-update-report.pdf?la=en&hash=0FDE7AF4554F5CE388E95FBFA48C914AD8101FCE.

Weston, L. (2013). Chapter 6 Shift work, in Craig R., Mindell J. (eds). *Health Survey for England 2013*. Volume 1: Health, social care and lifestyles. Health and Social Care Information Centre, Leeds, 2014. http://healthsurvey.hscic.gov.uk/media/1069/_6-shift-work_4th-proof.pdf.

## CHAPTER 10

# WellBeing Needs During Periods of Fasting

Rohit Sagoo

## KEY POINTS

1. There are some health and wellbeing benefits to intermittent fasting for nurses and midwives.
2. Fasting from religious and cultural perspectives has an emotional effect on nurses and midwives.
3. Controlling a diet with intermittent fasting can maintain a positive sense of wellbeing.
4. There are many health-promoting behaviours surrounding fasting, and it is important that you choose the right one for you.
5. Successful support for people who are fasting involves discussion, reassurance, support and respect.

## Introduction

This chapter will discuss a range of aspects that surround the practice of fasting among nurses and midwives, and how this affects their wellbeing. In the first instance, it is important to be clear about what is meant by the term *fasting*. The term is broad and can be referred to as a variety of programs of control around one's diet alongside dictating eating times during a day or longer. With this term borne in mind, we will not be discussing patient fasting in clinical practice, but we will be focusing on the personal aspects of nurses and midwives religiously or intermittently fasting during their clinical practice or working shift and how this impacts their wellbeing.

## How Do We Define WellBeing?

To begin with, it will be helpful to have a definition of wellbeing and how nurses and midwives perceive their own wellbeing. In the United Kingdom, the Courage of Compassion Report West et al. (2020) came about from an investigation in relation to supporting nurses and midwives during and after the COVID-19 pandemic, to ensure that health care professionals thrive in their working environment. The report clearly points out that the health and wellbeing of nurses and midwives is paramount to delivering optimum care for patients, and it is crucial that all sectors of health care support and invest in the wellbeing of nurses and midwives (Foster, 2020; Jones-Berry, 2013). Much of the literature around wellbeing for nurses focuses on supporting nurses and job satisfaction around various areas of work within a health or care environment, but unfortunately it does not focus on their personal wellbeing. Hence, a broader definition of wellbeing might be helpful in ascertaining what wellbeing may mean for nurses and midwives. Research has found that the wellbeing of nurses and midwives centres around positive emotions such as happiness and contentment, a sense of togetherness and good spirit, as well as effective communication in their clinical work. This resonates in practice from the notion of being happy in practice and supported positively. Taking these broad wellbeing perspectives into consideration, we must now ask how wellbeing is seen for nurses and midwives who are choosing to fast. Here is an example:

### The Individual Experience

Nurse A is 26 years old and works in a busy emergency department. He is a practicing Hindu and chooses to fast 2 days of the week. On this day of fasting, he is working. The senior nurse is unaware that he is fasting and asks him to take a break and get something to eat as the department has a busy day ahead, he tells the senior nurse that he is fasting, and she is curious to find out why. He tells her the reasons and states that fasting gives him a sense of oneness with God and that he can exercise self-control until it is time for him to break his fast. The senior nurse asks, 'How will you cope for all these hours on shift?' and 'How can we support you during your days of fasting?' He says, 'Sometimes I find it difficult with hunger pangs and a rumbling tummy, but as I have been fasting regularly for so long, I've got used to it. However, it can be challenging as I can feel fatigued and a little irritable by the end of my shift.'

## The Context and Practice of Fasting

The practice of fasting among nurses and midwives usually occurs within a religious context. There are many religions that observe fasting for varying amounts of time during the calendar year. These faith groups include Muslims, Jews, Buddhists, Roman Catholics, and Hindus. Here is a quick outline of the observation of fasts exercised by these religions:

- Islam: the holy month of Ramadan or Ramazan
- Judaism: Yom Kippur, the Day of Atonement, as well as 6 additional days in the Jewish calendar (e.g., Tish B'Av)
- Buddhism: according to the lunar calendar (usually on the days of a full moon) and any specific holidays or festivals
- Hinduism: commonly on new moon days and during festivals (e.g., Shivaratri, Saraswati, Puja)
- Roman Catholics: Ash Wednesday and Good Friday, and abstain from meat on all Fridays in Lent

As notable examples, it is widely known that for those of the Islamic faith, the observance of Ramadan constitutes fasting for a period of 1 month. Ramadan occurs annually, and Muslims are expected to abstain from eating/drinking and some other activities of daily living from the break of dawn until sunset. However, for Muslim nurses and midwives, what must be considered is the fact that fasting occurs from the break of dawn until sunset, during daylight hours, and how this impacts their wellbeing if they are working during this period. Studies have shown that fasting during Ramadan has physical and cognitive effects on Muslim health care professionals, and their wellbeing can be negatively affected in terms of lowered mood, increased stress, and higher levels of anxiety and depression. As such, there is a risk that clinical decision making may be impaired when Muslim nurses and midwives observe fasting during Ramadan. They might experience a slight deficit in attention and concentration and feel fatigued due to a lack of sleep or sleep disturbance. Sleep deprivation may also occur during Ramadan as Muslims are required to wake up at intervals during the night for mealtimes and/or prayer. This has clear implications for nursing practice.

TABLE 10.1 ■ Five Steps to WellBeing for Fasting

| Connect | Connect with the people around you: your family, friends, colleagues, and neighbours. Spend time developing personal and professional relationships. In the context of nursing practice this could mean building an understanding of cultural awareness within our profession. |
|---|---|
| Be Active | Find an activity that you enjoy and make it a part of your life. Swap inactive pursuits with active ones. |
| Keep Learning | Learning new skills can give you a sense of achievement and a new confidence, alongside underpinning learning about cultural awareness and fasting. |
| Give to Others | Small or larger acts of kindness, such as volunteering at your local community centre, can improve your mental wellbeing and help you build new social networks. |
| Be Mindful | Be more aware of the present moment, including your thoughts and feelings, your body, and the world around you. Some people call this awareness 'mindfulness'. It can positively change the way you feel about life and how you approach challenges. |

Another example of what is meant by religious fasting is fasting from the lens of Hinduism. Here, fasting is a frequent, but optional observation that may be carried out once a week on a specific day or on certain days of the lunar month, and during festivals and holy days. Hindus respectively believe that fasting is a symbolic ritual and sacrifice that establishes a deeper relationship with their spiritual being and devotion to God. This in turn signifies the purification of their soul and may play a part of penance for sin. Another significant aspect of fasting that we must consider is that, from a religious perspective, it goes hand in hand with prayer. Therefore, it is now necessary to explain the course of fasting and its effect on wellbeing. In some religions, fasting can also mean abstaining from eating only certain things for the sake of good health.

## Fasting and Wellbeing

In the United Kingdom, the Royal College of Nursing (RCN) developed the initiative Healthy Workplace, Healthy You after research suggested there was a rise in nurses engaging in unhealthy eating behaviours. The key to this RCN initiative was to embody a holistic view of healthy behaviours and a self-assessment tool that nurses can engage with, which encompasses many elements from the mind, body, spirit, and maintaining a balance between professional and personal life. Different authors have discussed the need for raising awareness about supporting nurses' wellbeing even more so in times of crisis when stress and pressures increase for all staff in the health care and social care sectors. There are many ways that wellbeing can be measured. Gilliver (2021) recognised two areas of wellbeing that could be incorporated into nursing: feeling good and functioning well. From this standpoint, Gilliver (2021) also identified the five ways model adopted by NHS England that incorporates five key messages to enhance patient and staff wellbeing (Table 10.1).

We will now apply this to fasting and wellbeing needs during periods of fasting. From Table 10.1 it is apparent that giving to others and being mindful lends itself to the notion of fasting and wellbeing, as fasting from a religious perspective is a form of giving to others in a spiritual sense and that being mindful is about the oneness we may feel about our self-image, self-concept, and self-esteem. This plays a key role in fasting as how we feel about ourselves directs us to whether we feel the need to fast. It could be that experiencing trauma, or an adverse event, triggers us to fast or that our body image has altered over time, and we feel the need to get back into shape, so what we learn and feel about ourselves defines whether we make the decision to fast. It is important to acknowledge that some nurses and midwives may choose to fast during their shifts, so the need for being more culturally aware is fundamental both within delivering patient care and in respecting differentiation between our work colleagues.

It is widely recognised that the roles of nurses and midwives today are increasingly emotionally and physically demanding. These job roles can be stressful and have the potential to cause anxiety, low mood, and even depression. Therefore, taking account of all the challenges faced in day-to-day roles, it is important to recognise that maintaining a positive wellbeing for nurses and midwives is paramount. Enhancing wellbeing in these professional groups has been a topic of discussion for quite some time, coupled with the demands of the increasing and ever-changing high expectations of nursing and midwifery care. For example, in the United Kingdom, a typical shift in nursing will last between 8 and 12 hours, and it may only include a couple of short breaks to rest, eat, and drink. Most breaks on a nursing shift may typically last 10 to 30 minutes; therefore one of the key areas of concern is having poor appetite during these short mealtimes or finding opportunities to eat and drink when on a break. On the other hand, nurses and midwives may have to adapt their shift pattern to fit in or make room for mealtimes and think carefully about the nutritional value and content of their meals so that it has a positive effect on their health and wellbeing. It is very often noted that nurses and midwives may not have time to eat or even think about eating or drinking during a busy shift. Healthy eating, hydration, and shift work are explained more fully elsewhere in this book. With these situations and infrequent breaks, it poses the question, are nurses and midwives naturally carrying out intermittent fasting without consciously knowing it?

As nurses and midwives may sometimes go without food or water for hours at a time before realising that they need to eat, it raises another question: is intermittent fasting a good thing? A considerable amount of general information has been published on intermittent fasting with a plethora of guidance to suggest that intermittent fasting in fact reduces cholesterol, blood pressure, and blood sugars. From the lens of a nurse's or midwife's wellbeing, intermittent fasting may be a positive approach to weight loss or diabetes prevention. Conversely, intermittent fasting may lead to food cravings or binge eating, especially if one is eating during day or night shift patterns. Given the nature of clinical practice, intermittent fasting may also increase stress in practice, and levels of the stress hormone cortisol may increase due to this.

Finally, for leaders in nursing and midwifery, one must be aware of the cultural diversity that surrounds fasting and acknowledge that some colleagues may choose to fast to improve their health, and some staff will fast as part of their religious practice. Both result in positive wellbeing.

**ACTIVITY**

1. What does your typical shift look like? Do you factor in mealtimes? How many hours might you go without eating?
2. Are you consciously or unconsciously fasting? And what does this do to your wellbeing? How do you feel?
3. What type of support is available in your organisation to improve staff wellbeing when fasting? Are there policies in your organisation to support staff who are religiously fasting?
4. If you choose to fast (or do so unconsciously), do you feel that accessing additional support during fasting would benefit you in any way?

**CASE STUDY 10.1**    **Observations From the British Sikh Nurses Association**

This case study arises from my personal observations of best practice, as leader of the British Sikh Nurses Association. The UK National Health Service (NHS) respects the observance of colleagues and patients of different faiths fasting at different points of their lives. Fasting can sometimes be a regular or periodic feature for some faiths, and some fasts may require abstinence from certain foods or food altogether. Fasting is a less well-noticed element of faith for nurses and midwives. However, in times of crisis, understanding more about fasting, and how to manage this, is particularly important. NHS England and NHS Improvement leads the NHS in England. FaithAction, a national network of faith-based and community organisations, has worked alongside NHS England and NHS Improvement to support faith groups during the COVID-19 pandemic. This partnership recognises the importance of cultural and spiritual needs of patients and health care professionals, and the positive influence of these needs on their mental health.

The All-Party Parliamentary Group (APPG) on Faith and Society was launched in 2012. The APPG's aims are to 'highlight the contribution to society by faith-based organisations, to identify best practice, and to promote understanding of the groups providing innovative solutions around the country.' The APPG published a report on how partnerships between local authorities and faith communities have strengthened during the COVID-19 pandemic. This report demonstrates how peers and leaders can work together in a collegiate way to support fasting in clinical practice. The report includes suggestions for supporting colleagues who are fasting that are relevant to both nurses and midwives:

- Working in partnership with nursing and midwifery leaders and staff of different faiths is an overwhelmingly positive experience and helps to deepen the relationship between all ranks of staff.
- Recognising religion or belief and the workplace (though there are NHS policies for protecting employees' faith and beliefs), it is beneficial for nurses and midwives to enhance the development of in-house polices by drawing on their own experiences and reflections of fasting. This enables a more sympathetic stance for employees who are fasting for a personal reason.
- Nurses and midwives who highlight experiences that are associated with the positive aspects of working in partnership with colleagues from different faith groups as opposed to the negative ones, better support learning and development.
- Spiritual and pastoral support from faith leaders in the hospital chaplaincy allows access to faith leaders for advice, guidance, and support and helps nurses and midwives to maintain a positive wellbeing whilst fasting during religious events.
- Working in harmony as a team ensures that no one has unreasonable extra burdens on them while fasting and recognises that people who are fasting may become fatigued with a heavy workload.

Over the years in my role as nurse and leader of the British Sikh Nurses Association, I have observed that the organisations that have most success in supporting staff with fasting tend to focus on these areas:

A Assng about the significance of fasting and what it means to them

B Reassuring peers and colleagues that it's okay to eat or drink in front of nurses who are observing a fast—it's okay!

C Supporting each other when a nurse is fasting—allowing some flexibility for nurses who are fasting as they may be agitated or cranky, and low on energy when fasting. Lunch beaks could be used to have a nap to reenergise oneself, being conscious of the physical activity and tasks that the nurse is undertaking during a shift

D Being respectful of all religions, cultural differences, and backgrounds regardless of what they are and the reasons for fasting.

## References

Banakhar, M. (2017). The impact of 12-hour shifts on nurses' health, wellbeing, and job satisfaction: A systematic review. *Journal of Nursing Education and Practice, 7*, 69. https://doi.org/10.5430/jnep.v7n11p69.

Foster, S. (2020). Supporting nurses' wellbeing. *British Journal of Nursing, 29*(20), 1223–1223.

Gilliver, C. (2021). The five ways to wellbeing model: A framework for nurses and patients. *Nursing Times, 117*(5), 48–52.

Jones-Berry, S. (2013). Too much pressure: NHS employers must invest in nurses' wellbeing. *Nursing Standard, 28*(2), 12–13. https://doi.org/10.7748/ns2013.09.28.2.12.s18.

Koushali, A. N., Hajiamini, Z., Ebadi, A., Bayat, N., & Khamseh, F. (2013). Effect of Ramadan fasting on emotional reactions in nurses. *Iranian Journal of Nursing and Midwifery Research, 18*(3), 232–236.

Tinsley, G. M., & La Bounty, P. M. (2015). Effects of intermittent fasting on body composition and clinical health markers in humans. *Nutrition Reviews, 73*(10), 661–674. https://doi.org/10.1093/nutrit/nuv041.

West, M., Bailey, S., Williams, E. (2020). The courage of compassion: supporting nurses and midwives to deliver high-quality care. The Kings Fund: London. Available at: https://www.kingsfund.org.uk/publications/courage-compassion-supporting-nurses-midwives.

## CHAPTER 11

# Mental WellBeing in Nursing and Midwifery Students

Anne Felton ■ Charlotte Halls

## KEY POINTS

1. Transitions throughout healthcare education are points of vulnerability for our mental health.
2. Finding balance whilst being a student is central to wellbeing.
3. Fostering connections and belonging to a professional community promote mental health.
4. It is important to access the resources that are available and ask for help.
5. Taking care of your mental wellbeing as a health professional is essential.

## Introduction

Student mental health has been in focus during recent years. New policy and practices have emerged amongst international recognition that rates of mental distress in the student body are growing. Changes in service and social structures have also made university more accessible to people who experience mental health problems. This has facilitated a welcome focus on how higher education institutions can best enable students to maintain positive mental health. Students studying to become health professionals are exposed to unique experiences which, whilst also rewarding, can create specific challenges for mental wellbeing.

In this chapter we explore pressure points for nursing and midwifery students that could impact negatively on their mental health. Strategies to maintain health and wellbeing will be considered to support students to navigate these challenges and achieve their potential at university. Throughout the discussion we recognise that nursing and midwifery careers attract students from a wide range of backgrounds, and there are many routes into the profession. The topics under discussion will also be relevant to those registered professionals returning to study and to all healthcare professionals supporting students in practice.

## Pressure Points

### TRANSITIONS

Transitions are an important part of the human experience. Changes in our physiologic, social or psychological situation create growth. Yet transitions can also disrupt our sense of safety and control as we are faced with new challenges, unfamiliar experiences and potential changes to our usual ways of coping. Times of transition can therefore pose a threat to mental health.

Nursing and midwifery education involves numerous transitions. The most visible are at the start and end of the programme. You will transition into becoming a student nurse or midwife and adapt to the higher education environment. After a few years, you will then move into the role of registered professional and transition to an employee within the health or social care setting. These significant transitions often receive the most attention. However, within a nursing or midwifery course there are several transition points. UK student mental health bodies (Student Minds, 2019) have recognised that progression between years of a university course and placements can be periods that students find stressful and therefore require specific support.

Embarking on nursing or midwifery courses entail a change in role, and with this comes a need to understand the expectations of that new role. Student nurses and midwives in many respects have a dual identity, as both a university student and a trainee health professional. Moving into this world therefore requires students to assimilate to the higher education setting and the healthcare setting, each with its own language and informal rules. Although an exciting time, the unfamiliarity of these roles and environments alongside the uncertainty of the new situation can create stress.

Universities are very aware of the importance of transitions for students. They will have considered this in the design of programmes and may have introduced specific initiatives to help students successfully manage these transitions. These could include learning approaches that help foster relationships between students such as small groups, buddying students up with each other in both theory and practice settings.

## UNIVERSITY AND HOME LIFE

Becoming part of an education setting can create a pressure point for psychological and emotional wellbeing. Like all changes there are opportunities and challenges in these new experiences. A sense of belonging is central to both mental wellbeing and successful studies (O'Keeffe, 2013). For those nursing and midwifery students moving away from family to a new place of study there can be pressure to fit in and conform to a stereotypical view of university life. It can be common for students, particularly during the first 6 months of a programme, to struggle to feel part of something. These challenges are not confined to those moving to a new place to study. Being part of a community can be hard for students who are distance learning or studying part time who have limited time spent with peers. For those coming back to studying after many years, there may be challenges in adapting to the language and systems of higher education, which can make people feel like they do not belong.

Being at university and studying in a healthcare programme impact on existing relationships, as students have new experiences and are exposed to different perspectives. The time commitment involved in becoming a nurse or midwife changes usual family routines, which may disrupt home life. Social networks and relationships are essential to wellbeing, and therefore tensions in these relationships can impact on mental health.

These examples highlight an important consideration when examining this pressure point: it is a common experience, not one confined to a certain pathway to university or a particular social demographic. Negative self-evaluation can become a further threat to wellbeing; therefore recognising that this can be a common experience is important. Nursing and midwifery programmes by their very nature foster relationships between students. Caring for people who are sick, vulnerable, disabled and in some cases dying can be a rewarding experience but one that places emotional demands on us. The shared experience of peers and team members on placement is one that draws people together and helps them begin to belong to a community of nurses and midwives. Practitioners within the healthcare setting can recognise and help students to become part of the team during placement experiences.

## PLACEMENTS

Integral to healthcare programmes is the learning that takes place in health and social care settings. Placements are for many the highlight of the course and offer unique and rewarding opportunities to make a difference as a student nurse or midwife. However, they are a significant transition accompanied by a weight of expectations. They are usually assessed, involve being in unfamiliar situations with new people, and taking on a responsible role. Increasingly for students, placements mean considerable time travelling in addition to full-time hours. Placements often involve shift work, with the resultant impact on health as discussed elsewhere in this book. Several of these factors can have an impact on wellbeing and make it harder to maintain positive mental health.

Being a nurse or midwife involves emotional demands for the professional as we care for individuals who may be in pain, suffering or distress alongside dealing with death and loss (Delgado et al., 2017). Part of the placement experience will involve learning how to deal with these emotional demands, understanding what may be personally difficult for you, and identifying the best ways to manage that. Healthcare and academic teams are very aware of these demands within the profession. Courses may include sessions on self-awareness and resilience to help individuals. Healthcare settings will also provide debriefing when particularly challenging situations have taken place.

## ASSESSMENTS

The pressure of assessment is an area many students will be familiar with. There may be multiple deadlines to contend with and assessments that are due during or after placement. Managing these workload pressures can be challenging and place real pressure on achieving a work-life balance that is essential for wellbeing. Being assessed is a stressful situation for most people, and our fears of being judged or failure are often present when approaching an assessment situation. Some people experience significant barriers, which can be paralysing when trying to write. Perfectionism, for example, can result in constant editing and reediting of each sentence and paralysis when constructing written work.

There are many practical tips that can help with managing stress related to assessments to promote wellbeing. Being clear about deadlines and planning ahead, and producing a study timetable creating guilt-free times with no study help us to feel more in control. They also create space for other activities that are important for managing stress such as exercise.

Higher education institutions provide significant resources on general study skills and assessment techniques, which often include individual meetings and drop-ins. Discussing assessments with lecturers can also be important. These resources are available to all students, any time, not only when you have problems. The next section explores some strategies that may help hold this in mind; however, blocking out the negative thoughts around assessments is important to keep focus, in that their purpose is to assess your learning on a module, not you.

## Survival Strategies

Recently, in *Nursing Times*, Mark Radcliffe writes, '...a failure to self-care is a failure to make the professions sustainable' (Radcliffe, 2020). Your time as a student at university is an excellent opportunity to start thinking about this concept. It is no secret that nursing and midwifery are challenging (yet wonderful!) careers, and the care you take of yourself will ensure your ability to care for others (service users and colleagues), and help ensure you have a long, fulfilling career. Following are some evidence-based techniques that, if regularly utilised, should provide a sound foundation for your mental health.

## MINDFULNESS

Buddhist-derived meditation interventions have been shown to be effective treatments for a broad range of physical and mental health illnesses, and a version of this, known as mindfulness, is now advocated by recognised healthcare bodies to promote good mental wellbeing.

Mindfulness is designed to bring us into the present moment by focusing on our thoughts, feelings, bodily sensations and/or the breath. Often when we are struggling, we focus on situations from our past or fears of the future. Mindfulness breaks this cycle to ensure we become rooted back in our present reality. It also provides us with a way to understand what an emotional state really is (e.g., we might tell others we are stressed, but we are likely to be experiencing a range of feelings, some of which may go unacknowledged in our busy lives).

The strength of mindfulness comes from a cumulative approach, where you begin building up a short, manageable daily practice. The best way to start is by using an app or resources that are freely available online, such as on YouTube. The UK National Health Service recommends the app Headspace, but there are others (e.g., Waking Up, Insight) that offer both free and paid-for content.

## SUPPORT NETWORK

Nursing and midwifery are careers that, at their core, centre around working with others. Although some areas, such as community roles, have an element of lone working, it is a team effort. Starting to build your support network while at university will also help sustain you throughout your career.

Knowing which family and friends you can talk to is one area of your support network. Certain people may not understand that you are not available as you once were (when doing shift work on wards, for example), but recognising those who support your goals is key to ongoing emotional resilience.

Due to the abovementioned thoughts, peer support, which is evidence based as a key component to good mental health (Mind, 2013), is invaluable because other students understand the pressures of nursing and midwifery training. You may make friends during seminars or placements, but there will also be peer support groups that already exist within university settings. You may find that your own experience is not reflected in your immediate cohort or seminar group, and so joining other peer support groups, such as the Disabled Students Network or the LGBTQI+ Students Network, can be beneficial. The sooner you make these connections (week 1 is a great time to start engaging with new groups!), the sooner you will start to feel more at home in this chapter of your life.

Another excellent resource to making connections during your course is through social media. It is important to understand the importance of e-professionalism to know how to present yourself on social media in a way that upholds the values of nursing. When used well, social media is a useful tool for making connections, engaging with the nursing and midwifery community as a whole, and influencing health issues (McGrath et al., 2019).

## UNIVERSITY SUPPORT

While there is much to look forward to when starting your course, it is also helpful to recognise that you are still having a human experience as a student and different challenges will arise, both internal and external to your studies. This can include issues such as bereavements, medical problems, financial worries, personality clashes, or accommodation difficulties.

Universities recognise that, in addition to ranking and research, robust student support systems are important to attracting and keeping students (GuildHE, 2018). Due to this, universities and student bodies have invested in developing services to specialise and advise on a range of needs a student may present with, and accessing the right one will help you make decisions that are best for you and your course. Tutors have some knowledge about the support systems in place, and the university website or app will have links and information. You can also ask at the student union centre or speak to your course representative (again, details will be available on your university's website). The main message is to not struggle alone when there are staff with a wealth of knowledge and experience available who can help you resolve your worries.

## COMMUNICATION

As suggested earlier, there may be times when you need to have conversations on sensitive issues with your university or placement team. Therefore it is worth preparing yourself for how you broach more difficult topics.

Often we become concerned that if we attempt to discuss issues we are struggling with, there might be an assumption made that we are not coping or cannot handle the requirements of the course. In reality the opposite is true: professional codes ask us as student nurses or midwives to act with honesty and integrity and to uphold our professionalism. Therefore being clear about your needs, and sometimes even your limitations, is evidence of professional conduct.

The recommended way of approaching more difficult conversations begins with the steps you may have already started to cultivate earlier. Decide who you need to approach. Typically this will be a personal tutor, although it may also be a mentor or manager in placement who is also appropriate. If you have a good rapport with another staff member or a seminar lead at university, either of these may be an option, too. Your university will have regulations governing different factors that impact student life (absences, bereavements, health issues), so familiarise yourself with this guidance. If you need help accessing these on the university website, your student union or student services should be able to help. Prepare a concise way to summarise the issue, considering the use of language and some suggestions for solutions, and what support you need.

Throughout your career it will be necessary to have conversations of this nature many times, especially if you intend to go into management. Instead of being fearful of them as a student, consider the opportunities to start practising your communication skills. Learning how to have conversations about mental health is covered in more detail elsewhere in this book.

## SPACE FOR YOURSELF

Nursing and midwifery is about balance: balancing the demands of your course/career, the needs of family and friends and time for yourself is a skill.

Begin to plan your weeks so you have a variety of ways to nurture your emotional health. Making time for mindfulness is a great way to begin, and you may want to incorporate some form of activity or exercise to support your body in what can be a physically demanding job. It is important that time for yourself also feels meaningful for you; when tired, it's easy to switch on the television and scroll through your phone, and sometimes that is not a problem. However, our minds are complex and need lots of different forms of stimulation to feel balanced, so make a list of different activities and find ways to fit this variety into your calendar. There will be some weeks when your plans do not come to fruition, but if there is an overall sense of balance over the weeks, months and years of your course, you will be in good stead for managing your emotional health and achieving your university and work goals.

Mental wellbeing is essential for all nurses and midwives, yet this can become overlooked with the focus of our role on caring for others. The time spent learning the profession poses several challenges for our wellbeing through the experiences gained at both university and in the healthcare setting. Yet the investment as a student in understanding our own wellbeing needs and how to address these within a busy role is essential. This establishes the foundation for a career of being able to care as effectively for ourselves as we do for other people.

**ACTIVITY**

Here is a short mindfulness session designed to help you connect with the present moment.

Begin by finding a comfortable, upright position and either close your eyes or maintain a soft focus on a spot in front of you.

Start to focus on your breath: breath into your abdominal space, then breathe out, slowing the breath down but not forcing it—let it feel natural. Do this for 10 rounds.

Next, start to notice the sensations in your body: is there any tension present? Focus on your feet, then draw your focus up your body through your lower legs, your upper legs, thighs, abdominal area, your chest, down into the arms and hands, back up through the neck, the jaw, the face and the top of your head. Where you encounter areas of tension, relax the muscles.

Return to five more rounds of noticing your breath drawing in and out.

Now, notice what is on your mind. Observe your thoughts, as they come and go like clouds in the sky. There is no need to pass judgement on them—your mind is doing what is natural by thinking—but also, do not attach any importance to the thoughts. Just notice. Where an emotion arises, see if you can name that emotion, then just notice it without judgement.

Bring your attention back to the breath, counting another five rounds. As you begin the sixth round, start to expand your awareness of your breath going from your lungs out to your whole body. See yourself as a human amid everything around you: connected but also having your own experience.

Now, bring your attention back to the room. If your eyes are closed, you can open them. Notice what you can see and what you can hear. Push your feet against the ground and, if it feels good, stretch. You are now ready to begin your day again.

---

**CASE STUDY 11.1**     **The Bridge Network**

Healthcare students can experience additional pressures that impact on mental wellbeing. Creative ways of ensuring that students who experience mental health difficulties are supported to manage their wellbeing and achieve their potential at university are of growing importance in this context. This case study provides an example of a pilot student mental health initiative to highlight an innovative development to promote wellbeing.

The Bridge Network is for healthcare students who experience mental health difficulties. The innovative development was cocreated between academics and students at a UK university. Student peer group facilitators draw on their own lived experience of mental distress or of being a carer to support others. Alumni funding was awarded by the university to enable student volunteers to access accredited training in peer support, active listening and self-disclosure.

The Bridge Network is based on a peer support model in which volunteer student peers who themselves have experienced mental health challenges provide group-based support for other students to promote mental wellbeing. Peer support entails the provision of support between individuals who have shared experience, promoting acceptance, respect and mutual empowerment. Peer supporters drawing on their own lived experience of mental distress to help others is what makes peer support distinctive.

The Bridge Network groups were founded on the following principles:
- It is for healthcare students by healthcare students.
- Run by students who share a mutual experience of being healthcare students and experiencing emotional challenges.
- Committed to providing a safe and supportive space for promoting and exploring mental wellbeing.
- Inclusivity: every student at the school who has an interest in mental wellbeing is welcome.
- As a healthcare professional to take care of other people, it is important to take care of yourself, and this group is about supporting students to do this.

Student peer group facilitators run group forums for students across the school of healthcare to meet and share experiences. Facilitators create an inclusive atmosphere, facilitating discussions on mental wellbeing or the student experience and signposting to support services. Volunteers have their own mental health experiences, which connect students with a shared but often hidden identity together. The training involved exploring these implications for practising as a healthcare professional and, through this mutuality, challenge internalised stigma. Giving or receiving peer support enhances self-confidence, empowerment, and self-identity. Support for peer facilitators was provided by academic staff and the counselling service.

CASE STUDY 11.1 **The Bridge Network—cont'd**

There have been some challenges to developing the network, most significantly the logistics of planning and facilitating groups for students on a demanding course with lengthy periods of time spent away from the university setting. Recruiting facilitators from different courses and different years was a means to address these challenges.

Student peer group facilitators from the Bridge Network have made wider contributions to mental health promotion and have led mental health awareness activities in the university in which student volunteers have role-modelled positive self-disclosure and openness, engaging with students across the faculty. The Bridge Network has an active Twitter page, using this platform to promote mental health self-care tips.

**ANNE FELTON ■ CHARLOTTE HALLS**

## References

Delgado, C., Upton, D., Ranse, K., Furness, T., & Foster, K. (2017). Nurses' resilience and the emotional labour of nursing work: An integrative review of empirical literature. *International Journal of Nursing Studies, 70*, 71–88.

GuildHE. (2018). *Wellbeing in higher education.* London. https://www.guildhe.ac.uk/wp-content/uploads/2018/10/GuildHE-Wellbeing-in-Higher-Education-WEB.pdf.

McGrath, L., Swift, A., Clark, M., & Bradbury-Jones, C. (2019). Understanding the benefits and risks of nursing students engaging with online social media. *Nursing Standard, 34*(10), 45–49.

Mind. (2013). *Mental health peer support in England: piecing together the jigsaw.* Mind: London. https://www.mind.org.uk/media/4096/piecing-together-the-jigsaw-full-version.pdf.

O'Keeffe, P. (2013). A sense of belonging: Improving student retention. *College Student Journal, 47*(4), 605–613.

Radcliffe, M. (2020). *A failure to self-care is a failure to make nursing sustainable.* Nursing Times. https://www.nursingtimes.net/opinion/mark-radcliffe/a-failure-to-self-care-is-a-failure-to-make-nursing-sustainable-03-12-2020/.

Student Minds. (2019). *Mental health charter.* http://universitymentalhealthcharter.org.uk.

## CHAPTER 12

# WellBeing and Late Career Nurses and Midwives

Sue Haines

## KEY POINTS

1. More proactive and innovative approaches are required to retain experienced late career professionals in the workplace, including a culture of flexible working, new roles and an earlier awareness of available options, well before retirement age.
2. Improving equality, diversity, and inclusion in the workplace is central to wellbeing and retention of late career nurses and midwives.
3. Learning is lifelong, and proactive career planning and continuing professional development are important at all stages of a career. At mid to late career, seek out a mentor or careers coach to help you reflect and consider your own personal situation, your strengths, talents, skills and work-life aspirations.
4. Let's talk more openly about menopause as an occupational health issue in the workplace and ensure employers, managers and staff are aware of support available to employees based on the best available evidence.
5. Financial worries can cause mental health anxiety, and pensions are complex, so take greater control of your financial situation. There is a need for employers to ensure access to advice about pension planning and finance for nurses and midwives.

## Introduction

This chapter focuses on wellbeing and support for late career nurses and midwives, recognising and valuing the importance and diversity of professional skills, knowledge and talents that nurses and midwives have and develop throughout their careers. In this context, late career is being described as the age when a nurse or midwife may be approaching or thinking of retirement, or alternative work-life options, often (but not exclusively) in their 50s or 60s. We will consider a range of issues that can impact on wellbeing at late career. Recommendations for individuals, employers and policymakers are proposed to value and retain late career nurses and midwives and maximise their wellbeing, motivation and job satisfaction.

## What Does Late Career Mean and Why Is This Important?

With an ageing nursing and midwifery workforce in many countries, the act of valuing and retaining older nurses and midwives has never been more important. However, research into the retention of older nurses and midwives and their experiences of wellbeing is limited, and definitions of late career vary internationally due to the diverse social and cultural contexts within which nurses and midwives work around the world. There are descriptions of how late career nurses and midwives with essential skills, knowledge, and professional expertise can often feel overlooked and undervalued at work, which can impact negatively on their psychological wellbeing and confidence.

Through my own research and experiences in professional development and careers coaching over many years, it is evident that nurses and midwives often do not recognise and value the talents they have, nor the transferability of their professional skills and knowledge to potentially new and different health and care roles. Traditionally career and development discussions at late career stage can be limited to the culture and expectations of a ward, a team or speciality service where the individual nurse or midwife is working, rather than being a proactive consideration of new opportunities to retain experienced nurses and midwives across wider organisations and/or care settings/systems. This limited perspective risks losing increasing numbers of nurses and midwives at a time when there are increasing health and social care needs of populations, globally. In addition, with growing numbers of newly qualified nurses, midwives and learners in the workplace, increasingly experienced practitioners are required to be supervisors and assessors to share their professional experience, knowledge and skills. Therefore retaining skilled nurses and midwives is also essential for training and developing the future workforce.

Meaningful career development and support from a proactive line manager is important at any stage of a nurse or midwife's career, although experiences of individual annual appraisals can sometimes feel like a tick box exercise. At mid to late career, conversations are often focused on finding out about an individual's retirement plans rather than considering career development or more flexible and alternative approaches to work. Consider the following questions:

- Have you considered your own career plan, financial situation and options? How far away are you from the age of retirement?
- How meaningful was your last annual performance appraisal or review?
- What time was spent focused on your own personal wellbeing and career development?
- How can you influence that experience to ensure your personal development needs are proactively considered in your next one-to-one with your line manager?
- Have you considered seeking support through a mentor or careers coach to help you reflect and develop a personalised approach to your own wellbeing and development plans?

There is a need to revisit our traditional career expectations, options and aspirations as individual nurses and midwives, as employers and as policymakers. We will now consider some of the main issues that impact on the wellbeing of mid to late career nurses and midwives.

# What Are the Issues That Can Impact on WellBeing of Late Career Nurses and Midwives?

## LACK OF RECOGNITION FOR CONTRIBUTION AND PROFESSIONAL EXPERIENCE

The lack of value of nursing as a profession is well documented; this is a result of the predominance of females within the nursing and midwifery workforce and a gendered perception of nursing work influencing pay and status (Clayton-Hathway et al., 2020). Within this context, late career nurses and midwives can often feel that their experience and knowledge is not adequately recognised by organisations and have reported feeling undervalued and invisible, with a lack of meaningful recognition or respect for their career experiences and achievements (Haines et al., 2021). This then can impact on levels of self-confidence; yet in the context of global shortages of nurses and midwives, there is an increasing focus on retention and emerging opportunities for experienced nurses and midwives to take on new roles that recognise their contribution and value their professional experience. Late career nurses and midwives I have spoken to often describe feeling frustrated at the lack of opportunities for career development and more flexible careers, and that training opportunities and courses are often not offered to them as an older member of the team. A UK Legacy Mentor nurse retention pilot project (Haines et al., 2021), built on evidence from a Canadian study (Clauson et al., 2011), utilises a focused development programme for late career nurses to value and retain their professional nursing knowledge, experience and skills and enables opportunities for knowledge transition in practice, with a positive impact on late career nurse participants (Case Study 12.1).

Rapid developments in technology are also resulting in changing skills required by nurses and midwives in many work environments. Generational differences and experience in utilising new technologies can cause apprehension and fear for nurses and midwives less familiar with digital technologies in practice. Building confidence and ensuring inclusive approaches to training and development are essential to ensure that these innovations are developed and implemented in partnership with experienced late career professionals.

Nurses and midwives require professional autonomy to feel valued, respected, engaged and able to develop. This helps to create positive work practice environments and enhance wellbeing, not only for late career nurses and midwives but across all generations of the professions. It is important to ensure line managers are trained and supported to have high-quality, individual appraisals and career conversations with staff to recognise and value individuals, their talents, potential and professional aspirations. Also, the ability for managers to develop and implement flexible work options and have greater awareness of new career development options available, both within and across organisations for late career nurses and midwives, helps to create innovative and positive career opportunities.

---

**CASE STUDY 12.1**    **Legacy Mentor Nurse Retention Pilot Project**

The Legacy Mentor pilot project (Haines et al., 2021) was developed and delivered in Nottinghamshire, United Kingdom during 2017-18 and was sponsored by the local integrated health and social care system's professional nursing and midwifery cabinet (a group of senior nurse and midwife leaders representing organisations and stakeholders from within the local health and care system). The project aimed to improve retention of late career registered nurses (RNs) who have professional nursing knowledge, experience and skills and enable opportunities for knowledge transition in practice. It built on evidence from a Canadian study (Clauson et al., 2011), which identified a focused mentorship intervention that retained skilled bedside RNs, developed pathways of knowledge transition, supporting and developing students, newly qualified RNs and other learners in practice.

Six experienced RNs were successfully appointed to Legacy Mentor roles (mentors) from across Nottinghamshire health and care organisations. The participating RNs had broad nursing experience from a range of settings, including acute hospital, health care of the older person, surgical, community, school nursing and outpatients. Participants included those who had retired and returned to practice, considering or about to commence retirement, and those later in their career.

All the mentors initially undervalued their own professional experience and expertise. The programme helped them to reflect on their years of nursing experience and recognise the wealth of professional knowledge they had. They were motivated to pass on their knowledge and skills to more junior staff and student nurses. Each mentor had an initial individual meeting with the project facilitator to discuss their personal development and to identify an area of practice where they had specific knowledge and experience and wanted to take forward as an educational project within their clinical area. The mentors attended two induction days where they also worked with the facilitator to coproduce the 6-month Legacy Mentor development programme, based on the learning needs they had identified for themselves as participants. The programme included protected time one day per week within clinical areas for the mentors to work on their individual educational projects. They participated in monthly facilitated development workshops, which included skills such as coaching, finance and pensions advice, and participated in individual career coaching sessions themselves with the programme facilitator.

The mentor projects included developing preceptorship resources in complex community roles (preceptorship is a period of structured transition to guide and support all newly qualified practitioners from

*Continued*

| CASE STUDY 12.1 | Legacy Mentor Nurse Retention Pilot Project—cont'd |
|---|---|

student to autonomous professional), education resources for continence assessment and care and pocket guides for students and new starters. Each of the projects delivered benefits by providing support and education for staff, students and other learners in the practice settings. The pilot project was evaluated and showed that participants built a supportive network, reported feeling energised by the mentor role, valued for their professional experience and knowledge, more confident, were learning new skills and had a renewed enthusiasm for nursing. The opportunity for cross-organisational working provided additional benefits building a community of practice, sharing of learning and wider understanding of the health and social care needs of patients, families and carers across care settings. The benefits are demonstrated by feedback comments from those who took part: 'When I'm in this project I'm beaming', 'I have regained my passion for nursing from the legacy mentor project', 'I feel meaningfully recognized', and 'I feel empowered and inspired to support others'.

In conclusion, the pilot project identified the critical importance in investing in late career nurses; valuing their professional expertise, knowledge and skills; and providing them with development opportunities, financial advice and career advice. This can both reenergise and retain experienced RNs, enabling them to share their knowledge and skills to enhance support for students and learners in increasingly complex and pressured clinical practice environments. The programme requires evaluation in other health and care settings, particularly considering the impact of the pandemic on late career nurses and their wellbeing needs and career intentions. It offers opportunities for new roles as part of a strategic approach to inclusive talent management and nurse retention.

**ELLEN CUTLER**

## PHYSICAL CHANGES OF AGEING

As nurse or midwife reading this, you will be aware of, or may have personal experience of, one or more of the physical changes associated with ageing. These can be very frustrating and difficult to manage at work, including back and joint pain, reduction in eye sight, hearing loss and the effects of other long-term conditions and disabilities. In addition, disrupted sleep patterns due to menopausal symptoms, or other long-term conditions can affect psychological and physical wellbeing. These can all cause a negative impact on personal confidence and pose increasing health challenges in certain work environments. For example, working variable shift patterns (including 12-hour shifts), night work requiring changes to sleep patterns, reduced visibility and wearing personal protective equipment (PPE) that poses physical, auditory and visual restrictions can be increasingly physically and psychologically demanding. There can be a lack of awareness of, or access to, opportunities for more flexible working and alternative roles, and yet there is an increasing need to retain experienced late career nurses and midwives in the workplace.

## IMPACT OF MENOPAUSE

The majority of nurses and midwives are women, and yet the impact of menopause and associated symptoms in the workplace has only recently been recognised as an occupational health issue. There is a need to ensure employers, managers and staff are aware of support available based on the best evidence. Symptoms vary, with some women experiencing little impact on their working life, whilst many women experience physical and psychological symptoms that can make functioning at work difficult. These include poor concentration, difficulty sleeping, tiredness, feeling low, hot flushes and urogenital problems such as frequency and urgency (Royal College of Nursing, 2020). If you are experiencing symptoms that are causing difficulties at work or home and feeling you are on your own, you are not! It is vital to seek specialist advice, which could be from your doctor, practice nurse or other health care professional, or talk to your manager and ask for a referral to occupational health where you can find support at work and receive information about self-help strategies to help alleviate symptoms.

## CULTURE OF FLEXIBLE WORKING

The majority of health and social care organisations have flexible working guidance or policies; however, implementation of these into practice varies. Opportunity for more flexible working has been identified as important for retention of employees, although many nursing and midwifery jobs are not routinely considered for part time or more flexible working hours. There are often expectations that to go part time or retire and return, experienced nurses and midwives will take roles with less responsibility and often on a lower pay scale. This does not recognise and value professional experience. Developing an organisational culture where all roles are identified as having potential for part time, job share and flexible working needs to become a normal expectation.

## MENTAL WELLBEING, BURNOUT, AND STRESS

It has long been recognised that increasing service pressures and the emotional labour of nursing and midwifery work result in stress and burnout. This has been further accentuated as a result of the recent pandemic with evidence of psychological impact on nurses and midwives, including post-traumatic stress, increasing anxiety and stress levels, and an increased intention to leave, particularly post the initial waves of a pandemic, for example, as exhaustion and burnout are evident. There are concerns that nurses and midwives approaching retirement age that may have stayed on at work for longer are now intending to leave due to the sustained pressures and stresses.

Consider the support mechanisms available to you and what best meets your professional and emotional wellbeing needs. Options can vary in different countries and between organisations and professions. For example, there are a diverse range of frameworks described for clinical supervision and support in nursing and midwifery globally.

- In the United Kingdom, this might include models of clinical supervision such as restorative clinical supervision (which contains elements of psychological support, including listening and supporting individuals to manage the emotional demands of their roles more effectively, helping reduce burnout and stress).
- Action learning sets are a small group of people who normally have a comparable level of responsibility or role within a workplace or professional context that meet with the specific intention of solving workplace problems.
- Multiprofessional Schwartz Rounds (these originated in the United States in the 1990s) are a group forum open to all staff, which focuses on reflection and sharing experiences of the emotional and social aspects of working in health care.
- Advice through professional unions, occupational health services, access to professional mentorship or coaching is helpful.
- The UK Professional Midwifery Advocates in the National Health Service (NHS) supports midwives in their clinical practice and advocates for women; more recently the Professional Nurse Advocates delivers training and restorative supervision for colleagues across England.

These are all means of supporting emotional wellbeing and can help to identify and sign post nurses and midwives to professional psychological support if required.

## FINANCIAL PRESSURES AND PENSIONS

Nursing and midwifery remain predominately female workforces, and often individuals have caring responsibilities either for children, grandchildren, elderly parents or others. Many work part time during their careers or take career breaks for caring responsibilities. Social expectations on carers can cause stress and pressure; in addition, part time working or career breaks can impact on personal finances, pensions and savings. Financial worries are the cause of much mental anxiety for many people and can cause relationship difficulties, which impact on wellbeing. Fair and equitable remuneration for nurses and midwives is recognised by the World Health Organisation as a global workforce priority, asking policymakers to ensure adequate investment to retain and motivate nurses and midwives.

As retirement approaches, nurses and midwives at late career who have not kept a close oversight of their finances may be disappointed as the reality of financial expectations is fully understood. Pensions are complex in different sectors and countries and often poorly understood by employees. It is important to understand your own personal situation; if you are unsure, then find out what financial advice your employer offers and attend a preretirement course if provided by your employer. Decisions about pensions can be complex, and what is right for your work colleague or friend may not be the best option for you; seek reputable professional advice early, know the facts about any debt, savings or pension you may have, and understand your options. Taking greater control of your financial situation is important for your wellbeing. Employers should ensure that nurses and midwives have access to professional financial advice to consider the best options for their personal situation and based on their expectations for their retirement.

## RACISM AND DISCRIMINATION IN THE WORKPLACE

The UK NHS recruitment processes have long been shown to disproportionately favour White applicants (Kline, 2015). For Black, Asian and Minority Ethnic nurses and midwives, evidence has identified experiences of underemployment, with larger numbers of ethnic minority nurses and midwives working at entry-level salaries later into their careers. This is often further compounded by lack of training and development opportunities (Pendleton, 2017).

Through my work in careers coaching, I have listened to experiences of late career Black, Asian and Minority Ethnic nurses (both UK trained and international nurses with years of skills and experience in their home country and in the UK NHS), who describe the frustration of being unsuccessful at interview and frequently seeing more junior, inexperienced White colleagues being promoted over them, with little constructive feedback on the rationale for decisions made. In England, the Workforce Race Equality Standard (WRES) captures data from across all NHS organisations on the experiences of Black, Asian and Minority Ethnic staff, and this shows evidence of bullying and harassment impacting on the wellbeing of nurses and midwives at all ages. Unconscious bias and discrimination impact negatively on both psychological and physical wellbeing of nurses and midwives. Creating inclusive team cultures, ensuring psychological safety (being able to speak up, raise concerns and question things without risk of punishment or humiliation), and taking meaningful action to ensure equality and diversity are central to decision making and career progression are critical priorities for wellbeing and improving retention in the workplace.

In summary, late career nurses and midwives have a wealth of skills, experience, knowledge and talents that are required within the global health and care workforce and are transferable across different work settings. Raising awareness of the needs of late career nurses and midwives enables potential for more focused support and recognition of the value of professional knowledge, experience and the safety critical roles that nurses and midwives provide across the full span and diversity of their careers.

## Wheel of Life

Regularly reviewing your own personal wellbeing and life-work balance can help to develop self-awareness and enable a clearer focus on your life priorities and wellbeing. It is important to reflect, review and recognise your own professional experiences, skills, strengths, hopes and career expectations alongside your personal life decisions. The Wheel of Life assessment tool is used in life and career coaching and attributed originally to Paul Meyers (The Coaching Tools Company, 2021).

Undertaking a Wheel of Life assessment is about taking positive action to feel more in control of your life (Fig. 12.1). This exercise can be undertaken either on your own or with the support of a trusted colleague, coach, mentor or friend. Use a notebook to record your thoughts and reflections.

- Draw a circle with eight segments; suggested headings can include Health, Home, Work, Money, Family and Friends, Hobbies and Social Life, Personal Growth and Development, and Professional Development. The section headings you include may be different; it depends on what is important to you in your life and may include different areas of focus that are priorities to you.
- The centre of the wheel = 0 and the edge of the wheel = 10. For each subject, score yourself out of 10 for your current situation by drawing a curved line across the segment at that level (10 being very satisfied and happy; 1 being very dissatisfied).
- How balanced does your wheel look?
- What would your ideal score be in each section?
- Consider and compare the current score with your ideal score and see where the gaps are. This helps to focus you on where you may wish to take actions to change the current life balance.
- Keep a diary for a couple of weeks to really reflect on your current situation and review your self-assessments.
- Consider what is available to help you, via your employer, your professional union, manager, clinical supervisor, professional work colleague, or consider a mentor or coach.
- Identify specific actions you are going to take. Keep a record and review regularly. You may find you need to seek some additional support and advice depending on what comes out as important for your wellbeing (e.g., specific career guidance or financial advice).

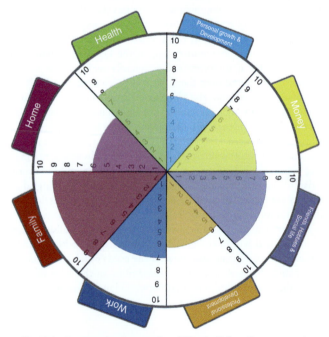

**Fig. 12.1**  An example of a completed Wheel of Life self-assessment.

## References

Clauson, M., Wejer, P., Frost, L., McRae, C., & Straight, H. (2011). Legacy mentors: Translating the wisdom of our senior nurses. *Nurse Education in Practice, 11*, 153–158.

Clayton-Hathway, K., Laure Humbery, A., Griffiths, H., McIlroy, R., & Schutz, S. (2020). *Gender and nursing as a profession—valuing nurses and midwives and paying them their worth.* Royal College of Nursing, London.

Haines, S., Evans, K., Timmons, S., & Cutler, E. (2021). A service improvement project of a legacy nurse programme to improve the retention of late career nurses and midwives. *Journal of Research in Nursing, 26*(7), 648–681. https://doi.org/10.1177/17449871211036172.

Kline, R. (2015). *Beyond the snowy white peaks of the NHS?* Better Health Briefing, 39. Race Equality Foundation: London. Available at: https://raceequalityfoundation.org.uk/wp-content/uploads/2018/02/Health-Briefing-39-_Final.pdf.

Pendleton, J. (2017). The experiences of black and minority ethnic nurses and midwives working in the UK. *British Journal of Nursing, 26*(1), 3742.

Royal College of Nursing. (2020). *RCN menopause and work guidance for RCN representatives.* www.rcn.org.uk.

The Coaching Tools Company. (2019). *The wheel of life: A complete guide for coaches!.* The Launchpad [blog]. https://www.thecoachingtoolscompany.com/wheel-of-life-complete-guide-everything-you-need-to-know/.

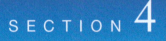

# Enhancing Wellbeing at Work

## CHAPTER 13

# Psychologically Safe Working Environments

Valerie James ■ Rebecca Thomas

## KEY POINTS

1. Psychological safety is 'a shared belief held by members of a team that the team is safe for interpersonal risk taking.' (Edmondson, 2018)
2. Psychological safety affects how teams collaborate and interact, and makes for a more inclusive, productive environment.
3. An emotional intelligence skill set is crucial to creating a culture of psychological safety in the workplace.
4. Emotions are neither positive nor negative; they may be pleasurable, like joy, or unpleasant, like anguish, but neither are bad or wrong. We need both in life to learn and grow.
5. Accurate awareness of your own emotions (self-awareness) and those of your colleagues (social awareness) helps you manage minor interactions, and manage major conflict too, making your workplace safer despite great pressures. This awareness is at the core of emotional intelligence.

## Introduction

The term *psychological safety* was first known to be mentioned by Schein and Bennis (1965). Psychological safety was defined as a group phenomenon that reduces interpersonal risk ('a person's anxiety about being basically accepted and worthwhile'). More recently, organisational behavioural scientist Amy Edmondson at Harvard Business School introduced the construct of 'team psychological safety' and defined it as 'a shared belief held by members of a team that the team is safe for interpersonal risk taking' (Edmondson, 2018).

In her book, *The Fearless Organisation*, Edmondson writes about an 'Epidemic of Silence' in which failing to speak up, dismissing warnings, and 'going along to get along' can be dire for organisations, as leaders who only welcome good news inadvertently create a fear of bad news.

Employees describe the following reasons why they feel fearful of sharing honest perspectives or personal challenges: 'Don't want to look ignorant? Don't ask questions… Don't want to look incompetent? Don't admit to mistakes or weaknesses… Don't want to be called disruptive? Don't make suggestions…' (Edmondson, 2018, p. 5).

Fostering psychologically safe workplace culture should be an organisational priority. It affects how teams collaborate and interact, and makes for a more inclusive, productive environment. Some managers and teams have a hard time acknowledging when they have a problem, instead putting the blame on a high turnover rate or change in leadership. Ignoring the issue, however, can have consequences. Psychological safety in teams is the cornerstone to building learning behaviours, avoidable harm reduction, shared decision making, better problem solving, and more creative solutions.

Taking this into consideration, how can nurses, midwives, and their colleagues feel psychologically safe at work? What does a safe environment look like? In our healthcare institutions, nurses and midwives are frequently seen as the advocates of patients' emotional wellbeing, and often this emotional labour is seen as lesser than the intellectual labour of medicine. Not only is this distinction unhelpful but it is not accurate. Goleman (2017) and others demonstrated some 25 years ago that emotional intelligence is just as vital as conventional intellectual intelligence—and that emotional intelligence, especially in a leader, is the more effective skill set of the two. This chapter will explore the concept of emotional literacy (emotional intelligence in action), what empathy is and is not, and how your own self-awareness—and your awareness of others—is crucial to good care and a healthier workplace. Nurses and midwives are often talented as patient advocates, and you can transfer this ability to how you look after yourself emotionally and care for your colleagues.

Do you sometimes feel your views are not valued, or even sought, at work? Do you find there can be uncomfortable standoffs with colleagues on some issues? Maybe you have a different set of guiding care principles, or you or your patient/s or clients are not being heard sometimes? How much do you encourage others to voice views different from yours and be genuinely interested in them? There is much an individual can do to make it easier for others to hear them out, to influence well, and to become an even better team member, such as being acutely focused on the goals that you do share. Then the workplace can become safer for all players, including service users and their families.

Psychological safety is underpinned by a commitment to, and investment in, developing emotional intelligence. If you truly understand your emotions, and those of your teammates, and you can really withhold judgements and be compassionate to those who you may disagree with, then the workplace becomes safer, more innovative, and greater fun! So, as your read this chapter, try to spot where you can still improve, both by finding deeper understandings of the usual myths about emotions and empathy and by experimenting with different ways of seeing common workplace issues.

A psychologically safe workplace is an infinitely complex reality, and this chapter cannot deal with the huge range of dimensions that it covers—from spoken to physical manipulation, bullying, coercions, or microaggressions relating to racism, sexism, homophobia, among others. There is also the impact of toxic cultures on staff and patients and the misuse or abuse of power and authority. All of these require excellent human resources (HR) support from the organisation and the independent support from confidential staff counselling services and listening services. Some HR departments also offer facilitation and mediation to colleagues. However, in any of these circumstances, key steps to empowering yourself, your teammates, and your clients/patients are still about having compassion for our human flaws and a willingness to engage emotionally but within clear, professional boundaries.

## What Are Emotions?

The root of the word *emotions* tells us: motion/emote/emotion/motivation. Emotions MOVE us. We experience them physically and we have chemical changes in the body that originate in the limbic system in the brain. We also know that being able to think and have strong feelings is often mutually exclusive in the moment because the amygdala in the limbic system floods us with adrenaline and cortisol. Everyone experiences this in stressful situations, such as when we are put on the spot in an interview. The good news is that we can improve on this throughout our lives, as Goleman (2017) has proven.

## What Is Emotional Intelligence?

In the 1990s, Daniel Goleman created an accessible model of emotions quotient (EQ)—as opposed to intelligence quotient (IQ), which is the traditional Western way of measuring intelligence. The concept of IQ has been much criticised as it only covers some aspects of intelligence such as verbal and numerical reasoning and abstract reasoning. Professors of psychology, such as Gardiner, have stated there are many other kinds of intelligence such as kinetic intelligence (dancers and racing drivers score well on this) that we do not test for—and we underestimate these qualities—such a loss of talent! And our Western notion of IQ does not apply to many cultures, leading to even greater exclusion of potential talents at work.

Goleman (2017) original model described five categories of emotional intelligence:

1. Self-awareness: of your moods, emotions, drives, and how they affect others
2. Self-regulation: to control or redirect disruptive moods or impulses, suspending judgement
3. Motivation: belief in reaching for a greater good with energy and tenacity
4. Empathy: ability to comprehend the emotional reactions of others and skill in dealing with them
5. Social skill: able to create rapport and connections with others, discerning common goals

Goleman (2017) says that unlike IQ, which is fixed in late adolescence, we can continue to improve our EQ all our lives. This is so hopeful! We know that some people truly mature as they age, and it is this ability to interact with others and learn to modify our own behaviour that helps us to deal more effectively with life and relationships and to enhance our professionalism.

## How Big Is Your Emotional Vocabulary?

As a psychologist and a nurse, when working with clinicians I often ask them to name the emotion/s that they are feeling—or guess what emotions their colleagues or patients are experiencing. Their most common responses reflect their thoughts or opinions, not their emotions. For example, I might ask a clinician what he feels about managers. He may reply that managers do not care enough about patient care. That is an opinion, a thought, a view. When I ask the same person what he feels about managers, he may finally express his emotions. He may be feeling powerless in meetings with managers, or threatened by managers, or supported by managers. Those emotions are different from the opinions/thoughts about managers. So, we work on expanding each person's vocabulary. The primary emotions are generally seen by most authors to be:

Anger
Grief
Curiosity
Wonder/awe
Love
Hatred
Disgust
Joy/excitement

If we take just one of these words, say anger, there are so many shades of anger. I like to think of those paint cards you find at a DIY store: if anger were a colour, it might be red, and there are so many shades of red, from the palest of pinks to deep flaming ruby. Look at these words that might describe the range of intensity:

Mild irritation (pale pink)
Annoyance
Exasperation
Anger
Fury
Outrage
Wrath (deep crimson)

Brown's (2021) *Atlas of the Heart* is a great way to explore your emotions with greater subtlety and deepen connections with friends, family, and colleagues. Her TED Talks and other books are excellent resources for understanding your own heart, personal power, and potential.

## Why Is Emotional Vocabulary So Important?

If we know we can name an emotion and say where we physically feel it in our body (and this is such an individual experience), then we can better contain or self-regulate that emotion and it is less likely to spill out inappropriately. When we can do this for ourselves, our ability to contain others—our colleagues, patients, families, and friends—improves. Our ability to guess with greater accuracy what it is like to be in the shoes of someone else improves, too. When this occurs, this person feels understood. What is most important, though, is that you describe and not evaluate or judge the other person's emotions. Emotions just ARE. They are neither right nor wrong.

People often talk about positive and negative emotions, as if trying to get rid of the negative ones. This is deeply unhelpful, so I like to talk about pleasurable and unpleasurable emotions instead. It is the unpleasurable emotions (grief, envy, fear, etc.) that help us grow as people because we are confronted with needing to decide what we really value in life. I believe that what is most important is being real—not positive or negative—but in the middle of the two. In my work with clinicians, my colleague and I often use the phrase 'building hope and facing reality'. A person needs to do both. If too positive, the person can alienate colleagues who are having a tough time because of failing to acknowledge the team's reality. Yet it is vital to hold on to hope and point to even small reasons to keep others motivated, such as common goals, vision, and professional standards. So, emphasise with what is difficult at work and point to the potential for hope, too.

Emotions make us human, and usually there is no logical reason for someone to react in such a manner. The person is entitled to feel that way, but not necessarily to act on that emotion (e.g., think of rage). You cannot stop feeling it, but you can self-regulate and not punch someone in the nose! That would be called 'acting out the emotion'. This acting out may be completely inappropriate. However, there are times when our emotions save us (e.g., the fear and adrenaline rush that enables us to flee from a menacing person in a dark alley).

The more you can safely describe your emotions, the more self-regulation is possible and the less likely that your emotions will have you. Nurses and midwives are often more skilled in doing this when they are with patients and service users, but it is a trickier challenge to do this with peers and other colleagues.

## Are You Empathic? Or Sympathetic?

In working with thousands of clinicians over 30 years, I have found that empathy is often a misunderstood concept. Empathy itself is not an emotion. It is a state of being: you empathise with the emotion of the other person, not the situation. Why? People can have totally different emotional responses to the same situation, even if experienced at the same time. When we relate to the situation, and assume our reactions are the same, that is sympathy, not empathy. It is vital that we respect the other person's experience, which may be different to ours, but neither experience is better or more accurate, just different.

For example, I heard a nurse say to another, 'Oh, I'm so sorry about your father's death. My father died 4 years ago, and my grief was terrible.' However, the recently bereaved nurse had been abused by her father, and her emotional reaction to her father's death was relief not grief! So, to truly empathise, you need to find out (or be an accurate guesser!) the emotion/s from the other person, not the situation. Then connect with your memories of that emotion in yourself. It is like resounding/echoing in your own body with a time when you felt that emotion, too, bringing that connection to the both of you in the moment. It is such a humane and compassionate thing to do, to be beside someone in their pain or their joy! So, the nurse in the previous example could connect with a time when she felt relief when others around her expected her to feel grief, and how shaming that might also have felt for her.

What is also important is that you never assume that you know how people feel; rather, check it out. That phrase 'I know just how you feel' is just not true. Your experiences of grief, for example, might be very different from the person grieving in front of you. Remembering that your emotions are not the same as another's—we do not match exactly—helps us hold a degree of objectivity and stops us drowning in the other person's experience. It is truly respectful of the uniqueness of every single one of us.

## Empathy and Agreement Are Not the Same Thing

Another key point is that when you empathise with others you do not necessarily agree with them. You are respecting their right to their emotional response, their view, and their experience. Try this out at work: when a colleague says something you do not agree with, instead of countering with your view, simply summarise what the colleague said—listen deeply—and ask if your summary is accurate. You can say, 'Let me check out whether I understand your view…(summary). Is that correct?' Allow yourself to be corrected if necessary. Your colleague is likely to be delighted that she is allowed to have her view. Then you are in a strong position to voice your own views/emotional responses, equally. Rogers (2021; Rogers & Mani, 2016), a world-class workplace coach, teaches many practical ways to help people listen to each other at a deep and respectful level.

We cannot be free of our individual judgements, but we can know when we are judging another and suspend our judgements through a conversation. This allows us to become better at recognising and suspending, and ultimately a superb team player.

## Conclusion

Creating a fully and psychologically safe workplace is an impossible task for nurses or midwives in charge. Too many factors are out of their control, such as workforce numbers, professional-patient ratios, and organisational power dynamics. Even when there are excellent formal HR systems and procedures that work well, such as good rota principles and helpful mediation services, each of us still needs to take responsibility for managing our own emotional responses in each encounter with patients/clients and colleagues. Indeed, even with ourselves, our ability to self-regulate becomes a highly valuable skill set, valuable in every interaction.

First Lady Michelle Obama said in 2020 that empathy is the cornerstone of emotional intelligence and that recognition of others' experiences as valid is often what we try to teach our children (Obama, 2020). You will no doubt have many opportunities to enable others to their best team behaviours, starting with leading by example, being your very best and most generous self, and cocreating a psychologically safer workplace.

**ACTIVITY**

1. Think of a time at work that was difficult. Name the emotions you experienced at the time. Guess at the emotions of the other people in the situation. How was the situation difficult for you? How was the situation difficult for them? What common goal did you share even though you were having a difficult time together? Write notes.
2. Think of a time when you and a colleague had a strong difference about what should happen next at work. Write down your view. Write down the colleague's view as if you were neutral about it, using no judgements, just describing and summarising the colleague's view without agreeing or disagreeing.
3. Think of a time when you felt able to share your views without fear of a negative consequence. What conditions were present that enabled you to do that? For example, how was the conversation facilitated? Was there an implicit or explicit shared understanding that created trust within the interaction? What did you agree to do following the interaction that helped you feel confident it would not result in a negative outcome?

## CASE STUDY 13.1    Raising Awareness of Psychological Safety

For many years I have observed and talked about experiences of a cultural climate that cultivates fear, blame, and ultimately paralysis in decision making and accountability. Then I heard about this thing called psychological safety (PS)—at last a term I could use to articulate these observations. And so, I started to use it…a lot!!!

My reading on the topic made me think about how I needed to speak up and find a way to share my learning with others by raising awareness of PS and how we might start to cultivate it in our teams.

On World Patient Safety Day in 2021, I delivered my first awareness session on PS. The session was open to the entire organisation and was run virtually through MS Teams. I had prepared a PowerPoint presentation as a visual aid with some salient key points to help prompt my thinking. I used examples of real experiences whilst ensuring anonymity of those involved. Opportunities for wider discussion were limited, mainly due to time restrictions, but participants were encouraged to submit any questions that they had through the chat function. Most of what came through was congratulations for a job well done with some reflections of how the session was thought provoking and left some participants wanting to go off and find out more.

This session, however, led to further requests for me to deliver something to senior and lead nurses in a nearby health board. These sessions were to be face to face and for 2 hours. In order that I tailor my session and maximise the benefits to the participants, I first had a planning conversation with the director of nursing (DON) who had requested the sessions)) to understand what she hoped that her teams would get from attending the sessions and was able to build the session to align with this.

I opened the session with an activity to ground everyone in the room. I did this by providing several coloured photographs and asked them to choose the photograph that most spoke to them. I then paired them up and asked them to tell each other why they had chosen the photograph they had. They then fed back as a larger group. This set the stage by letting everyone share and put the principle of equality in conversational turn-taking front and centre.

The activity generated conversations around the realities of current working and how participants were feeling. Unsurprisingly, there was a consistent theme of pressure, guilt, and helplessness. To show that I was actively listening I would provide feedback about what was just said and invite others to contribute (e.g., Was this something that had resonated with others in the group?) whilst ensuring I was sensitive to how people may be feeling based on their tone of voice, their expressions, and other nonverbal cues. All of this, I believe, helped to build a safe environment for everyone allowing space for honesty, inclusion, asking questions, and a sense of feeling valued/included. Creating psychological safety so that people feel comfortable trying, and perhaps failing, is partially my responsibility as a facilitator; however, it's still up to the participants to take that final leap to vulnerability, to show their true authentic selves, and to go all in on the exercises that we do. Establishing this safe environment early on helped me to continue to have honest conversations about everyone's experiences of PS or lack of it.

The main session involved a blended approach of traditional didactic learning and inquiry-based learning where we underwent the learning together. As facilitator, I fostered some exploration of PS in the participants' workplace, linking it back to the theory. The group agreed that they had PS with their immediate mangers (who were in the room), and this was evident during the session, but not always in the context of the broader organisation, leading to discussions around leadership and what leaders can do to foster a climate of PS in their teams.

I found these sessions incredibly powerful, especially as the DON and deputy were in attendance, which for me spoke of the absence of hierarchy status in the room. The individuals reported, honestly, their reflections and experiences and we took some time to explore what they might be able to do differently back in the workplace. These ideas were recorded, and the DON and deputy were asked to commit to enabling the ideas where practically feasible. I have since been asked to deliver a workshop for the Royal College of Nursing Wales.

To bolster the learning experience of those who attend the awareness sessions I have curated all my research resources into a Padlet, an online bulletin board that can be used as a collaborative learning tool. Moving forward I will continue to engage in conversations whenever I can to raise staff awareness of psychological safety in teams in the hope that these small repetitive actions will grow into better workplace cultures where there is demonstrable psychological safety.

**BECKY THOMAS**

## *References*

Brown, B. (2021). *Atlas of the heart: Mapping meaningful connection and the language of human experience.* Vermillion, London.

Edmondson, A. C. (2018). *The fearless organization: Creating psychological safety in the workplace for learning, innovation, and growth.* John Wiley & Sons, Hoboken, New Jersey.

Goleman, D. (2017). What makes a leader. *Harvard Business Review Press,* Boston, Massachusetts.

Obama, M. (2020). *Michelle Obama's DNC speech is a powerful example of emotional intelligence.* https://www.inc.com/minda-zetlin/michelle-obama-dnc-speech-emotional-intelligence-empathy.html.

Rogers, J. (2021). *Are you listening? Stories from a coaching life.* Penguin, London, England.

Rogers, J., & Mani, A. (2016). *Coaching for health: Why it works and how to do it.* McGraw Hill, Open University Press, United Kingdom.

Schein, E. H., & Bennis, W. G. (1965). *Personal and organizational change through group methods: The laboratory approach.* Wiley & Sons, New York.

Zhi, Q., & Su, M. (2015). Enhance collaborative learning by visualizing process of knowledge building with Padlet. In *International Conference of Educational Innovation through Technology (EITT)* 10.1109/EITT.2015.54. (pp. 221–225).

## CHAPTER 14

# Clinical Supervision and WellBeing

Jess Sainsbury ■ Tony Butterworth

## KEY POINTS

1. Clinical supervision can be practiced with value at any stage in the career of a registered nurse or midwife, to mitigate the pressures experienced by the professions.
2. Both HEIs and practice providers need to work collaboratively and innovatively to embed clinical supervision into the preregistration experience of nursing students and midwives.
3. Early career nurses (those in the first 5 years of independent practice) can be utilised to facilitate clinical supervision for students while simultaneously developing their own professional practice.
4. Organisations may wish to consider including clinical supervision as a component of their preceptorship programmes as a method of attracting applicants.
5. Mature learners at all stages in their careers may find it difficult to expose their practice to others, and therefore clinical supervisors must be sensitive to experience, self-esteem, and anxiety.

## Introduction

Clinical supervision is a formal process of professional support, reflection, and learning that contributes to individual development and support. Nurses and midwives work with people who are likely to be in physical and/or psychological pain. This creates demands and pressures on nurses that can be both testing and cumulative. Clinical supervision can offer support to new and experienced practitioners alike in their daily work.

Clinical supervision in psychological therapies is well established, but the emergence of clinical supervision for nurses and midwives began in earnest in the United Kingdom and Australia in the 1990s. The publication of a first textbook for nurses in 1992 (Butterworth & Faugier, 1992) was followed by a series of papers and surveys over the next 2 decades looking at the benefits of and difficulties in implementing clinical supervision. The UK Department of Health funded a national review of clinical supervision to try and determine its usefulness (Butterworth et al., 1996), and several textbooks and seemingly endless review papers have followed since then adding to the debate. Although embraced quickly by nurses in mental health settings, it was less widely adopted in general nursing care. Where there was reluctance to engage with clinical supervision, time, opportunity, and suitable expertise of the supervisors were frequently cited barriers.

The measurable evidence base as to the usefulness of outcomes of clinical supervision is growing constantly (Butterworth et al., 2008). Recent events relating to the work of nurses during the COVID-19 pandemic has underscored the need for support for all health professionals. There are strategies now in place across the United Kingdom to experience clinical supervision through the development of professional advocates who, as part of their role, have experienced an additional professional training development course that enables them to offer clinical supervision to the nurse and midwife workforce. The ambition of the PNA programme is to have 1 in 20 nurses qualified to offer clinical supervision by 2024 (Oxtoby, 2022). This policy push is likely to cement the place of clinical supervision within the professional practice of nurses and midwives in the United Kingdom.

Some of the reasons for a renewed interest in clinical supervision are explored in this chapter.

# What Does the Research Tell Us?

Significant and repeated research has been undertaken into clinical supervision globally for more than 20 years. There should now be sufficient confidence in its utility and usefulness in developing professional practice to see it in everyday use, particularly in the United Kingdom. If, as noted earlier, there is now UK government policy to develop clinical supervision and to evaluate its implementation, then we may proceed with greater confidence. Evaluation studies have reported on levels of engagement with clinical supervision processes as an educational and supportive intervention, the effects on patients and families, and any personal and organisational challenges. There are some unproductive debates often lamenting poor takeup, which offer no practical ideas as to how this might be improved. It is the view of the authors that there is now a renewed energy affecting the implementation of clinical supervision that will be realised through the work of nurse advocates and similar measures in other UK countries.

## SOME WORKING PRINCIPLES

In 2020, an expert group convened by the UK Florence Nightingale Foundation agreed to a list of working principles when nurses and midwives engage with clinical supervision (be it facilitating or receiving). These include the following:

1. Education providers should be introducing nursing and midwifery students to the experience of clinical supervision during their professional preparation and build expectation in them that they will continue thereafter into their everyday practice.
2. Clinical supervision should embrace elements that include restorative (supporting personal wellbeing), formative (assisting knowledge development), and normative (that which explores organisational accountability).
3. To sustain appropriate professional and cultural sensitivity, nurses and midwives should preferably receive their clinical supervision from other suitably registered health care professionals.
4. Nurses and midwives require regular clinical supervision to ensure the highest patient safety in their work.
5. Employers and educators should be aware that a supportive and sympathetic organisational culture is necessary for regular and purposeful clinical supervision.
6. It may be necessary to explain and demonstrate the value of clinical supervision to nonclinicians who may be unfamiliar with its processes and benefits.
7. It is important to differentiate between managerial oversight (performance related (e.g., appraisals)), educational assessment (competency related (e.g., clinical skill sign-off)) and clinical supervision; they are not the same.

The list is by no means complete but a good starting point when considering clinical supervision and its implementation.

# Clinical Supervision as a Key Component of the Curriculum

Despite the benefits of clinical supervision for the student population being identified by the UK Department of Health in the early 1990s, it remains an optional part of the preregistration (student) nurse education curriculum. Many nursing students believe that clinical supervision is a practice reserved for those in mental health settings, as this is where it has been more commonly practiced, aligning it to a field within the profession rather than the profession as a whole. This has led to disparity of not only access to, but understanding of, clinical supervision across the four UK nations.

The Nursing and Midwifery Council requires the basic format of nurse education programmes in the United Kingdom to take place 50% in practice and 50% in higher education institutions (HEIs), encouraging continuous self-reflection, promotion of reflection, contribution toward team reflection activities, and critical reflection on incidents within its standards of proficiency for registrants. With such a strong requirement of reflective practice within the proficiencies from the regulator and clear political support, why, nearly 30 years later, do preregistration education programmes not include clinical supervision teaching and practice?

But it is not solely the responsibility of the HEI to encourage the practice of clinical supervision within the student communities, as practice providers play a huge role in the educational experience of nursing students. In many clinical settings there are practice education teams who are responsible for the overall learning experiences of students. The scope of practice for these educators varies, but they are in a prime position to role model and facilitate clinical supervision for students on placement with them. This could be in the format of group supervision or when visiting clinical areas utilising other members of the clinical team.

It is worth considering who is best placed to take on the role of clinical supervisor, as some students may be comfortable with a direct member of the clinical team that they are on placement with, whereas other students may prefer an independent clinical supervisor. Students may wish to seek out clinical supervision following a particularly traumatic clinical experience or even simply a first-time experience, and the practice of clinical supervision will help them to process what has happened and identify what went well and areas for improvement. This empowers students to learn from their placement experiences and develop as practitioners in a psychologically safe space. In addition, allowing time for clinical supervision in the clinical environment encourages students to process and seek clarification in the work setting rather than taking it home.

It is not surprising that a common misunderstanding students experience with regard to clinical supervision is that they confuse educational competency sign-off with the critical reflection required in true clinical supervision. Nursing students are faced with a complex task of achieving their clinical competencies to the required standard of their regulatory body, all while orientating themselves to a new clinical environment on a regular basis, navigating local cultures and politics, and sometimes with additional academic work to complete simultaneously. Is it any surprise that nursing students themselves are not advocating for regular clinical supervision? Are they being overloaded, and is clinical supervision a solution to this?

# Clinical Supervision and the Early Career Nurse

The transition from nursing student to newly registered and early career nurse is well known to be a difficult experience. Not only due to the change in status from supernumerary learner (supernumerary means that students cannot be counted as part of the workforce when they are learning on placement in a clinical setting) to accountable registered professional, but also the awareness of simply how much there is yet to learn of the art and science of nursing.

Although not mandated, with the ongoing staffing crisis, an organisation running an exceptional preceptorship programme (a package of support and education during the transition to independent practice) is often a favourable deciding factor for newly registered nurses when confirming their first registered nursing position. Both authors would encourage those shaping preceptorship programmes to consider including teaching sessions regarding clinical supervision: education on what it is and is not, as well as advice for how to facilitate it.

Many early career nurses step forward to support nursing students as they are all too aware of the challenges students face throughout their nurse education, and while they may not immediately step into formal assessor roles, they are in an ideal position to become clinical supervisors for students. It is, however, important that the early career nurses themselves are aware of the differences between clinical supervision, educational competency sign-off, and managerial supervision.

There are a growing number of virtual support networks run by nursing students and early career nurses that demonstrate there is not only a need for peer support but a desire to facilitate it. While clinical supervision is much more advanced than a volunteer-run peer support network, should the profession not utilise this passion for supporting one another, and encourage and educate early career nurses to facilitate clinical supervision for others?

# Clinical Supervision and the Experienced Practitioner

The confident and experienced nurse and midwife may well find it difficult to expose their practice to others. They are likely to be mature learners and may well find the process of clinical supervision difficult to begin with. There is a great deal of literature on mature learners and approaches that can be taken to engage with them

## CHARACTERISTICS OF THE MATURE LEARNER

It is often stated that mature learners will need to know the what and the why of their learning. They will have already developed personal values and preconceptions that are important to them. In introducing clinical supervision, it is important to be challenging and yet sensitive to those personal values and preconceptions that the learner may hold dear.

Experienced practitioners are likely to have a definite and strong self-image in the work that they do. If adult learners believe that they are being respected, then they are likely to learn better. Conversely if they feel that their experiences are of little value, they will resist any attempts to their ways of working and sharing.

The positive contribution that life and extensive practice experience can bring to clinical supervision is important, and the effective supervisor should be able to use those experiences to good effect. It is often reported that mature learners will adapt and change best when they are not under time pressure.

## SIX PRINCIPLES OF ANDRAGOGY

Knowles (1984) is well known for his use of the term *andragogy*, which he uses to describe six characteristics of mature learners that can be applied to the process of clinical supervision. Some small case vignettes are offered here as examples.

1. **Need to know why they are being asked to learn.** In the context of clinical supervision this can be explained through the component parts of normative, formative, and restorative processes that might benefit their practice.
   *Case example:* A supervisee sees little point in the supervision session as she is worn out and sees no way to release the pressure on her working day. Engagement is critical here, and the supervisor will need sensitivity and care to explain the potential advantages offered by clinical supervision without suggesting it is a panacea for all ills!
2. **Mature learners come with experience.** The clinical supervisor should be able to tie those experiences to any new material or explanations of the processes involved.

*Case example:* In the context of a clinical supervision session the supervisee states that he has tried to make time in his day to offer learning opportunities for students, but the pressures on his practice are worsening, and any suggestions for supervision time are rebuffed by managers. The supervisor will be in something of a dilemma in this situation but might suggest approaching the partner university or encouraging the learner to do so instead.

3. **Self-concept.** Mature learners have a need for self-direction and often like to be responsible for their learning decisions.

   *Case example:* Mature learners, working in a European country, experience difficulty when trying to find clinical supervision as it is not common within their country. With encouragement from a group supervisor, they established an e-learning platform on which they support each other online. When unanswerable difficulties arise, they call on an external expert supervisor to give support and direction (Butterworth & Trifkovic, 2014).

4 and 5. **Readiness and Problem orientation.** Motivation increases in mature learners when there is an immediate problem to solve.

   *Case example:* Nurses caring for a group of people damaged by serious and enduring mental illness were told that the organisation wanted to introduce a model of early intervention and family-focused approach. They felt themselves to be unready for this and tested by the approach. Their clinical supervisor challenged their low expectations of patient recovery and how easily new interventions could be learned and become part of their practice (Bradshaw et al., 2007).

6. **Intrinsic motivation.** Intrinsic motivation (where motivation to act is driven by internal rewards) and feeling better about oneself is an important part of more positive learning. When experienced practitioners recognise a need to learn within themselves, they become an easy target for clinical supervision.

   *Case example:* In this situation the supervisor might find it easier to deal with as the intrinsic motivations are quite high. In circumstances such as seeking promotion or undertaking professional re-registration, engagement will be relatively easy but anxiety levels high. Using clinical supervision with mature and experienced practitioners carries some different responsibilities for the supervisor. Sensitivity to experience, self-esteem, and anxiety are clearly important issues for proficient practitioners.

## ACTIVITY

There are different models of clinical supervision. Research them and find out which you prefer. Having a supervision model as your framework will help guide your clinical supervision. Write it here with a brief explanation why you think this model would work best for you.

_____

_____

_____

_____

Now it is time to find yourself a clinical supervisor. List three qualities you would like in a clinical supervisor. Next, reach out to someone who you believe embodies these essential qualities.

   1.
   2.
   3.

Clinical Supervisor Name:

It may be helpful to keep a log of themes and topics discussed during clinical supervision. Use this space to do so.

_____

_____

_____

_____

_____

---

## CASE STUDY 14.1   Resilience-Based Clinical Supervision

In 2021, commissioned by Health Education England, the Foundation of Nursing Studies (FoNS) virtually facilitated a Resilience-Based Clinical Supervision (RBCS) programme for 24 nursing students in England to equip them with the skills to develop both personally and professionally and ultimately to improve recruitment and retention of nursing staff. The commitment from each nursing student was 14 hours, which included preparation, attendance at a virtual masterclass, reflection, and evaluation.

Treasure, a nursing student who participated in the programme, shared her reflections with the authors regarding the impact the programme has had on her. Treasure shared that despite being a mental health nursing student, she had not experienced clinical supervision before commencing the FoNS RBCS programme, only mindfulness training. The reason she applied to participate is she was hopeful the programme would have a positive impact on her practice and university experience.

Treasure described the period in which she participated in the RBCS programme as difficult due to the ongoing COVID-19 pandemic and the uncertainties about her education and training as a nursing student. Undeterred by this, she wanted to help not only herself but her peers with any skills she could learn because of undertaking the programme. She described the group as 'united online' despite their diverse backgrounds, universities, fields of nursing, and stages in nurse education. Topics discussed during the programme included experiences on placement but also personal issues. Treasure shared that the group helped one another during a time where they would otherwise feel isolated. She shared that as well as having a better theoretical knowledge, she felt that the RBCS programme opened her eyes to the practice of clinical supervision. It helped her immediately when on a clinical placement as she was not only able to practice clinical supervision but felt confident to request it from registrants when she needed it. Treasure pointed out that it is common for students to be rostered to work opposite shifts to one another, in an attempt to make access to learning experiences equitable; however, this results in students not receiving peer support. This is an additional reason, according to Treasure, why registrants in practice should offer students clinical supervision.

There was, however, a drawback to participating in the programme in that Treasure felt disappointed that registrants from her previous clinical placements had not offered her clinical supervision, particularly when she had faced complex clinical situations. She reflected that she would ensure that in the future when supporting students herself she would offer them clinical supervision.

Upon completion of the programme, Treasure believes that clinical supervision should be taught as part of the curriculum, and while nursing students are on clinical placements, they should be allocated protected time to participate in it meaningfully. The reason? She felt that it made her stronger, taught her to open up, and know her own limits—all to be a safe and competent health care professional.

JESS SAINSBURY   ■   TONY BUTTERWORTH   ■   GRACE COOK

---

## References

Bradshaw, T., Butterworth, T., & Mairs, H. (2007). Does workplace based clinical supervision during psychosocial education enhance outcomes for mental health nurses and the service users they work with? *Journal of Psychiatric and Mental Health Nursing, 14,* 4–12.

Butterworth, T., & Faugier, J. (1992). *Clinical supervision and mentorship in nursing.* London: Chapman and Hall.

Butterworth, T., & Trifkovic, K. (2014). *Slovenian students' experiences of clinical supervision using Facebook—innovation in action.* Foundation of Nursing Studies Open Access Library.

Butterworth, T., Bell, L., Jackson, C., & Pajnkihar, M. (2008). Wicked spell or magic bullet? A review of the clinical supervision literature 2001–2007. *Nurse Education Today, 28*(3), 264–272.

Butterworth, T., Bishop, V., Carson, J. (1996). First steps towards evaluating clinical supervision in nursing and health visiting. Theory, policy, and practice. A review. *Journal of Clinical Nursing, 5*(2), 127–132.

Knowles, M. (1984). *Andragogy in action.* San Francisco: Jossey-Bass.

Oxtoby, K. (2022). A new, powerful source of support. *Independent Nurse.* https://www.independentnurse.co.uk/professional-article/a-new-powerful-source-of-support/245915/.

## CHAPTER 15

# Developing Teamwork and Social Support Across Occupational Boundaries

Stefan Schilling ■ Maria Armaou

## KEY POINTS

1. Interprofessional (IP) teamwork directly impacts upon staff wellbeing and patient outcomes.
2. IP teamwork can be hindered by organisational structures and hierarchies and impacted by stereotypes about team members' abilities and skills.
3. IP teamwork benefits from frequent and open communication, inclusion of team members, clarity of roles, and a shared understanding of tasks.
4. Social support protects against negative mental health outcomes and aids in coping with job stressors and traumatic situations.
5. Socially supportive teams invest in frequent giving and asking for help to create a mutually supportive network.

## Introduction

This chapter will address teamwork and social support in teams, consisting of personnel from different occupational backgrounds, by examining some of the factors that make collaboration in such teams more difficult and providing examples of how teamwork and social connectedness can be nurtured and maintained. In today's health care environment, nurses and midwives are regularly asked to work alongside or in collaboration with other health care professionals. Interprofessional (IP) teams, where members of different health care professions work together to deliver care (e.g., mental health nurse, pharmacist, psychologist, physician), as well as multi- (or inter-) disciplinary teams, where members from different occupational pathways work together (e.g., midwife, neonatal nurse, children's nurse), are increasingly common. However, being part of such a team can often be daunting and fraught with challenges, especially without prior exposure to each other.

## What Is Teamwork and Why Is It So Important?

IP teamwork, defined as the combined, collaborative action of a group of people from different occupational backgrounds, has repeatedly been linked to positive patient outcomes, better team performance, and higher levels of staff wellbeing. For example, IP teamwork has been found to increase patient satisfaction and decrease mortality and readmission rates, length of inpatient stay, and clinical error rates (Courtenay et al., 2013). Integration of a wider skill mix into teams can also improve patient survival and cardiac arrest rates, and reduce adverse drug events

(Almost et al., 2016; Aufegger et al., 2019). Simultaneously, as team members bring different ideas, expertise, and skills to the table, such teams are found to be more efficient and innovative than teams from a single occupation and have beneficial effects on staff satisfaction, retention, and wellbeing (Morley & Cashell, 2017). Feeling connected to staff members and contributing to a common goal can also increase trust within a team and reduce stress and risks of burnout (Deneckere et al., 2013). However, despite these benefits, developing effective teamwork and supportive working environments is more difficult in IP and interdisciplinary teams as they tend to face a range of challenges that teams from a similar occupational background are not exposed to.

## Us and Them—Occupational Stereotypes and Professional Hierarchies

Unlike teams from similar backgrounds, IP team members often are unaware of the exact skills and abilities colleagues bring to the team and may demonstrate different procedures and ways of communicating. Lacking detailed knowledge about someone's actual professional competence, team members rely on common stereotypes about colleagues' occupational skills and the perceived benefit of their occupation to the wider team as a mental shortcut to evaluate ability. As such, when team members first meet they go through a short process of introducing each other to develop an idea of someone's skills, abilities, and trustworthiness. For example, it is assumed an oncology nurse is familiar with infection control, cytotoxic drugs, and intravenous lines.

While relying on stereotypes is a valuable and useful tool to quickly assess someone's perceived fit, stereotypes can also lead to confusion and misperceptions about someone's actual role and responsibilities especially when the knowledge about colleagues' ability is based on imperfect and unhelpful labels (e.g., 'Radiographers are more interested in algorithms than patients'). In fact, research has repeatedly shown that misperceptions of roles and responsibilities are some of the main reasons for conflict and negative patient outcomes in IP teams. While conflict in IP teams results in less incivilities or rude behaviour than in teams from similar backgrounds (Keller et al., 2020), such conflict increases the risk of division of the team into occupational identities, such as 'us nurses' versus 'those therapists.'

Retreat into such occupational identities or formal hierarchies all too often causes grievances and conflict in IP teams. For example, due to stereotypes about physicians as clinically superior, it is not uncommon for nurses and midwives—even those with years of experience—to defer to doctors' expertise and not share opinions during bedside rounds or handovers. Similarly, stereotypes about nurses and midwives as communal, social, and caring may run the risk of minimising their role as being responsible for dealing with emotional and psychosocial aspects of care. This neglects that, because of longer and more frequent exposure to patients, nurses can play a key role in the diagnostic process. Conversely, individual team members themselves may also cling on to stereotypes of their own occupation and thus insist on processes to be done in a particular way. This can undermine the development of a shared understanding of the team's tasks and responsibilities (technically referred to as shared mental models). Allowing personnel to feel they are, so to speak, on the same page, singing the same song, or contributing to a common goal is a crucial component of effective teamwork and a good working environment. Here are some valuable steps IP teams can do to increase teamwork.

- **Ask, do not assume. Emphasise the contribution of each team member to develop trust and collaboration.** As IP teams are amalgamated for their skill mix, it is important to make time for short introductions, asking people about their prior experiences to clarify roles and responsibilities and establish trust in their abilities. Be aware that team members often have subject-matter expertise beyond their occupational role, from which the team might benefit. The more information staff members have, the easier it is to go beyond occupational stereotypes and integrate a new team member into the team.

- **Get everyone on the same song sheet and develop a shared identity based on what the team has in common.** Creating a shared identity in IP teams relies mostly on a shared understanding of responsibilities, tasks, and goals. As such, previous occupational identities and their inherent stereotypes should as far as possible be deemphasised in favour of common teamwide purpose and tasks. Establishing such a shared identity based on the common goal requires the active integration of all team members into the process of developing it.

## Personalities and the Importance of Leadership

IP teams are usually assembled to cover a particular skill mix, but with different skills come different personalities, and personalities are at risk of clashing. While individual personalities (e.g., confidence, emotional intelligence, ability to reflect, or communication style) influence the working environment in any team (Almost et al., 2016), teams from different backgrounds are especially prone to disturbances and conflict due to more opportunities for misunderstandings. For one, IP colleagues have often different experiences and professional training. Some might have participated in interdisciplinary simulation training, others are more inclusive because they changed medical pathways, but many will not have had such opportunities. Personal or professional experiences can therefore not only influence how a colleague interprets certain team dynamics but also how they react to stressors in a team. As such IP personnel need to learn to bond and be more mindful of colleagues' background. Regular informal discussions to get to know each other, simulation training, and short rotations in different wards are ways to clarify job roles and expectations and to experience different ways of working. This is especially important for older or long-term members of staff who tend to be more settled and require a bit of shaking out of their comfort zone.

In such an environment team leaders and managers play a vital role in assigning roles and responsibilities, managing work expectations and resources and, most importantly, setting the tone for how team members are treated. Unfortunately, IP teams are often characterised by unclear leadership, which undermines a collaborative work environment. For example, team members may be expected to report to an IP team leader as well as their own occupational department leader. Simultaneously, leaders in IP teams, unlike in teams from the same background, seldom have professional expertise in every one of the team's various occupations, which, if not addressed, can hinder the development of trust and familiarity between team members. Collaborative or shared leadership styles, where leaders integrate and empower team members from different backgrounds, have been found to be useful in improving team performance, allowing for more inclusive working environments and better information exchange in IP teams. On the other hand, not listening to staff members' concerns, lack of fairness, not being inclusive of team members, or not working in the interest of one's team can make it difficult for IP teams to effectively work together. Here are some tips to address interpersonal problems and challenges to leadership.

- **Develop clear leadership structures.** It is important to set up clearly defined leadership structures within the team. Given that IP team leaders seldom have professional expertise in all the team's occupations, leaders are advised to deemphasise their own occupational identity and focus on the team's common goals, while treating staff fairly, developing standards collaboratively, and taking care of and mentoring their staff. If responsibilities are clearly assigned, IP teams may even benefit from shared leadership, utilising dual management structures between clinical and managerial leaders.
- **Practice collaborative leadership and empower team members.** Considering the skill mix in IP teams, it is useful to empower those with subject-matter expertise relevant to the team's tasks. Sometimes this merely requires flattening the hierarchy within the team, using inclusive language, and emphasising knowledge exchange; at other times it means creating a

space where individuals with a particular subject-matter expertise can take informal leadership roles. In any case, involving team members across the occupational spectrum will help them to feel included and valued.

- **Enhance IP exposure.** Staff members and leaders alike are often caught up in their own departmental bureaucracy and lack exposure to other departments. Exchange of leaders into a ward or department outside of their direct professional expertise not only benefits cross-departmental collaboration by familiarising them with different procedures and working environments, but it can also promote more empathic reactions to new colleagues by reminding personnel of how daunting it felt to start somewhere new.

## Setting the Scene—What the Organisation Can Do to Facilitate Teamwork

While many organisations value IP or interdisciplinary teamwork, facilitating teamwork requires planning and resources to ensure that staff members do not get sucked back into their previous hierarchies. As IP teams are embedded into complicated hospital structures, decisions about skill mix and team structure, where the team is located, or what their working hours will be, can have pivotal impact. For example, teamwork demands spaces in which team members can congregate for meetings or breaks. If IP team members are asked to fill out their patient reports in a separate location, it will inevitably result in feeling like they are not seen as an integral part of it. In the spirit of 'out of sight, out of mind', such team members are also more likely to be forgotten during handovers or informal chats. As much of the daily decisions about patient care occur in informal settings (i.e., quick chats in the corridor), dislocation can further inhibit information flow and reduce reaction times in urgent situations. In fact, in one of our recent studies, physiotherapists reported higher identification with IP colleagues and were more likely to aid in patient care responsibilities if they were in the same area as nurses and incorporated into the bedside rounds.

Similarly, wider organisational decisions, such as design of a staff rota without consideration of IP team members, can impact on teamwork and information exchange. As communication during handovers or during breaks is crucial to develop both a sense of shared contribution to medical decision making and familiarity between colleagues, it is important to take different working patterns and contracts into account. For example, medication rounds coinciding with bedside rounds or restricted work hours of staff members encumber information sharing and may make personnel feel excluded and not valued. Frequent staff turnover requires longer periods of getting to know each other and thus undermines the development of fluid work and communication processes visible in teams that are familiar with each other. Here are some organisational suggestions that can help alleviate the aforementioned pitfalls.

- **Increase opportunities for information exchange to increase shared understanding.** It is important to provide opportunities for formal and informal communication to increase shared understanding of tasks and responsibilities. For example, regular shared handovers, IP ward rounds, impromptu huddles—which encourage all members to participate and contribute—are good opportunities to develop shared understanding and strengthen communication and collaboration. Similarly, whiteboards, patient care checklists, goal sheets, scripts, and health records can improve role clarity and increase accountability.
- **Optimise provision of communal spaces and departmental layout.** In many hospitals providing communal spaces and time outside of direct patient contact (e.g., common break rooms or office space available for all IP staff) can be difficult to achieve due to limitations on estates or staffing; however, colocation of staff is a crucial factor in maintaining information exchange, team cohesion, and familiarity.

## BUILDING AND PRESERVING A SUPPORTIVE WORK CLIMATE

Effective teamwork and high levels of team cohesion not only impact on patient outcomes, but the feeling of personally making a valuable contribution to a common goal alongside like-minded people also has beneficial effects on increased life satisfaction and positive health outcomes by creating a socially supportive working environment. In the health care setting, social support—depending on both the recognition of a team as a socially supportive network and the actual reception of support from colleagues—has been repeatedly linked to job satisfaction and wellbeing, a reduction of conflict, and recovery from traumatic experiences (Aufegger et al., 2019). Furthermore, through formal debriefs and informal chats, team members can make sense of their experiences and take an active role in constructing and reconstructing collective experiences providing an important source of group-based interpretations of complex situations.

However, IP staff are often temporary and may face difficulties if divisions in the team increase social isolation and stress. In particular, junior personnel have less established social or family networks due to starting new positions or being on rotations and so rely more on collegial support than older staff members. Additionally, staff members may feel cut off, unable to reflect and share their experiences with people who 'have been there,' especially if the work in the subsequent role differed from the work in the IP team. Given that personnel in other IP contexts routinely report higher levels of negative mental health outcomes after leaving a team, it is important to support team members after they leave the team. The following tips highlight a few ways that can aid teams to stay connected.

- **Organise frequent team-bonding events to increase social support.** It is important to develop interpersonal ties with team members to develop a socially supportive network. Team-bonding events, such as a challenging training activity or a sports day, will require staff members to work together. Nothing breaks down the ice faster than overcoming a difficult situation as a team and then having social time to reminisce, get to know each other, and recognise each other as similar.
- **Encourage formal and nonformal debriefs to facilitate sensemaking.** Debriefs—be they informal or formal—allow staff to share their experience, create a sense of commonality and shared hardship, and assist in feeling socially supported by colleagues. Whilst after traumatic incidents a formal meeting (facilitated by a psychologist or a trained peer) can be beneficial, staff members often value more localised support: a shared space to retreat, debriefs, or time to decompress alongside colleagues.
- **Encourage giving and asking for social support.** Many staff members, especially in IP teams, are reluctant to ask for help or provide unsolicited support. Such support often starts with small gestures. Help with small tasks or checking up on staff can make a difference (e.g., asking how they are 'really' doing; helping with making beds or emptying a urinary drainage bag).

Teamwork is a crucial aspect of IP and interdisciplinary health care provision, with direct repercussions for patient outcomes and staff wellbeing. Social support provided by IP team members and leaders can provide important benefits for staff members and protect against job stressors and traumatic experiences. This chapter has addressed some of the main challenges for teamwork in IP teams, provided examples of how teamwork and trust can be developed, addressed the importance of social support in IP and interdisciplinary teams, and offered some examples to aid team members to stay connected and supportive.

1. Write down how you felt when you entered your first ward and what small gestures and behaviours from colleagues and leaders made you feel welcome and included in the team. Which of these behaviours can you apply in your team?
2. Reflect upon the skill sets colleagues from other teams bring to the table. If you only know their occupation, ask them about important experiences for them and special skills they have acquired. Use their experience when developing a joint vision for your team.

---

**CASE STUDY 15.1**  **An Interprofessional Community Response and Rehabilitation Team**

The Newcastle upon Tyne Hospitals Community Response and Rehabilitation Team (CRRT) is a citywide interprofessional (IP) service created to support admission avoidance and facilitate early discharge from hospital. The service has grown since its inception 10 years ago and now has a 68 full-time equivalent strong workforce. The team is comprised of the following:

1. Registered adult nurses
2. Physiotherapists
3. Occupational therapists
4. Podiatrists
5. Community psychiatric nurses
6. Care support staff and administrative support teams

The team is high performing and known locally and regionally for delivering high-quality patient care through IP. However, since the creation of the team there have been several challenges in achieving effective IP working, which have required focused and continued intervention.

Initially, there were challenges in developing team identity and cohesiveness. Attention was paid to recognising individual professional expertise as well as clinical and professional commonality and shared skills. This subsequently led to the development of core clinical processes and documentation so that in certain cases, any professional can be involved in certain parts of the patient assessment process. Clinical documentation is team documentation and not individual professional documentation. Visits to patients are undertaken jointly, which ensures problem solving is collaborative and naturally leads to IP handovers and clinical huddles (regular short discussions regarding the clinical caseload). This has helped the team develop a unified identify and shared purpose whilst still celebrating the uniqueness each profession brings to the patient journey.

To build and preserve the IP work climate and team identity, the team share clinical and rest space. Over the years this has led to the building of IP social networks past the traditional professional boundaries and has led to CRRT being seen as a cohesive team rather than a collection of different professional groups.

Whilst facilitating the need for IP working, it has been important to develop individuals within their own professional roles. Training and education are facilitated both for the IP team collectively and for independent professions. This approach balances the need for IP connectedness with the need to develop professional individuality, recognising that each profession brings a new perspective. This has supported the development of the team and prevented it becoming stagnant in its view.

There has been a consistent leadership presence throughout the 10 years with the leader coming from one of the professional groups. Line management and leadership responsibility is clear, and individual professions still have clear professional support outside of the team structure. It is recognised that having a clear leader has been important to foster team identity. The leader is seen as just that, a leader, rather than the professional group they come from.

Whilst several factors have been effective in supporting IP working in the CRRT, it is important to acknowledge that constant attention is required. In recent years, team stability has been challenged as new issues have arisen. More recently, working patterns and hours were reviewed and the different professions came with quite different professional norms and therefore different expectations. Whilst challenging, this was addressed but highlighted that inherent individual professional nuances may remain.

**IAN JOY**

## References

Almost, J., Wolff, A. C., Stewart–Pyne, A., McCormick, L. G., Strachan, D., & D'Souza, C. (2016). Managing and mitigating conflict in healthcare teams: An integrative review. *Journal of Advanced Nursing, 72*(7), 1490–1505. https://doi.org/10.1111/jan.12903.

Aufegger, L., Shariq, O., Bicknell, C., Ashrafian, H., & Darzi, A. (2019). Can shared leadership enhance clinical team management? A systematic review. *Leadership in Health Services (Bradford, England), 32*(2), 309–335. https://doi.org/10.1108/lhs-06-2018-0033.

Courtenay, M., Nancarrow, S., & Dawson, D. (2013). Interprofessional teamwork in the trauma setting: A scoping review. *Human Resources for Health, 11*(1), 57. https://doi.org/10.1186/1478-4491-11-57.

Deneckere, S., Euwema, M., Lodewijckx, C., Panella, M., Mutsvari, T., & Sermeus, W. (2013). Better interprofessional teamwork, higher level of organized care, and lower risk of burnout in acute health care teams using care pathways. *Medical Care, 51*(1), 99–107.

Keller, S., Yule, S., Zagarese, V., & Parker, S. H. (2020). Predictors and triggers of incivility within healthcare teams: A systematic review of the literature. *BMJ Open, 10*(6), e035471. https://doi.org/10.1136/bmjopen-2019-035471.

Morley, L., & Cashell, A. (2017). Collaboration in health care. *Journal of Medical Imaging and Radiation Sciences, 48*(2), 207–216. https://doi.org/10.1016/j.jmir.2017.02.071.

## CHAPTER 16

# Enhancing Health and WellBeing Through Shared Governance

Louise Bramley ■ Aquiline Chivinge

## KEY POINTS

1. Shared governance is also known as collective leadership, shared decision making, or professional decision making.
2. Nurses and midwives are a vital and valuable part of health care, and their voice should be represented in decision making in all health care settings.
3. Shared governance is designed to engage, empower, and unify those working in frontline roles, through to executive level individuals in a bid to improve the quality of care that patients and service users receive.
4. Shared governance is voluntary, inclusive, and can give new skills in project and change management, chairing meetings, presentations skills, networking, and sharing good practice.
5. Using shared governance as a framework to promote autonomy, contribution, and belonging at work can help nurses and midwives to flourish, ensure their wellbeing, and minimise their stress at work.

## Introduction

As a nurse or midwife, chances are that at one time or another you will have felt that you do not have a say in the decisions that are being made and that you are disconnected to senior leaders within your workplace. Nurses and midwives are a vital and valuable part of health care and exist at every level in every health care setting across the globe; yet, as a community, their voice, especially of those who work on the frontline, is often missing from debates and decision making. Recent work carried out by the Kings Fund in 2020 identified that autonomy, contribution, and belonging are the three core needs that must be met for nurses and midwives to flourish, ensure their wellbeing, and minimise their stress at work (West et al., 2020).

## What Is Shared Governance?

Shared governance, also known as collective leadership or shared/professional decision making, is a form of distributed leadership that is designed to engage, empower, and unify nurses and midwives, from those working in frontline roles through to executive level individuals in a bid to improve the quality of care that patients and service users receive. This chapter aims to describe how engaging staff in shared governance can help to establish a culture at an individual, clinical area, and organisational level that puts nurses and midwives at the heart of decision making and gives them the sense of autonomy, contribution, and belonging that is required to help them flourish, ensure wellbeing, and minimise stress at work.

Shared governance originated in the business and management literature as an antidote to the traditional top-down, hierarchical style of leadership. It focused more on the relationships that employees had with their leaders, working on the principle of happy staff, and emphasising that the success of business was down to the commitment and ownership of those who work in it. Shared governance made its way into the nursing literature in the United States in the late 1970s and early 1980s. Early adopters such as Drs Tim Porter-O'Grady and Robert Hess recognised that nurses' dissatisfaction was down to the institutions within which they worked as opposed to the profession itself and set about developing structures and processes that focused on culture change, thus empowering nurses to take greater ownership of decision making. They and others recognised that shared governance empowering nurses and developing their knowledge, skills, and commitment to continuous quality improvement had the potential to improve patient outcomes, promote longevity of employment, and increase nurse and patient satisfaction (Swihart & Hess, 2018). Although this initial work was done with nursing, it is also relevant and has been successful where midwifery services coexist alongside nursing.

## Making It Work in a Health Care Setting: The Principles of Shared Governance

Changing cultures, however, is not an easy task. Implementing shared governance in health care systems means a shift from traditional and well-established models of centralised decision making. In addition to this, health care systems are complex, traditionally bureaucratic in nature, and dependent on size may even have a variety of leadership styles operating within them.

When implementing shared governance, it is not a case of designing, implementing, and evaluating change via a project. Making a change of this magnitude requires senior leaders to recognise the benefits that a model of shared governance can bring to nurses and midwives as well as other professional groups within their organisations. Culture change takes time, resources, and commitment by individual teams and their leaders. It is also something that is an ongoing process, the starting point of which needs to include consultation and listening to what nurses and midwives need to help improve their health and wellbeing and help them flourish at work.

Starting with consultation sets the tone for shared governance and is the start of engaging with the four overarching principles of shared governance that emerged from Porter-O'Grady's (2009) work: partnership, equity, accountability, and ownership. It is important when beginning the process of implementation that nurses and midwives at all levels work in partnership and take accountability and ownership of the decisions to be made about which model (Table 16.1) of shared governance to adopt. This approach, promotes the development of a direct relationship and two-way communication with senior nursing and midwifery and other executive level health care leaders.

Most contemporary experiences of shared governance are aligned to the councilor model. Our own experience of this model of shared governance and distributed leadership has provided a framework/structure that enables shared leadership, with the main principle being that this makes nurses and midwives feel more empowered to make decisions about the care they deliver. This in turn has promoted a positive and innovation culture, where nurses and midwives feel like they can contribute and have greater job satisfaction. It is this element of shared governance that has promoted the health and wellbeing of our, not only at individual but also organisation levels (Quek et al., 2021).

## Shared Governance Promoting Autonomy, Contribution, and Belonging

Shared governance is voluntary and inclusive, and being part of council gives new skills in project and change management, chairing meetings, presentations skills, networking, and sharing good practice.

TABLE 16.1   **Models of Shared Governance**

| Model of Delivery | Key Feature |
| --- | --- |
| Councillor Model | The councillor model is the most common shared decision-making model for Shared Governance. Councils are founded at ward and specialty level, and these report into a coordinating council that oversees the structure and process of the councils. Within this model, the Chief Nurse/Director of Nursing/Midwifery can interact with frontline workers and engage in professional debate and decision making. It is also an opportunity for councils to share and celebrate their successes and debate and trouble shoot challenges. Depending on the size of the organisation there may be several localised coordinating councils that feed into an overarching council as well as several central councils that focus on areas of interest e.g. research and innovation. |
| Congressional Model | One of the first founded models, the congressional model features an elected staff senate, with a chair working alongside staff from the frontline and leaders from across the organisation. Committees are then formed around areas of strategic importance and report back to the senate. |
| Administration Model | The administrative model follows the more traditional organisation leadership and management structures and for that reason, it is rarely used in contemporary shared governance. |

One of the elements of shared governance is to bring together groups of nurses and midwives with a commonality to work together to bring change that impacts on patient care and staff experience and wellbeing. Shared governance celebrates good practice, and councils decide on an area of importance to invest their time in. Being part of a shared governance culture can have an impact on nurses' and midwives' wellbeing by being part of a council, but it also extends beyond this and often results in launching initiatives where the need is greatest to support staff wellbeing. Examples of this have been around supporting shielding staff during the COVID-19 pandemic and increasing staff morale with reward and recognition initiatives and campaigns to promote capital investment in rest areas, mindfulness initiatives and ensuing colleagues take breaks and stay hydrated.

Shared governance is a structure that facilitates the process of shared decision making and promotes the principles of distributed leadership and shared accountability. It embodies many compassionate leadership elements that are promoted as being essential to ensure wellbeing and motivation at work. This in turn can create a sense of belonging and minimise workplace stress that is described in the Kings Fund report (West et al., 2020). The focus on equity as one of its core principles encourages and supports staff to contribute within the scope of their practice as part of the team. Shared governance promotes inclusion of different cultures, and its focus is on the largest frontline staff group within organisations. It does not discriminate and encourages a learning environment that includes diversity of learners, and where this is lacking, encourages and empowers nurses and midwives to take action to address it (Case Study 16.1).

Although in the first instance shared governance is often focused on nursing and midwifery, engaging wider with the multidisciplinary teams at council level is pivotal to its success. This often means that nurses and midwives are collaborating with wider members of the health care team (e.g., strategy leads, finance colleagues, data analysts and other healthcare professionals). Engaging and establishing partnerships with the patients and public is also encouraged and central to its success.

Internationally, many health care organisations have adopted distributed leadership models. The chances are that if you already work in an organisation that has adopted shared governance, you will hear about it, and there will be evidence around the organisation that it is part of the culture of decision making for nurses and midwives. Students are often encouraged to be involved, too, so you may already be aware if you have been on placement in an area that has a council. If you are new to an area, look around and have a look on the website as there are often displays and information as to how you can get involved. You could also ask your manager, the clinical educator, or the senior nursing and midwifery leaders where you work. Shared governance promotes leadership at all levels and encourages all nurses and midwives to see themselves as leaders. If you work somewhere that it does not exist yet, then maybe your questions will prompt leaders to act.

This chapter considers shared governance as a culture within which nurses and midwives can feel empowered and contribute to decision making within their organisations. It demonstrates that feeling empowered can create a greater sense of and promote health and wellbeing at both individual and organisational levels. Our experience has produced many examples that show shared governance can offer a framework that promotes being part of an innovative and positive culture. It is this aspect that can lead to greater job satisfaction and encourage much needed and highly skilled nurses and midwives to be retained within the profession.

## ACTIVITY

1. Consider the leadership styles within your current work environment. How do these impact on your health and wellbeing at work?
2. Consider the principles of shared governance (accountability, equity, partnership, and ownership). How would they fit within your organisation?

## CASE STUDY 16.1   Black Asian Minority Ethnic Shared Governance Council at Nottingham University Hospitals NHS Trust

The Black Asian Minority Ethnic (BAME) Shared Governance Council was formed in April 2018 in response to staff feedback about lack of career progression and development and a low representation of ethnic minority nurses at ward and specialty council level within my organisation (Chivinge et al., 2021). The council was designed to promote engagement, promote the equality and diversity agenda within the organisation, give a safe space to explore areas of dissatisfaction, promote autonomy, and listen and act on ethnic minority patient and staff feedback. This work has played an important part in supporting ethnic minority staff wellbeing as well as in my personal life. I joined the BAME Shared Governance Council and volunteered to become the vice chair. Although I needed to learn and build on some skills, I was relaxed as I was amongst friends. Since then, shared governance has been very pivotal in my career, and I am a true example of how shared governance can empower staff.

Before joining the council I was on the verge of leaving the nursing profession. However, shared governance turned my negative experiences into opportunities for growth. It has also redirected my career and has seen me progress to chair of the BAME Council and gain a permanent post within the shared governance team as clinical educator. More recently I have been successful in gaining a promotion to practice development lead (leadership), and I have enrolled in the Professional Nursing Advocate training to continue to support colleagues' health and wellbeing across the Trust. With constant practice I now feel confident speaking and teaching at big events. There was support from inspirational colleagues, the chief nurse, the shared governance educators, and the senior nurses within my organisation. Shared governance also gave me the opportunity to become a staff nurse representative at the highest nursing and midwifery decision-making board within the organisation.

We have also made great progress with patient initiatives. These include ensuring that the food we serve in hospital takes account of the diversity of the patient population and holding events in the community to promote and offer services such as breast screening, career advice, dementia awareness, smoking cessation, nutrition, cervical screening, and research participation. From the feedback we have received so far, the community members have started attending their breast screening and cervical screening appointments and are now encouraging others to attend their appointments and participate in research. Although there is still some way to go, at organisational level, we now have greater representation of ethnic minority staff on our councils, the number of senior leaders from diverse backgrounds is growing, and we have success at local and national fellowships especially with clinical academic careers.

The ultimate aim is to dissolve the council once integration and representation is achieved to the level that is representative of the population we represent.

ONYINYE ENWEZOR

## References

Chivinge, A., Enwezor, O., Haines, S., & Cooper, J. (2021). Setting up a Black, Asian and minority ethnic (BAME) shared-governance council in an acute hospital trust. *Nursing Times, 117*(7), 18–22.

Porter-O'Grady, T. (2009). *Interdisciplinary shared governance: Integrating practice, transforming health care.* Jones & Bartlett Learning.

Quek, S. J., Thomson, L., Houghton, R., Bramley, L., Davis, S., & Cooper, J. (2021). Distributed leadership as a predictor of employee engagement, job satisfaction and turnover intention in UK nursing staff. *Journal of Nursing Management, 29*(6), 1544–1553.

Swihart, D., & Hess, R. (2018). *Shared governance: A practical approach to reshaping professional nursing practice.* HCPro Inc.

West, M., Bailey, S., & Williams, E. (2020). *The courage of compassion supporting nurses and midwives to deliver high-quality care.* Kings Fund.

## CHAPTER 17

# Acknowledging the Emotional and Social Challenges of Nursing and Midwifery Through Schwartz Rounds

Aggie Rice

## KEY POINTS

1. For you to provide compassionate care for your patients, you must feel cared for and offered compassion, too.
2. Schwartz Rounds are a way for organisations to provide compassionate care to staff by offering a space for you to share experiences of the emotional impact of your work.
3. Being able to attend Rounds may help you to feel less stressed, less isolated, and more connected to your colleagues and your organisation.
4. Though not intended to change practice, the Rounds can shift the culture in your health care organisations to one that is more open and more connected.
5. It may be difficult for you to find time to attend Rounds, but support from senior colleagues to rota space in, or the use of innovations such as Pop-Up Rounds and Team Time, will lead to easier-to-access spaces for reflection.

## Introduction

The community nurse tells her story on the theme of 'a day in the life of…'. In a moving account of the emotional impact of doing her home visits, she talks of the anguish, helplessness, sadness, and guilt she feels when entering and leaving houses of her often isolated and lonely patients. Describing how hard it is knowing that she is likely to be the only person to have talked with these patients for days, she encounters conflict in wanting to stay and provide that compassionate company they crave. She knows that every moment the clock is ticking faster, and she is getting later and later for her next appointment. With care and generosity she tells of the cumulative impact of these home visits and the guilt she feels when she comes in running late for her afternoon clinic, knowing that the receptionist has been fielding angry patients and getting frustrated and distressed herself.

Her colleagues, in particular the receptionist, are in the Schwartz Round hearing this story, and for the first time they have gained insight into what it is really like for the community nurse in her work. The receptionist speaks of feeling moved and ashamed of her own stress and anger each time the nurse reenters the clinic. She wants now to be more patient and understanding and to greet the nurse, not with paperwork and frustration, but instead with space to breathe.

In my role as a Schwartz Round facilitator, mentor, and trainer with the Point of Care Foundation in the United Kingdom, I have heard hundreds of stories from nurses and midwives.

Stories of hurt, pride, anguish, and guilt; stories of joy, stress, and love; and stories of both hope-lessness and hope. Stories that would mostly otherwise have gone untold.

Schwartz Rounds carve that necessary space in which, amidst a pressurised and stretched sys-tem, to share and listen to these stories centred on the emotional impact of working in health care.

## What Are Schwartz Rounds?

Schwartz Rounds (Rounds) can offer a structured space for staff to come together regularly to discuss the emotional and social aspects of their work. The purpose is not to problem-solve or to learn how to be or do things better; instead, it is to provide space and time to come together and to share stories about the emotional impact of work. Rounds provide a chance for nurses, midwives, and other care staff to change pace, slow down, and together create connection, understanding, and insight into each other's roles and daily world. The underlying premise is that compassion shown by staff makes all the difference to a patient's experience; yet, to do that, staff must also feel supported in their work.

Schwartz Rounds originated in Boston, Massachusetts (United States), following the death of Health Attorney Kenneth Schwartz. During his time in hospital, he wrote extensively on his experience of care. What he was most struck by in those final months, was not the excellent medi-cal care he experienced and observed but the small acts of kindness from his caregivers that 'made the unbearable bearable' (Schwartz, 2012). He also noted, however, that there were times when it became impossible for staff to offer these, either through fatigue or through working under pres-sure in a system with scarce time or capacity. Schwartz wanted to create space within health care institutions where staff, in being asked to provide compassionate care to patients, were at the same time offered compassion and humanity themselves.

Rounds are intended to run on a routine, regular monthly basis, not as a response to significant events or corporate agendas. Often they are based on a particular theme, for example: 'Being thrown in at the deep end', 'A patient I will never forget', 'The day I nearly walked out', or 'When a thank-you goes a long way'. The model is unchanging each time; this ensures the psychological safety of the space (meaning that those involved feel free to speak up and share their story). In recent years, adjusted versions of Rounds (Team Time and Pop-Up Rounds) (see Case Study 17.2) have emerged to ensure frontline staff, particularly nurses, are able to attend this form of reflective practice.

## Why Are They Needed?

Providing compassionate care can take its toll. In their book *Intelligent Kindness*, Ballatt and Campling (2011) explore the conflict between kindness and compassion, and self-preservation. They draw words from Czech writer Milan Kundera on the conflict of compassion: 'There is nothing heavier than compassion. Not even one's own pain weighs so heavy as the pain one feels for someone [else] … pain intensified by the imagination and prolonged by a hundred echoes.' In caring for patients, nurses and midwives are constantly having to establish 'the necessary balance of kindness and professional detachment, to perform the most intimate tasks imaginable' (Ballatt & Campling, 2011, p. 54). It often becomes another thing to have to get right: to somehow know instinctively, every time, where that line is drawn between caring compassionately and retaining a sense of professional detachment. Certainly the ability to provide compassionate care and to understand the form it may take is impossible when there is no compassionate care offered to staff.

Schwartz Rounds are intended as one way to try and make sense of this. To be able to reflect on and understand experiences of providing often painful care, Ballatt and Campling (2011) note that as caregivers 'the struggle of feelings of helplessness and hopelessness in the face of suffering cannot be avoided' (p. 54). While they cannot be avoided, at the very least they can be discussed, shared, and ultimately normalised and validated.

Rounds provide the space to tell stories that may otherwise go untold and offer a chance to make sense of and reframe experience as the stories are heard and validated by others. They shift from feelings of failure to a recognition that the best was done in difficult circumstances.

Storytelling can be a powerful experience for all staff but particularly impactful for nursing and midwifery staff who often feel unheard. Feeling that expertise goes unacknowledged and carrying the burden of responsibility without any of the power means many end up 'voting with their feet'. One midwife mentioned that feelings of frustration, powerlessness over decision making, and changes in practice may be leading many to leave; ironically, this is the only way in which they feel heard. Storytelling in Rounds therefore enables this space to be heard and provides the chance to own the narrative in a way that is difficult to achieve elsewhere. It also leads to a shift in culture to one that is more open, that recognises the inherent uncertainty in the provision of care, and that values and legitimises this vulnerability and uncertainty; it reveals something of the person behind the professional.

It is not a surprise that during the COVID-19 pandemic I have heard many stories from nurses about moral injury, from having to act or make decisions in ways that conflict with their values. One that stands out is the hospice nurse who described the painful conflict of having to prevent distressed and frustrated family members from seeing a dying relative to keep within the COVID-19 infection control requirements. In Rounds, as one attendee has put it, 'I think you realise more and more that there is no true right and wrong' (Maben et al., 2018). What Rounds offer, in the telling and hearing of stories of moral injury, is the space to reflect on and to reframe the experience. Feelings of shame, guilt, and disgust emerge as human in those uncertain and chaotic situations that may be entirely beyond the control of individuals.

## How Can They Help?

The Rounds process provides the opportunity to begin to see the person behind the professional, for hierarchies to be flattened, and silos to be dismantled. Staff begin to feel less isolated, knowing their reactions to their work are normal and shared. A sense emerges of solidarity and of us 'all being in this together, regardless of seniority, length of time in role or professional status' (Maben et al., 2018). In the often-tribal environment of health care, staff members can understand more deeply the world each other occupies and why they do the things they do.

There is a substantial evidence base for the effectiveness of the Rounds as a support for staff. A recent evaluation showed people who attend Rounds regularly experience significantly less psychological distress than their peers who do not attend regularly. They describe improved teamwork, a reduction of feelings of stress and isolation, and increased empathy and compassion for patients, colleagues, and (crucially) themselves (Maben et al., 2018). Rounds should never therefore be seen as a forum to solve specific problems or change practice, but stories of small but significant shifts in culture and behaviours are often the result. Rounds have the power to shift culture toward being more open and compassionate. In creating this space where staff can come together to share and listen to stories, they begin to see, rather than badges and professional roles, the human within each other.

## How Can They Be Accessed?

As nurses and midwives, particularly newly qualified, you may experience some challenge in accessing Schwartz Rounds. Being able to manage your own time in unpredictable, fast-paced shift work, alongside staff shortages and an overstretched workforce, may make it difficult to attend. Being aware of the space and encouraging more senior staff to allow junior staff access can help. Many Trusts have created innovative mechanisms to ensure that Rounds remain, in practice as well as theory, as accessible as possible—particularly to those, like you, as newly qualified nurses, and midwives, who may need this space the most.

Rounds and the role of storytelling within them are successful when they become a routine practice of an organisation, where everyone's story—from the chief executive officer to the most junior member of staff—can be heard. It is often the case that a widely held culture of openness and compassion develops. Within this culture of openness and compassion it becomes easier for newly qualified staff to allow for uncertainty, to disclose mistakes, and to connect to senior, perhaps more intimidating, colleagues. Senior staff within Rounds, in disclosing stories of fallibility and vulnerability, likewise benefit from beginning to appear more approachable and more human. Attending Rounds may be able to help you, as newly qualified staff, feel more connected to colleagues and to your own values, and to why you came into this work in the first place.

**ACTIVITY**

1. Does your organisation run Schwartz Rounds? We can help you find out and get connected to the team there. You may want to join the Schwartz Round steering groups or offer to tell your story in a Round. What story might you tell?
2. If your organisation does not run Schwartz Rounds, get in touch with us, The Point of Care Foundation, for more information and help in getting started.

**CASE STUDY 17.1** | **Basildon and Thurrock University Hospitals NHS Foundation Trust (BTUHFT): Staff Shortages Schwartz Round**

A senior nurse, a senior member of the finance team, a junior doctor, and a recruitment lead tell their stories of the emotional impact of staff shortages from their own perspective.

The senior nurse describes her feeling of dread walking round the wards and the pervading sense of failure she feels in not providing the resources for her staff who are 'running ragged' to meet the needs of their patients. She talks of her sleepless nights haunted by the images of the faces of her team. And reflects that 'this was not why I came into nursing.'

She then passes on to the senior finance member who begins his story by remarking, 'I never realised how much you took this home with you' to the nurse. He goes on to talk about why he came to work for the National Health Service (NHS): because of the values it holds and so he can help clinical colleagues to deliver the best care for patients. He reflects on the worry he and his colleagues have over what they ask of staff and the relentless pressure they are under. He exclaims it has become too much and announces his last day at the hospital. For the first time in his career, he has thought about leaving the NHS. Tears roll down his cheeks. He hands over to the junior doctor who describes a demanding shift where she is beholden to a relentlessly buzzing bleep. She shares feelings of frustration and irritation as patients shout at her or 'tut' in earshot. She describes feeling alone and out of her depth. Onto the final storyteller, the recruitment lead, who begins to tell her story through tears. She describes the difficulties of her work in the current climate of national shortages and Brexit. Watching what her clinical colleagues are facing drives her and her team to work late into the evening and on weekends to recruit. She ends her story on a note of optimism and pride in wanting to show new staff the joys of working in the organisation and to welcome them in. The participants begin their responses, and the emotions move from sadness to anger to compassion to a sense of pride. Pride in the fact that the organisation is filled with people who are committed to finding ways to deliver the best services they can in difficult circumstances. And through support and understanding of each other, feel more hopeful, resilient, and optimistic.

**REBECCA MYERS, BTUHFT SCHWARTZ TEAM AND AGGIE RICE**

| CASE STUDY 17.2 | **Ashford and St. Peter's Pop Up Rounds** |

While Rounds were proving popular and impactful, the Schwartz team were mindful that there were often staff who were unable to attend Rounds. They noticed that while specialist nurses, clinical staff with lunch breaks, nonclinical staff, and allied health professionals were often present, other staff groups at the Trust, who would benefit hugely, were underrepresented. So, the team decided to take the Rounds on tour; that is, bring the Rounds to them instead. A new, additional form of Rounds to target staff who were underrepresented was created. Nurses and midwives who attended Pop-up Rounds remarked that 'the Round helped me understand and accept what is happening a little better', and 'the discussion helped me deal with my emotions.' Pop-up Rounds offered a space to give a voice to staff who find it difficult to get away, staff who work on busy wards, emergency departments, and operating theatres in particular.

This case example was inspired by Harriet Barker, Farhana Nargis, and the Ashford and St. Peter's team.

**AGGIE RICE**

### References

Ballatt, J., & Campling, P. (2011). *Intelligent Kindness Reforming the Culture of Healthcare.* UK: RCPsych Publications.

Maben, J., Taylor, C., Dawson, J., et al. (2018). A realist informed mixed methods evaluation of Schwartz Centre Rounds in England. *Health Services and Delivery Research*, 6(37).

Schwartz, K. (2012). A patient's story. *The Boston Globe.* https://www.bostonglobe.com/magazine/1995/07/16/patient-story/q8ihHg8LfyinPA25Tg5JRN/story.html.

## CHAPTER 18

# Supporting Distressed Colleagues Using Psychological First Aid

Kerry Sheldon ■ Emma Coyne

## KEY POINTS

1. Psychological first aid (PFA) is first aid for emotions.
2. PFA gives structure to peer-to-peer supportive conversations.
3. Learning to listen is an important part of PFA.
4. Colleagues are more likely to recover from distressing work events when they feel safe, connected to others, calm, and hopeful, plus when they have access to social, physical, and emotional support.
5. To provide PFA, learning to care for yourself is a priority.

## Introduction

This chapter covers what is meant by psychological first aid (PFA) and how it can operate as a mechanism for the peer-to-peer support of health care colleagues during or after an adverse event. It details the skills of paying attention to reactions, normalising distress, addressing basic needs, reintroducing safety and hope, consoling, promoting healthy coping, and signposting to further services. First coined at the end of World War II, PFA has a long history and is now the globally recommended training and guidance for supporting people during and in the aftermath of emergencies, natural disasters, and pandemics (Blake et al., 2021; Wang et al, 2021; World Health Organisation [WHO] et al., 2011). So, what, if any, relevance does it have for health care workers such as nurses, midwives, porters, doctors, surgeons or receptionists? Health care workers face stressful, traumatic or difficult work situations every day, and therefore we see PFA acting as a potential buffer against the negative psychological impact of daily occupational stresses. Training health care workers in PFA has the potential to enable employees to develop their skills and confidence in providing immediate support to their colleagues following any stressful event(s) at work and is a useful adjunct to supporting the wellbeing of health care employees.

### WHAT DO WE MEAN BY PFA?

There is no universally accepted definition of PFA, but in a nutshell think of it as first aid for someone's emotions or a useful first thing you might do with a distressed colleague immediately following a highly stressful event or even a few days or weeks after (Australian Psychological Society [APS] & Australian Red Cross [ARC], 2013). It is caring, listening and showing empathy. Empathy (unlike sympathy) requires taking a moment to step outside of our normal patterns of thinking and feeling to imagine what it feels like to be the colleague in front of us and using this knowledge to guide how we support them. Moreover, despite being mental health professionals, we do not believe PFA is something that only mental health professionals do, because it is not psychotherapy nor is it labelling or diagnosing a colleague with a mental health condition. That is because most of us do not develop serious mental health issues after a stressful event but recover well with some simple support (APS & ARC, 2013), such as PFA, especially when that support is offered by a kind, attentive colleague who helps us feel safe, connected, and calm, and, if required, helps us to access advanced support.

Our experience is that most health care employees have the potential skill set to offer PFA, but they require training or guidance through the process. We have been delivering group training on PFA (adapted from National Health Service (NHS) Education Scotland, 2020) to all clinical and nonclinical hospital staff via remote platforms since early 2020, and more recently face-to-face training with more advanced skill workshops. Anecdotal feedback from hospital staff concurs with early research, which suggests that PFA is relevant and useful and that its simplicity can facilitate wellbeing conversations (Blake et al., 2021). The model outlines a format of seven core components (Fig. 18.1). The use of the word *model* suggests rigid application (i.e., start at point 1 and end at point 7). Instead, see the model more like a toolbox containing helpful actions to potentially adopt when supporting a distressed colleague. You may use two with one person and all seven with another, depending on need/circumstances. These actions, we believe, are transferable to any job role as well as in our home lives. So next we describe what these core PFA components might look like in action and what someone trained in PFA skills might do.

## Educate About Normal Responses

When any of us endures a serious stressor there is the potential to experience a wide range of reactions. You may recognise some in yourself, as follows:

- *Physical effects:* numbness, fatigue/sleep difficulties, increased heartbeat, nausea, lightheadedness, headaches, stomach complaints, sweating, shaking, shortness of breath, easily startled, decreased/increased appetite or sex drive
- *Feelings:* rage, anger, frustration, irritability, anxiety, uncertainty, fear, terror, guilt, sadness, relief, hopelessness, helplessness, frustration, disinterest, resentment
- *Thoughts:* self-blame, questioning own/other's competence, difficulty making decisions and comprehending complex information, lowered attention span, forgetfulness, confusion, intrusive thoughts, memories and flashbacks, distortion to sense of time, changes in spiritual/faith beliefs
- *Behaviour:* crying spells, angry outbursts, withdrawal and avoidance of people/places/tasks, increased risk taking, changes in work functioning, or inattention to self-care

The attributes of the stressful event and our personal characteristics may also influence our distress responses (WHO et al., 2011). For example, we may find a work situation more intense or frightening when:

- It is unexpected (e.g., the suicide of a colleague).
- There is no opportunity for us to prepare or we do not have the necessary training to deal with the situation.
- It happens on a night shift.
- It is ongoing (e.g., a pandemic or repeated staff shortages).
- It involves children, serious injury, death, or the loss of our working infrastructure such as a hospital fire.

Our personal characteristics and our experience of the event may also influence our individual stress responses or vulnerability. For instance, we may feel more upset if:

- We are closer to a stressful event (e.g., we were the responding paramedic to a child's death).

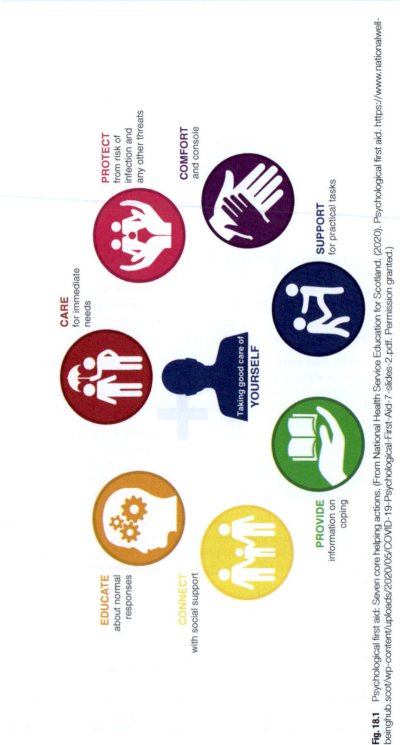

**Fig. 18.1** Psychological first aid: Seven core helping actions. (From National Health Service Education for Scotland. (2020). Psychological first aid. https://www.nationalwell-beinghub.scot/wp-content/uploads/2020/05/COVID-19-Psychological-First-Aid-7-slides-2.pdf. Permission granted.)

- There was a delay in receiving appropriate support, such as no-one asking us how we are until the following week.
- Our pre-crisis stress levels are already high due to personal circumstances such as financial difficulty, divorce proceedings, bereavement, or health conditions.
- Our connectedness with others is limited in some way (e.g., our family members live abroad and thus we rarely see them, we are new to the team/redeployed, there is existing conflict with supervisors/colleagues).

Key here is that reactions like those mentioned are natural human responses to scary and unpredictable threats and events. They are adaptive; they protect us, warn us. There is no right or wrong way to respond. The way we respond is not an indication of a failure in us or that we are not capable or are not up to the job.

One phrase that really helps us in delivering this core component of PFA is the aim to 'normalise worry, fear, and other emotions.' We often say to colleagues not to underestimate the importance of validating (i.e., confirming or authenticating) and naming another person's reactions. So, consider how would you normalise a colleague's feelings/thoughts to a stressful event. How would you prefer your emotions to be validated? There are countless ways, but here are just some examples heard in practice:

'Yes, that would be confusing.'

'In this situation, your reaction is quite natural.'

'It's okay to feel scared; I'd feel scared, too.'

'It makes sense that you think....'

'When you go home don't be surprised if you suddenly start crying.'

'Would it be helpful to know that it's not unusual to feel...when...?'

Sound easy? You will be surprised at the difference it makes.

## Care for Immediate Needs

Healthcare work is a physically and emotionally demanding profession. Shift work, long working hours, and a lack of rest breaks, all exacerbated by low staffing levels, can make it extremely challenging for colleagues to self-care. During a crisis, colleagues may further neglect their basic needs as distress can impair attention and decision-making abilities. So when supporting a colleague offer, direct them to, or encourage rest (e.g., sitting down, sleep, compensatory break), rehydration (e.g., drink), and refueling (e.g., food). Pay attention to their safety and security by allowing them to deal with any health concerns they may have, to take any necessary medication, or support them to meet any protection needs, such as torn protective equipment might need replacing. Importantly before providing support ask yourself if you can be there safely and without harming others; if not, can you support and communicate from a safe distance? Do not be afraid to seek emergency and/or medical assistance if necessary.

## Protect From Further Threat and Distress

We know across cultures that strong reactions can continue even when the crisis has passed. Equally when safety is reintroduced distress gradually reduces over time (APS & ARC, 2013). Creating safety for our colleague means communicating to their brain's fight-or-flight system that the stressful situation is over. How might we achieve this safety? Consider the following:

- Can you take your colleague away from or reduce exposure to the crisis, including the sights, sounds, smells, and other reminders? Is there a quiet, safe, private place for you both to talk undisturbed? Maybe even be a short walk outside?
- You may need to repeat information, ensure it is simple and accurate and whether it needs to be written (e.g., card with a listening helpline number on it) and verbal.

- We can be reassured by the presence of another, so be mindful if you are leaving your colleague alone. Stay with or close by until the person's reactions pass or try to ensure the person has someone kind nearby to help if you need to leave.
- Remind persons that they are safe and the danger has passed if that is the case.
- Try some grounding techniques (International Federation of Red Cross and Red Crescent Societies, 2019) by asking the colleague to describe all the things that are different now compared to the time of the stressor; you might say, 'Describe five things you can see around the room.'

Misinformation and rumours can intensify distress so only say what you know; if you do not know an answer it is okay to say so, but try saying, 'We can find some answers together.' Given the intensity of health care work, we can be caught off guard and unaware of how we are relating to our colleagues. Frustrations rise and we can be impolite without meaning to be. If you find you have said something you wish you had not, then apologise. You might express your apology using statements like the following:

'I'm sorry I didn't let you finish what you were saying.'

'I'm sorry if I hurt your feelings.'

## COMFORT AND CONSOLE

You do not have to wait for your colleague to approach you if you see this person is distressed; simply state, 'You seem upset. May I help?'

Such persons may want to tell their story, or they may not. If they appear to not want to connect with you, then accept that and do not pressure them to describe what happened. This is different from psychological debriefing, where you directly encourage a survivor to talk about and analyse the experience. If possible, make yourself available so they can connect with you later: 'I can see that maybe now is not the time to talk about how you feel but when you are ready my door is always open.'

Sometimes being physically present can be comfort enough: 'I can see how difficult it has been for you; I can sit here with you quietly until you feel able to carry on.'

For those who do wish to talk, active listening can be a great support. This means making a conscious effort to hear not only the words that your colleague is saying but, more importantly, the message that is being communicated. Most of us when we are upset want an active listener before being offered advice and resources, but proper listening takes time, concentration, and practice! So, consider Table 18.1, which illustrates both helpful and less helpful approaches to listening.

## Support for Practical Tasks

There may come a point in your conversation where you believe that your colleague needs practical suggestions or information about or links to other avenues of support. Depending on the origin of the distress, signposting made be necessary to services within and outside your place of work. It can be challenging to signpost a colleague to services, so think of it as facilitating access. Let us give you some examples:

'If I provide a list of available support, shall we look at it together?'

'You can read it in your own time, and we can review in a couple of days.'

'Shall we look through this website and see whether anything looks helpful for you at the moment?'

'Is there anything I can do to help you make that phone call to the listening service/your GP, etc?'

TABLE 18.1    **Listening Is an Action**

| What Might Help | What Might Not Help |
|---|---|
| Gentle eye contact, calm tone of voice, politeness, patience<br>Sitting at a slight angle same eye level<br>'Mm,' 'Yes,' nods<br>Minimise distractions | Staring, head down, standing over someone<br>Checking emails/answering phone/looking around<br>Touching the person (e.g., hugging) without asking first |
| Asking...<br>'Tell me a bit about what upsets you.'<br>'It looks as if you have something on your mind.' | Assuming...<br>'I know exactly how you feel. It happened to me last week.' |
| Providing space...<br>Resist the urge to fill silences; slow down. They might need courage for the next part of their story, or time to process their thoughts/feelings. | Hurrying...<br>Clock watching, talking fast, interrupting, finishing their sentences |
| Acknowledging...<br>'I'm sorry it's hard for you.'<br>'It's okay to feel as you do.' | Belittling...<br>'But it's been 2 weeks since that happened, correct?'<br>'That doesn't sound so bad. You should hear what happened to....'<br>Mentally rehearsing a rebuttal or judging<br>'I'm surprised you're upset by that.' |
| Paraphrasing...<br>'What I'm hearing is that you're feeling worried about....'<br>'Sounds like what you are saying is....'<br>If you are right, they are likely to feel heard. If you are wrong, they can correct you. | Fixing/resolving....<br>'What I would do is....'<br>'Look on the positive side. At least....'<br>Rushing to give advice/problem solving too early, false reassurances/promises |
| Emotional labelling...<br>'You seem sad...' | Ignoring...<br>'Don't feel ... (guilty/bad, etc.).' |
| Reflecting/mirroring...<br>Repeating back a key word/phrase used<br>'Work is difficult.' | Platitudes...<br>'Well, it's for the best.'<br>'It will all come good.' |

## PROVIDE INFORMATION ON COPING

Distress reactions may interfere with your colleague's adaptive coping strategies—strategies that lessen their unpleasant feelings and help them get through the bad times. The more disorientating the situation, the harder it may be for them to access usual helpful coping methods. There are options, however, to help them reconnect with healthy strategies and adjust to what has happened and plan for the future.

You might ask what is most important to them at that moment. This will help them work out their priorities. Consider the following:

'Is there something you need to do first?'

'What can I help you with right now?'

'How are you going to care for yourself in the next half hour?'

Being able to manage one or two issues and to reflect on managing in the short term can help enhance a sense of control and mastery in the situation and reduce feelings of helplessness that sometimes come with a distressing event. Maybe help your colleague reflect on previous occasions when the person has successfully managed adversity, as follows:

'There will have been tough times in the past, what did you do to help you get through them? How can you use those same strategies now?'

'What are you doing at the moment to care for yourself when you get home?'

If there are no usual strategies, suggest to the colleague activities designed to help people relax or focus on the present, such as exercise, being outside in nature, or mindful breathing. Or discuss helpful versus less helpful coping strategies, such as calming self-talk versus withdrawing from social activities.

We find acknowledging strengths and how the colleague has positively helped oneself beneficial. It looks something like this: 'That was an upsetting ward emergency today, you said you phoned your partner afterwards, that's a good thing, it's not a sign of weakness, it's what we do, to rely on others.'

You can keep things even simpler and ask if the colleague would like to talk to someone who can help with coping strategies (e.g., a work-based staff wellbeing team).

## Connecting With Social Support

From our clinical practice and research (APS & ARC, 2013) people who are connected to their family, friends and colleagues are likely to cope with, and recover better, following a traumatic stressor at work. It is also the strongest predictor of resilience, or the ability to bounce back from adversity, because others support our sense of self-worth, wellbeing, confidence, and hope. It allows for emotional understanding, shared knowledge and information, normalisation of reactions, and opportunity for problem solving (NHS Education for Scotland, 2020). We find the following are particularly helpful ways to promote connectedness for our distressed colleagues:

- Facilitate their access to a phone/other methods of communication, such as email.
- Encourage colleagues to routinely stay in touch with primary networks such as family and friends and wider support networks such as neighbours, clinical supervisors, or work-based support groups. If these are not easily available, encourage people to stay in touch with those closest and most readily available.
- Where religious/spiritual practice is helpful, we try to connect them with services within and outside the workplace, such as a hospital-based chaplain.

Also, do not be afraid of asking questions about those who might help:

'Who helps you feel better when you are upset?'

'Who takes your mind off your problems at least for a little while?'

'Who do you speak to when you feel low?'

'Can I help you contact anyone right now?'

'You said you've used the work-based listening service before. How might it help you now?'

'Our work-based counsellors are trained to help colleagues manage stress, including helping you manage the challenges you are facing right now. Would you like to talk to someone from the service?'

## Risk Factors

For most, stress reactions begin to subside within a short period of time (<1 month) and PFA will feel helpful and sufficient. Conversely, sometimes PFA is not enough, and a minority of colleagues have more complex emotional reactions. It is important to recognise this, and when necessary, make referrals or facilitate access to more advanced assistance. Complex reactions may include (APS & ARC, 2013):

- **Panic attacks:** feeling of sudden and intense anxiety, with fast heartbeat, shortness of breath, chest pain, sweating, dizziness, etc.

- **Hallucinations:** seeing, hearing, smelling, tasting, or feelings things that do not exist outside of the mind
- **Delusions:** unshakeable belief(s) in something untrue
- **Self-harm:** cutting or attempting suicide, for example
- **Harmful coping methods:** self-medicating with drugs, alcohol, or medication, for example
- **Violence:** becoming violent or aggressive or hurting others or endangering the lives of others
- **Separation:** keeping oneself completely apart from other people
- **Prolonged grief reactions:** feeling stuck in the grief and causing significant distress and functional impairment
- **Sleeping problems:** lengthy periods of no or little sleep
- **Flashbacks:** feeling as if one is back in the original stressful event, which can cause confusion and intense fear
- **Intense or prolonged feelings (≥1 month)** that do not resolve as expected and/or are having significant impact on daily functioning

This list might look scary, but hold in mind that your role is to escalate to services that can actively assist in managing the risk and support your colleague's longer term recovery. This can include medical (e.g., family doctors) and/or (crisis) mental health or emergency services (e.g., with suicide/self-harm attempts), or an employer assistance programme or occupational health service.

## Taking Care of Yourself

This chapter has considered practical examples and key actions when providing PFA to a distressed colleague. Moreover, it is important to acknowledge that providing support to a colleague can be stressful, tiring, and even upsetting. You may feel frustration or inadequacy when you cannot help others with their problems or feel responsible for their care. You may hear stories of their emotional pain and may have even witnessed or directly experienced the same stressful event as your colleague. A misconception is that health care staff are meant to endure in the face of adversity and that because we are health care staff we are immune to the distress and the emotional labour of supporting others. But it is how we restore ourselves that helps us face the challenges brought by another working day. The good news is that most of us are resilient in the face of stresses, if we take the right steps to protect and restore ourselves. So, ask yourself: 'How can I take time to rest, recover and reflect? How can I know my limits when supporting colleagues?'

Importantly, remember that you are not responsible for solving all your colleague's problems. It is about being a supportive listener, doing what you can to empower the person, and facilitating further support if required. Reflect on and acknowledge what you were able to do to help, even in small ways, how you might support differently next time, and the likely limits of what you could do in the circumstances. Take some time, if possible, to rest and relax before resuming other work duties and have colleagues check in on you. NHS Education for Scotland (2020) presents a useful way of reflecting on self-care in such situations. Thinking about how to self-care is important not only for your own wellbeing but so that you can be more effective in providing PFA.

## ACTIVITY

### Scenario

A colleague who you do not know particularly well is standing in the hospital corridor and is clearly upset. You know it has been a very busy shift today, where there have been several patients displaying challenging behaviour. There has been a patient whom it was suspected has mental health difficulties who was trying to leave the department. You heard that colleagues tried to de-escalate and encourage this patient to stay in the department, but the patient was verbally aggressive and may have lashed out and hit a staff member, although you do not know who this was. Your colleague is clearly very upset. You cannot see any injuries on the colleague. You also know the department is short staffed, and in such circumstances your colleagues tend to be very reluctant to admit when they are finding work challenging.

*What Could You Do or Say?*

Educate about, and normalise, their reactions

Care for immediate needs

Protect from further threat and distress

Comfort and console, and listen

Provide information on coping

Provide support for practical tasks

Connect with social supports

Any risks to be considered?

Identify ways to self-care, during or after, providing psychological first aid

---

**CASE STUDY 18.1    Behind the Mask. Seeing the Person, Hearing the Person's Words: Providing Psychological First Aid in Practice During COVID-19 Pandemic**

In 2020, right at the beginning of the COVID-19 pandemic, I was working as a practice development nurse in critical care. With previous experience as a ward manager, I rejoined the team providing direct nursing care and leadership. My initial thoughts were focused on how we were going to best support our teams. I reached out to see what was available, after which a colleague introduced me to psychological first aid (PFA).

There were key points I learnt from PFA that I was able to put into everyday practice. First and foremost, I had to try and slow things down and take time to see the person in front of me, what this person was telling me verbally and nonverbally. Noticing the clues that someone needs psychological support isn't without its challenges, particularly in COVID-19 areas. Faces are hidden behind visors, voices disguised by masks. I became better equipped to have a focused wellbeing conversation and to put supportive measures into action.

At times, colleagues would need some time out of the clinical area, a quiet place, a space to talk, or a space to be silent. Within the areas I was working, due to time and distance, we were struggling to access the Trust wellbeing rooms. Re-purposing nearer, appropriate spaces, we created our own. Supported by different funds and donations, we transformed these spaces into quiet areas with comfortable chairs, refreshments, and information about how to support our wellbeing.

I recall one of the times I put PFA into action utilising this space, an extremely difficult time during the pandemic. I was working in a COVID-19 area, and it was clear to me that a colleague was struggling. I noticed this person's body language. When I asked if the colleague was okay, I could see a tearful look and hear a broken voice responding 'No.'

I guided the colleague to the wellbeing room, made a warm drink, and sat with this person. I didn't rush things, and we sat together in silence for some time with our drinks. I asked if the colleague wanted

*Continued*

| CASE STUDY 18.1 | **Behind the Mask. Seeing the Person, Hearing the Person's Words: Providing Psychological First Aid in Practice During COVID-19 Pandemic—cont'd** |
|---|---|

me to be there. My colleague welcomed the quiet time together. I didn't fill the silence. I gave eye contact and facial expressions that signaled I was ready to talk when ready. When the colleague did talk, I actively listened.

Noticing words such as 'overwhelmed' and 'anxious,' I repeated them back, paraphrasing sentences. The colleague nodded and confirmed I had understood. I acknowledged this person's feelings and reassured: 'It's okay to be feeling like this. We've never been here before. All eyes are on us, and everyone is telling us that this is the most pressure we've ever been under.' I identified this as a way of normalising these feelings.

The colleague didn't feel capable of continuing work that day. We looked at the next days at work and discussed if time away was needed. I also enquired how the colleague would be getting home and who would be there. We agreed to have regular contact, and we discussed other means of support that were available, both internally and externally.

Afterwards, I continued to check in with the colleague, who expressed gratitude for the support I had provided. The PFA framework has equipped me with a toolkit and the confidence to have wellbeing conversations like this in practice.

**NIKKI SARKAR**

## *References*

Australian Psychological Society, & Australian Red Cross. (2013). *An Australian guide to supporting people affected by disaster.* https://www.psychology.org.au/for-the-public/Psychology-topics/Disasters/Recovering-from-disasters/Psychological-first-aid-supporting-people-disaster.

Blake, H., Gupta, A., Javed, M., Wood, B., Knowles, S., & Coyne, E. (2021). COVID-well study: Qualitative evaluation of supported wellbeing centres and psychological first aid for healthcare workers during the COVID-19 pandemic. *International Journal of Environmental Research and Public Health, 18,* 3626. https://doi.org/10.3390/ijerph18073626.

International Federation of Red Cross and Red Crescent Societies. (2019). *A short introduction to psychological first aid for Red Cross and Red Crescent Societies.*

National Health Service (NHS). (2020). *Education for Scotland.* Psychological first aid. https://www.nationalwellbeinghub.scot/wp-content/uploads/2020/05/COVID-19-Psychological-First-Aid-7-slides-2.pdf.

Wang, L., Norman, I., Xiao, T., Li, Y., & Leamy, M. (2021). Review psychological first aid training: A scoping review of its application, outcomes and implementation. *International Journal of Environmental Research and Public Health, 18,* 4594. https://doi.org/10.3390/ijerph18094594.

World Health Organisation, War Trauma Foundation, and World Vision International. (2011). *Psychological first aid: Guide for field workers.* WHO: Geneva.

# Being Physically Active

Richard Kyle

## Introduction

Nurses and midwives are always on the move. Think back to your last shift. How far do you reckon you walked? The answer might surprise you. During a typical 12-hour shift you would probably walk between 4 and 5 miles. Let's assume that you work three 12-hour shifts a week; that is equivalent to walking the distance of two marathons every single month. Nurses and midwives are clearly being physically active. But is walking at work enough to make a positive difference to you, your patients and the population? These are the questions we will answer in this chapter.

## What Are the Benefits of Physical Activity?

If I asked you to list the benefits of exercise you would probably start from your own experience: what you feel when you move and why you get up and go in the first place. For me, as a runner, the rhythmic contact of my shoes on tarmac calms a racing mind. My motivation to run is mainly the need to support my mental health. For others, the drive to be active is about fitness, physical conditioning, social interaction, or a sense of accomplishment.

We know from evidence that physical activity has wide-ranging and indisputable benefits for our physical and mental health. The World Health Organization (WHO) has summarised the benefits of physical activity for adults aged 18 to 64 years old. These include reduced risk of cardiovascular disease, cancer, hypertension, type 2 diabetes, obesity, anxiety and depression, as well as improved cognitive health and sleep. Based on this evidence, WHO makes recommendations for how much exercise people should do. They recommend that all adults should do some physical activity and ideally at least:

- 150 to 300 minutes of moderate-intensity aerobic physical activity, or
- 75 to 150 minutes of vigorous-intensity aerobic physical activity, or
- An equivalent combination of moderate- and vigorous-intensity activity throughout the week.

These recommendations form the basis of physical activity guidelines issued by governments and public health agencies around the world, but the focus WHO places on the intensity of physical activity is important. Guidelines distinguish between moderate-intensity physical activity, such as brisk walking, cycling, and dancing, and vigorous physical activity, like running, swimming, and aerobic workouts. We have already seen that nurses and midwives walk several miles every shift, but does that bring you the health benefits of physical activity?

This is a question that a group of Australian researchers explored through a systematic review of international studies of nurses' occupational physical activity (Chappel et al., 2017). They concluded that low-intensity physical activity, such as standing and slow walking, made up most of the a nurse's physical activity during a shift, with some periods of moderate-intensity physical activity. What this means is that walking at work may not be enough for you to meet physical activity guidelines.

Research from the United Kingdom confirms this. In Scotland, a study showed that 46% of nurses reported not meeting physical activity guidelines (Schneider et al., 2019). It is a similar picture for student nurses. A study in England found that 48% of student nurses were not meeting physical activity guidelines, and exercise levels were lower among nursing students than medical students (Blake et al., 2017). This begs another important question: if almost half of registered and student nurses tell us that they are not meeting physical activity guidelines, what gets in the way?

# What Gets in the Way of Nurses and Midwives Being Physically Active?

Behavioural scientists help us understand what influences what we do or do not do and why. They often use psychological models (i.e., simplifications of complex human behaviour) to think through the different factors that could lead to a change in a specific behaviour, such as physical activity. One of the most commonly used models is COM-B. The COM-B model has three components, each with two parts, that influence **behaviour** (B):

- **Capability** (C): how what we know (psychological capability) and what we can do (physical capability) influences our ability to do something
- **Opportunity** (O): how our environment, like time and location (physical opportunity) and how our relationships with others (social opportunity) shapes our behaviour
- **Motivation** (M): how our plans and goals (reflective motivation) or desires and impulses (automatic motivation) lead us to do what we do.

Researchers who used this model to understand what gets in the way of Scottish student nurses doing physical activity and other healthy behaviours found that four factors were important: knowledge (Capability), culture (Opportunity), shift work (Opportunity), and stress (Motivation) (Bak et al., 2020). English students said similar things: finding time to exercise alongside the busyness of studying and placements, and lack of facilities, were key challenges (Blake et al., 2017).

Overcoming these barriers is essential so that nurses and midwives can gain the benefits of regular intense exercise. Setting aside these potential benefits for your own health, however, a crucial question remains: how does encouraging and enabling nurses and midwives to be physically active support first-class clinical care?

# Why Does It Matter to Patients if Nurses and Midwives Are Physically Active?

Take a moment to think back to the range of activities you did on your last shift. We have discovered that you did a lot of walking, but you likely did a lot of talking, too. During those discussions you will have given or clarified information, provided emotional support to patients and their families, and offered advice and education.

Nurses have long been encouraged to develop their role in health promotion, that is, helping people to take more control over or improve their health. One way this is often encouraged is through so-called teachable moments. These are opportunities that open up in practice, perhaps prompted by a direct question from a patient or something you hear in passing, that allow you to share some information that can help to guide, advise or educate someone toward making changes to their behaviour. Making Every Contact Count (MECC) is an approach to this used in the United Kingdom by the National Health Service (NHS) to enable and equip health and social care professionals to seize these teachable moments and point people to services that can help them make and sustain lifestyle change, such as exercise referral schemes.

Nurses are particularly well placed to have these conversations. Not only do nurses work in a diverse range of settings, which means they encounter many different people, but national and international surveys repeatedly show that people trust nurses more than any other professional group. In the United Kingdom, the survey company Ipsos MORI publishes an annual veracity index. In 2021 nurses topped the list, with 94% of the public saying that they trust nurses to tell the truth (13 percentage points higher than professors and 75 percentage points higher than politicians!). Nurses' words matter. They carry considerable weight and potential impact. So, whether it is a commonplace bedside interaction with a patient or their family, an impromptu chat between a midwife and a soon-to-be parent, a nurse talking with a child at school, a nursing academic supporting students or a chief nursing officer shaping nursing policy for a nation, conversations that nurses have with patients and the public can lead to positive changes and improved health.

But this is where we face a problem. Studies have also found that nurses who are less physically active are also less likely to initiate conversations with patients about physical activity (Bright et al., 2021). The main reasons were a lack of time and space to have conversations, worry that they might offend, and, for some, feeling hypocritical because of their own lifestyle (Bright et al., 2021). What this research shows is that there is a link between nurses' own health behaviours and their motivation to promote healthy behaviours for others. And just as having these conversations can make a significant positive difference to people's lives, missing these teachable moments means nurses are not able to fully realise their potential to impact the health of individuals and communities.

# Why Does It Matter to the Population if Nurses and Midwives Are Physically Active?

Concern for the health of communities has long been part of the nursing profession. Florence Nightingale, alongside being famed for nursing soldiers during the Crimean War and laying the foundation for nursing education at St. Thomas' Hospital in London on her return, was a social reformer. Nightingale used her statistical prowess to advocate for public health legislation that improved sanitation and saved lives by reducing the spread of infectious diseases. Almost 150 years later, the COVID-19 pandemic has once again forcefully fused together nursing and public health.

Before the pandemic, levels of physical activity around the world were already low, with an estimated one in four adults (27.5%) doing insufficient levels of physical activity (Guthold et al., 2018). One impact of the pandemic and national lockdown measures is further reduced physical activity levels. Nurses' role at the forefront of health promotion is needed now more than at any other time in the profession's history, and never in the profession's history has nurses' potential to make a difference to global health through their health promotion role been greater.

Nurses are not only the most trusted professionals, but they are also the largest group of health professionals in the world. In 2020, the International Year of the Nurse and Midwife, WHO published the *State of the World's Nursing* report. It showed that 59% of all health care professionals are nurses. That's 28 million nurses. There is no other group of professionals that has greater potential to make a difference to the lives and health of people around the world. Think about it: every day millions of nurses or midwives just like you can talk to patients and families and encourage them to take steps to improve their health. Take that one chat and multiple it by millions, and talking about health has potential to change the health of communities and entire countries. But where do we start?

## What Is the Next Step?

In this chapter we have explored the difference that being physically active can make to you, your patients and the wider population. The next step is surprisingly simple: a chat in a snatched moment of time with people you care for.

Supporting each other to have these conversations, however, is crucial. We have discovered that nurses struggle to start this discussion with patients because they worry about being hypocritical, which if we are honest usually starts with us being hypercritical of ourselves. That needs to change. Caring about you is just as important as caring for others. Being physically active so that you get the health and wellbeing benefits of exercise is equally as vital as doing it to make a difference for patients and the population—even more so. You cannot care for others unless you first care for yourself.

However, we have also seen how many things get in the way of this: having time and space to exercise, feeling stressed, the culture of our organisations and knowing what to do. The Activity at the end of this chapter will help you to reflect on and overcome these barriers. The Case Study from Fiona McQueen, a former chief nursing officer for Scotland, shows how small steps can make a big difference for you and others.

So, as we reach the end of our walk through the reasons why being physically active is important for you and others, it is important to make one last point: you are not doing this alone. There is a community of nurses around the world who are part of the #NursesActive and #MidwivesActive movements on Twitter. Through daily posts of cycles, swims, workouts—and the occasional marathon *outside* working hours!—nurses and midwives encourage and inspire one another to be more physically active. Let's take the first step to being more physically active together, encourage each other along the way and then crucially talk about it. That way we will see the difference around the world we have discovered only nurses and midwives can make.

**ACTIVITY**

We have explored some of the things that get in the way of being more physically active. I would now like to encourage you to reflect on what these barriers are for you and then identify the next step that you could take to break these down. Once you have thought through how to overcome personal barriers to physical activity, I would then like you to consider what gets in the way of you talking about physical activity with your patients and how these too can be overcome.

Using the COM-B framework we discussed earlier as a guide, copy out and complete the following table. I have included an example based on the evidence we have explored to get you started.

| Question | Capability | Opportunity | Motivation |
|---|---|---|---|
| **Considering You** | | | |
| 1(a) What gets in the way of you being more physically active? | | "I can't find time to fit physical activity into my busy day." | |
| 1(b) What single step could you take to overcome this barrier? | | Search #NursesActive and #MidwivesActive on Twitter to find out how other nurses and midwives balance work and being physically active. | |
| **Considering Your Patients** | | | |
| 2(a) What gets in the way of you talking about physical activity with patients? | "I don't know how to begin this conversation with patients." | | |
| 2(b) What single step could you take to overcome this barrier? | Search for Making Every Contact Count resources at www.makingevery contactcount.co.uk | | |

| CASE STUDY 19.1 | A Personal Story of Weight Management |

"A journey of a thousand miles begins with a single step." That saying encapsulated the way I felt when in my former role as chief nursing officer for Scotland I was reflecting on how my leadership could help support the health and wellbeing of nurses and midwives. The evidence on the health and wellbeing of nurses relative to the general population did not make happy reading. At that time, the Scottish Government was launching consultation on a diet and obesity strategy. Like many nurses and midwives across the country, I struggled with weight management, and like most nurses and midwives, whether in a leadership role or public facing, I found my role demanding of my time and emotional energy. So, what to do?

I passionately believed that the health and wellbeing of nurses and midwives was inextricably linked with the health and wellbeing of the nation (given the reach of the profession) and that action needed to be taken from a policy perspective. However, that would take time.

Inspired by the work of Richard Kyle, when he was a lecturer in Edinburgh Napier University, on the health of nurses, as well as some innovative work carried out by the lecturing team and nursing undergraduates at the University of West Scotland in Dumfries, I knew I had to do something. And that something was starting with myself.

So, in addition to looking more carefully at my nutrition, I picked up my physical activity, and the dread, shock, and horror that I worked through led me to enjoy classes at the local gym. I felt, though, I needed something more and, importantly, more accessible. That was, to have regular physical activity throughout my day. So, what better way than walking briskly for periods throughout the day? Others were interested and encouraged to do the same; they were keen to hear my story of how I increased my physical activity and how others were approaching such an important area both in the curriculum and in their personal lives. For me, increased physical activity opened up nonjudgemental dialogue about health and wellbeing—both obesity and mental health—in a positive way. So how could I connect with the nurses and midwives of Scotland in a similar fashion?

Paths for All, a Scottish nonprofit, ran a Step Count Challenge event twice a year. The challenges ask for either individual or work-based team participation. The power of social media certainly worked in our professions' favour; interest grew, not to mention the competitive genes coming out, and we paced each other to excellence. Using social media (principally Twitter) and slotting into an already established brand of Paths for All and the Step Count Challenge, how many steps we had taken became an easy conversation starter. The stories, the camaraderie, and encouragement kept coming with many others picking up local leadership for the Step Count Challenge, which also blossomed into other areas. Instead of the conversation revolving around what we couldn't do, it became what we could do—even that smallest step.

FIONA C. MCQUEEN

## References

Bak, M. A., Hoyle, L. P., Mahoney, C., & Kyle, R. G. (2020). Strategies to promote nurses' health: A qualitative study with student nurses. *Nurse Education in Practice, 48*, 102860.

Blake, H., Stanulewicz, N., & Mcgill, F. (2017). Predictors of physical activity and barriers to exercise in nursing and medical students. *Journal of Advanced Nursing, 73*, 917–929.

Bright, D., Gray, B. J., Kyle, R. G., Bolton, S., & Davies, A. R. (2021). Factors influencing initiation of health behaviour conversations with patients: Cross-sectional study of nurses, midwives, and healthcare support workers in Wales. *Journal of Advanced Nursing, 77*, 4427–4438.

Chappel, S. E., Verswijveren, S. J. J. M., Aisbett, B., Considine, J., & Ridgers, N. D. (2017). Nurses' occupational physical activity levels: A systematic review. *International Journal of Nursing Studies, 73*, 52–62.

Guthold, R., Stevens, G. A., Riley, L. M., & Bull, F. C. (2018). Worldwide trends in insufficient physical activity from 2001 to 2016: A pooled analysis of 358 population-based surveys with 1.9 million participants. *Lancet Global Health, 6*, e1077–e1086.

Schneider, A., Bak, M., Mahoney, C., Hoyle, L., Kelly, M., Atherton, I. M., et al. (2019). Health-related behaviours of nurses and other healthcare professionals: A cross-sectional study using the Scottish Health Survey. *Journal of Advanced Nursing, 75*, 1239–1251.

## CHAPTER 20

# Healthy Eating, Diet, and Obesity

Jane Wills

## KEY POINTS

1. Nurses' and midwives' own health status is important to be able to do a physically and emotionally demanding job.
2. Organisational factors such as long working hours and shift work are significant barriers to a healthy diet.
3. Social factors (e.g., eating practices with colleagues or eating alone in a rush), and personal characteristics (e.g., motivation to eat healthily, knowledge about a healthy diet) play a role in determining nurses' healthy eating behaviours in the workplace.
4. The social and physical environment can also influence healthy eating by, for example, increasing the availability of fresh food for evening/night shift workers and providing adequate food preparation and storage facilities.
5. To eat healthily at work requires planning and careful decision making.

## Introduction

Across the world obesity rates in the general population have been increasing in recent years, a trend that has also been seen among nurses and midwives. Alongside the negative health effects of obesity such as type 2 diabetes mellitus and cardiovascular disease, obesity affects an individual's ability to work and results in increasing rates of absenteeism. This chapter discusses how obesity and healthy eating can affect the nursing role, as well as examining leadership and management practices that can support healthy eating in the workplace.

The former chief executive of the National Health Service (NHS), Simon Stevens claimed that obesity in the United Kingdom (UK) is a 'slow motion car crash' that could be financially disastrous for the health service. The NHS is now spending more on bariatric surgery for obesity, for example, than on the national rollout of the intensive lifestyle intervention programmes. The health service must 'get its own act together' on obesity by helping staff to lose weight. Stevens claimed that more than half of the NHS's 1.3 million staff are overweight or obese. Whilst the source of the figure is not known, the latest Health Survey for England states that a quarter of adults are obese (24% of men and 26% of women), while 65% of men and 58% of women are overweight or obese. Research by London South Bank and Edinburgh Napier Universities has shown that about a quarter of nurses in England are obese, which is about the same level as in the general population (Kyle et al., 2017). Indeed, the prevalence of obesity amongst health and social care workers mirrors the inequalities and opportunities of general society. In other words, the poorest of the workforce, care workers, are three times more likely to be obese than doctors. Such figures are mirrored globally with a survey of national leaders of nurse associations ranking obesity alongside mental health as a significant priority to be addressed. Obesity does matter. It matters because obesity is harmful to individuals and, as we see through the COVID-19 pandemic, is a risk factor for more severe COVID-19 infection. Eating well reduces your risk of developing cancer, heart disease, diabetes, and stroke regardless of what you weigh.

## Explanations for Rates of Obesity in Nurses and Midwives

Weight-related problems are strongly related to economic factors, but so too is the difficult task of rectifying them. We all make decisions about food and what we eat every day, but for nurses and midwives their long hours, shift work, low pay, and the work itself of caring for others all make it particularly challenging to address personal health and maintain a healthy diet. Many of the decisions we make are automatic food choices where we unconsciously eat without considering what or how much food we select and consume. Individuals who make the most decisions about food are those who are either of normal weight, or who are considering how to maintain their weight, or those who are obese. Nurses and midwives, on the other hand, need to be thinking about when to eat, what to eat, where it is coming from, and with whom or where they will eat. Yet many nurses and midwives do not make active food decisions.

## Impact of Working Life on Food Choices and Healthy Eating

Shift patterns disrupt metabolism and make it harder to eat regularly and healthily. In addition, long shifts where it can be difficult to take a break make it far more likely to just grab a snack just to keep going. Stress and high levels of emotion can also prompt a person to go for a comforting food such as chocolate or alcohol at the end of the shift. After a long night, the last thing anyone wants to do is eat, and often those working night shifts will do chores and perhaps get children ready for school before eating. It is best not to skip eating before going to bed. Develop a routine for this recurring food decision situation and adhere to a 24-hour intake so you are avoiding hunger. For example, a light breakfast of yogurt and fruit or even porridge followed by a good meal before going to work again will help to maintain blood sugar levels. During the night, try not to snack but heat up homemade soup or a stew you have decided on the day before. Eating healthy fats and protein such as avocado, nuts, and eggs will help night shift workers feel full for longer and will stave off the snack craving.

Those in the acute sector and those in the community all report the difficulties of accessing healthy food whilst on duty, on the road or at night. In a survey for the Royal College of Nursing in 2017, most nurses wanted free fruit to be available and for healthier options to be subsidised. It took the pandemic to highlight how important nutritious food is to health care workers as numerous organisations set out to deliver meals to hospitals and the public donated £1.8 million to Meals for the NHS. Despite attempts to improve the food offered to patients, what is offered to staff in workplace canteens rarely meets criteria for a healthy meal (Department of Health and Social Care [DHSC], 2020), and there is little available for those on night shifts other than vending machines. Those working in the community are not necessarily in a better position, as many report buying food at a local garage or petrol station or mini supermarket and eating by the side of the road. This lack of access to nutritious food and drink can contribute to feelings of stress and lack of control in the workplace. Facilities where staff can store and prepare food (using fridges, toasters, microwaves) can make all the difference. Innovative hospital Trusts provide meals from the restaurant that can be reheated overnight or provide food for staff on patient food trolleys at the end of the day.

# Strategies for Healthy Eating: Individual Level

Obesity is a product of the slow drip-drip effect of poor diet and sedentary lifestyles. The behaviours that lead to obesity become routine, unconscious, and resilient to change.

From surveys and interviews with nurses and midwives who are obese or struggle with excess weight, we know that for some it is a really important issue that can make a person unhappy, embarrassed or depressed and others see it almost as an inevitable consequence of the job and/or ageing about which they are not particularly bothered. We also know that motivation varies as do feelings about one's own self-efficacy and confidence in being able to address excess weight. For most, tackling obesity is not a value for health but rather to improve functioning in daily life, both in relation to work demands and for others such as family or a partner. So, what works for those who are aware of their obesity but unsure what next steps to take and those who are very well informed but are dispirited by frequent weight loss attempts?

Eating to manage a long shift requires planning; there can be a lot of triggering factors that can contribute to unhealthy choices before work even starts. Once you start your working day or night, it can often seem that you have been at work for hours, and how are you going to get through the day/night? Midway through your working shift it can seem that the day will go on forever, and at the end of the day you may be absolutely exhausted and then that can cause unhealthy choices. Think about your arrival at work: did you have time to eat beforehand? Is the hospital canteen open at the start of your shift? So, what do you normally do—not eat at all, eat lots of biscuits on a break, grab an unhealthy snack from a fast-food outlet on the way to work? Does it sound familiar? What could you do instead? Perhaps buy a bag of nuts and weigh it into small portions to take to work every morning or evening. You could soak oats overnight for a ready-to-eat porridge or take some fruit or even keep some at work. The main thing is to recognise your patterns and decisions and set yourself a goal.

Canteens often cook high-fat foods, so opt for salads, pulses and lower calorie options when these are signposted if possible. Because it is often difficult to take full breaks or canteens may be quite far away, try to bring food with you that you have prepared so as to avoid the vending machine or grabbing a quick snack of crisps or chocolate. Examples of foods that you could bring with you include whole-grain pasta dishes, whole-grain sandwiches, hardboiled eggs, almonds, kimchi fried rice, tray bake roasted vegetables, natural yogurt, and homemade curries. Keeping hydrated is vital: begin the shift with 2 cups of warm water, then keep a bottle at your station that you continuously fill. Think about what you ate the last time you were at work: during that 24 hours you should have had at least three servings of vegetables, two of fruit, grains such as bread or rice, and some protein from meat, fish, tofu, eggs, or nuts.

There is an unspoken expectation that having a healthy lifestyle is part of professional duty. Health care staff who become obese are often judged harshly by society with the expectation that 'they should know better' and that the general public will be reluctant to attempt to do something about their own weight if given advice by health care professionals who appeared to have an unhealthy lifestyle. Whilst the public—and nurses and midwives themselves—expect them to be role models for healthier living, there is as yet no evidence that less credence is given to their advice if they happen to be obese. Indeed, nurses and midwives themselves argue that any struggles they may have with their weight make them more able to empathise, support, and communicate with patients or members of the public experiencing the same thing (Kelly et al., 2016).

Nurses and midwives are well placed to provide dietary advice and to encourage improvements in eating behaviours and risk factors in individuals with lifestyle-related chronic disease. They have regular contact with large numbers of individuals, which also provide opportunities for referral to specialist services such as dietitians when required. Despite this, there is evidence that not only is nutritional advice rarely offered but the levels of knowledge about a healthy diet are also lacking. Despite the centrality of nutrition to health, it remains insufficiently attended to in health care education (Crowley et al., 2019). Making Every Contact Count (https://www.makingeverycontactcount.co.uk/) is a national UK initiative to train nurses and midwives to find out what motivates people and to work out with them what are the best steps they personally can take to improve their own health. Yet this kind of health promotion is also rare to observe in practice. Numerous studies report that health care professionals find weight a sensitive conversation topic, and midwives in particular find it challenging to strike a balance between being woman centred and empathetic and yet alerting women to the potential risks of obesity in pregnancy (Foster & Hirst, 2014). This may be because nurses and midwives think advice on weight would not be welcome or that it may damage a good relationship between the health care professional and patient but also because their own weight may make them reluctant to raise the issue.

## Strategies for Healthy Eating: Employers

A recent report into hospital food in the UK (DHSC, 2020) highlighted that the whole food environment of the hospital needs to make healthy eating easier, which includes onsite shops, cafés, canteens and vending machines, and the spaces where staff can prepare their own meals. Healthy and low-calorie options need to be available and labelled as such, and there should be widespread availability of water with no restrictions on opportunities to hydrate. Staff areas should have fridges and microwaves for those who want to bring in healthy food. The NHS uses an incentive scheme, called the Commissioning for Quality and Innovation (CQUIN) payment framework introduced in 2009, which makes some of the funding for a hospital conditional on demonstrating quality improvements. A CQUIN indicator (1b) was introduced in 2017 to improve the commissioning and provision of healthy food. It included bans on the advertisement or price promotion of foods high in fat, sugar, and salt and includes strict specifications for the sale of such foods. Retail outlets and canteens act as key profit generators for the NHS, so alteration to the products that can be sold and promoted is contentious. At one hospital, staff on the busiest wards are offered excess, unserved food from the hospital restaurant at the end of the day, which is a great initiative to reduce waste and provide staff with hot meals.

A review of existing workplace interventions to address obesity in the health care workforce (Kelly & Wills, 2018) identified interventions targeted at individuals such as weight management (currently offered to all NHS staff via a 12-week digital weight management programme), motivational interviewing or coaching, community and team-based challenges such as the Global Corporate Challenge, and organisational interventions such as walking meetings, workplace awards, and healthy canteens. The review concluded that the most effective interventions to improve employees' health behaviours combine individual and environmental strategies such as pairing personalised messages with environmental support and reinforcement. The evidence is inconclusive as to whether targeting a specific behaviour such as physical activity or weight is more effective than a healthy lifestyle approach. Many of the case studies from NHS settings noted that support and buy-in from board members and senior management was essential to programme success.

## Conclusion

Being a nurse or midwife is a demanding job, both physically and mentally. So, it is important to understand the importance of caring for your own body and maintaining a balanced diet and healthy weight. Many studies have shown (e.g., Nicholls et al., 2016) that there are organisational and environmental barriers that make healthy eating difficult. Yet there are behaviour change techniques that can help individuals to better manage their diet and weight. Food choice decisions based on food as fuel rather than a way to preserve or improve health (e.g., snacking on high-calorie junk food because of the perceived energising effect or as an emotional coping strategy) may be easier in health care environments. Self-monitoring and planning are key, however, to incorporating healthy eating into work life.

Healthy eating, diet, and obesity in the health care workforce is not, however, solely an individual responsibility. The pandemic showed the importance of healthy food and proper nutrition for COVID-19 outcomes, and improving the nation's health and tackling health inequalities means we must address food provision and insecurity. The UK government has published a new obesity strategy (https://www.gov.uk/government/publications/tackling-obesity-government-strategy/tackling-obesity-empowering-adults-and-children-to-live-healthier-lives) with the aim of improving the nation's diet and supporting us to lose weight. The UK National Food Strategy (https://www.nationalfoodstrategy.org/) also features a commitment to improve public sector procurement of food and drink to make it more healthy, sustainable and accessible.

## ACTIVITY

Think about what you ate the last time you were at work. Make a list of what you ate, when, with whom, and where. Start from before you arrived at work and continue to when you went to bed.

Look at the list. Would you say it was healthy? Does it, for example, include fruit and vegetables? Does it include lots of high-fat or sugary foods? What could you have added or done without?

Why did you eat the high-fat or sugary foods? Was it because you were rushed, stressed, with someone else eating those foods?

## CASE STUDY 20.1 | Supporting Weight Management at Nottingham University Hospitals NHS Trust, Nottingham, UK

Tackling obesity is a complex area that is not just related to how we behave or look. We need to provide multiple ways for tackling obesity and weight management, and this needs to include support for emotional factors that influence eating habits, a strong educational component, engaging managers about the ultimate benefits to patient care and addressing the obesogenic culture of the estate.

Nottingham University Hospitals NHS Trust launched its staff wellbeing programme in 2005, which has expanded over the years to become a wide-ranging programme supporting staff from all occupational groups (including nurses and midwives) across three hospital sites. I managed this programme for over a decade. Healthy eating and weight management were important components of our work.

The overall programme was driven by a multistakeholder steering group, a Trust-wide staff wellbeing strategy and a dedicated staff wellbeing lead. Much of the work was delivered in partnership with internal departments and external partners. It was thanks to these partnerships that we were able to offer two pilot weight management initiatives working in collaboration with two external partners: Slimming World (an internationally known weight loss and maintenance programme) and Notts County Football in the Community (a regional sports development charity serving the people of Nottinghamshire). The former provided staff with the opportunity to take part in a Slimming World group for 12 weeks, whilst the latter provided an onsite physical activity session with nutritional advice.

It was successful and led to further collaboration between the staff wellbeing lead and a specialist senior dietitian to develop our own in-house 12-week diet and weight loss programme. This included education sessions about food groups and portion sizes alongside a weekly weigh-in. Although it was extremely popular with staff, there were limitations on how much could be offered in-house due to clinical demands on the dietician's time.

When our hospital Trust was one of a handful in England to be selected as a site for the NHS England Healthy Workforce pilot in 2016, the Trust received some government funding that was to be dedicated to specific staff wellbeing initiatives. The 12-week in-house weight management programme was identified as a key activity. This led to a staff dietitian being employed to support our work in this area.

*Continued*

> ### CASE STUDY 20.1 | Supporting Weight Management at Nottingham University Hospitals NHS Trust, Nottingham, UK—cont'd
>
> Benefits of the programme included:
> - Participants who completed at least 10 of 12 sessions lost 5% or more of their body weight.
> - Staff changed their behaviours in relation to diet and exercise. More of them were eating '5 portions a day' of fruits and/or vegetables, they were more aware of portion sizes, and were more physically active.
> - Reports of improved sleep, having more energy, and better mental health.
> - Reports of fewer aches and pains and needing less medication for chronic conditions; one person reported long-standing foot pain had disappeared!
>
> In England, the Commissioning for Quality and Innovation (CQUIN) framework supports improvements in the quality of services and the creation of new, improved patterns of care. A CQUIN was introduced for Trusts to reduce the amount of high-fat and high-sugar foods available onsite. The staff wellbeing lead, estates colleagues, dietetics, and the catering provider worked closely together to improve access to healthy foods onsite.
>
> Today, the offer has expanded to include:
> - A 12-week nutrition and physical activity weight management initiative
> - Drop-in weight management clinics
> - Food and wellbeing seminars covering a wide range of topics
> - Eating with mindfulness workshops
> - Onsite physical activity opportunities
> - Advice and education for tackling obesity for the occupational health teams
> - Healthy options available in the onsite catering outlets
>
> **STEPH KNOWLES**

## References

Crowley, J., Ball, L., & Hiddink, G. J. (2019). Nutrition in medical education: A systematic review. *Lancet Planet Health*, *3*, e379–e389. https://doi.org/10.1016/S2542-5196(19)30171-8.

Department of Health and Social Care. (2020). *Report of the independent review of NHS hospital food*. https://assets.publishing.service.gov.uk/government/uploads/system/uploads/attachment_data/file/929234/independent-review-of-nhs-hospital-food-report.pdf.

Foster, C. E., & Hirst, J. (2014). Midwives' attitudes towards giving weight-related advice to obese pregnant women. *British Journal of Midwifery*, *22*(4), 254–262.

Kelly, M., & Wills, J. (2018). Systematic review: What works to address obesity in nurses? *Occupational Medicine*, *68*(4), 228–238. https://doi.org/10.1093/occmed/kqy038.

Kelly, M., Wills, J., Jester, R., & Speller, V. (2016). Should nurses be role models for healthy lifestyles? Results from a modified Delphi study. *Journal of Advanced Nursing*, *73*(3), 665–678.

Kyle, R. G., Wills, J., Mahoney, C., Hoyle, L., Kelly, M., & Atherton, I. M. (2017). Obesity prevalence among healthcare professionals in England: A cross-sectional study using the Health Survey for England. *BMJ Open*, *7*(12), e018498. https://doi.org/10.1136/bmjopen-2017-018498.

Nicholls, R., Perry, L., Duffield, C., Gallagher, R., & Pierce, H. (2016). Barriers and facilitators to healthy eating for nurses in the workplace: An integrative review. *Journal of Advanced Nursing*, *73*(5), 1051–1065. https://doi.org/10.1111/jan.13185.

## CHAPTER 21

# The Impacts of Dehydration and Staying Hydrated at Work

Kathryn Halford

**KEY POINTS**

1. Ensure that all staff and patients have access to drinks throughout their period of work.
2. When developing a policy, ensure that all stakeholders are involved.
3. Provide a dedicated space for the water bottles to be keep during the period of work.
4. Ensure that the team decides when additional drinks should be taken (e.g., during handovers).
5. Be flexible if there is a significant infection control issue that prevents staff drinking.

## Introduction

For humans to survive, they must eat and drink regularly. It is possible to survive for about 3 days without water and about 1 week without food. All the latest research is clear that if you drink regularly, you will function better, your memory is better, you feel better, and your health improves. The need to replace fluid at the rate it is lost is also noted to be important.

The European Food Safety Authority (2010) panel on dietetic products, nutrition, and allergies recommends a daily fluid intake of 2 L for women and 2.5 L for men.

In the United Kingdom, this is supported by 'Rest, Rehydrate, Refuel—A Resource to Improve the Working Environments for Nursing' (Royal College of Nursing, 2018), Hydration for Health (2017), and NHS Choices (2015) recommendations.

Against this backdrop of beliefs, health care workers have historically been unable to drink whilst in the clinical environment, with infection control being cited as the reason.

There is no evidence to confirm that drinking in a clinical area has an impact on infection control nor would it have been the case historically. Having partly drunk cups of tea and coffee lying around on the wards would have an impact as mould can grow, but if tided away promptly there is no reason to say they pose an infection control risk.

It is more likely that in the past there was not enough space in the wards for cups to be safely left. The long Nightingale Wards used to have a small central desk where the nurses would sit and there would be no space for drinks to be left. In addition, the senior staff on the wards had sitting rooms attached to the wards where they would have the opportunity to have food and drinks.

Over the years the layout of wards and shift patterns have changed, but the rules linked to drinking and eating in the clinical area have not, and it is time to challenge this.

## PATTERNS OF WORK AND BREAKS

The UK National Health Service (NHS) began life in 1948 when most local hospitals that had traditionally been run by a variety of organisations were pulled together under one name, the NHS. The hospitals had a variety of rules and regulations, which again differed depending on which organisation the individual was working in.

One rule that was consistently applied was that no staff should eat or drink in the clinical areas under any circumstances. Usually, again, the reason for this was infection control.

At that time, the shift patterns were short shifts with an overlap in the afternoon between early and late shifts. This meant that the morning staff had a coffee break off the ward and then when the late staff arrived, they had lunch together. Not only did this mean that all staff had a break, but it also meant that there was time to discuss the work on the ward during the morning and debrief informally with team members.

Once the morning shift returned from lunch there was time for teaching whilst the late staff had afternoon tea off the ward. In the evening they then had a short meal break, known as supper. This meant that in an 8-hour shift there were two breaks built in usually about 3 to 4 hours apart, giving staff the opportunity of making sure they had drinks on a regular basis.

At night, the acuity of the patients meant that the ward was quiet, and it was not uncommon to see groups of nurses sitting in the middle of a Nightingale Ward doing their knitting! Breaks at night were also regulated, so everyone had two breaks taken in the canteen, which was open all night to ensure that staff could access food and drinks. For those less familiar with these terms, a Nightingale Ward is a type of hospital ward that contains one large room without subdivisions for patient occupancy.

During the last 40 years, the working pattern of nurses and midwives has changed, and the acuity of the patients has increased. This means there is a reduction in the opportunities for staff to leave the ward and have some food and a drink regularly during the shift. In most organisations the canteen is not open during the night, further reducing opportunities for staff to have a drink or some food.

Most wards do have staff rooms where staff can sit and have a break; they are usually equipped with a microwave for people to heat food. As in earlier years, the staff can spend the time debriefing from the shift, but not everybody would be able to have a break at the same time, which is entirely different from earlier times.

During the late 1980s and early 1990s there was a move to working longer shift patterns, usually of 12 hours. Initially when people were working these long shifts, there were very regimented shift breaks: 20 minutes for coffee, 45 minutes for lunch, 20 minutes for afternoon tea, 15 minutes for a supper break, and two breaks during the night. This meant that you stayed hydrated and only had 3 to 4 hours between each break.

Today this regimented approach to break times seems to have stopped. Staff often have one or two breaks, which means the opportunity to ensure that they are well hydrated and have eaten is reduced, at night there is often no food available, and use of the vending machine is the default position.

## Why Change?

Over the past few years there has been lots of research that suggests if you drink regularly and keep well hydrated your level of concentration improves and general health improves. All the literature states that you should drink regularly, and water should be freely available to everyone from children in school to adults at work.

Working in the NHS today is exhausting; it is physically demanding, with the work often undertaken in hot conditions with heavy uniforms being worn. It is recognised that nurses often do not take their breaks. This is sometimes because people are so busy they cannot leave their ward, and at other times people feel that they cannot leave their colleagues and therefore choose not to leave the ward. Whatever the reason this results in staff not taking their breaks and not always having enough to drink or eat.

More recently, hospital wards have had to deal with patients with coronavirus (COVID-19), which has impacted still further on staff being able to leave the wards for breaks. Hospitals have been split into separate zones, those for patients who are COVID-19 positive, negative, or unknown. In the first wave of COVID-19 in the United Kingdom, staff could not move between zones (due to COVID-19 hospital policy). Therefore, if there was no canteen in the zone where they were working, food and drinks were not readily available unless there was a vending machine nearby. This further reduced opportunities for staff to ensure they were well hydrated and nourished.

For all organisations there is an imperative to ensure that staff are well looked after and can have adequate food and drink breaks during their shift. However, this is not always possible in times of stress on wards where there are shortages of staff (e.g., during a pandemic or other crisis). It is important to recognise that whilst this is not ideal, sometimes it is the reality of working in busy clinical areas.

The need to change is to recognise the latest research that demonstrates that well-hydrated staff can function more effectively, are fitter, stay healthier, and in turn are less likely to have time off sick.

## Regulatory Responsibility

All Trusts are committed to the health and wellbeing of staff and to meeting its obligations under the UK Working Time Regulations (1998). These regulations set limits on daily and weekly working hours and provision of rest breaks within those working hours. The Regulations state that when a shift lasts 6 hours or more, the worker is entitled to an uninterrupted 20-minute break away from the workstation.

Adequate rest breaks are essential to prevent excessive tiredness and fatigue and to prevent dehydration when working in a physically demanding role. Good hydration contributes to staff health and safety as even mild levels of dehydration can adversely affect both mental and physical performance and contribute to sickness or musculoskeletal injury. Ultimately, if staff do not remain hydrated, patient care may be adversely affected leading to mistakes such as drug errors or failure to recognise subtle changes in a patient's condition.

Conversely, staff who are hydrated have better concentration and mental performance, and are less likely to develop illness such as urinary tract infection and chronic disease. They are more refreshed, have better job satisfaction, and can provide a safer improved patient experience.

## Managing Change

Having reviewed the latest research and taken advice from clinical staff who are working in busy clinical areas, a decision may be reached to change from the traditional rule of 'no drinks on the ward' to one of supporting staff wellbeing and introducing a policy that supports staff to have drinks in the clinical environment.

But there are some considerations:

How many and how often will drinks be taken on the wards? Will hydration breaks occur in addition to regulated rest breaks as defined in the UK Working Time Regulations (1998)? Should only water be allowed on the ward or would other drinks such as coffee and tea also be acceptable?

Service provision and patient care must not be compromised because of hydration breaks. If staff have water bottles readily available, they will be able to have a quick drink as they are working.

So, what does good practice look like?

The senior sister/charge nurse/lead nurse/matron/manager will agree the most appropriate place for hydration breaks to occur based on the individual patient group and area layout, considering maintenance of patient safety; these are called hydration stations.

Drinking bottles stored in hydration stations should be easily accessible and clearly labeled and should be cleared away at the end of each shift ready for the next group to store their water bottles. During exceptionally busy periods when breaks cannot be taken, then the senior members of staff should decide if a tray of drinks may be prepared and put in the staff hydration station making sure they are cleared away promptly.

Many staff have long journeys to work and may not have been able to eat prior to starting their shift; the handover period is usually 10 to 15 minutes, so the team may decide that this is a suitable time to have a drink, and the whole multidisciplinary team can be involved.

Whilst leaders should ensure that breaks are taken and drinks are available during shifts, the individual staff are responsible for ensuring they drink enough to maintain hydration for their own wellbeing and to raise concerns when this is not possible to ensure that action is taken. They are also responsible for ensuring that patient need is attended to if required during their hydration breaks.

## WHERE ARE WE AT?

For over 100 years the accepted rule in clinical environments is that there is no eating or drinking—except of course chocolates left by patients as a thank-you! Some staff will be cautious about having drinks on the ward due to a prior, strict understanding that they should never drink on the ward due to infection control concerns. To ensure that staff understand the importance of the change, which includes nurses, midwives, wider teams, doctors and administrators, they should be fully involved in implementing any changes and understanding the rationale for that. Throughout this chapter infection control teams have been referenced as the team that prevents drinks being available in the clinical area. They too will have worked in an environment where drinking has not been allowed, and although there is no infection control reason to not have drinks on the wards, psychologically they may also be concerned that drinks should not be on the wards. The only exception to this is where there is a real infection control issue, such as during a pandemic when the source of transmission was not entirely clear; however, these circumstances are very rare and should not stop the introduction of a new policy that allows drinking on the wards. Clinical areas should be clean and tidy so it may be sensible to consider designating a specific area with hydration station clearly marked in each area. This not only prevents visitors or inspectors negatively commenting about drinking on the wards but positively reinforces the need to support staff keeping hydrated at work.

Hydration stations should not be an excuse for staff not being allowed to take their regulatory breaks. It should be clear that both are required, and this should be regularly reviewed, and the shift leader should make sure that staff are using the station and feel able to take regular drinks in addition to their breaks. In implementing a new policy, the staff employed there at the time need to be fully aware of the change, and when new staff join the team it is important to make sure they understand the importance of drinking regularly, which includes all members of the multidisciplinary team.

---

**ACTIVITY**

1. Have you ever gone a long time without a drink at work? What were the reasons for this? How did it make you feel? Were there any impacts on how you carried out your job?
2. Find out whether the place you work has a policy for staff around hydration at work. If not, start a conversation with your colleagues and manager about this. How can you make a difference?

| CASE STUDY 21.1 | Hydration Policy at the Barking, Havering, and Redbridge University Hospitals NHS Trust |
|---|---|

As the chief nurse of a large district general hospital in the United Kingdom, I became increasingly concerned about the health and wellbeing of the staff working on the wards, and specifically the nursing staff who were least able to leave the wards at times of greatest pressure. In 2016, in consultation with the senior nursing team, we agreed that we needed to act; the result was the organisations Staff Hydration and Hydration Breaks Guidance, which has most recently been amended in 2021.

When developing the new policy, it was imperative that the key stakeholders were involved, in this circumstance the infection control team had a view. They were clear that there is a difference between bottles of water and lots of cups scattered around, and they were supportive of the clinical teams having water bottles readily available in a specific place. Having dispelled the myth that infection control would stop nursing staff drinking on the ward, we were able to develop our guidance.

We have designated drink stations with named water bottles in each ward area. We encouraged teams to share a cup of tea, coffee, or cold drink whilst they are at the board huddles, with those being cleared away immediately when the drinks were finished. Our aim is for each member of staff to have at least five drinks per shift in addition to those taken during their breaks. In addition to the infection control team, other key stakeholders supported the need for hydration stations to ensure that hydration of staff was maintained throughout the day.

When this was first introduced it was with some nervousness that staff brought their bottles and put them on the trays on the ward. Today, this is just part of the ward routine. We have of course occasionally had to remind people that a take-away coffee cup on the notes trolley during the ward round is not acceptable, but this is rare.

The infection control team is happy with the water stations and agrees that it is important to ensure that staff remain hydrated.

During peaks of very hot weather, the Estates team ensures that the wards have additional water and ice lollies; of course the patients are offered the same, to make sure staff and patients stay hydrated.

The Hydration Breaks Guidance that was developed supports staff to remain hydrated during working hours. This includes the use of supplementary hydration for hydration purposes only and taken in the staff member's ward/work area. They occur at a time and in an area of the ward that has been agreed locally. These breaks are in addition to rest breaks, which staff are entitled to in accordance with UK Working Time Regulations (1998).

During our latest Care Quality Commission inspection, we took the opportunity to explain our policy, which we as an organisation support. To date, various regulatory inspectors have approved of this approach.

Our staff have told us via several media and forums that they value the hydration stations and recognise that this is part of the organisation supporting their wellbeing.

Thanks to Gary Etheridge, Director of Nursing, Barking, Havering, and Redbridge University NHS Trust who developed the initial guidance.

**KATHRYN HALFORD**

## References

European Food Safety Authority. (2010). Panel on Dietetic Products, Nutrition and Allergies: Scientific opinion on dietary reference values for water. *EFSA Journal, 8*(3), 1459. https://doi.org/10.2903/j.efsa.2010.1459.

Hydration for Health. (2017). *Everyday hydration.* http://www.h4hinitiative.com/everyday-hydration/water-requirements-daily-life.

NHS Choices. (2015). *Water, drinks, and your health.* https://www.nhs.uk/Livewell/Goodfood/Pages/water-drinks.aspx.

Royal College of Nursing. (2018). *Rest, rehydrate, refuel—a resource to improve the working environments for nursing staff.* RCN: London.

Working Time Regulations. (1998). http://legislation.gov.uk/uksi/1998/1833/contents/made.

## CHAPTER 22

# The Challenge of Health and Wellbeing in a Crisis

Holly Blake ■ Joanne Cooper

## KEY POINTS

1. The health and wellbeing of the nursing and midwifery workforce is critical to the future of health care services globally.
2. Crisis situations such as the COVID-19 pandemic generate unique pressures, often for an extended period, with impacts on health and wellbeing extending far beyond the duration of the crisis itself.
3. It is normal to experience emotional impacts during and after a crisis situation such as the COVID-19 pandemic.
4. Mitigation strategies can help to minimise the impact of a crisis on nurses and midwives; interventions have been implemented with some agility at organisational and policy level, by leaders and managers, within teams, and by individuals.
5. Forward-thinking health care employers invest routinely in staff health and wellbeing as prevention, not just reactively during a crisis.

## Introduction

In this chapter, we set the context of a contemporary global crisis and the impact of challenging times on the wellbeing of nurses and midwives. We examine specific wellbeing issues arising in or from crisis situations and provide selected examples of efforts to mitigate the psychological impact of a crisis on workforce health and wellbeing.

## Public Health Crisis: The Outbreak of Disease

Through history, healthcare workers have responded to the outbreak of disease that affects many individuals at once and spreads very rapidly. In simple terms, outbreaks can occur in particular communities, geographic locations, or across countries and are known as epidemics (where there is an increase, often suddenly, in the number of cases of an infectious disease above what is normally expected in a localised population) or pandemics (epidemic that has spread over several countries or even continents). For example, cholera, bubonic plague, smallpox, influenza, and HIV/AIDS have been widely spread with a huge toll on human life and health.

A contemporary global crisis is the emergence of coronavirus disease 2019 (COVID-19), caused by the severe acute respiratory syndrome coronavirus 2 (SARS-CoV-2) and declared a pandemic by the World Health Organisation (WHO) in March 2020. The COVID-19 pandemic is the third recorded outbreak of a coronavirus, following epidemics of sudden acute respiratory syndrome in 2002 (SARS, SARS-CoV-1 or SARS-CoV) and the Middle East respiratory syndrome in 2012 (MERS or MERS-CoV).

The COVID-19 pandemic has impacted work and employment across the globe. Workplace closures and measures taken to curb the spread of the virus have led to changes in people's working relationships, job roles, work patterns, place of work, income, and job losses for some. The devastating impact of the pandemic on public health has worsened existing health inequalities and put untenable pressures on health and care services worldwide.

## What Is the Impact on the Healthcare Workforce?

The COVID-19 pandemic brings more than a public health emergency. It exacerbates an existing problem in the public sector: severe staffing shortages. Globally, WHO estimated a projected shortfall of 18 million health workers by 2030, with the greatest impacts seen in low and lower-middle income countries. Across all countries, it is predicted that there will be continued difficulties in the future with education, employment, deployment, retention, and performance in the health and care workforce.

Let's look at the situation in England, as an example. Here, our largest employer is the National Health Service (NHS) with almost 1.2 million full-time equivalent staff employed across hospital and community services. According to a report by the Kings Fund (2021), 'NHS hospitals, mental health services and community providers are now reporting a shortage of nearly 84,000 FTE (full-time equivalent) staff, severely affecting key groups such as nurses, midwives, and health visitors.' Unfilled vacancies are increasing stress levels, sickness absence, and turnover rates and there is an urgent need to retain the skilled workforce and increase the number of nurses and allied health professionals in training.

Added to this, the psychological impact of the pandemic on health and care workers is profound. Many nurses and midwives have been worried about their risk of contracting COVID-19 and getting ill or passing the virus to their colleagues and loved ones. Due to their proximity to others and higher exposure to the virus, health care workers are at increased risk of contracting COVID-19 through their everyday work and of falling ill with more severe forms of the virus. Exposure to COVID-19 has been greater for women because they account for a greater proportion of the healthcare workforce (there are more women working as nurses, midwives, and carers) (International Labour Organisation, 2021). Some have even experienced social stigma and abuse due to their high exposure to COVID-19 and public fears about contracting the virus.

Nurses and midwives have reported feeling anxious about shortages of personal protective equipment (PPE), and access to PPE has varied at different stages of the pandemic and in different geographic regions. Many nurses and midwives have worked significantly longer hours, with higher workloads, sometimes in unfamiliar clinical roles. For many, this has been coupled with worries about the health of their own families and balancing caregiving responsibilities at home with high pressures at work.

Dealing with escalating cases of COVID-19, hospitalisations and deaths has taken its toll; many healthcare workers have seen colleagues (and patients) die from the virus. Through this physical and mental exhaustion, nurses and midwives have been tasked with providing the best possible care through uncertain times—a level of care sometimes in conflict with their moral code due to high pressures and limited resources, often leading to the experience of moral dilemmas, moral injury, and guilt.

We must acknowledge that a crisis, such as the COVID-19 pandemic, will turn people's lives upside down. Nurses and midwives have been dealing with unprecedented demand for an extended period, with risks to their own health that will extend well beyond the most urgent phases of the pandemic. It is not surprising, therefore, that research has identified high levels of stress, anxiety, and depression in the healthcare professions, particularly frontline care workers, although it should be emphasised that these reactions are to some extent, normal in the face of a pandemic. But, the COVID-19 pandemic has been long lasting, and there is evidence of burnout and emerging signs of posttraumatic stress disorder in healthcare workers worldwide. The prevalence of mental health disorders is likely to increase over time, and being prepared for this is essential because mental ill health in health care workers can have serious implications for individuals, organisations, care quality, and patient safety. Protecting the welfare of health care workers must be a priority for healthcare employers.

In the early stages of the pandemic, at the University of Nottingham in the United Kingdom (UK), we conducted a programme of research to explore the impacts of COVID-19 on healthcare workers (Blake et al., 2021a) and healthcare trainees (Blake et al., 2021b). In qualitative interviews, following the first wave of COVID-19 in the UK, nurses, midwives and students (among other professionals) shared the stark reality of the pandemic, particularly for frontline workers: the impact on their job roles (or studies), the personal sacrifices, the emotional highs and lows. They spoke of the privilege, reward and satisfaction gained from contributing to the national (and global) effort, the camaraderie, and pulling together as a team.

These discussions highlighted the dedication and commitment of nurses and midwives (and students) to the profession and to the NHS.

At the same time, our data showed widespread psychological impacts on the workforce. Nurses spoke about experiencing a deep sense of guilt when they were unable to take what they viewed to be the appropriate course of action due to organisational or resource constraints. These health care professionals spoke at length about the worry, fear, anxiety and expectation that they or their colleagues would at some point experience burnout or even trauma from what they had seen and experienced.

## What Can Be Done to Help?

The most powerful indicator of workforce wellbeing is the context of the organization: policies and organisational strategies for employee wellbeing, the cultural norms, leadership styles, patterns of communication, work patterns, safety considerations and rapid establishment of precautionary measures, peer support and psychologically safe working environments where people feel empowered to speak up without fear of retribution. With appropriate organisational structures and culture in place, individuals can then take additional actions themselves to support their own health and wellbeing (i.e., self-compassion, self-care).

We advocated for the mobilisation of early psychological support to mitigate the impact of COVID-19 on healthcare workers and trainees. This was based on the normalisation of psychological responses during a crisis and encouragement of self-care and help-seeking behaviour. Our conceptual model (Fig. 22.1) published in Blake, Mahmood, et al, 2021 draws together the core areas for targeting strategies, interventions and initiatives. Here we provide four Case Studies of successful initiatives that were implemented during the COVID-19 pandemic that draw on core areas of the model.

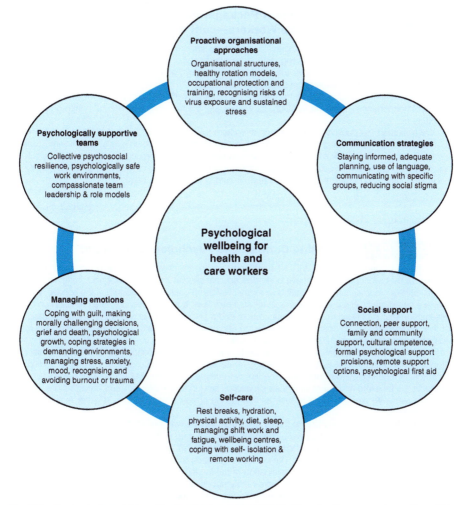

**Fig. 22.1** Conceptual model for mitigating the impacts of COVID-19 on health care workers. (From Blake, Mahmood, Dushi et al, 2021b.)

<table>
<tr><td>CASE STUDY 22.1</td><td>**Digital Support Package: Psychological Wellbeing for Health Care Workers**</td></tr>
</table>

During a crisis, the amount of information circulating can be overwhelming. We have all at some point experienced the feeling of information overload. Within 3 weeks of the outbreak of COVID-19 in the UK in March 2020, we developed and released a digital support package aimed at mitigating the psychological impact of COVID-19 on health care workers (Blake & Bermingham, 2020). This was the first digital support package of its kind, globally, and by December 2021 it had already been accessed by over 72,000 healthcare workers around the world.

Content of the package draws on the principles of positive psychology by focusing on strengths that allow individuals and communities to thrive. It provides guidance and advice related to the following:
  (a) *The organisation*: proactive organisational structures and approaches, communication strategies and approaches to reducing social stigma, prioritising staff wellbeing
  (b) *Leaders and teams*: actions that can be taken to create psychologically safe spaces for staff, compassionate leadership and role modelling, team collaboration, building team resilience, peer support, and signposting others to support through psychological first aid

| CASE STUDY 22.1 | Digital Support Package: Psychological Wellbeing for Health Care Workers—cont'd |
|---|---|

(c) *Individuals*: building self-worth, practising self-care (importance of sleep, rest, and work breaks, managing shifts and fatigue, engaging in healthy lifestyle behaviours), staying connected with others and managing emotions (moral injury, coping, guilt, grief, fear, anxiety, depression, recognising signs of burnout, and psychological trauma).

The e-package includes advice from experts in mental wellbeing as well as those with direct pandemic experiences from the frontline, as well as signposting to public mental health guidance (Blake et al., 2020a).

We evaluated the package with health care workers (Blake et al., 2020a) and health care trainees (Blake et al., 2021b), including nurses and midwives, and they found it to be relevant, meaningful, and useful. Given this positive evaluation and widespread uptake, we recommend distribution of this package to nurses and midwives (and indeed all professional groups) to augment strategies to support the health and wellbeing of health care workers through and beyond the pandemic.

HOLLY BLAKE

| CASE STUDY 22.2 | Wellbeing Centres and Psychological First Aid |
|---|---|

From the early stages of the COVID-19 pandemic, healthcare organisations rapidly created respite spaces for their workforce. These have been described in several ways (e.g., wobble rooms, time-out rooms, chill-out rooms, safe rooms, rainbow rooms, wellbeing centres). The nature of the spaces, what they are called, and the provisions available for staff may vary, but essentially they are premised on the assumption that staff need rest and recouperation, and a place where this can happen, ideally outside of their clinical area. Such spaces are intended to encourage staff to take work breaks, provide quiet spaces for rest and relaxation, areas to eat and drink, and opportunities to socialise with peers and access support—albeit physical distancing maybe be required during a pandemic. Some organisations provide sensory items such as low-level lighting, stress balls, aromatic oils, and lava lamps, in addition to wellbeing resources and signposting. The aim is to create a positive atmosphere that helps staff to deal with the pressure and stress of a crisis situation. Through these spaces, many organisations have provided staff with pastoral support such as counselling or psychological support either face-to-face or by video link.

The UK Nottingham University Hospitals NHS Trust led the way with staff wellbeing support in the early weeks of the pandemic; two wellbeing centres were set up in April 2020, providing high-quality rest spaces and peer-to-peer psychological support from staff volunteers (wellbeing buddies) who were trained in psychological first aid. The centres were open to all staff from any job group, including nurses and midwives. We led the first evaluation of the implementation of supported COVID-19 staff wellbeing centres globally. The centres were highly accessed; over 17 weeks during the first wave of COVID-19 in the United Kingdom, we recorded almost 15,000 facility visits across the two facilities (Blake et al., 2020b). Our qualitative research showed that the wellbeing centres and access to psychological first aid was valued by staff who viewed the provisions as critical to the wellbeing of hospital employees during and after the first surge of COVID-19 in the UK (Blake et al., 2021a). The impacts were wide ranging, as attendees of the wellbeing centres reported benefits for individual staff members (e.g., personal wellbeing), teams (e.g., teamwork, camaraderie, improved team cohesion), the health care organisation (e.g., potential to prevent sickness absence through timely support), and patient care quality (e.g., through improved individual/team wellbeing supporting productivity and compassion). Our research highlighted the importance of managerial support and role modelling in staff wellbeing service access. Staff told us that they were more likely to access the wellbeing centres and psychological support if they felt that it was sanctioned (or even better, role modelled and advocated) by their line managers and colleagues. Although we have much to learn from the rapid implementation of these facilities for healthcare workers during the COVID-19 pandemic, it should be emphasised that rest, recouperation, and access to psychological support are essential elements of supporting staff wellbeing always, not just in a crisis.

HOLLY BLAKE

## CASE STUDY 22.3  Understanding the Uncertainties of Care Home Managers and Staff Expressed in Response to COVID-19

It is important for us to consider proactive organisational approaches and resilience across acute, primary, and social care settings in supporting staff wellbeing during a crisis. Uncertainties about how to respond to the COVID-19 pandemic were felt not only in acute care settings but also in the care home sector. As practitioners, we are in an ideal position to understand more fully what these might be. Spilsbury et al. (2021), for example, tackled these issues directly during the first stages of the pandemic (March-June 2020), working in partnership with care home managers and staff via a self-formed closed WhatsApp discussion group. Together they identified and examined the important care and organisational questions of concern and considered what information was essential in the short, medium, and long term. Key areas included the support required by residents, relatives, and staff, many of whom you may feel are pertinent to your practice and are worthy of further discussion with colleagues and teams.

JOANNE COOPER

## CASE STUDY 22.4  Effective Communication Strategies and Support During Practice Transitions

Effective communication strategies during a crisis are critical to creating the best practice environment, team cohesion, and best outcomes for patients and families. Positive examples have maximised the benefits of existing local communication strategies, such as regular team huddles, multidisciplinary team meetings, training activities, sharing of best practice through printed communication in staff areas, and in-reach specialist teams to share expert knowledge. Undoubtedly, communication strategies have adapted rapidly in response to the COVID-19 pandemic. In part, this was due to changes in physical distancing requirements, cohorting of patients within COVID-specific clinical areas, and movement of staff across clinical specialties. Refresher training, local inductions, and supporting resources are essential for orientating and welcoming staff to a clinical team, not only in support of safe care but for the psychological safety of staff within new areas and during times of transition in practice.

Communication and support to students is also essential, as shown by Godbold et al. (2021) whose qualitative study examined the experiences of nursing students undertaking an extended placement during the first wave of the pandemic. They reiterate how we must attend to the welfare and support of students, including preparation for placement, resilience, provision of e-learning, and opportunities for learning at the frontline. Pivotal to this is close partnership working between higher education institutions and practice areas to ensure ongoing communication, training, and clinical supervision is offered, often using online forms of communication and e-learning to suit the needs of learners.

Importantly, we have seen that access to up-to-date, accurate communication about COVID-19 has been both essential and at times contentious. Effective leadership, role modelling and decision making during this time have played key roles in communicating rapidly changing information as learning from the pandemic has developed. Visible leadership based on a distributed model (where leaders are given the autonomy to make key decisions in their own areas of responsibility) is effective in promoting shared decision making, understanding the views and concerns of those at the point of care, and maximising the key messages to be shared.

JOANNE COOPER

## CASE STUDY 22.5  Pandemic Support in Response to Its Impact on Race and Health

From the early stages of the COVID-19 pandemic, the disproportionate impact on mortality and morbidity for individuals belonging to certain ethnic minority groups became apparent. Timely organisational responses were therefore critical to supporting the physical and psychological wellbeing of staff. These responses were aimed at minimising the risk of adverse outcomes from COVID-19 within the context of an emergent condition and in the absence of an established vaccine programme.

In the UK, Nottingham University Hospitals NHS Trust implemented a strategic approach to understanding and addressing concerns of staff from ethnic minority populations, working in partnership with an established Black, Asian, and minority ethnic (BAME) staff network, BAME shared governance council, and newly formed BAME COVID-19 operational group.

| CASE STUDY 22.5 | **Pandemic Support in Response to Its Impact on Race and Health—cont'd** |

Using the increased communication opportunities from newly available online platforms, the BAME staff network convened an online meeting to engage with members about the early evidence about COVID-19 and its increased impact on ethnic minority populations. This formed the basis for regular meetings to discuss other areas of interest and concern and has latterly informed the development of the Trust's strategic response to BAME staff support and development.

The BAME shared governance council, comprised mainly of nurses and support staff, spearheaded community engagement activities to understand more fully the concerns of local ethnic minority populations about the impact of the pandemic and associated risks. More recently this has included specific activities to support vaccinations within community settings and role modelling vaccination uptake, using videos and online messaging, to help alleviate fears among staff members of ethnic minority communities. The council has also played a key role in supporting international nursing staff joining the Trust with challenging travel restrictions and requirements for isolation.

The BAME COVID-19 operational group was chaired by the chief people's officer, with representation across professional groups and corporate teams. At weekly meetings, the group defined what data was required to understand the impact of the pandemic on staff absence due to COVID-19, risk assessment compliance for protected characteristics, preparation for vaccination services, and opportunities for engagement with the wider Trust community. These were informed by the BAME staff network and ongoing communication with staff across professional groups and roles.

Priorities identified by staff included key areas of action relating to the following:

(a) *Communication and coproduction*: Trust-related communication was examined and codesigned to ensure equality, diversity, and inclusivity are addressed in messaging and approach. A blended delivery was deemed essential, recognising many clinical and support staff do not have access to email communication during work hours, and that verbal, written, and other forms of online media were required.

(b) *Understanding and influencing the emerging evidence*: A dedicated research engagement event was led by the National Institute for Health Research Biomedical Research Centre (NIHR BRC): Nottingham Digestive Diseases Centre. This was facilitated by the BAME staff network and BAME shared governance council, where current evidence in relation to COVID-19 and ethnic minority populations was shared, and the design of a research study in grant development was informed by over 80 attendees via a mixture of online meeting platform and a socially distanced in-person meeting.

(c) *Workforce data and risk assessment processes*: A locally driven COVID-19 staff risk assessment tool was developed in advance of nationally designed tools, with particular sensitivity to data capture and monitoring at ward, divisional, and organisational level. Weekly meetings examined comparative data for risk assessment completion, sickness and absence, and shielding according to reported ethnic group.

JOANNE COOPER

**ACTIVITY**

The COVID-19 pandemic is a contemporary global crisis. We would like you to take a moment to reflect on how the pandemic has impacted on your health and wellbeing and that of others.

1. What were your own experiences during the COVID-19 pandemic? How has the pandemic made you feel? Note any changes or disruptions that occurred to your work, studies, or home life.

2. How did your peers or colleagues react during that time? What were the impacts for nurses and midwives? Or for other occupational groups?

3. What initiatives did your employer put in place to support the health and wellbeing of nurses and midwives during this crisis? How were they implemented? Or if you are a student, was specific support offered to healthcare students during this time? What was helpful? What could be done differently in the future?

## References

Blake, H., & Bermingham, F. (2020). *Psychological wellbeing for healthcare workers: Mitigating the impact of CO-VID-19*. The University of Nottingham, Nottingham. https://www.nottingham.ac.uk/toolkits/play_22794.

Blake, H., Bermingham, F., Johnson, G., & Tabner, A. (2020a). Mitigating the psychological impact of CO-VID-19 on healthcare workers: A digital learning package. *International Journal of Environmental Research and Public Health, 17*(9), 2997. https://doi.org/10.3390/ijerph17092997.

Blake, H., Gupta, A., Javed, M., et al. (2021a). COVID-well study: Qualitative evaluation of supported wellbeing centres and psychological first aid for healthcare workers during the COVID-19 pandemic. *International Journal of Environmental Research and Public Health, 18*(7), 3626. https://doi.org/10.3390/ijerph18073626.

Blake, H., Mahmood, I., Dushi, G., Yildirim, M., & Gay, E. (2021b). Psychological impacts of COVID-19 on healthcare trainees and perceptions towards a digital wellbeing support package. *International Journal of Environmental Research and Public Health, 18*(20), 10647. https://doi.org/10.3390/ijerph182010647.

Blake, H., Yildirim, M., Wood, B., et al. (2020b). COVID-well: Evaluation of the implementation of supported wellbeing centres for hospital employees during the COVID-19 pandemic. *International Journal of Environmental Research and Public Health, 17*(24), 9401. https://doi.org/10.3390/ijerph17249401.

Godbold, R., Whiting, L., Adams, C., Naidu, Y., & Pattison, N. (2021). The experiences of student nurses in a pandemic: A qualitative study. *Nurse Education in Practice, 56*, 103186. https://doi.org/10.1016/j.nepr.2021.103186.

International Labour Organisation. (2021). *World employment and social outlook: Trends, 2021*. International Labour Office, Geneva. https://www.ilo.org/wcmsp5/groups/public/---dgreports/---dcomm/---publ/documents/publication/wcms_795453.pdf.

Spilsbury, K., Devi, R., Griffiths, A., Akrill, C., Astle, A., Goodman, C., et al. (2021). Seeking answers for care homes during the COVID-19 pandemic (COVID SEARCH). *Age Ageing, 50*(2), 335–340.

The Kings Fund. (2021). *NHS workforce: Our position*. https://www.kingsfund.org.uk/projects/positions/nhs-workforce.

## CHAPTER 23

# The Future of Health and Well-Being at Work

Holly Blake  ■  Gemma Stacey

## Introduction

Is health and well-being important for nurses and midwives? Have you ever wished you were healthier, happier, or better supported? What is the impact of this on how you feel and how you do your job? Can health care organisations survive without a healthy and happy workforce? What does 'getting it right' look like?

The aim of this text was to provide practical and accessible guidance to nurses and midwives on managing their well-being at work. So, what have we learned, and where do we go next?

## Moving On From Here

There is no doubt that fostering a healthy and happy workforce is good for everyone. Employers have a duty of care to protect the health and well-being of their employees, and globally, employee wellness is becoming a hot topic that is high on many organisational agendas.

Promoting and supporting well-being at work makes good business sense (Hassard et al., 2021) because there is growing evidence that healthy and happy employees are less likely to take time off work and are more likely to feel valued, motivated, engaged, and productive at work. As with any area of health, prevention is better than cure. Reactive approaches are essential for managing issues arising from ill health. Examples include sickness absence management, occupational health services, and employee assistance programmes, which are confidential counselling services offered by employers to their employees to support their well-being in the workplace and in their personal lives. Rates of sickness absence and presenteeism (coming to work when unwell) are higher in nurses and midwives than other professions (Taylor et al., 2022).

Reactive approaches play a vital role, but there is evidence to suggest that preventative approaches offer a greater return on investment. That is, the gains from preventative initiatives are higher than the costs of doing it, and the gains of prevention are more than gains generated from reactive approaches. Preventative approaches might include health and well-being awareness raising, educational initiatives, leadership and line manager training, review of organisational policies, workloads and structures, risk assessments, coaching, mentoring, and health promotion programmes, incorporating physical and mental health and well-being. Research shows that there is a link between pre-registered nurses' and midwives' own health (ie., body composition, diet) and their attitudes towards, and confidence in, health promotion practice (Blake et al., 2021). So, promoting health may have implications for care provision. Workplace health promotion programmes in healthcare settings can be beneficial (Blake et al., 2013; Blake & Lloyd, 2008). Promoting healthy behaviours such as diet or exercise and delivering workplace interventions to reduce stress can have positive outcomes for nurses (Stanulewicz et al., 2019). However, initiatives to promote wellbeing need to go beyond individually targeted programmes and look to the complex issues within organisations that influence wellbeing, like job design, teams, and work environment.

There is no a one-size-fits-all approach to employee well-being, and strategies should be targeted to the organisation and the needs of the workforce, across job role, levels of experience, cultures, and communities. The health and care workforce is diverse. It is made up of multiple races, ages, genders, ethnicities, and orientations. Recognising this diversity and creating equality of opportunity for nurses and midwives will help everyone in the workforce to achieve their full potential, deliver a more inclusive and compassionate service, and ultimately improve the care of patients or services users. Indeed, research has identified that staff wellbeing is linked to staff-reported care performance, and patient-reported patient experience (Maben et al., 2012). This is further 'food for thought', in terms of recognising the knock-on effects of poor wellbeing at work.

The success of health and well-being strategies depends critically on organisational culture, which refers to the shared values, expectations, and practices that guide and inform the actions of all team members. This could mean a clear prioritisation of the workforce, a robust organisational framework that supports employee well-being, a culture where people can speak openly. Knowing how to have conversations with people about their mental wellbeing is important for establishing and maintain an open culture around wellbeing. The buy-in of senior leaders is vital for setting the precedent for a healthy workforce from the top down. Our leaders should champion health and well-being and take action when it is needed. There are many ways this can be achieved, but research shows us that, when it is done well, providing staff with a safe, reflective and confidential space to talk and support one another can increase empathy and compassion for colleagues and patients and lead to positive changes in practice (Maben et al., 2021).

Through this book we have taken you on a journey, starting with the business case for why organisations should invest in the health and well-being of their workforce and embed well-being into their organisational policies and practice. We introduced some key areas of health and well-being and provided strategies for the actions we can take to maximise physical and mental health and support the well-being of ourselves and others. We have discussed health and well-being in the specific context of the nursing and midwifery roles across the whole professional career, even through the most challenging of times, such as a global public health crisis. At all times, we have asked you to think more about the issues raised in our chapters by engaging with activities involving reflecting or planning. Through our case studies we want to inspire you by showcasing innovations implemented by individuals, teams, or organisations across the health and care sector.

So, how can you use this information to make a difference where you work or study? Individual people are not just passive recipients of health and well-being initiatives. YOU play a key role (either now or in the future) in creating and sustaining environments where people feel supported and can flourish. Environments that foster well-being are needed right from the early days, transitioning through higher education and into nursing and midwifery roles, throughout the whole career pathway. What have you learned? Will you seek out help when you need it? How can you help others? What can you do to advocate well-being and improve the work environment for your peers, patients, and clients?

In short, health and well-being at work should no longer be viewed as nice to have, but as an organisational priority across the public, private, and third sectors. A workforce health and well-being strategy is essential to fostering an organisational culture that allows employees and employers to thrive.

### References

Blake, H., Watkins, K., Middleton, M., & Stanulewicz, N. (2021). Obesity and diet predict attitudes towards health promotion in pre-registered nurses and midwives. *Int J Environ Res Public Health*, *18*(24), 13419.

Hassard, J., Teoh, K., Thomson, L., & Blake, H. (2021). Understanding the cost of mental health at work: an integrative framework. In T. Wall, C. Cooper, & P. Brough (Eds.), *The SAGE Handbook of Organisational Wellbeing (9–25)*. SAGE Publications Ltd. https://dx.doi.org/10.4135/9781529757187.n2.

Maben, J., Taylor, C., Reynolds, E., McCarthy, I., & Leamy, M. (2021). Realist evaluation of schwartz rounds® for enhancing the delivery of compassionate healthcare: Understanding how they work, for whom, and in what contexts. *BMC Health Serv Res, 21*, 709.

Maben, J., Peccei, R., Adams, M., Robert, G., Richardson, A., Murrells, T., et al. (2012). *Exploring the relationship between patients' experiences of care and the influence of staff motivation, affect and wellbeingNIHR Service Delivery and Organisation programme.* Final report https://njl-admin.nihr.ac.uk/document/download/2008618.

Stanulewicz, N., Knox, E., Narayanasamy, M., Shivji, N., Khunti, K., & Blake, H. (2019). Effectiveness of lifestyle health promotion interventions for nurses: A systematic review. *Int J Environ Res Public Health, 17*(1), 17.

Taylor, C., Mattick, K., Carrieri, D., Cox, A., & Maben, J. (2022). 'The WOW factors': Comparing workforce organization and well-being for doctors, nurses, midwives and paramedics in England. *British Medical Bulletin, 141*(1), 60–79.

*Note*: Page numbers followed by *f* indicate figures and *t* indicate tables.

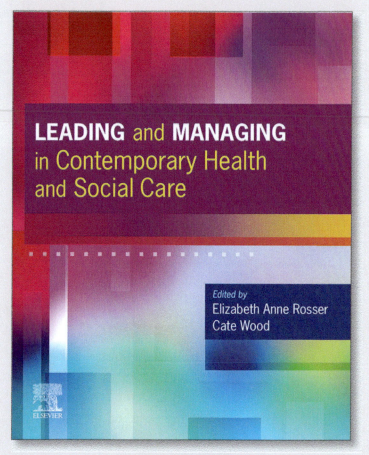

CPI Antony Rowe
Eastbourne, UK
February 12, 2024

# Contributors

**Rashid Ali**
School of Intelligent Mechatronics Engineering, Sejong University, Seoul, Republic of Korea

**Majed Alsadhan**
Department of Computer Science, Kansas State University, Manhattan, KS, United States

**Emmanuel Ayodele**
School of Electronic and Electrical Engineering, University of Leeds, Leeds, United Kingdom

**Praveen Chakravarthy Bhallamudi**
Lumirack Solutions, Chennai, India

**Dilip Kumar Choubey**
Department of Computer Science & Engineering, Indian Institute of Information Technology, Bhagalpur, India

**Giuseppe Ciaburro**
Department of Architecture and Industrial Design, Università degli Studi della Campania Luigi Vanvitelli, Aversa, Italy

**Anup Das**
Electrical and Computer Engineering, Drexel University, Philadelphia, PA, United States

**Apurba Das**
Department of CSE, PES University; Computer Vision (IoT), Tata Consultancy Services, Bangalore, India

**Jaydeep Das**
Advanced Technology Development Center, Indian Institute of Technology Kharagpur, West Bengal, India

**Parneeta Dhaliwal**
Department of Computer Science and Technology, Manav Rachna University, Faridabad, India

**Haytham Elmiligi**
Computing Science Department, Thompson Rivers University, Kamloops, BC, Canada

**Ahmed A. Ewees**
Department of Computer, Damietta University, Damietta, Egypt; Department of e-Systems, University of Bisha, Bisha, Saudi Arabia

**O.K. Fasil**
Department of Computer Science, Central University of Kerala, Kerala, India

**Marwa A. Gaheen**
Department of Computer, Damietta University, Damietta, Egypt

**Pardeep Garg**
Department of Electronics and Communication Engineering, Jaypee University of Information Technology, Solan, India

**Isel Grau**
Artificial Intelligence Lab, Free University of Brussels (VUB), Brussels, Belgium

**Rahul Gupta**
National Institute of Technology, Hamirpur, Himachal Pradesh, India

**Sunil Kumar Hota**
DIHAR, Defense Research & Development Organization, Leh, Jammu & Kashmir, India

**William H. Hsu**
Department of Computer Science, Kansas State University, Manhattan, KS, United States

**Enas Ibrahim**
Department of Computer, Damietta University, Damietta, Egypt

**Muhammad Taimoor Khan**
Medical Department, University of Debrecen, Debrecen, Hungary

**Sung Won Kim**
Department of Information and Communication Engineering, Yeungnam University, Gyeongsan, Republic of Korea

**Dipesh Kumar**
Department of ECE, IIT(ISM), Dhanbad, India

**Vijay Kumar**
National Institute of Technology, Hamirpur, Himachal Pradesh, India

**Yugal Kumar**
Department of CSE & IT, JUIT, Solan, Himachal Pradesh, India

**Seshadri Sastry Kunapuli**
Xinthe Technologies PVT LTD, Visakhapatnam, India

**Deepti Lamba**
Department of Computer Science, Kansas State University, Manhattan, KS, United States

**Theodore V. Maliamanis**
HUman-MAchines INteraction Laboratory (HUMAIN-Lab), Department of Computer Science, International Hellenic University, Kavala, Greece

**Nirupama Mandal**
Department of ECE, IIT(ISM), Dhanbad, India

**Des McLernon**
School of Electronic and Electrical Engineering, University of Leeds, Leeds, United Kingdom

**Pradeep Kumar Naik**
School of Life Sciences, Sambalpur University, Sambalpur, Orissa, India

**Ali Nauman**
Department of Information and Communication Engineering, Yeungnam University, Gyeongsan, Republic of Korea

**Muhammad Hassan Nawaz**
Electrical Engineering Department, University of Debrecen, Debrecen, Hungary

**Ann Nowe**
Artificial Intelligence Lab, Free University of Brussels (VUB), Brussels, Belgium

**George A. Papakostas**
HUman-MAchines INteraction Laboratory (HUMAIN-Lab), Department of Computer Science, International Hellenic University, Kavala, Greece

**Advika Parthvi**
School of Computer Science and Engineering, Vellore Institute of Technology, Vellore, Tamil Nadu, India

**Yazdan Ahmad Qadri**
Department of Information and Communication Engineering, Yeungnam University, Gyeongsan, Republic of Korea

**Rakesh Raja**
Department of Computer Science and Engineering, Birla Institute of Technology, Mesra, Ranchi, India

**R. Rajesh**
Department of Computer Science, Central University of Kerala, Kerala, India

**Kartik Rawal**
School of Computer Science and Engineering, Vellore Institute of Technology, Vellore, Tamil Nadu, India

**Riya Sapra**
Department of Computer Science and Technology, Manav Rachna University, Faridabad, India

**Bikash Kanti Sarkar**
Department of Computer Science and Engineering, Birla Institute of Technology, Mesra, Ranchi, India

**Jane Scott**
School of Architecture, Planning and Landscape, Newcastle University, Newcastle, United Kingdom

**Dipankar Sengupta**
PGJCCR, Queens University Belfast, Belfast, United Kingdom; Artificial Intelligence Lab, Free University of Brussels (VUB), Brussels, Belgium

**Isha Sharma**
National Institute of Technology, Hamirpur, Himachal Pradesh, India

**Sunil Datt Sharma**
Department of Electronics and Communication Engineering, Jaypee University of Information Technology, Solan, India

**Vijay Kumar Sharma**
DIHAR, Defense Research & Development Organization, Leh, Jammu & Kashmir, India

**Rohit Shukla**
Department of Biotechnology and Bioinformatics, Jaypee University of Information Technology (JUIT), Solan, Himachal Pradesh, India

**Vaibhav Shukla**
Tech Mahindra Ltd., Mumbai, Maharastra, India

**S.S. Shylaja**
Department of CSE, PES University, Bangalore, India

**Tiratha Raj Singh**
Centre of Excellence in Healthcare Technologies and Informatics (CHETI), Department of Biotechnology and Bioinformatics, Jaypee University of Information Technology (JUIT), Solan, Himachal Pradesh, India

**Ravi B. Srivastava**
DIHAR, Defense Research & Development Organization, Leh, Jammu & Kashmir, India

**Wenhan Tan**
Electrical and Computer Engineering, Drexel University, Philadelphia, PA, United States

**Abdalrahman Tawhid**
Computing Science Department, Thompson Rivers University, Kamloops, BC, Canada

**Tanya Teotia**
Computing Science Department, Thompson Rivers University, Kamloops, BC, Canada

**Arvind Kumar Yadav**
Department of Biotechnology and Bioinformatics, Jaypee University of Information Technology (JUIT), Solan, Himachal Pradesh, India

**Syed Ali Raza Zaidi**
School of Electronic and Electrical Engineering, University of Leeds, Leeds, United Kingdom

**Zhiqiang Zhang**
School of Electronic and Electrical Engineering, University of Leeds, Leeds, United Kingdom

# Preface

Medical informatics, also known as healthcare analytics, is a useful tool that can assess and monitor health-related behavior and conditions of individuals outside the clinic. The benefits of medical informatics are significant, including improving life expectancy, disease diagnosis, and quality of life. In many individual situations, a patient requires continuous monitoring to identify the onset of possible life-threatening conditions or to diagnose potentially dangerous diseases. Traditional healthcare systems fall short in this regard.

Meanwhile, rapid growth and advances have occurred in the digitization of information, retrieval systems, and wearable devices and sensors. Our times demand the design and development of new effective prediction systems using machine learning approaches, big data, and the Internet of Things (IoT) to meet health and life quality expectations. Furthermore, there is a need for monitoring systems that can monitor the health issues of elderly and remotely located people. In recent times, big data and IoT have played a vital role in health-related applications, mainly in disease identification and diagnosis. These techniques can provide possible solutions for healthcare analytics, in which both structured and unstructured data are collected through IoT-based devices and sensors. Machine learning and big data techniques can be applied to collected data for predictive diagnostic systems. However, designing and developing an effective diagnostic system is still challenging due to various issues like security, usability, scalability, privacy, development standards, and technologies. Therefore machine learning, big data, and IoT for medical informatics are becoming emerging research areas for the healthcare community.

## Outline of the book and chapter synopses

This book presents state-of-the-art intelligent techniques and approaches, design, development, and innovative uses of machine learning, big data, and IoT for demanding applications of medical informatics. This book also focuses on different data collection methods from IoT-based systems and sensors, as well as preprocessing and privacy preservation of medical data. We have provided potential thoughts and methodologies to help senior undergraduate and graduate students, researchers, programmers, and healthcare industry professionals create new knowledge for the future to develop intelligent machine learning, big data, and IoT-based novel approaches for medical informatics applications. Further, the key roles and great importance of machine learning, big data, and IoT techniques as mathematical tools are elaborated in the book. A brief and orderly introduction to the chapters is provided in the following paragraphs. The book contains 23 chapters.

Chapter 1 presents a survey of machine learning and predictive analytics methods for medical informatics. This chapter focuses on deep neural networks with typical use cases in computational medicine, including self-supervised learning scenarios: these include convolutional neural networks for image analysis, recurrent neural networks for time series, and generative adversarial models for correction of class imbalance in differential diagnosis and anomaly detection. The authors then continue by assessing salient connections between the current state of machine learning research and data-centric healthcare analytics, focusing specifically on diagnostic imaging and multisensor integration as crucial research topics within predictive analytics. Finally, they conclude by relating open problems of machine learning for prediction-based medical informatics surveyed in this article to the impact of big data and its associated challenges, trends, and limitations of current work, including privacy and security of sensitive patient data.

Chapter 2 presents a proposed model for geolocation aware healthcare facility with IoT, Fog, and Cloud-based diagnosis in emergency cases. An end-to-end infrastructure has been modeled for the healthcare system using geolocation-enabled IoT, fog, and cloud computing technology to identify the nearest hospital or medical facility available to the patient. It has also achieved 25%–27% less delay and 27%–29% less power consumption than the cloud-only environment.

Chapter 3 aims to capture the status of medical computer vision threats and the recent defensive techniques proposed by researchers. This chapter intends to shed light on the vulnerability of machine learning models in medical image analysis, e.g., disease diagnosis, and to become a guide for any researcher working in medical image analysis toward the development of more secure machine learning-based computer-aided diagnosis systems.

Chapter 4 demonstrates a model for skull stripping and tumor detection from brain images using 3D U-Net. The demonstrated model has been tested over 373 MRIs of the LCG Segmentation Dataset, showing good standard performance over metrics of dice coefficient, and the accuracy results are competitive with the existing methods.

Chapter 5 addresses the issue of corrupted laparoscopy video by haze, noise, oversaturated illumination, etc., in minimally invasive surgery. To effectively address the issue, the authors have proposed a novel algorithm to ensure the enhancement of video with faster performance. The proposed $C^2D^2A$ (Cross Color Dominant Deep Autoencoder) uses the strength of (a) a bilateral filter, which addresses the one-shot filtering of images both in the spatial neighborhood domain and psycho-visual range; and (b) a deep autoencoder, which can learn salient patterns. The domain-based color sparseness has further improved the performance, modulating the classical deep autoencoder to a color dominant deep autoencoder. The work has shown promise toward providing a generic framework of quality enhancement of video streams and addressing performance. This, in turn, improves the image/video analytics like segmentation, detection, and tracking the objects or regions of interest.

Chapter 6 presents an alternative way of estimating respiratory rate from ECG and PPG by using machine learning to improve estimation accuracy. The proposed methods are based on respiratory signals extracted from raw signals and use a support vector machine (SVM) and neural network (NN) to estimate respiratory rate. The proposed methods achieve comparable accuracy to current methods when the number of classes is low. Once the number of classes increases, the accuracy drops significantly.

Chapter 7 serves as an introductory guideline to address the challenges and opportunities while designing machine learning-enabled Healthcare Internet of Things (H-IoT) networks. It provides a discussion on traditional H-IoT, challenges, and opportunities in the Network 2030 paradigm. It also discusses potential machine learning techniques compatible with H-IoT and points out open issues and future research directions.

Chapter 8 presents a skin lesion segmentation approach based on the Elitist-Jaya optimization algorithm. The proposed method contains two stages: image preprocessing and edge detection. The experimental sample consists of a set of 320 images from the skin lesion dataset. The outcomes proved that the proposed approach improved the segmentation accuracy of the affected skin lesion area and outperformed the compared methods.

Chapter 9 provides its readers with an all-encompassing review that will enable a clear understanding of the current trends in glove-based gesture classification and provide new ideas for further research. The authors have analyzed deep learning approaches in terms of their current performance, advantages over classical machine learning algorithms, and limitations in specific classification scenarios. Furthermore, they present other deep learning approaches that may outperform current algorithms in glove-based gesture classification.

Chapter 10 presents an ensemble approach for evaluating the cognitive performance of the human population at high altitude. The authors identify the key multidomain cognitive screening test (MDCST) and clinical features among the lowlander ($\leq 350$ m) and highlander ($\geq 1500$ but $<4300$ m) populations, staying at an altitude $\geq 4300$ m for a prolonged duration. A goodness-of-fit test was applied to the two population cohorts for identifying significant independent measures. Rule-based mining was followed to discover associative rules between the clinical, behavioral, and cognitive screening parameters. Conclusively, a unique set of association rules have been identified with at least 30% support and more than 60% confidence in behavioral and clinical features associated with the cognitive parameters.

Chapter 11 presents the role of machine learning in expert systems for disease diagnostics in human healthcare. The authors discuss essential existing expert systems for human disease diagnosis in detail. They also provide a brief evaluation of various techniques used for the development of expert systems.

Chapter 12 presents an entropy-based hybrid feature selection approach for medical datasets. A stable linear-time entropy-based ensembled feature selection approach is introduced, mainly focusing on medical datasets of several sizes. The suggested approach is validated using three state-of-the-art classifiers, namely C4.5, naïve Bayes, and JRIP, over 14 benchmark medical datasets (drawn from the UCI machine learning repository). The empirical results achieved from the datasets demonstrate that the proposed ensemble model outperforms the selected learners.

Chapter 13 shows how to utilize machine learning algorithms to create models that can predict healthcare systems' critical issues. The chapter's discussion relates to the COVID-19 pandemic and highlights the solutions offered by machine learning in such scenarios. The chapter also highlights the significance of feature engineering and its impact on machine learning models' accuracy. The chapter ends with two case studies. The first case study shows how to build a prediction model that can predict the number of diabetic patients who will visit certain hospitals in a specific geographic location in future years. The second case study analyzes health records during the COVID-19 pandemic.

Chapter 14 presents an interpretable semisupervised classifier for predicting cancer stages. Authors illustrate the self-labeling gray-box applications on the omics and clinical datasets from the cancer genome atlas. They show that the self-labeling gray-box is accurate in predicting cancer stages of rare cancers by leveraging the unlabeled instances from more common cancer types. They discuss insights, the features influencing prediction, and a global representation of the knowledge through decision trees or rule lists, which can aid clinicians and researchers.

Chapter 15 presents an overview of applications of blockchain technology in smart healthcare. The authors overviewed the fundamental blockchain concepts and applications to be used for different aspects of the smart healthcare industry and proposed a live patient monitoring system by deploying blockchain technology in the model. Keeping an eye on recent technologies in connected healthcare, they finally presented various research factors and potential challenges where blockchain technologies can play an outstanding role in realizing the concept of smart optimization in the healthcare industry.

Chapter 16 focuses on clustering and classification techniques for the prediction of leukemia. The proposed work consists of Phase I, which will be dealing with the collection of datasets and visualization of datasets, whereas Phase II will be dealing with the machine learning and data mining techniques for the prediction of leukemia disease. The authors claim that the proposed techniques would give higher performance than the existing techniques.

Chapter 17 presents a performance evaluation of fractal features toward seizure detection from electroencephalogram signals. The authors have evaluated the ability of three well-known fractal dimension feature extraction methods (the Katz fractal dimension, Higuchi fractal dimension, and Petrosian fractal dimension) to classify epileptic and nonepileptic electroencephalogram signals. The features are fed to an SVM classifier for the classification of epileptic and nonepileptic electroencephalogram signals. The SVM classifier results show that the fractal features are good measures to characterize the complex information of epileptic signals.

Chapter 18 presents an integer period discrete Fourier transform-based algorithm to identify tandem repeats in the DNA sequences. The authors have discussed the importance of tandem repeats in diverse applications. They proposed an integer period discrete Fourier transform (IPDFT)-based algorithm to detect the tandem repeats in DNA sequences. A comparison of the proposed algorithm's performance has also been made with existing methods.

Chapter 19 discusses the scope, applicability, and usage of blockchain technology to preserve patients' sensitive medical data. A framework is also proposed that allows patients and hospitals to store medical records. The framework allows patients to share the information by providing access to their data and by invoking smart contracts for automatic payments for their medical claims.

Chapter 20 presents a novel approach to securing e-health applications in the cloud environment. The authors provide an algorithm to secure data in e-health applications in the cloud environment. A new architecture for e-health applications in the cloud environment is proposed, which will provide application-level security and server-level security using certificates.

Chapter 21 presents different ensemble learning algorithms and explains how these algorithms can be used to classify health disorders. The authors have discussed an ensemble classifier approach for thyroid disease diagnosis using the AdaBoostM algorithm.

Chapter 22 presents a review of the latest artificial intelligence research in this immense medical science field, including various architectures and approaches, with special attention given to brain tumor analysis. The authors discuss various deep learning architectures used to diagnose brain tumors and compare results with existing architectures. They have examined case studies from basic clustering techniques such as K-means clustering to fuzzy and neurotrophic C-means clustering techniques and kernel graph cuts (KGC) to advanced artificial intelligence techniques such as deep convolution neural networks (DCNs), atrous convolution neural networks (ACNs), and unit architectures to find the area of interest in the coherent/incoherent regions.

Finally, Chapter 23 focuses on machine learning in precision medicine. An overview of how machine learning is used in precision medicine and its potential use in the detection, diagnosis, prognosis, risk assessment, therapy response, and discovery of new biomarkers and drug candidates is presented in this chapter.

We especially thank the Intelligent Data-Centric Systems: Sensor Collected Intelligence Series Editor, Prof. Fatos Xhafa, for his continuous support and insightful guidance.

We would also like to thank the publishers at Elsevier, in particular, Chiara Giglio, Editorial Project Manager, and Sonnini Ruiz Yura, Acquisitions Editor–Biomedical Engineering, for their helpful guidance and encouragement during this book's creation.

We are sincerely thankful to all authors, editors, and publishers whose works have been cited directly/indirectly in this manuscript.

## Special acknowledgments

The first editor gratefully acknowledges the authorities of the Jaypee University of Information Technology, Waknaghat, Solan, Himachal Pradesh, India, for their kind support for this book.

The second editor gratefully acknowledges the authorities of the Jaypee University of Information Technology, Waknaghat, Solan, Himachal Pradesh, India, for their kind support for this book.

The third editor would like to acknowledge the Natural Sciences and Engineering Research Council of Canada and Thompson River University, Kamloops, Canada, for their kind support of his research on this book.

**Dr. Pardeep Kumar**
Solan, India

**Dr. Yugal Kumar**
Solan, India

**Dr. Mohammad A. Tawhid**
Kamloops, BC, Canada

# Predictive analytics and machine learning for medical informatics: A survey of tasks and techniques

**Deepti Lamba, William H. Hsu, and Majed Alsadhan**

*Department of Computer Science, Kansas State University, Manhattan, KS, United States*

## Chapter outline

Machine Learning, Big Data, and IoT for Medical Informatics. https://doi.org/10.1016/B978-0-12-821777-1.00023-9

# 1 Introduction: Predictive analytics for medical informatics

*Medical informatics* is a broad domain at the intersection of technology and health care which aims to (1) make medical data of patients available to them and to healthcare providers, thus enabling them to make timely medical decisions; and (2) manage this data for educational and research purposes. According to Morris Collen, the first articles on medical informatics appeared in the 1950s (Collen, 1986). However, it was first identified as a new specialty in the 1970s (Hasman et al., 2014).

This section surveys goals, the state of practice, and specific task definitions for machine learning in medical fields and the practice of health care. These sectors produce an enormous amount of data which is highly complex and comes from heterogeneous sources: electronic health records (EHRs) (Thakkar and Davis, 2006), medical equipment and devices, wearable technologies, handwritten notes, lab results, prescriptions, and clinical information. The application of predictive analytics to this data offers potential benefits such as improved standards of care for patients, lower medical costs, and higher resultant patient satisfaction with healthcare providers.

## 1.1 Overview: Goals of machine learning

*Predictive analytics* is a branch of data science that applies various techniques including statistical inference, machine learning, data mining, and information visualization toward the ultimate goal of forecasting, modeling, and understanding the future behavior of a system based on historical and/or real-time data. This chapter focuses on machine learning (Samuel, 1959; Jordan and Mitchell, 2015) algorithms for building predictive models. In addition, we will survey applications of machine learning to automation and computer vision, especially image classification, which in some medical domains has achieved accuracy comparable to that of a human expert (Esteva et al., 2017). Sidey-Gibbons and Sidey-Gibbons (2019) provided an introduction to machine learning using a publicly available data set for cancer diagnosis. In recent years, deep learning (LeCun et al., 2015; Goodfellow et al., 2016) has attained technical success and scientific attention in application domains including medicine (Miotto et al., 2018) and health care (Kwak and Hui, 2019). Deep neural networks such as convolutional neural nets (*ConvNets* or *CNNs*) have become the predominant state-of-the-art method for analysis of images such as magnetic resonance imaging (MRI) scans, to predict diseases such as Alzheimer's disease (Liu et al., 2014).

Deep learning models face several challenges in medical domains which hinder their acceptability to the medical community—temporality of data, domain complexity, and lack of interpretability (Miotto et al., 2018). According to Miotto et al. (2018), the most used deep architectures in the health domain, briefly discussed in Section 3, include recurrent neural networks (RNNs) (Schuster and Paliwal, 1997), ConvNets (Lawrence et al., 1997), restricted Boltzmann machines (Nair and Hinton, 2010; Fischer and Igel, 2012), autoencoders (Baldi, 2012; Baxter, 1995), and variations thereof. This chapter focuses on five tasks of medical informatics: differential diagnosis (Sajda, 2006), prediction (Chen and Asch, 2017), therapy recommendation (Gräßer et al., 2017), automation of treatment (Mayer et al., 2008a), and analytics in integrative medicine (Kawanabe et al., 2016).

## 1.2 Current state of practice

A trend forecast study (Healthcare, 2021) published by the Society of Actuaries indicates a growing usage of predictive analytics for health care. In 2019, 60% of healthcare organizations were already using predictive analytics, and 20% indicated that they would be using the same in the following year. Among those that currently use predictive analytics, 39% reported a decrease in healthcare costs and 42% improvement in patient satisfaction. These statistics demonstrate the interest of organizations in using predictive analytics in medical domain for improving their services.

## 1.3 Key task definitions

This section provides an overview of machine learning goals in health informatics. The goals of prediction are introduced in Section 1.1.

### 1.3.1 Diagnosis

*Differential diagnosis* is defined as the process of differentiating between probability of one disease versus that of other diseases with similar symptoms that could possibly account for illness in a patient. A technical series published by World Health Organization (WHO) in 2016 states that the most important task performed by primary care providers is diagnosis (World Health Organization, 2016). Machine learning tools have been used primarily for disease diagnosis throughout the history of medical informatics. Graber et al. (2005) conducted a study to determine the causes of diagnostic errors and to develop a comprehensive taxonomy for the classification of these errors.

Miller (1994) provided a representative bibliography of the state of the art and history of medical diagnostic decision support systems (MDDSS) at the time. These systems can be divided into several subcategories, among which expert systems have been used most often (Shortliffe et al., 1979). Many of the earliest rule-based expert systems (Giarratano and Riley, 1998) were developed for medical diagnosis. Shortliffe (1986) gave insights into the design of expert systems for diagnostic medicine developed during the 1970s and 1980s, including: (1) MYCIN (Shortliffe and Buchanan, 1985; Shortliffe, 2012), which focused on infectious diseases; (2) INTERNIST-1 (Miller et al., 1982); (3) QMR (Miller and Masarie, 1989; Rassinoux et al., 1996); (4) DXplain (Barnett et al., 1987; mghlcs, n.d.; Bartold and Hannigan, 2002), a diagnostic decision support system developed continuously between 1986 and the early 2000s.

The most prominent limitation of expert systems was the acquisition of knowledge (Gaines, 2013) or building a knowledge base, which is both, time-consuming and a complex process that requires access to expert domain knowledge. In addition, updating the knowledge base requires significant human effort. These systems were usually designed to support users with an expert level of medical knowledge. A more recent review of expert systems is presented by Abu-Nasser (2017). Expert systems are still around but their limitations led to advances in rule learning and classification for differential diagnosis. Salman and Abu-Naser (2020) developed a diagnostic system for COVID-19 using medical websites for the knowledge base. COVID-19 is a novel viral disease that has affected millions of people around the world. The system was tested by a group of doctors and they were satisfied with its performance and ease of use. Another expert system for COVID-19 was built by Almadhoun and Abu-Naser (2020) for helping patients determine if they have been infected with COVID-19. The system gives instructions to the user based on the symptoms. The knowledge base was compiled using medical sites such as NHS Trust.

Kononenko (2001) provided an historical overview of ML methods used in medical domain and a discussion about state-of-the-art algorithms: Assistant-R and Assistant-I (Kononenko and Simec, 1995), lookahead feature construction (Ragavan and Rendell, 1993), naïve Bayesian classifier (Rish et al., 2001), seminaïve Bayesian classifier (Kononenko, 1991), k-nearest neighbors (k-NN) (Dudani, 1976), and back propagation with weight elimination (Weigend et al., 1991). The paper's experimental findings show that most classifiers have a comparable performance which makes model explainability a deciding factor behind the choice of classifier.

### 1.3.2 Predictive analytics

*Prognosis* is defined as a forecast of the probable course and/or outcome of a disease. It is an important task in clinical patient management. Cruz and Wishart (2006) outlined the focal predictive tasks of prognosis/predictions for cancer. Based on these predictive tasks, the general definition of the prognosis task comprises these variants: (1) prediction of disease susceptibility (or likelihood of developing any disease prior to the actual occurrence of the disease); (2) prediction of disease recurrence (or predicting the likelihood of redeveloping the disease after its resolution); and (3) prediction of survivability (or predicting an outcome after the diagnosis of the disease in terms of life expectancy, survivability, disease progression, etc.).

Ohno-Machado (2001) defined prognosis as "an estimate of cure, complication, recurrence of disease, level of function, length of stay in healthcare facilities, or survival for a patient." The author focused on techniques that are used to model prognosis—especially the *survival analysis methods*. A detailed discussion of survival analysis methods is beyond the scope of this chapter. We refer the interested readers to the book (Cantor et al., 2003) and a review of survival analysis techniques (Prinja et al., 2010). Prognostic tasks are categorized as (1) prediction for a single point in time and (2) time-related predictions. Methods used to build prognostic models include Cox proportional hazards (Cox and Oakes, 1984), logistic regression (LR) (Kleinbaum et al., 2002), and neural networks (Hassoun et al., 1995).

Mendez-Tellez and Dorman (2005) published an article that states that intensive care units (ICUs) have increased the critical care being provided to injured or critically ill patients. However, the costs for the ICU treatments are very high, which has given rise to prediction models, which are classified as disease-specific or generic models. These systems work by employing a scoring system that assigns points according to illness severity and then generate a probability estimate as an outcome of the model. We do not discuss scoring systems in this chapter. We refer the interested reader to a compendium of scoring systems for outcome distributions (Rapsang and Shyam, 2014). A few of the outcome prediction models used for intensive care predictions include Mortality Probability Model II (Lemeshow et al., 1993), Simplified Acute Physiology Score (SAPS) II (Le Gall et al., 1993), Acute Physiology and Chronic Health Evaluation (APACHE) II (Knaus et al., 1985), and APACHE III (Knaus et al., 1991). These systems build LR models to predict hospital mortality by using a set of clinical and physiology variables.

Another important application of learning is cancer prognosis and prediction. Early diagnosis and prognosis of any life-threatening disease, especially cancer, presents crucial real-time requirements and poses research challenges. Machine learning is being used to build classification models for categorization of cases by risk level. This is essential for clinical management of cancer patients. Kourou et al. (2015) reviewed methods that have been used to model the progression of cancer. The methods used for this task include artificial neural networks (ANNs) (Hassoun et al., 1995) and decision trees (Brodley and Utgoff, 1995), which have been used for three decades for cancer detection. The authors also noticed a growing trend of using methods such as support vector machines (SVMs) (Suykens and Vandewalle, 1999; Vapnik, 2013) and Bayesian networks (BN) (Friedman et al., 1997) for cancer prediction and prognosis.

### 1.3.3 Therapy recommendation

A classic example of a machine learning application is a recommender system (Portugal et al., 2018; Melville and Sindhwani, 2010). *Recommender systems* are widely used to recommend items, services, merchandise, and users to each other based on similarity. However, the use of recommender systems in health and medical domain has not been widespread. The earliest article on recommender system in health is from the year 2007 and by 2016 only 17 articles were found for the query "recommender system health" in web of science (Valdez et al., 2016).

Valdez et al. (2016) argued that the lack of popularity of recommender systems in the medical domain is due to several reasons: (1) the benchmarking criteria in medical scenarios, (2) domain complexity, (3) the different end-user groups. The end users or target users for recommender systems can be patients, medical professionals, or people who are healthy. Recommender systems can be designed to recommend therapies, sports or physical activities, medication, diagnosis, or even food or other nutritional information. This chapter also outlines major challenges faced by recommender systems in the medical domain. Challenges include a lack of clear task definition for recommender systems in the health domain. The definition depends on the target user and the item being recommended.

Wiesner and Pfeifer (2014) proposed a health recommender system (HRS) that recommend relevant medical information to the patient by using the graphical user interface of the personal health record (PHR) (Tang et al., 2006). The HRS uses the PHR to build a user profile and the authors argued that collaborative filtering is an appropriate approach for building such a system.

Gräßer et al. (2017) proposed two methods for recommending therapies for patients suffering from psoriasis: a collaborative recommender and a hybrid demographic-recommender. The two are compared and combined to form an ensemble of recommender systems in order to combat drawbacks of the individual systems. The data for the experiments were acquired from University Hospital Dresden. Collaborative filtering (Sarwar et al., 2001; Su and Khoshgftaar, 2009) is applied, where therapies are items and therapy responses are treated as user preferences.

Stark et al. (2019) presented a systematic literature review on recommender systems in medicine that covers existing systems and compares them on the basis of various features. Some interesting finds from the review include the following observations: (1) most studies attempt to develop the general-purpose recommender systems (i.e., one system for all diseases); (2) disease-specific systems focus on drug recommendation for diabetes. The review points to several future research directions that include building a recommender system for recommending dosage of medicine and finding highly scalable solutions. Recommender systems can be used to suggest drugs for treatment. A popular commercial solution is IBM's AI machine Watson Health (IBM Watson AI Healthcare Solutions, 2021), which is used by healthcare providers and researchers to make suitable decisions about providing treatment to patients based on insights from the system.

### 1.3.4 Automation of treatment

In surgical area, research focus has been on automating tasks such as surgical suturing, implantation, and biopsy procedures. Taylor et al. (2016) presented a broad overview of medical robot systems within the context of computer integrated surgery. This article also provides a high-level classification of such systems: (1) surgical CAD/CAM systems and (2) surgical assistants. The former refers to the process of preoperative planning involving the analysis of medical images and other patient information to produce a model of the patient. This article presents examples of both kinds of robotic systems.

Mayer et al. (2008b) developed an experimental system for automating recurring tasks in minimal invasive surgery by extending the learning by demonstration paradigm (Schaal, 1997; Atkeson and Schaal, 1997; Argall et al., 2009). The system consists of four robotic arms which can be equipped with minimally invasive instruments or a camera. The benchmark task selected for this work is minimally invasive knot-tying.

Moustris et al. (2011) presented a literature review of commercial medical systems and surgical procedures. This work solely focuses on systems that have been experimentally implemented on real robots. Automation has also been used for simulating treatment plans on virtual surrogates of patients called phantoms (Xu, 2014). The phantoms represent the anatomy of a patient but they are too generic and hence cannot accurately represent individuals. These phantoms are especially used in pediatric oncology to study the effects of radiation treatment and late adverse effects. Virgolin et al. (2020) proposed an approach to build automatic phantoms by combining machine learning with imaging data. The problem of structuring a pediatric phantom is divided into three prediction tasks: (1) prediction of a representative body segmentation, (2) prediction of center of mass of the organ at risk, and (3) prediction of representative segmentation. Machine learning algorithms used for all three prediction tasks are least angle regression (Efron et al., 2004), least absolute shrinkage and selection operator (Tibshirani, 1996), random forests (RFs) (Breiman, 2001), traditional genetic programming (GP-Trad) (Koza, 1994), and genetic programming—gene pool optimal mixing evolutionary algorithm (Virgolin et al., 2017).

### 1.3.5 Other tasks in integrative medicine

The Consortium of Academic Health Centers for Integrative Medicine (imconsortium, 2020) defines the term *integrative medicine* as "an approach to the practice of medicine that makes use of the best-available evidence taking into account the whole person (body, mind, and spirit), including all aspects of lifestyle." There are many definitions for integrative medicine in the literature, but all share the commonalities that reaffirm the importance of focusing on the whole person and lifestyle rather than just physical healing. According to Maizes et al. (2009), integrative medicine gained recognition due to the realization that people spend only a fraction of time on prevention of disease and maintaining good health. The authors presented a data-driven example to promote the importance of integrative medicine—walking every day for 2 h for adults afflicted with diabetes reduces mortality by 39%. It is important to note that integrative medicine is not synonymous with complementary and alternative medicine (CAM) (Snyderman and Weil, 2002). We refer interested readers to Baer (2004), which chronicles the evolution of conventional and integrative medicine in the United States.

CAM refers to medical products and practices that are not part of standard medical care. Ernst (2000) presented examples of techniques used in CAM which include but are not limited to the following: acupuncture, aromatherapy, chiropractic, herbalism, homeopathy, massage, spiritual healing, and traditional Chinese medicine (TCM).

Zhao et al. (2015) presented an overview of machine learning approaches used in TCM. TCM specialists have established four diagnostic methods for TCM: observation, auscultation and olfaction, interrogation, and palpation. This article explains each of the four diagnostic methods and provides a list of machine learning methods used for each task. The most common methods are kNNs and SVM. Other methods include decision trees, Naïve Bayes (NB), and ANNs.

## 1.4 Open research problems

A recently published editorial by Bakken (2020) highlights five clinical informatics articles that reflect a consequentialist perspective. One of the articles that we discuss here focuses on a methodological concern, that is, predictive model calibration (Vaicenavicius et al., 2019). Predictive models are an important research topic as discussed in Section 1.3.2, but many studies continue to focus on model discrimination rather than calibration. Ghassemi et al. (2020) outlined several promising research directions, specifically highlighting issues of data temporality, model interpretability, and learning appropriate representations. Machine learning models in most of the existing literature have been trained on large amount of historical data and fail to account for temporality of data in the medical domain, where patient symptoms and or treatment procedures change with time. The authors cited Google Flu Trends as an example of the need to update machine learning models to account for this data temporality, as it persistently overestimated flu (Lazer et al., 2014). Another promising research area is model interpretability (Ahmad et al., 2018; Chakraborty et al., 2017). The authors suggested many directions toward the achievement of this goal: (1) model justification to justify the predictive path rather than just explaining a specific prediction; (2) building collaborative systems, where humans and machines work together. A final research topic is representation learning, which can improve predictive performance and account for conditional relationships of interest in the medical domain.

### 1.4.1 Learning for classification and regression

*Classification* is the identification of one or more categories or subpopulations to which a new observation belongs, on the basis of a training data set containing observations, or instances. In the data sciences of statistics and machine learning, classification may be supervised (where class labels are known) (Caruana and Niculescu-Mizil, 2006), unsupervised (where they are not and assignment is based on cohesion and similarity among instances) (Ghahramani, 2003), or semisupervised. Dreiseitl and Ohno-Machado (2002) surveyed early work using LR (particularly the binomial logit model) and ANNs (particularly multilayer perceptrons or MLP) for dichotomous classification, also known as binary classification or concept learning, on diagnostic and prognostic tasks from 72 papers in the existing literature. In parallel with this broad study of discriminative approaches to diagnosis and prognosis, Dybowski and Roberts (2005) compiled a comprehensive anthology of probabilistic models primarily for generative classification.

In contrast with these broad surveys, which are included for completeness and historical breadth, application papers tend to focus on specific use cases for classification, such as prediction of mortality. Eftekhar et al. (2005) presented one such paper which addresses the task of predicting head trauma mortality rate based on initial clinical data, and focuses methodologically on LR and MLP, as do Dreiseitl and Ohno-Machado (2002).

*Regression* is the problem of mapping an input instance to a real-valued scalar or tuple, which in data science is defined as an estimation task. In medical informatics, many predictive applications can be formulated as risk analysis tasks, that is, tasks requiring estimation of syndrome probability, given data from electronic medical records. Typical examples include estimating risk of a particular form of cancer, such as in a study by Ayer et al. (2010), where they use LR and MLP to estimate risk of breast cancer. In some additional use cases, the predictive task requires estimation of a continuous value such as the size (widest diameter) of a cancer mass, rather than a probability of occurrence. Royston and Sauerbrei (2008) presented a methodological introduction to numerical estimation methods for such tasks.

### 1.4.2 Learning to act: Control and planning

Another general category of tasks falls under the rubric of *learning to act*, or intelligent control and planning in engineering terminology. This includes the application of machine learning to the overlapping subarea of *optimal control*, the branch of mathematical optimization that deals with maximizing an objective function such as cost-weighted proximity to a target.

One example of an optimal control task, which was investigated by Vogelzang et al. (2005), is maintaining a patient's blood glucose level via automatic control of an insulin pump. The functional requirement of the system is to regulate the change in pump rate as a function of past pump rate, target glucose level, and past blood glucose measurements. The Glucose Regulation in Intensive care Patients (GRIP) system developed by Vogelzang et al. (2005) used a fixed weighted optimal control function based on previous clinical studies. Other optimal control tasks include prolonging the onset of drug resistance in treatment applications such as chemotherapy, a task studied by Ledzewicz and Schättler (2006), who formulated a dynamical system for the development of drug resistance over time and applied ordinary differential equation solvers to the task. Such numerical models can also be developed for therapeutic objectives such as minimizing tumor volume as a function of angiogenic inhibitors administered over time, an optimal control task studied by Ledzewicz et al. (2008).

By formulating parametric models for problems such as maintaining a patient's healthcare characteristics (e.g., blood glucose level, tumor size) within desired ranges while minimizing the total cost of doing so, optimization methods from industrial engineering and operations research, such as control charts, can be used. For example, Dobi and Zempléni (2019) applied Markov chain models and a variety of control charts to this cost-optimal control task (Dobi and Zempléni, 2019).

Yet another family of intelligent control approaches originates from classical planning, particularly the inverse problem of *plan recognition* (mapping from observed action sequences to individual plan steps, preconditions, and desired postconditions) and the problem of plan revision, which entails modifying a plan (such as a course of drug therapy) due to an identified complication (such as a toxic episode or other adverse reaction or interaction). Such systems are discussed by Shahar and Musen (1995). Plan revision may be necessitated as a consequence of historical observation (case studies), predictive simulation, or inference using a domain theory.

Finally, *enterprise resource planning* (ERP) is an integrative planning task of managing business processes (in health care, these include sales and marketing, patient services, provider human resources, specialist referrals, procurement of equipment and materials, treatment, billing, and insurance). van Merode et al. (2004) surveyed ERP requirements and systems for hospitals.

### 1.4.3 Toward greater autonomy: Active learning and self-supervision

Machine learning depends on availability of a training experience, but this experience needs not come in the form of labeled data, which is expensive to acquire even with copious available resources such as expertise and nonexpert annotator time, whose cost may be reduced by gamification or other means of crowd sourcing to volunteers. In this section, we survey three species of learning without full supervision that help to free machine learning users from some aspects of these data requirements and other experiential requirements. These are

1. *active learning* (Settles, 2009), the problem of developing a learning system that can seek out its own experiences;
2. *transfer learning* (Pan and Yang, 2009), training on a set of experiences for one or more tasks or domains and using the resulting representations to facilitate learning, reasoning, and problem solving in new tasks and domains; and
3. *self-supervised learning* (Ross et al., 2018), the generalized task of learning with unlabeled data and inducing intrinsic labels by discovering relationships between subcomponents of the training input (such as views or parts of an object in computer vision tasks).

Active learning in medical informatics spans a gamut of experiential domains from text to case studies, to controllers and policies. An example of active learning in text is the work of Druck et al. (2009), who applied categorical feature labels to words. This is a typical methodology in biomedical texts, where domain lexicons are organized into syndromic, pharmaceutical, and anatomical hierarchies, among others. Chen et al. (2012) used active learning with labels on two text categorization tasks. The first of these is at the sentence level, on the ASSERTION data set, a clinical healthcare text corpus for the 2010 i2b2/VA natural language processing (NLP) challenge. The second is at the whole-document level, on the NOVA data set, an email corpus with labels corresponding to a generic "religion versus politics" topic classification task. In subsequent work, Chen et al. (2017) applied a conditional random field (CRF)-based active learning system to the corpus of the 2010 i2b2/VA NLP challenge to show how annotation time could be reduced: by using latent Dirichlet allocation for sentential topic modeling (sentence-level clustering) and by bootstrapping the process of set expansion for the named entity recognition (NER) task using active learning. Dligach et al. (2013) also developed an active learning system for the i2b2 task, but focused on document-level phenotyping (prefiltering of ICD-9 codes, CPT codes, laboratory results, medication orders, etc. followed by category labeling). In their work, a document consists of EHRs and all associated data for a given patient, which may be generated at multiple stages of an admission and treatment workflow.

Transfer learning is typically defined as task to task or domain to domain but what constitutes a domain in medical informatics can vary. Wiens et al. (2014) investigated interhospital transfer learning by training on subsets of 132,853 admissions at three different hospitals, among which 1348 positive cases of *Clostridium difficile* infection were diagnosed, to boost hospital-specific precision and recall as measured holistically using the area under the receiver operating characteristic curve. As with active learning, transfer learning can be based on natural language features, typically at the word, sentence, or document level for medical informatics. For example, Lee et al. (2018) outlined a neural network approach to deidentification in patient notes, which is an instance of NER and crucial for compliance with patient confidentiality laws such as the Health Insurance Portability and Accountability Act in the United States. They applied a long short-term memory (LSTM), a type of deep learning neural network for sequence modeling, to classify named entities that represented protected health information. The transfer learning task, training on a large labeled data set to a smaller one with fewer labels, is another case of interdomain transfer. Yet another NER transfer learning problem for EHRs is defined and studied by Wang et al. (2018), who applied a bidirectional LSTM (Bi-LSTM) on a shared training corpus to create a shared representation (specifically, a word embedding) for text classification that is then fine-tuned for source and target domains by training a CRF model with labeled training data as available, to achieve label-aware NER. The experimental corpus, in this case, is a Chinese-language medical NER corpus (CM-NER) consisting of 1600 anonymized EHRs across four departments: cardiology (500), respiratory (500), neurology (300), and gastroenterology (300). Wang et al. (2018) demonstrated effective interdepartmental NER (domain-to-domain) transfer through experiments on CM-NER. Similar deep learning approaches for NLP are applied by Du et al. (2018), who demonstrated transfer using RNNs from clinical notes on psychological stressors to tweets on Twitter, to detect posts by users at risk of suicide. New architectures for implementing transfer are demonstrated by Peng et al. (2019), who used the deep bidirectional transformers BERT and ELMo to achieve cross-domain transfer among 10 benchmarking data sets from the Biomedical Language Understanding Evaluation (BLUE) compendium.

Self-supervised learning consists of generating labels by means of (1) comparing objects (e.g., clustering), (2) extracting relationships, or (3) designing experiments (especially model selection). The first approach applies similarity or distance metrics over entire instances (unlabeled examples) and has traditionally been similar to unsupervised learning for classification tasks in general, while the second involves using relational patterns and/or probabilistic inference over structured data models to capture new relationships, and the third involves generating multiple candidate models (by random sampling or parameter optimization methods such as identifying support vectors for large margin discriminative classifiers), and then applying model selection.

Hoffmann et al. (2010) took the second approach, introducing LUCHS, a self-supervised, relation-specific system for information extraction (IE) from text. Roller and Stevenson (2014) also used a relation-specific, ontology-aware approach to relation extraction; rather than being based on lexicon expansion, however, it uses the curated Unified Medical Language System, a biomedical knowledge base.

Stewart et al. (2011) presented an application of the third approach to the task of event detection in the domain of social media-based epidemic intelligence, where self-supervised learning consists of tokenizing text corpora, namely ProMED-Mail and WHO outbreak reports, to obtain bag of words (BOW or word vector space) embeddings. An SVM classifier is then trained, to which the authors applied model selection, testing the result against an avian flu text corpus.

As Blendowski et al. (2019) noted, self-supervision in medical imaging applications is a necessity because of the comparatively high cost of supervision for medical images and video versus general computer vision and video. In medical domains, annotation may require specialization in radiology and other medical subdisciplines, whereas generic images and videos may be annotated via microwork systems such as Amazon Mechanical Turk, or even via volunteer crowdsourcing. Blendowski et al. presented a modern, deep learning-based approach to self-supervision, applying convolutional neural networks (CNNs) to capture 3D context features.

## 2 Background

### 2.1 Diagnosis

#### 2.1.1 Diagnostic classification and regression tasks

Nadeem et al. (2020) presented a very comprehensive survey on classification of brain tumor. Jha et al. (2019) evaluated 32 supervised learning methods across 17 classification data sets (in domains that include cancer, tumors, and heart and liver diseases) to determine that decision tree-based methods perform better than others on these data sets. Mostafa et al. (2018) used three classification methods (decision trees, ANNs, and NB) to determine the presence of Parkinson's disease by using features extracted from human voice recordings, reaching a similar conclusion that decision trees performed best on this data set.

Polat and Güneş (2007) presented a binary classification task for categorizing breast cancer as malignant or benign. The authors used least square support vector machine (LS-SVM) (Suykens and Vandewalle, 1999) for classification.

Another machine learning task used for diagnosis is regression. Kayaer et al. (2003) used general regression neural network (GRNN) (Specht et al., 1991) for diagnosing diabetes using the Pima Indian diabetes data set (http://archive.ics.uci.edu/ml). The results show that it performs better than standard MLP and radial basis function (RBF) feedforward neural networks (Broomhead and Lowe, 1988) that have been used by other studies using the same data set. Hannan et al. (2010) have also used GRNN and RBF for heart disease diagnosis. Jeyaraj and Nadar (2019) proposed a regression-based partitioned deep CNN for the classification of oral cancer as malignant or benign. The network obtains accuracy comparable to that of a human expert oncologist.

### 2.1.2 Diagnostic policy-learning tasks

Yu et al. (2019b) presented the first comprehensive survey of reinforcement learning (RL) applications in health care. The aim of the survey is to provide the research community with an understanding of the foundations, methodologies, existing challenges, and recent applications of RL in healthcare domain. The range of applications vary from dynamic treatment regimes (DTRs) in chronic diseases and critical care, automated clinical diagnosis, to other tasks such as clinical resource allocation and scheduling.

Early RL systems for medical informatics were predominantly designed for medical image processing and analysis (as a specialized application of computer vision). Sahba et al. (2006) developed such a system, based on Q-learning, for ultrasound image analysis, focusing on tasks such as local thresholding, feature extraction, and segmentation of organs (in this case, the prostate gland). In subsequent work, Sahba et al. (2007) extended this Q-learning system for organ segmentation to an adversarial framework that they termed "Opposition-Based Learning." This framework allowed for more flexible formulation of utility gradients for RL problems such as balancing exploration versus exploitation.

Peng et al. (2018) introduced REFUEL, a deep Q-network (DQN)-based system for reward shaping and feature construction ("rebuilding") in differential diagnosis of diseases. Such systems are examples of reinforcement-based metalearning and can potentially incorporate aspects of both self-supervision and active learning of representation. DQN has also been used by researchers such as Al and Yun (2019) to learn policies for recognizing anatomical landmarks in X-ray-based computerized tomography (CT) and MRI images. In addition, DQN has recently been applied to learn control policies for clinical decision support tasks such as guiding a healthcare professional or first responder, especially an emergency medical technician, in obtaining ultrasound images as a remote sensing step before administering treatment. Milletari et al. (2019) presented a novel application of this method to Point of Care Ultrasound (POCUS) for scanning the left ventricle of the heart.

Utility functions for deep RL in medical informatics may be tied to anatomical mapping and other automation tasks of internal medicine. Examples of such mapping include the context maps of Tu and Bai (2009), which are based on learning, i.e., parameter estimation, in Markov random fields and CRFs.

In this work, the authors trained and applied inference using these models to solve high-level vision tasks such as image segmentation, configuration estimation (orientation), and region labeling of 3D brain images.

A key family of RL applications is that of control policies for medical treatment. Weng et al. (2017) described a deep RL method using a sparse autoencoder for glycemic control in septic patients. While experimental validation of this system was performed using historical data, the RL framework presented can include medical devices and mixed-initiative systems.

Finally, RL can also be applied to interactive differential diagnosis using natural language (i.e., dialogue). Liu et al. (2018) described a dialogue-based system for disease phenotype identification (eliciting observable characteristics or traits of diseases, such as the presentation and development of symptoms, morphology, biochemical or physiological properties, or patient behavior). The dialogue policy formulated here is a Markov decision process (MDP). The RL problem is that of detecting symptoms of any or all four known pediatric diseases by simulating query-based dialogue using an annotated corpus. The authors showed that DQN for dialogue outperforms SVM for supervised classification learning, random dialogue generation, and a rule-based dialogue agent.

### 2.1.3 Active, transfer, and self-supervised learning

Sánchez et al. (2010) proposed a computer aided diagnosis (CAD) (Castellino, 2005) system for diabetic retinopathy screening using active learning approaches. There are four components that constitute the DR screening process: quality verification, normal anatomy detection, bright lesion detection, and red lesion detection (Niemeijer et al., 2009). The findings from these four components need to be fused in order to generate an outcome for a patient. The outcome is in the form of a likelihood that the patient will be referred to an ophthalmologist. The output from the four components of the DR screening are used to extract some features which are further used to train a kNN classifier. Active learning is applied in the training phase to select an unlabeled sample from the pool of samples and pose a query to the expert in order to acquire a label for the sample. This is an iterative process that only stops when a stopping criterion has been reached. This work used two different query functions: uncertainty sampling (Lewis and Gale, 1994) and query-by-bagging (QBB) sampling (Abe, 1998).

Apostolopoulos and Mpesiana (2020) used a transfer learning approach for the classification of medical images to diagnose COVID-19. This study uses publicly available thoracic X-rays of healthy people as well as patients suffering from COVID-19 to build an automatic diagnostic system. The aim of their work is to evaluate the effectiveness of state-of-the-art pretrained CNN models for the diagnosis of COVID-19. The CNN used for this study include VGG19 (Simonyan and Zisserman, 2015), Mobile-Netv2 (Sandler et al., 2018), Inception (Szegedy et al., 2015), Xception (Chollet, 2017), and Inception-ResNet v2 (Szegedy et al., 2017). The study formulates the task as a multiclass classification problem with three classes: normal people, pneumonia patients, and COVID-19 patients. The study does accomplish its goals of establishing the benefits of transfer learning by using state-of-the-art CNN models.

Bai et al. (2019) used a semisupervised approach for learning features from unlabeled data for the task of cardiac MR image segmentation. This segmentation is important for characterizing the function of the heart. The authors discussed the different angulated planes at which the MR images are acquired. For brevity, we refer the readers to Bai et al. (2019). Specific views of the scans and their labels have been traditionally used to train a network from scratch. The authors used a standard U-Net architecture (Ronneberger et al., 2015) with three variations to it. The results of their work show that by using self-supervised learning even a small data set is able to outperform a standard U-Net that has been trained from scratch.

## 2.2 Predictive analytics

### 2.2.1 Prediction by classification and regression

We start by discussing *prediction of disease susceptibility*: Kim and Kim (2018) tried to predict an individual's susceptibility to cancer by using genomic data. The authors used kNN for building a multi-class classification model.

Next we move on to *prediction of survivability*: Choi et al. (2009) proposed a hybrid ANN and BN model to predict 5-year survival rates for breast cancer patients. The model combines the best of both worlds using black box ANN for their higher accuracy and BNs for their explainability.

The survivability of a cancer patient depends on the stage of cancer, which is based on tumor size, location, spread, and other factors. Machine learning models that predict survivability in breast cancer research usually use breast cancer stage as a feature for training the model. Kate and Nadig (2017) referred to such a model as a joint model. Their work used the SEER data set (SEER Incidence Database—SEER Data & Software, 2021), which classifies cancer into four stages: in situ, localized, regional, and distant.

Mobadersany et al. (2018) proposed an approach called Survival Convolutional Neural Network (SCNN), which uses a CNN integrated with Cox survival analysis technique for the task of survivability prediction for patients with brain tumors. The CNN includes a Cox proportional hazards layer that models overall survival. The proposed approach surpasses the prognostic accuracy of human experts.

The final task that we discuss is *prediction of recurrence*: The task involves correctly predicting the recurrence of disease with a binary outcome. Abreu et al. (2016) presented a literature review to evaluate the performance of machine learning methods for the task of predicting breast cancer recurrence. The review covers literature during the years 2007–14 and find that the key algorithms used for the task include: decision trees, LR, ANN, NB, K-Means, RFs, and kNN. These algorithms are discussed in Section 3. The authors outlined a few challenges based on their review that make this task less popular: (1) lack of publicly available data of reasonable size—most of the studies have used local data sets usually with a small number of patients; (2) data imbalance is not handled in most cases; (3) feature selection was performed manually in most studies with the help of domain experts—there is no agreement on variables that are important for the study of breast cancer recurrence; (4) accuracy as evaluation metric for classification performance which is not appropriate for imbalanced data sets; and (5) lack of model interpretability of machine learning models—these challenges provide a scope for future research in the area. A more recent review was published by Zhu et al. (2020) who covered the usage of deep learning for the task of cancer prognosis. The study also presents similar challenges encountered by deep learning models in the domain as were pointed by Abreu et al. (2016). Some of the challenges listed include: (1) availability of small data sets; (2) handling data imbalance; (3) handling sparse and missing data; (4) handling high-dimensional sequencing data; and (5) need of researchers with expertise in both, machine learning and biomedical domain.

### 2.2.2 Learning to predict from reinforcements and by supervision

The advent of institution-wide terascale to petascale data mining, considered "big data" as of 2020, has brought machine learning for predictive analytics to the fore in many clinical domains. Shah et al. (2018) presented a commentary piece on the state of the field in data mining for predictive analytics in medical informatics. It cites the $CHA_2DS_2 - VASc$ score as an example of a predictive rule regarding the doubling of thromboembolic risk in atrial fibrillation as a function of congestive heart failure, hypertension, age, diabetes, and previous stroke or transient ischemic attack, citing it as a use case of predictive models with consequence for finely balanced treatment decisions, which the authors note are commonplace. Rajkomar et al. (2019) reviewed a broader set of diagnostic and prognostic applications, along with best practices for using machine learning as an augmentative technology for clinicians. Shameer et al. (2018) surveyed the field of artificial intelligence (AI) in medicine even more broadly, discussing the species of machine learning surveyed in this chapter and the actionable products thereof, from classification rules and regression formulas to annotated images and policies from RL.

Many predictive analytics applications involve estimating risk of adverse effects, or detecting imminent adverse outcomes in time for preventative or anticipatory measures. For example, Kendale et al. (2018) developed an LR-based system for predicting hypotension in patients after surgical anesthesia.

Just as supervised learning finds precedent in rule-based expert systems for differential diagnosis, RL finds precedent in both educational technology and early automation for the practice of internal medicine and general surgery. Examples are surveyed in Section 4. One general use case of RL for predictive analytics is given by Khurana et al. (2018), who cast feature engineering for predictive applications as an RL task where the policy is defined in terms of data transformations.

Taking such diverse use cases as a whole, a major consideration in medical predictive analytics, which overlaps with AI, ethics, and society (AIES), as well as with AI safety and security, is how to determine appropriate regulatory standards of clinical benefit. Parikh et al. (2019) discussed meaningful minimum standards of functionality and interoperability, in the context of endpoints (clinical outcomes), appropriate benchmarks, and the importance of associating predictive systems with interventions.

### 2.2.3 Transfer learning in prediction

Gliomas are a type of tumors that are found in the brain. They are of different types and are usually graded from I to IV with grade IV being the most aggressive type. MRI images are used for grading gliomas into two categories: lower-grade glioma (LGG), which is grade II and III and higher-grade glioma, which is a grade IV. Cabezas et al. (2018) proposed a model using CNN for classifying LGG and HGG by analyzing MRI images. Two CNN architectures were explored for this purpose, namely: AlexNet and GoogLeNet. These two architecture are discussed in Section 3.3.2. The results indicate that with transfer learning and fine-tuning the performance improved for both deep learning architectures (DLAs). Yang et al. (2018) presented a transfer learning approach to segment the gliomas and its subregions and use the results along with other clinical features to predict patient survival. The approach is divided into two main tasks, where the first task focuses on segmentation of glioma using a 3D U-Net (Ronneberger et al., 2015). The second task segments the tumor subregions using a small ensemble net (Kamnitsas et al., 2017). Their work uses a VGG-16 network, which is discussed in Section 3.3.2.

## 2.3 Therapy recommendation

### 2.3.1 Supervised therapy recommender systems

Therapy recommendation remains a common use case of supervised learning, beyond diagnosis. General-purpose models for classification such as nearest-neighbor and rule-based classification are often effective, particularly when explainability is desired. Zhang et al. (2013) discussed supervised learning for therapy recommendation in the domain of physical therapy, where class imbalance is a frequent issue, and derive both a modified rule-learning algorithm (ARIPPER) and an application of the selective minority oversampling technique (SMOTE) for this task.

Mental health and wellbeing are major health issues in the world. There is a growing research effort to alleviate the symptoms of depression. Rohani et al. (2020) built a recommender system for the mental health domain. The authors cited the motivation behind such systems stemming from research that suggests that when participants regularly participate in a pleasant activity then it has a beneficial impact on the mental health of the individual (MacPhillamy and Lewinsohn, 1982; Fredrickson, 2000). An effective treatment for depression has been the pleasant event scheduling system (Lewinsohn and Libet, 1972). Wahle et al. (2016) described multiuser and personalized variants of an affective recommender system developed using data from two mobile health applications for both clinically depressed users and nonclinical users. Mood ratings for activities are predicted using trained NB and SVM models. These classification-based predictions enable personalized treatment recommendations using a mobile app.

## 2.4 Automation of treatment

### 2.4.1 Classification and regression-based tasks

Learning in the presence of hybrid training data (consisting of continuous and discrete or nominal variables) is a frequent and typical necessity in medical AI applications. Schilling et al. (2016) described the use of Classification and Regression Trees (CART) to identify thresholds for cardiovascular disease. Such hybrid tasks can also be addressed using binary response models such as probit models, but as the authors note, three distinct strengths of CART are that: (1) its hierarchical structure makes it more human comprehensible than linear or LR models; (2) it can capture nonlinearity in response and some multivariate interactions; and (3) it has more expressiveness than regression models.

For some predictive applications, accuracy, precision, and recall are of highest significance and may be considered more important than explainability by diagnosticians. Taylor et al. (2018) presented a task where regression methods, gradient boosting improvements, and committee machines such as bagged RFs and Adaboost are highly effective. In some cases, association rule mining and basic NLP methods suffice: De Silva et al. (2018) described a social media mining task, analytics of online social groups for cancer patients, where the technical objective is to extract information about user demographics in relation to terms indicating patient age, cancer stage, side effects reported, and sentiments.

### 2.4.2 RL for automation

An essential task in automation of surgical tasks is optimal path planning to avoid collisions between tool and surrounding tissue before resection automation. Baek et al. (2018) aimed to create a global path to cut a tissue during surgery without colliding with the surrounding tissue. The generated path was simulated on APOLLON, which is a Single Incision Laparoscopic Surgery system developed by KAIST Telerobotics and Control Lab (Medical Robot|KAIST Telerobotics and Control Lab, 2021). Their work uses a popular path planning method called probabilistic roadmap (RPM) (Kavraki et al., 1998), which creates a path from a static environment to a desired point and Q-learning (Watkins and Dayan, 1992), an RL technique.

### 2.4.3 Active learning in automation

In a hospital setting, hand hygiene is one of the most important factors for the prevention of infectious diseases. Monitoring hand hygiene could be vital in reducing any outbreak within an operating room (OR). Kim et al. (2020) proposed a fully augmented automatic hand hygiene monitoring tool for monitoring the anesthesiologists on OR video. The aim is to identify the alcohol-based hand rubbing actions of anesthesiologists in the OR presurgery and postsurgery. The proposed approach uses a 3D CNN for classification task with two classes: rubbing hands and other actions. The data were collected from a hospital over a span of 4 months from a single OR. Additional data were generated by simulating a situation in OR for synthetic data. The proposed approach uses I3D model, an Inception v1 architecture that inflates 2D convolutions into 3D convolutions to train three models: I3D networks for RGB, I3D networks for optical flow inputs, and a joint model. Transfer learning approach is employed by pre-training the CNN on Kinetics-400 (Carreira and Zisserman, 2017) data set. The I3D for RGB outperforms the other two models.

## 2.5 Integrating medical informatics and health informatics

This section surveys machine learning at the interface of medical informatics and health informatics, particularly clinical health and medical informatics (HMI).

### 2.5.1 Classification and regression tasks in HMI

Ralston et al. (2007) discussed patient web services in integrated delivery system portals, which provide access to EHRs as well as financing and delivery of other healthcare products such physician consultation, medical devices, and prescription medicines. These comprise point of care (POC) and post-POC services, which serve as both information retrieval and EHR compilation mechanisms that can produce data for subsequent machine learning and data science. Data integration is a key requirement of such systems (Ralston et al., 2007). As underscored by the work of Oztekin et al. (2009) on predicting heart-lung transplant survival using a combination of case data, elicited subject matter expertise, and commonsense reasoning from a basic domain theory, the most effective learning strategy is sometimes to incorporate all available data sources and then use algorithms for feature selection and construction on these. Furthermore, Holzinger and Jurisica (2014) advocated for an integrative and interactive approach to knowledge discovery and data mining in biomedical informatics (BMI)—specifically, one that is informed by objectives of both human-computer interaction and knowledge discovery in databases.

### 2.5.2 Reinforcement learning for HMI

Medical informatics is a field where medical practitioners have traditionally used mixed-initiative AI, especially human-in-the-loop systems. In such systems, performance elements of machine learning are used for recommendation and decision support rather than for full automation at the POC. Holzinger (2016) discussed this general practice and its rationale in modern interactive POC systems, specifically when humans in the loop are beneficial. They note that there are specific usage contexts where humans are good at spotting irrelevant features, assessing novelty and anomaly in annotation, and behavioral modeling of adversaries in security and safety contexts (such as anonymity and privacy of patient data in HMI systems). This is an important consideration for mixed-initiative HMI because the interactive machine learning (iML) framework they advocate is rooted in RL.

RL is not limited to Q-learning and its dynamic programming relatives, the temporal differences and SARSA family of algorithms, but can include complex adaptive systems such as multiarmed bandits and contextual bandits. Yom-Tov et al. (2017) explored the problem of generating physical activity reminders to diabetes patients using RL in a contextual bandit. They show a slightly positive slope in reduction of hemoglobin A1c (HbA1c) for experimental users of this system over a 6-month period, compared to a slightly negative slope for a control group.

Deep RL (DRL) systems for HMI often frame treatment tasks as optimal control problems as outlined in Section 1.4.2. Raghu et al. (2017) gave one example of such a DRL application: the administration of intravenous fluids and vasopressors in septic patients. Their DQN-based approach calculates discounted return from off-policy (historical) data rather than by directly controllable reinforcements. Liu et al. (2017) applied DQN to a high-dimension space of (about 270) actions corresponding to medicines given to acute myeloid leukemia (AML) patients who received hematopoietic cell transplantation (HCT), with the goal of preventing acute graft versus host disease (GVHD). The training data set consists of historical medical registry data for 6021 AML patients who underwent HCT between 1995 and 2007; these data are sequential but asynchronous (with standard follow-up forms collected at 100 days, 6 months, 12 months, 2 years, and 4 years). The authors demonstrated value enhancement of up to 21.4% using DQN and note that a larger training data set compiled by the Center for International Blood and Marrow Transplant Research (CIBMTR) can potentially be used for DRL.

*Inverse reinforcement learning (IRL)* is the problem of inferring the reward function of an observed agent, given its behavior as reflecting a policy. Yu et al. (2019c) addressed the IRL task of capturing the reward functions for mechanical ventilation and sedative dosing in ICUs from the Medical Information Mart for Intensive Care (MIMIC III), an open data set containing records of demographics, vital signs, laboratory tests, diagnoses, and medications for nearly 40,000 adult and 8000 neonatal ICU patients. The authors demonstrated that IRL from this critical care data is feasible using a Bayesian inverse Q-learning algorithm (fitted Q-iteration) applied to an MDP representation.

An MDP is also used by Yu et al. (2019a) in a direct RL application. Here, they incorporate causal factors between options of anti-HIV drugs and observed effects into a model-free policy gradient RL learning algorithm, to learn DTRs for human immunodeficiency virus (HIV). This approach is shown to facilitate direct learning of causal policy gradient parameters without requiring a model-based intermediary, a finding which has potential relevance to DRL and IRL as well.

### 2.5.3 Self-supervised, transfer, and active learning in HMI

Qiu and Sun (2019) applied this paradigm to RL in vision, for iterative refinement of tomographic images and in order to improve diagnostic image classification. The specific type of imaging is called *optical coherence tomography*.

Self-supervision is also used in other deep learning representations. Among the earliest of these to be developed were CNNs, which in HMI are designed to perform visual phenotyping. Gildenblat and Klaiman (2019) developed a Siamese network for segmentation of pathological images (e.g., into regions corresponding to stromata, tumors infiltrating lymphocytes, blood vessels, fat, healthy tissue, necrosis, etc.). Sarkar and Etemad (2020) used a CNN to learn relevant patterns from electrocardiograms for emotion recognition.

Another self-supervised learning representation is found in word embedding models in NLP. Meng et al. (2020) used BERT to classify radiology reports by urgency, learning a contextual representation rather than using more traditional sentiment analysis or other methods requiring word-level grading or subjective annotation of the training corpus.

Yet another self-supervised learning architecture is the generative adversarial network (GAN), which has been applied to create artificial images (DeepFakes) and achieve style transfer from drawings and paintings to photographic images. Tachibana et al. (2020) used a GAN to improve the electronic cleansing process to remove fecal artifacts in CT colonoscopy images.

# 3 Techniques for machine learning

## 3.1 Supervised, unsupervised, and semisupervised learning

We provide a very brief description of each of the machine learning methods that have been used in the medical informatics literature.

### 3.1.1 Shallow

A *decision tree* (Brodley and Utgoff, 1995) is a directed tree model that is used as a rule-induction system where each node represents a feature (univariate decision tree) and following a path of features (represented as nodes in the tree) leads to a specific classification.

*NB* (Rish et al., 2001) is a probabilistic classifier used for binary or multiclass classification problems. It is based on the poor assumption of conditional independence among the features and uses Bayes' theorem.

*ANNs* (Hassoun et al., 1995) are inspired by biological neural network and the brain's ability to process massive amount of information in parallel that allows it to recognize and classify the world around it. Researchers introduced ANN that can be created using a weighted directed graph to process information in parallel where nodes of the graph are connected together in a similar way the neurons in the brain are connected.

*SVMs* (Suykens and Vandewalle, 1999) use a mathematical function called kernel that transforms linearly inseparable data to linearly separable by finding the hyper-plane (decision boundary) that maximizes distance from data points on either side of the plane.

*RFs* (Breiman, 2001) are initially a group of decision trees where each tree randomly selects a sample from the data set. Once the trees (forest) have been built, each tree produces a class prediction, which is used in the vote for the most popular class. The majority vote is used as the final classification of an input example.

*kNN* (Dudani, 1976) is a supervised, nonparametric, and lazy learning algorithm that is used for classification and regression problems. A kNN implementation has three important components—training and test data set; an integer value $K$; and a distance metric such as Euclidean, Manhattan, or Hamming.

### 3.1.2 Deep

*Convolutional neural networks* Tajbakhsh et al. (2016) explained CNNs as a special class of ANNs where each neuron from one layer does not fully connect to all neurons in the next layer. CNNs work by using convolutional layers that are mainly for detecting certain local features in all locations of their input images. A set of convolutional kernels is responsible for learning a set of local features within input images, which results in a feature mapping. Anwar et al. (2018) showed that CNNs are wildly used in medical imaging which help to achieve the following tasks: segmentation, detection and classification of abnormality, computer-aided detection or diagnosis, and medical image retrieval.

A *U-Net* (Ronneberger et al., 2015) is a CNN network that consists of a contracting path to capture context, and a symmetric expanding path that enables precise localization (class label is supposed to be assigned to each pixel). The architecture of the network resembles a U-shaped network of CNNs where the left side of the U-shape consists of a contracting path and the right side consists of an expansive path.

*Stacked denoising autoencoders (SDAE)* (Vincent et al., 2010) are multilayered denoising autoencoders that are stacked together for training purposes. These networks are trained by adding noise to the raw input, which is then fed to the first denoising autoencoder in the stack. After minimizing the loss (convergence), the information in the hidden layer (latent features) is obtained and again noise is added, and the resulting features are fed to the next denoising autoencoder in the stack. This process continues for all denoising autoencoders in the stack.

*GANs* (Goodfellow et al., 2014) consist of two models—a generative model and a discriminative model that are simultaneously trained. The generative model captures the data distribution by producing fake data, and the discriminative model determines if a sample comes from the real training data or from the generative model (fake data). The training goal is to maximize the probability of the discriminative model making a mistake.

*RNNs* (Übeyli, 2010) are a special type of neural network where the output from previous step is fed as input to the current step. The most important feature of RNN is their internal states which allow the network to have the ability of remembering information about a sequence of inputs. This is especially useful when trying any kind of prediction that relies on information that can be viewed as a sequence, such as an EEG signal.

## 3.2 Reinforcement learning

### 3.2.1 Traditional

*Q-learning* (Watkins and Dayan, 1992) is a simple RL algorithm that given the current state, seeks to find the best action to take in that state. It is an off-policy algorithm because it learns from actions that are random (i.e., outside the policy). The algorithm works in three basic steps: (1) the agent starts in a state and takes an action and receives a reward; (2) for the next action, the agent has two choice—either reference the Q table and select an action with the highest value or take a random action; and (3) agent updates the Q-values (i.e., Q[State, Action]). A Q-table is a reference table for the agent to select the best action based on the Q-value.

### 3.2.2 Deep RL

The *Deep Q-Network (DQN) model* by Sorokin et al. (2015) combine Q-learning (discussed earlier) with a deep CNN. The goal of this model is to train a network to approximate the value of the Q function which maps state-action pairs to their expected discounted return. The inputs to the neural network are the state variables and the outputs are the Q-values.

## 3.3 Self-supervised, transfer, and active learning

### 3.3.1 Traditional

Although the term "self-supervised" dates back to learning systems that used shallow representations rather than deep neural networks and similar representations (Hoffmann et al., 2010; Stewart et al., 2011; Roller and Stevenson, 2014), we can see from the distinct purpose and methodology used to achieve self-supervision that deep learning has emerged as a paradigm that facilitates new forms of self-supervised learning. Transfer learning has similarly been studied extensively since the advent of deep learning, but compared to self-supervision, is better understood as an independent task. A broad and comprehensive overview of the problem is provided by Torrey and Shavlik (2010).

### 3.3.2 Deep

*AlexNet* (Krizhevsky et al., 2012) is an eight-layered CNN network of five convolutional layers followed by three fully connected layers with 60 million parameters and 650,000 neurons. The authors trained this network using a subset of the popular *ImageNet* image corpus.

*VGG* (Simonyan and Zisserman, 2015) is a very deep CNN for large-scale image recognition developed as part of the Large-Scale Visual Recognition Challenge (ILSVRC).

*ResNets* (He et al., 2016), or residual neural networks, are a type of deep neural net architecture modeled on pyramidal cells (high-connectivity cortical neurons). To alleviate the difficulty of training deeper neural networks, ResNets contain shortcut (skip) connections that propagate activations forward by one or more layers; these activation blocks are referred to as *residual blocks* and this structure reformulates a baseline plain network into its counterpart residual version. ResNets have a typical depth of 50 to over 150 layers (ResNet-152), which is very big compared to VGG.

*SqueezeNet* (Iandola et al., 2016) is another CNN architecture which was mainly developed to achieve a similar accuracy to AlexNet, but with far less number of parameters and size. It maintains an accuracy on ImageNet data set that is comparable to that of AlexNet.

*DenseNet* (Huang et al., 2017) was developed based on the observation that CNNs can be deeper, more accurate, and very efficient to train if they contain shorter connections between layers close to the input and those close to the output. DenseNet consists of dense blocks where each block connects each layer to every subsequent layer in that block. The advantages of DenseNet include avoiding the vanishing-gradient problem, strengthening feature propagation, feature reuse, and reduce the number of training parameters.

## 4 Applications

We now survey selected popular test beds for medical predictive analytics.

## 4.1 Test beds for diagnosis and prognosis

The most used data set for breast cancer diagnosis is the Breast Cancer Wisconsin (Diagnostic) Data Set 2.1.1 (http://archive.ics.uci.edu/ml). This data set is publicly available from the University of California Irvine (UCI) Machine Learning Repository.

Data sets used for the task of predicting breast cancer recurrence (Abreu et al., 2016) include: (1) The Wisconsin prognostic breast cancer (WPBC) data set from the UCI ML repository (http:// archive.ics.uci.edu/ml) and (2) the data set from the SEER database (SEER Incidence Database— SEER Data & Software, 2021; Choi et al., 2009).

An RNA-seq data set for cancer prediction (Xiao et al., 2018) is freely available from The Cancer Genome Atlas (TCGA) program database (The Cancer Genome Atlas Program, 2021). TCGA is a cancer genomics program that has generated over 2.5 petabytes of genomic, epigenomic, transcriptomic, and proteomic data. These data have been used to facilitate improvements in the diagnosis, treatment, and the prevention of cancer.

### 4.1.1 New test beds
We refer the interested reader to work by Deserno et al. (2012), Murphy et al. (2015), and Svensson-Ranallo et al. (2011), and the guidelines of the National Heart, Lung, and Blood Institute (NHLBI) for preparation of clinical study data (Guidelines for Preparing Clinical Study Data Sets for Submission to the NHLBI Data Repository, 2021).

## 4.2 Test beds for therapy recommendation and automation
We refer the interested reader to relevant work by Valdez et al. (2016), Son and Thong (2015), and Thong et al. (2015).

### 4.2.1 Prescriptions
We refer the interested reader to work by Galeano and Paccanaro (2018), Kushwaha et al. (2014), Zhang et al. (2015), Bao and Jiang (2016), Bhat and Aishwarya (2013), and Guo et al. (2016).

### 4.2.2 Surgery
We refer the interested reader to relevant work by Ciecierski et al. (2012), Petscharnig and Schöffmann (2017), Wang and Fey (2018), and Shvets et al. (2018).

## 5 Experimental results
### 5.1 Test bed
As an experimental example, we include a test bed introduced by Fanconi (2019) in this chapter. This consists of a subset of 3600 pictures extracted from the data set in the International Skin Imaging Collaboration Archive (ISIC), which contains more than 23,000 mole pictures. The test bed contains balanced cases of malignant (1) and benign (0) skin moles. Here, we present a simple performance comparison between different pretrained DLAs that classify a skin mole as being malignant or benign.

This data set has been used by several recent publications (Zhang et al., 2019; Tschandl et al., 2019; Nida et al., 2019; Mahbod et al., 2019).

**Table 1  Classification of skin cancer: accuracy, precision, recall, and F1-score for deep learning neural networks.**

| Network | Acc wtd. | Precision benign | Precision malignant | Recall benign | Recall malignant | F1 benign | F1 malignant |
|---|---|---|---|---|---|---|---|
| AlexNet | 0.87 | 0.91 | 0.85 | 0.87 | 0.89 | 0.89 | 0.87 |
| VGG11_bn | 0.85 | 0.91 | 0.81 | 0.82 | 0.90 | 0.86 | 0.85 |
| Resnet18 | 0.83 | 0.92 | 0.77 | 0.78 | 0.91 | 0.84 | 0.84 |
| SqueezeNet | 0.85 | 0.92 | 0.80 | 0.81 | 0.92 | 0.86 | 0.85 |
| DenseNet | 0.84 | 0.90 | 0.80 | 0.81 | 0.89 | 0.85 | 0.84 |

## 5.2 Results and discussion

We use weighted accuracy, precision, recall, and F1-score to test the performance of the DLAs. Table 1 shows the performance of the different DLAs used in this comparison. In terms of weighted accuracy, AlexNet have achieved the best accuracy. SqueezeNet and Resnet-18 achieved the best precision score when classifying a mole as benign, but the worst precision score when classifying a mole as malignant. AlexNet has the best precision score when classifying a mole as malignant and the best F1-score as well. We can also see that the difference in the performance of the DLAs is only marginal and we believe that different data set would yield different performance between the tested DLAs.

# 6  Conclusion: Machine learning for computational medicine

This chapter has introduced machine learning tasks for diagnostic medicine and automation of treatment, comprising supervised, self-supervised, and RL. After surveying task definitions, we outlined existing methods for diagnosis, predictive analytics, therapy recommendation, automation of treatment, and integrative HMI. We now look forward to current and continuing work in applied machine learning for medical applications.

## 6.1 Frontiers: Preclinical, translational, and clinical

Machine learning has developed into a cross-cutting technology across areas of medical informatics, from theory, education, and training (*preclinical*) aspects to the observation and treatment of patients (*clinical* computational medicine), to *translational* medicine, which aims toward bridging experimental tools and treatments to deployed ones used in clinical practice. For preclinical surveys, we refer the interested reader to the following: Prashanth et al. (2016), who discussed experimental Parkinson's treatments (Prashanth et al., 2016; Kolachalama and Garg, 2018) surveyed machine learning as a subarea of AI, particularly in medical education (Kolachalama and Garg, 2018); and Bannach-Brown et al. (2018) reviewed natural language learning and text mining in medical informatics. Ravì et al. (2016) surveyed deep learning in translational health informatics; Weintraub et al. (2018) reviewed translational text analytics; and Shah et al. (2019) broadly examined machine learning and AI in translational medicine, from sensors and medical devices to drug discovery. Finally, Savage (2012) provided an early survey of big data for improving clinical medicine, while Char et al. (2018) addressed ethical considerations.

## 6.2 Toward the future: Learning and medical automation

As of this writing in 2020, the coronavirus disease SARS-Cov-2 is of pervasive interest as a highly time-critical use case of intelligent systems for improved diagnosis and epidemiological modeling, as discussed by Randhawa et al. (2020), and for understanding etiology toward vaccine discovery, as discussed by Alimadadi et al. (2020). The (Stanford HAI (2021)) conference surveys broad methods for combatting Covid-19 and future pandemics. More generally, the fields of diagnostic medicine and predictive analytics have grown significantly since the early work of Kononenko (2001) and the health informatics applications of Pakhomov et al. (2006), but there are deep technical gaps and significant challenges remaining before the "eDoctor" envisioned by Handelman et al. (2018) becomes a reality. Meanwhile, AI safety concerns, as mapped out by Yampolskiy (2016) in both historical and anticipatory contexts of risks and remedies, loom large.

## References

Abe, N., 1998. Query learning strategies using boosting and bagging. In: Proc. 15th Int. Conf. Machine Learning (ICML98), pp. 1–9.

Abreu, P.H., Santos, M.S., Abreu, M.H., Andrade, B., Silva, D.C., 2016. Predicting breast cancer recurrence using machine learning techniques: a systematic review. ACM Comput. Surv. 49 (3), 1–40. https://doi.org/10.1145/2988544.

Abu-Nasser, B., 2017. Medical expert systems survey. Int. J. Eng. Inf. Syst. 1 (7), 218–224.

Ahmad, M.A., Eckert, C., Teredesai, A., 2018. Interpretable machine learning in healthcare. In: Proceedings of the 2018 ACM International Conference on Bioinformatics, Computational Biology, and Health Informatics, pp. 559–560.

Al, W.A., Yun, I.D., 2019. Partial policy-based reinforcement learning for anatomical landmark localization in 3D medical images. IEEE Trans. Med. Imaging 39 (4), 1245–1255.

Alimadadi, A., Aryal, S., Manandhar, I., Munroe, P.B., Joe, B., Cheng, X., 2020. Artificial Intelligence and Machine Learning to Fight COVID-19. American Physiological Society, Bethesda, MD.

Almadhoun, H.R., Abu-Naser, S.S., 2020. An expert system for diagnosing coronavirus (COVID-19) using SL5. Int. J. Acad. Eng. Res. 4 (4), 1–9.

Anwar, S.M., Majid, M., Qayyum, A., Awais, M., Alnowami, M., Khan, M.K., 2018. Medical image analysis using convolutional neural networks: a review. J. Med. Syst. 42 (11), 226. https://doi.org/10.1007/s10916-018-1088-1.

Apostolopoulos, I.D., Mpesiana, T.A., 2020. Covid-19: automatic detection from X-ray images utilizing transfer learning with convolutional neural networks. Phys. Eng. Sci. Med., 1. https://doi.org/10.1007/s13246-020-00865-4.

Argall, B.D., Chernova, S., Veloso, M., Browning, B., 2009. A survey of robot learning from demonstration. Robot. Auton. Syst. 57 (5), 469–483. https://doi.org/10.1016/j.robot.2008.10.024.

Atkeson, C.G., Schaal, S., 1997. Robot learning from demonstration. In: ICML, vol. 97, pp. 12–20.

Ayer, T., Chhatwal, J., Alagoz, O., Kahn Jr., C.E., Woods, R.W., Burnside, E.S., 2010. Comparison of logistic regression and artificial neural network models in breast cancer risk estimation. Radiographics 30 (1), 13–22. https://doi.org/10.1148/rg.301095057.

Baek, D., Hwang, M., Kim, H., Kwon, D.-S., 2018. Path planning for automation of surgery robot based on probabilistic roadmap and reinforcement learning. In: 2018 15th International Conference on Ubiquitous Robots (UR), pp. 342–347.

Baer, H.A., 2004. Toward an Integrative Medicine: Merging Alternative Therapies With Biomedicine. Rowman Altamira.

Bai, W., Chen, C., Tarroni, G., Duan, J., Guitton, F., Petersen, S.E., Guo, Y., Matthews, P.M., Rueckert, D., 2019. Self-supervised learning for cardiac MR image segmentation by anatomical position prediction. In: International Conference on Medical Image Computing and Computer-Assisted Intervention, pp. 541–549.

Bakken, S., 2020. Hot Topics in Clinical Informatics. Oxford University Press, https://doi.org/10.1093/jamia/ocaa025.

Baldi, P., 2012. Autoencoders, unsupervised learning, and deep architectures. In: Proceedings of ICML Workshop on Unsupervised and Transfer Learning, pp. 37–49.

Bannach-Brown, A., Przybyła, P., Thomas, J., Rice, A.S.C., Ananiadou, S., Liao, J., Macleod, M.R., 2018. The use of text-mining and machine learning algorithms in systematic reviews: reducing workload in preclinical biomedical sciences and reducing human screening error. BioRxiv, 255760. https://doi.org/10.1101/255760.

Bao, Y., Jiang, X., 2016. An intelligent medicine recommender system framework. In: 2016 IEEE 11th Conference on Industrial Electronics and Applications (ICIEA), pp. 1383–1388.

Barnett, G.O., Cimino, J.J., Hupp, J.A., Hoffer, E.P., 1987. DXplain: an evolving diagnostic decision-support system. Jama 258 (1), 67–74. https://doi.org/10.1001/jama.1987.03400010071030.

Bartold, S.P., Hannigan, G.G., 2002. DXplain. J. Med. Libr. Assoc. 90 (2), 267.

Baxter, J., 1995. Learning internal representations. In: Proceedings of the Eighth Annual Conference on Computational Learning Theory, pp. 311–320.

Bhat, S., Aishwarya, K., 2013. Item-based hybrid recommender system for newly marketed pharmaceutical drugs. In: 2013 International Conference on Advances in Computing, Communications and Informatics (ICACCI), pp. 2107–2111.

Blendowski, M., Nickisch, H., Heinrich, M.P., 2019. How to learn from unlabeled volume data: self-supervised 3D context feature learning. In: International Conference on Medical Image Computing and Computer-Assisted Intervention, pp. 649–657, https://doi.org/10.1007/978-3-030-32226-7_72.

Breiman, L., 2001. Random forests. Mach. Learn. 45 (1), 5–32. https://doi.org/10.1023/A:1010933404324.

Brodley, C.E., Utgoff, P.E., 1995. Multivariate decision trees. Mach. Learn. 19 (1), 45–77. https://doi.org/10.1023/A:1022607123649.

Broomhead, D.S., Lowe, D., 1988. Multivariate functional interpolation and adaptive networks. Complex Syst. 2, 321–355.

Cabezas, M., Valverde, S., González-Villà, S., Clérigues, A., Salem, M., Kushibar, K., Bernal, J., Oliver, A., Lladó, X., 2018. Survival prediction using ensemble tumor segmentation and transfer learning. In: Multimodal Brain Tumor Segmentation Challenge 2018 (BRATS) in Medical Imaging. MICCAI 2018.

Cantor, A., et al., 2003. SAS Survival Analysis Techniques for Medical Research. SAS Institute.

Carreira, J., Zisserman, A., 2017. Quo vadis, action recognition? A new model and the kinetics dataset. In: Proceedings of the IEEE Conference on Computer Vision and Pattern Recognition, pp. 6299–6308.

Caruana, R., Niculescu-Mizil, A., 2006. An empirical comparison of supervised learning algorithms. In: Proceedings of the 23rd International Conference on Machine Learning, pp. 161–168.

Castellino, R.A., 2005. Computer aided detection (CAD): an overview. Cancer Imaging 5 (1), 17.

Chakraborty, S., Tomsett, R., Raghavendra, R., Harborne, D., Alzantot, M., Cerutti, F., Srivastava, M., Preece, A., Julier, S., Rao, R.M., et al., 2017. Interpretability of deep learning models: a survey of results. In: 2017 IEEE SmartWorld, Ubiquitous Intelligence & Computing, Advanced & Trusted Computed, Scalable Computing &

Communications, Cloud & Big Data Computing, Internet of People and Smart City Innovation (SmartWorld/SCALCOM/UIC/ATC/CBDCom/IOP/SCI), pp. 1–6.

Char, D.S., Shah, N.H., Magnus, D., 2018. Implementing machine learning in health care—addressing ethical challenges. N. Engl. J. Med. 378 (11), 981.

Chen, J.H., Asch, S.M., 2017. Machine learning and prediction in medicine-beyond the peak of inflated expectations. N. Engl. J. Med. 376 (26), 2507. https://doi.org/10.1056/NEJMp1702071.

Chen, Y., Mani, S., Xu, H., 2012. Applying active learning to assertion classification of concepts in clinical text. J. Biomed. Inform. 45 (2), 265–272. https://doi.org/10.1016/j.jbi.2011.11.003.

Chen, Y., Lask, T.A., Mei, Q., Chen, Q., Moon, S., Wang, J., Nguyen, K., Dawodu, T., Cohen, T., Denny, J.C., et al., 2017. An active learning-enabled annotation system for clinical named entity recognition. BMC Med. Inform. Decis. Mak. 17 (2), 35–44. https://doi.org/10.1186/s12911-017-0466-9.

Choi, J.P., Han, T.H., Park, R.W., 2009. A hybrid Bayesian network model for predicting breast cancer prognosis. J. Korean Soc. Med. Inform. 15 (1), 49–57. https://doi.org/10.4258/jksmi.2009.15.1.49.

Chollet, F., 2017. Xception: deep learning with depthwise separable convolutions. In: Proceedings of the IEEE Conference on Computer Vision and Pattern Recognition, pp. 1251–1258.

Ciecierski, K., Raś, Z.W., Przybyszewski, A.W., 2012. Foundations of recommender system for STN localization during DBS surgery in Parkinson's patients. In: International Symposium on Methodologies for Intelligent Systems, pp. 234–243, https://doi.org/10.1007/978-3-642-34624-8_28.

Collen, M.F., 1986. Origins of medical informatics. Western J. Med. 145 (6), 778–785.

Cox, D.R., Oakes, D., 1984. Analysis of Survival Data. vol. 21 CRC Press.

Cruz, J.A., Wishart, D.S., 2006. Applications of machine learning in cancer prediction and prognosis. Cancer Inform. 2, 59–77.

De Silva, D., Ranasinghe, W., Bandaragoda, T., Adikari, A., Mills, N., Iddamalgoda, L., Alahakoon, D., Lawrentschuk, N., Persad, R., Osipov, E., et al., 2018. Machine learning to support social media empowered patients in cancer care and cancer treatment decisions. PLoS One 13 (10), e0205855. https://doi.org/10.1371/journal.pone.0205855.

Deserno, T.M., Welter, P., Horsch, A., 2012. Towards a repository for standardized medical image and signal case data annotated with ground truth. J. Digit. Imaging 25 (2), 213–226.

Dligach, D., Miller, T., Savova, G., 2013. Active learning for phenotyping tasks. In: Proceedings of the Workshop on NLP for Medicine and Biology Associated With RANLP 2013, September, INCOMA Ltd. Shoumen, BULGARIA, Hissar, Bulgaria, pp. 1–8.

Dobi, B., Zempléni, A., 2019. Markov chain-based cost-optimal control charts for health care data. Qual. Reliab. Eng. Int. 35 (5), 1379–1395. https://doi.org/10.1002/qre.2518.

Dreiseitl, S., Ohno-Machado, L., 2002. Logistic regression and artificial neural network classification models: a methodology review. J. Biomed. Inform. 35 (5–6), 352–359. https://doi.org/10.1016/S1532-0464(03)00034-0.

Druck, G., Settles, B., McCallum, A., 2009. Active learning by labeling features. In: EMNLP '09. Proceedings of the 2009 Conference on Empirical Methods in Natural Language Processing, vol. 1, Association for Computational Linguistics, USA, pp. 81–90.

Du, J., Zhang, Y., Luo, J., Jia, Y., Wei, Q., Tao, C., Xu, H., 2018. Extracting psychiatric stressors for suicide from social media using deep learning. BMC Med. Inform. Decis. Mak. 18 (2), 43. https://doi.org/10.1186/s12911-018-0632-8.

Dudani, S.A., 1976. The distance-weighted k-nearest-neighbor rule. IEEE Trans. Syst. Man Cybern. SMC-6 (4), 325–327. https://doi.org/10.1109/tsmc.1976.5408784.

Dybowski, R., Roberts, S., 2005. An anthology of probabilistic models for medical informatics. In: Probabilistic Modeling in Bioinformatics and Medical Informatics, Springer, pp. 297–349.

Efron, B., Hastie, T., Johnstone, I., Tibshirani, R., et al., 2004. Least angle regression. Ann. Stat. 32 (2), 407–499.

Eftekhar, B., Mohammad, K., Ardebili, H.E., Ghodsi, M., Ketabchi, E., 2005. Comparison of artificial neural network and logistic regression models for prediction of mortality in head trauma based on initial clinical data. BMC Med. Inform. Decis. Mak. 5 (1), 1–8. https://doi.org/10.1186/1472-6947-5-3.

Ernst, E., 2000. The role of complementary and alternative medicine. Bmj 321 (7269), 1133. https://doi.org/10.1136/bmj.321.7269.1133.

Esteva, A., Kuprel, B., Novoa, R.A., Ko, J., Swetter, S.M., Blau, H.M., Thrun, S., 2017. Dermatologist-level classification of skin cancer with deep neural networks. Nature 542 (7639), 115–118. https://doi.org/10.1038/nature21056.

Fanconi, C., 2019. Skin Cancer: Malignant vs. Benign. https://www.kaggle.com/fanconic/skin-cancer-malignant-vs-benign. (June).

Fischer, A., Igel, C., 2012. An introduction to restricted Boltzmann machines. In: Iberoamerican Congress on Pattern Recognition, pp. 14–36.

Fredrickson, B.L., 2000. Cultivating positive emotions to optimize health and well-being. Prev. Treat. 3 (1), 1a. https://doi.org/10.1037/1522-3736.3.1.31a.

Friedman, N., Geiger, D., Goldszmidt, M., 1997. Bayesian network classifiers. Mach. Learn. 29 (2–3), 131–163. https://doi.org/10.1023/A:1007465528199.

Gaines, B.R., 2013. Knowledge acquisition: past, present and future. Int. J. Hum. Comput. Stud. 71 (2), 135–156. https://doi.org/10.1016/j.ijhcs.2012.10.010.

Galeano, D., Paccanaro, A., 2018. A recommender system approach for predicting drug side effects. In: 2018 International Joint Conference on Neural Networks (IJCNN), pp. 1–8.

Ghahramani, Z., 2003. Unsupervised learning. In: Summer School on Machine Learning, pp. 72–112.

Ghassemi, M., Naumann, T., Schulam, P., Beam, A.L., Chen, I.Y., Ranganath, R., 2020. A review of challenges and opportunities in machine learning for health. AMIA Summits Trans. Sci. Proc. 2020, 191.

Giarratano, J.C., Riley, G., 1998. Expert Systems. PWS Publishing Co.

Gildenblat, J., Klaiman, E., 2019. Self-supervised similarity learning for digital pathology. CoRR abs/1905.08139.

Goodfellow, I., Pouget-Abadie, J., Mirza, M., Xu, B., Warde-Farley, D., Ozair, S., Courville, A., Bengio, Y., 2014. Generative adversarial nets. In: Advances in Neural Information Processing Systems, pp. 2672–2680.

Goodfellow, I., Bengio, Y., Courville, A., 2016. Deep Learning. MIT Press.

Graber, M.L., Franklin, N., Gordon, R., 2005. Diagnostic error in internal medicine. Arch. Intern. Med. 165 (13), 1493–1499. https://doi.org/10.1001/archinte.165.13.1493.

Gräßer, F., Beckert, S., Küster, D., Schmitt, J., Abraham, S., Malberg, H., Zaunseder, S., 2017. Therapy decision support based on recommender system methods. J. Healthcare Eng. 2017. https://doi.org/10.1155/2017/8659460.

Anon., 2021. Guidelines for Preparing Clinical Study Data Sets for Submission to the NHLBI Data Repository. https://www.nhlbi.nih.gov/grants-and-training/policies-and-guidelines/guidelines-for-preparing-clinical-study-data-sets-for-submission-to-the-nhlbi-data-repository. (Accessed 16 March 2021).

Guo, L., Jin, B., Yao, C., Yang, H., Huang, D., Wang, F., 2016. Which doctor to trust: a recommender system for identifying the right doctors. J. Med. Internet Res. 18 (7), e186. https://doi.org/10.2196/jmir.6015.

Handelman, G.S., Kok, H.K., Chandra, R.V., Razavi, A.H., Lee, M.J., Asadi, H., 2018. eDoctor: machine learning and the future of medicine. J. Intern. Med. 284 (6), 603–619.

Hannan, S.A., Manza, R.R., Ramteke, R.J., 2010. Generalized regression neural network and radial basis function for heart disease diagnosis. Int. J. Comput. Appl. 7 (13), 7–13. https://doi.org/10.5120/1325-1799.

Hasman, A., Mantas, J., Zarubina, T., 2014. An abridged history of medical informatics education in Europe. Acta Inform. Med. 22 (1), 25. https://doi.org/10.5455/aim.2014.22.25-36.

Hassoun, M.H., et al., 1995. Fundamentals of Artificial Neural Networks. MIT Press.

He, K., Zhang, X., Ren, S., Sun, J., 2016. Deep residual learning for image recognition. In: Proceedings of the IEEE Conference on Computer Vision and Pattern Recognition, pp. 770–778.

Anon., 2021. Healthcare. https://healthcare-analytics.soa.org/. (Accessed 17 March 2021).

Hoffmann, R., Zhang, C., Weld, D.S., 2010. Learning 5000 relational extractors. In: Proceedings of the 48th Annual Meeting of the Association for Computational Linguistics, July, Association for Computational Linguistics, Uppsala, Sweden, pp. 286–295.

Holzinger, A., 2016. Interactive machine learning for health informatics: when do we need the human-in-the-loop? Brain Inform. 3 (2), 119–131. https://doi.org/10.1007/s40708-016-0042-6.

Holzinger, A., Jurisica, I., 2014. Knowledge discovery and data mining in biomedical informatics: the future is in integrative, interactive machine learning solutions. In: Interactive Knowledge Discovery and Data Mining In Biomedical Informatics, Springer, pp. 1–18.

Huang, G., Liu, Z., Van Der Maaten, L., Weinberger, K.Q., 2017. Densely connected convolutional networks. In: Proceedings of the IEEE Conference on Computer Vision and Pattern Recognition, pp. 4700–4708.

Iandola, F.N., Han, S., Moskewicz, M.W., Ashraf, K., Dally, W.J., Keutzer, K., 2016. SqueezeNet: AlexNet-level accuracy with $50\times$ fewer parameters and $<0.5$ MB model size. CoRR.

Anon., 2021. IBM Watson AI Healthcare Solutions. https://www.ibm.com/watson-health. (Accessed 16 March 2021).

imconsortium, 2020. Introduction. The Academic Consortium for Integrative Medicine & Health. https://imconsortium.org/about/introduction/. (Accessed 16 March 2021).

Jeyaraj, P.R., Nadar, E.R.S., 2019. Computer-assisted medical image classification for early diagnosis of oral cancer employing deep learning algorithm. J. Cancer Res. Clin. Oncol. 145 (4), 829–837.

Jha, S.K., Pan, Z., Elahi, E., Patel, N., 2019. A comprehensive search for expert classification methods in disease diagnosis and prediction. Expert Syst. 36 (1), e12343. https://doi.org/10.1111/exsy.12343.

Jordan, M.I., Mitchell, T.M., 2015. Machine learning: trends, perspectives, and prospects. Science 349 (6245), 255–260. https://doi.org/10.1126/science.aaa8415.

Kamnitsas, K., Bai, W., Ferrante, E., McDonagh, S., Sinclair, M., Pawlowski, N., Rajchl, M., Lee, M., Kainz, B., Rueckert, D., et al., 2017. Ensembles of multiple models and architectures for robust brain tumour segmentation. In: International MICCAI Brainlesion Workshop, pp. 450–462.

Kate, R.J., Nadig, R., 2017. Stage-specific predictive models for breast cancer survivability. Int. J. Med. Inform. 97, 304–311. https://doi.org/10.1016/j.ijmedinf.2016.11.001.

Kavraki, L.E., Kolountzakis, M.N., Latombe, J.C., 1998. Analysis of probabilistic roadmaps for path planning. IEEE Trans. Robot. Autom. 14 (1), 166–171. https://doi.org/10.1109/70.660866.

Kawanabe, T., Kamarudin, N.D., Ooi, C.Y., Kobayashi, F., Mi, X., Sekine, M., Wakasugi, A., Odaguchi, H., Hanawa, T., 2016. Quantification of tongue colour using machine learning in Kampo medicine. Eur. J. Integr. Med. 8 (6), 932–941. https://doi.org/10.1016/j.eujim.2016.04.002.

Kayaer, K., Yildirim, T., et al., 2003. Medical diagnosis on Pima Indian diabetes using general regression neural networks. In: Proceedings of the International Conference on Artificial Neural Networks and Neural Information Processing (ICANN/ICONIP), vol. 181, p. 184.

Kendale, S., Kulkarni, P., Rosenberg, A.D., Wang, J., 2018. Supervised machine-learning predictive analytics for prediction of postinduction hypotension. Anesthesiol. J. Am. Soc. Anesthesiol. 129 (4), 675–688. https://doi.org/10.1097/ALN.0000000000002374.

Kim, B.-J., Kim, S.-H., 2018. Prediction of inherited genomic susceptibility to 20 common cancer types by a supervised machine-learning method. Proc. Natl. Acad. Sci. 115 (6), 1322–1327.

Khurana, U., Samulowitz, H., Turaga, D., 2018. Feature engineering for predictive modeling using reinforcement learning. In: Proceedings of the AAAI Conference on Artificial Intelligence, vol. 32, no. 1.

Kim, M., Choi, J., Kim, N., 2020. Fully automated hand hygiene monitoring in operating room using 3D convolutional neural network. CoRR.

Kleinbaum, D.G., Dietz, K., Gail, M., Klein, M., Klein, M., 2002. Logistic Regression. Springer.

Knaus, W.A., Draper, E.A., Wagner, D.P., Zimmerman, J.E., 1985. APACHE II: a severity of disease classification system. Crit. Care Med. 13 (10), 818–829.

Knaus, W.A., Wagner, D.P., Draper, E.A., Zimmerman, J.E., Bergner, M., Bastos, P.G., Sirio, C.A., Murphy, D.J., Lotring, T., Damiano, A., et al., 1991. The APACHE III prognostic system: risk prediction of hospital mortality for critically III hospitalized adults. Chest 100 (6), 1619–1636. https://doi.org/10.1378/chest.100.6.1619.

Kolachalama, V.B., Garg, P.S., 2018. Machine learning and medical education. npj Digit. Med. 1 (1), 1–3. https://doi.org/10.1038/s41746-018-0061-1.

Kononenko, I., 1991. Semi-Naive Bayesian classifier. In: European Working Session on Learning, pp. 206–219.

Kononenko, I., 2001. Machine learning for medical diagnosis: history, state of the art and perspective. Artif. Intell. Med. 23 (1), 89–109. https://doi.org/10.1016/S0933-3657(01)00077-X.

Kononenko, I., Simec, E., 1995. Induction of decision trees using RELIEFF. In: Proceedings of the ISSEK94 Workshop on Mathematical and Statistical Methods in Artificial Intelligence, pp. 199–220.

Kourou, K., Exarchos, T.P., Exarchos, K.P., Karamouzis, M.V., Fotiadis, D.I., 2015. Machine learning applications in cancer prognosis and prediction. Comput. Struct. Biotechnol. J. 13, 8–17. https://doi.org/10.1016/j.csbj.2014.11.005.

Koza, J.R., 1994. Genetic programming as a means for programming computers by natural selection. Stat. Comput. 4 (2), 87–112. https://doi.org/10.1007/BF00175355.

Krizhevsky, A., Sutskever, I., Hinton, G.E., 2012. ImageNet classification with deep convolutional neural networks. In: Advances in Neural Information Processing Systems, pp. 1097–1105.

Kushwaha, N., Goyal, R., Goel, P., Singla, S., Vyas, O.P., 2014. LOD Cloud mining for prognosis model (Case study: Native app for drug recommender system). Adv. Internet Things 2014. https://doi.org/10.4236/ait.2014.43004.

Kwak, G.H.-J., Hui, P., 2019. Deephealth: deep learning for health informatics. In: ACM Transactions on Computing for Healthcare.

Lawrence, S., Giles, C.L., Tsoi, A.C., Back, A.D., 1997. Face recognition: a convolutional neural-network approach. IEEE Trans. Neural Netw. 8 (1), 98–113. https://doi.org/10.1109/72.554195.

Lazer, D., Kennedy, R., King, G., Vespignani, A., 2014. The parable of Google Flu: traps in big data analysis. Science 343 (6176), 1203–1205. https://doi.org/10.1126/science.1248506.

Le Gall, J.-R., Lemeshow, S., Saulnier, F., 1993. A new simplified acute physiology score (SAPS II) based on a European/North American multicenter study. Jama 270 (24), 2957–2963. https://doi.org/10.1001/jama.270.24.2957.

LeCun, Y., Bengio, Y., Hinton, G., 2015. Deep learning. Nature 521 (7553), 436–444. https://doi.org/10.1038/nature14539.

Ledzewicz, U., Schättler, H., 2006. Drug resistance in cancer chemotherapy as an optimal control problem. Discrete Contin. Dyn. Syst. B 6 (1), 129. https://doi.org/10.3934/dcdsb.2006.6.129.

Ledzewiecz, U., Marriott, J., Maurer, H., Schättler, H., 2008. The scheduling of angiogenic inhibitors minimizing tumor volume. J. Med. Inform. Technol. 12. https://doi.org/10.3934/dcdsb.2009.12.415.

Lee, J.Y., Dernoncourt, F., Szolovits, P., 2018. Transfer learning for named-entity recognition with neural networks. In: Proceedings of the Eleventh International Conference on Language Resources and Evaluation (LREC 2018).

Lemeshow, S., Teres, D., Klar, J., Avrunin, J.S., Gehlbach, S.H., Rapoport, J., 1993. Mortality probability models (MPM II) based on an international cohort of intensive care unit patients. Jama 270 (20), 2478–2486. https://doi.org/10.1001/jama.1993.03510200084037.

Lewinsohn, P.M., Libet, J., 1972. Pleasant events, activity schedules, and depressions. J. Abnorm. Psychol. 79 (3), 291. https://doi.org/10.1037/h0033207.

Lewis, D.D., Gale, W.A., 1994. A sequential algorithm for training text classifiers. In: SIGIR'94, pp. 3–12.

Liu, S., Liu, S., Cai, W., Pujol, S., Kikinis, R., Feng, D., 2014. Early diagnosis of Alzheimer's disease with deep learning. In: 2014 IEEE 11th International Symposium on Biomedical Imaging (ISBI), pp. 1015–1018.

Liu, Y., Logan, B., Liu, N., Xu, Z., Tang, J., Wang, Y., 2017. Deep reinforcement learning for dynamic treatment regimes on medical registry data. In: 2017 IEEE International Conference on Healthcare Informatics (ICHI), pp. 380–385.

Liu, Q., Wei, Z., Peng, B., Tou, H., Chen, T., Huang, X.-J., Wong, K.-F., Dai, X., 2018. Task-oriented dialogue system for automatic diagnosis. In: Proceedings of the 56th Annual Meeting of the Association for Computational Linguistics (vol. 2: Short Papers), pp. 201–207.

MacPhillamy, D.J., Lewinsohn, P.M., 1982. The pleasant events schedule: studies on reliability, validity, and scale intercorrelation. J. Consult. Clin. Psychol. 50 (3), 363. https://doi.org/10.1037/0022-006X.50.3.363.

Mahbod, A., Schaefer, G., Ellinger, I., Ecker, R., Pitiot, A., Wang, C., 2019. Fusing fine-tuned deep features for skin lesion classification. Comput. Med. Imaging Graph. 71, 19–29.

Maizes, V., Rakel, D., Niemiec, C., 2009. Integrative medicine and patient-centered care. Explore 5 (5), 277–289. https://doi.org/10.1016/j.explore.2009.06.008.

Mayer, H., Gomez, F., Wierstra, D., Nagy, I., Knoll, A., Schmidhuber, J., 2008a. A system for robotic heart surgery that learns to tie knots using recurrent neural networks. Adv. Robot. 22 (13–14), 1521–1537.

Mayer, H., Nagy, I., Burschka, D., Knoll, A., Braun, E.U., Lange, R., Bauernschmitt, R., 2008b. Automation of manual tasks for minimally invasive surgery. In: Fourth International Conference on Autonomic and Autonomous Systems (ICAS'08), pp. 260–265.

Anon., 2021. Medical Robot|KAIST Telerobotics and Control Lab. http://robot.kaist.ac.kr/medical-robots/. (Accessed 16 March 2021).

Melville, P., Sindhwani, V., 2010. Recommender systems. Encyclopedia Mach. Learn. 1, 829–838. https://doi.org/10.1007/978-0-387-30164-8_705.

Mendez-Tellez, P.A., Dorman, T., 2005. Predicting patient outcomes, futility, and resource utilization in the intensive care unit: the role of severity scoring systems and general outcome prediction models. In: Mayo Clin. Proc., vol. 80, pp. 161–163.

Meng, X., Ganoe, C.H., Sieberg, R.T., Cheung, Y.Y., Hassanpour, S., 2020. Self-supervised contextual language representation of radiology reports to improve the identification of communication urgency. AMIA Summits Trans. Sci. Proc. 2020, 413.

mghlcs, n.d. DXplain. The Laboratory of Computer Science. http://www.mghlcs.org/projects/dxplain.

Miller, R.A., 1994. Medical diagnostic decision support systems—past, present, and future: a threaded bibliography and brief commentary. J. Am. Med. Inform. Assoc. 1 (1), 8–27. https://doi.org/10.1136/jamia.1994.95236141.

Miller, R.A., Masarie Jr., F.E., 1989. Quick medical reference (QMR): an evolving, microcomputer-based diagnostic decision-support program for general internal medicine. In: Proceedings of the Annual Symposium on Computer Application in Medical Care, p. 947.

Miller, R.A., Pople Jr., H.E., Myers, J.D., 1982. Internist-i, an experimental computer-based diagnostic consultant for general internal medicine. N. Engl. J. Med. 307 (8), 468–476. https://doi.org/10.1056/NEJM198208193070803.

Milletari, F., Birodkar, V., Sofka, M., 2019. Straight to the point: reinforcement learning for user guidance in ultrasound. In: Smart Ultrasound Imaging and Perinatal, Preterm and Paediatric Image Analysis, Springer, pp. 3–10.

Miotto, R., Wang, F., Wang, S., Jiang, X., Dudley, J.T., 2018. Deep learning for healthcare: review, opportunities and challenges. Brief. Bioinform. 19 (6), 1236–1246. https://doi.org/10.1093/bib/bbx044.

Mobadersany, P., Yousefi, S., Amgad, M., Gutman, D.A., Barnholtz-Sloan, J.S., Vega, J.E.V., Brat, D.J., Cooper, L.A.D., 2018. Predicting cancer outcomes from histology and genomics using convolutional networks. Proc. Natl. Acad. Sci. 115 (13), E2970–E2979. https://doi.org/10.1073/pnas.1717139115.

Mostafa, S.A., Mustapha, A., Khaleefah, S.H., Ahmad, M.S., Mohammed, M.A., 2018. Evaluating the performance of three classification methods in diagnosis of Parkinson's disease. In: International Conference on Soft Computing and Data Mining, pp. 43–52.

Moustris, G.P., Hiridis, S.C., Deliparaschos, K.M., Konstantinidis, K.M., 2011. Evolution of autonomous and semi-autonomous robotic surgical systems: a review of the literature. Int. J. Med. Robot. Comput. Assist. Surg. 7 (4), 375–392. https://doi.org/10.1002/rcs.408.

Murphy, S.N., Herrick, C., Wang, Y., Wang, T.D., Sack, D., Andriole, K.P., Wei, J., Reynolds, N., Plesniak, W., Rosen, B.R., et al., 2015. High throughput tools to access images from clinical archives for research. J. Digit. Imaging 28 (2), 194–204. https://doi.org/10.1007/s10278-014-9733-9.

Nadeem, M.W., Ghamdi, M.A.A., Hussain, M., Khan, M.A., Khan, K.M., Almotiri, S.H., Butt, S.A., 2020. Brain tumor analysis empowered with deep learning: a review, taxonomy, and future challenges. Brain Sci. 10 (2), 118. https://doi.org/10.3390/brainsci10020118.

Nair, V., Hinton, G.E., 2010. Rectified linear units improve restricted Boltzmann machines. In: ICML, pp. 807–814.

Nida, N., Irtaza, A., Javed, A., Yousaf, M.H., Mahmood, M.T., 2019. Melanoma lesion detection and segmentation using deep region based convolutional neural network and fuzzy C-means clustering. Int. J. Med. Inform. 124, 37–48.

Niemeijer, M., Abramoff, M.D., Van Ginneken, B., 2009. Information fusion for diabetic retinopathy CAD in digital color fundus photographs. IEEE Trans. Med. Imaging 28 (5), 775–785. https://doi.org/10.1109/TMI.2008.2012029.

Ohno-Machado, L., 2001. Modeling medical prognosis: survival analysis techniques. J. Biomed. Inform. 34 (6), 428–439. https://doi.org/10.1006/jbin.2002.1038.

Oztekin, A., Delen, D., Kong, Z.J., 2009. Predicting the graft survival for heart-lung transplantation patients: an integrated data mining methodology. Int. J. Med. Inform. 78 (12), e84–e96. https://doi.org/10.1016/j.ijmedinf.2009.04.007.

Pakhomov, S.V.S., Buntrock, J.D., Chute, C.G., 2006. Automating the assignment of diagnosis codes to patient encounters using example-based and machine learning techniques. J. Am. Med. Inform. Assoc. 13 (5), 516–525. https://doi.org/10.1197/jamia.M2077.

Pan, S.J., Yang, Q., 2009. A survey on transfer learning. IEEE Trans. Knowl. Data Eng. 22 (10), 1345–1359. https://doi.org/10.1109/TKDE.2009.191.

Parikh, R.B., Obermeyer, Z., Navathe, A.S., 2019. Regulation of predictive analytics in medicine. Science 363 (6429), 810–812. https://doi.org/10.1126/science.aaw0029.

Peng, Y.-S., Tang, K.-F., Lin, H.-T., Chang, E., 2018. REFUEL: exploring sparse features in deep reinforcement learning for fast disease diagnosis. In: Bengio, S., Wallach, H., Larochelle, H., Grauman, K., Cesa-Bianchi, N., Garnett, R. (Eds.), Advances in Neural Information Processing Systems 31. Curran Associates, Inc, pp. 7322–7331.

Peng, Y., Yan, S., Lu, Z., 2019. Transfer learning in biomedical natural language processing: an evaluation of BERT and ELMo on ten benchmarking datasets., https://doi.org/10.18653/v1/w19-5006.

Petscharnig, S., Schöffmann, K., 2017. Deep learning for shot classification in gynecologic surgery videos. In: International Conference on Multimedia Modeling, pp. 702–713.

Polat, K., Güneş, S., 2007. Breast cancer diagnosis using least square support vector machine. Digit. Signal Process. 17 (4), 694–701. https://doi.org/10.1016/j.dsp.2006.10.008.

Portugal, I., Alencar, P., Cowan, D., 2018. The use of machine learning algorithms in recommender systems: a systematic review. Expert Syst. Appl. 97, 205–227. https://doi.org/10.1016/j.eswa.2017.12.020.

Prashanth, R., Roy, S.D., Mandal, P.K., Ghosh, S., 2016. High-accuracy detection of early Parkinson's disease through multimodal features and machine learning. Int. J. Med. Inform. 90, 13–21.

Prinja, S., Gupta, N., Verma, R., 2010. Censoring in clinical trials: review of survival analysis techniques. Indian J. Community Med. 35 (2), 217. https://doi.org/10.4103/0970-0218.66859.

Qiu, J., Sun, Y., 2019. Self-supervised iterative refinement learning for macular OCT volumetric data classification. Comput. Biol. Med. 111, 103327. https://doi.org/10.1016/j.compbiomed.2019.103327.

Ragavan, H., Rendell, L.A., 1993. Lookahead feature construction for learning hard concepts. In: ICML, pp. 252–259.

Raghu, A., Komorowski, M., Celi, L.A., Szolovits, P., Ghassemi, M., 2017. Continuous state-space models for optimal sepsis treatment—a deep reinforcement learning approach. In: Proceedings of the 2nd Machine Learning for Healthcare Conference, PMLR, vol. 68, pp. 147–163.

Rajkomar, A., Dean, J., Kohane, I., 2019. Machine learning in medicine. N. Engl. J. Med. 380 (14), 1347–1358. https://doi.org/10.1056/NEJMra1814259.

Ralston, J.D., Carrell, D., Reid, R., Anderson, M., Moran, M., Hereford, J., 2007. Patient web services integrated with a shared medical record: patient use and satisfaction. J. Am. Med. Inform. Assoc. 14 (6), 798–806. https://doi.org/10.1197/jamia.M2302.

Randhawa, G.S., Soltysiak, M.P.M., El Roz, H., de Souza, C.P.E., Hill, K.A., Kari, L., 2020. Machine learning using intrinsic genomic signatures for rapid classification of novel pathogens: COVID-19 case study. PLoS One 15 (4), e0232391.

Rapsang, A.G., Shyam, D.C., 2014. Scoring systems in the intensive care unit: a compendium. Indian J. Crit. Care Med. 18 (4), 220. https://doi.org/10.4103/0972-5229.130573.

Rassinoux, A.M., Miller, R.A., Baud, R.H., Scherrer, J.-R., 1996. Modeling principles for QMR medical findings. In: Proceedings of the AMIA Annual Fall Symposium, p. 264.

Ravì, D., Wong, C., Deligianni, F., Berthelot, M., Andreu-Perez, J., Lo, B., Yang, G.-Z., 2016. Deep learning for health informatics. IEEE J. Biomed. Health Inform. 21 (1), 4–21. https://doi.org/10.1109/JBHI.2016.2636665.

Rish, I., et al., 2001. An empirical study of the naive Bayes classifier. In: IJCAI 2001 Workshop on Empirical Methods in Artificial Intelligence, vol. 3, pp. 41–46.

Rohani, D.A., Springer, A., Hollis, V., Bardram, J.E., Whittaker, S., 2020. Recommending activities for mental health and well-being: insights from two user studies. IEEE Trans. Emerging Topics Comput. https://doi.org/10.1109/TETC.2020.2972007.

Roller, R., Stevenson, M., 2014. Self-supervised relation extraction using UMLS. In: International Conference of the Cross-Language Evaluation Forum for European Languages, pp. 116–127.

Ronneberger, O., Fischer, P., Brox, T., 2015. U-Net: convolutional networks for biomedical image segmentation. In: International Conference on Medical Image Computing and Computer-Assisted Intervention, pp. 234–241.

Ross, T., Zimmerer, D., Vemuri, A., Isensee, F., Wiesenfarth, M., Bodenstedt, S., Both, F., Kessler, P., Wagner, M., Müller, B., et al., 2018. Exploiting the potential of unlabeled endoscopic video data with self-supervised learning. Int. J. Comput. Assist. Radiol. Surg. 13 (6), 925–933. https://doi.org/10.1007/s11548-018-1772-0.

Royston, P., Sauerbrei, W., 2008. Multivariable Model-Building: A Pragmatic Approach to Regression Analysis Based on Fractional Polynomials for Modelling Continuous Variables. vol. 777 John Wiley & Sons, https://doi.org/10.1002/9780470770771.

Sahba, F., Tizhoosh, H.R., Salama, M.M.A., 2006. A reinforcement learning framework for medical image segmentation. In: The 2006 IEEE International Joint Conference on Neural Network Proceedings, pp. 511–517.

Sahba, F., Tizhoosh, H.R., Salama, M.M.M.A., 2007. Application of opposition-based reinforcement learning in image segmentation. In: 2007 IEEE Symposium on Computational Intelligence in Image and Signal Processing, pp. 246–251.

Sajda, P., 2006. Machine learning for detection and diagnosis of disease. Annu. Rev. Biomed. Eng. 8, 537–565. https://doi.org/10.1146/annurev.bioeng.8.061505.095802.

Salman, F.M., Abu-Naser, S.S., 2020. Expert system for COVID-19 diagnosis. Int. J. Acad. Inf. Syst. Res. (IJAISR) 4 (3), 1–13.

Samuel, A.L., 1959. Some studies in machine learning using the game of checkers. IBM J. Res. Dev. 3 (3), 210–229. https://doi.org/10.1147/rd.33.0210.

Sánchez, C.I., Niemeijer, M., Abràmoff, M.D., van Ginneken, B., 2010. Active learning for an efficient training strategy of computer-aided diagnosis systems: application to diabetic retinopathy screening. In: International Conference on Medical Image Computing and Computer-Assisted Intervention, pp. 603–610.

Sandler, M., Howard, A., Zhu, M., Zhmoginov, A., Chen, L.-C., 2018. Mobilenetv2: inverted residuals and linear bottlenecks. In: Proceedings of the IEEE Conference on Computer Vision and Pattern Recognition, pp. 4510–4520.

Sarkar, P., Etemad, A., 2020. Self-supervised ECG representation learning for emotion recognition. IEEE Trans. Affect. Comput. https://doi.ieeecomputersociety.org/10.1109/TAFFC.2020.3014842.

Sarwar, B., Karypis, G., Konstan, J., Riedl, J., 2001. Item-based collaborative filtering recommendation algorithms. In: Proceedings of the 10th International Conference on World Wide Web, pp. 285–295.

Savage, N., 2012. Better medicine through machine learning. Commun. ACM 55 (1), 17–19. https://doi.org/10.1145/2063176.2063182.

Schaal, S., 1997. Learning from demonstration. In: Advances in Neural Information Processing Systems, pp. 1040–1046.

Schilling, C., Mortimer, D., Dalziel, K., Heeley, E., Chalmers, J., Clarke, P., 2016. Using classification and regression trees (CART) to identify prescribing thresholds for cardiovascular disease. Pharmacoeconomics 34 (2), 195–205. https://doi.org/10.1007/s40273-015-0342-3.

Schuster, M., Paliwal, K.K., 1997. Bidirectional recurrent neural networks. IEEE Trans. Signal Process. 45 (11), 2673–2681. https://doi.org/10.1109/78.650093.

Anon., 2021. SEER Incidence Database—SEER Data & Software. https://seer.cancer.gov/data/. (Accessed 12 March 2021).

Settles, B., 2009. Active Learning Literature Survey. Department of Computer Sciences, University of Wisconsin-Madison.

Shah, N.D., Steyerberg, E.W., Kent, D.M., 2018. Big data and predictive analytics: recalibrating expectations. Jama 320 (1), 27–28. https://doi.org/10.1001/jama.2018.5602.

Shah, P., Kendall, F., Khozin, S., Goosen, R., Hu, J., Laramie, J., Ringel, M., Schork, N., 2019. Artificial intelligence and machine learning in clinical development: a translational perspective. npj Digit. Med. 2 (1), 1–5. https://doi.org/10.1038/s41746-019-0148-3.

Shahar, Y., Musen, M.A., 1995. Plan recognition and revision in support of guideline-based care. In: Working notes of the AAAI Spring Symposium on Representing Mental States and Mechanisms, pp. 118–126.

Shameer, K., Johnson, K.W., Glicksberg, B.S., Dudley, J.T., Sengupta, P.P., 2018. Machine learning in cardiovascular medicine: are we there yet? Heart 104 (14), 1156–1164. https://doi.org/10.1136/heartjnl-2017-311198.

Shortliffe, E.H., 1986. Medical expert systems—knowledge tools for physicians. Western J. Med. 145 (6), 830.

Shortliffe, E., 2012. Computer-Based Medical Consultations: MYCIN. vol. 2 Elsevier.

Shortliffe, E.H., Buchanan, B.G., 1985. Rule-Based Expert Systems: The MYCIN Experiments of the Stanford Heuristic Programming Project. Addison-Wesley Publishing Company.

Shortliffe, E.H., Buchanan, B.G., Feigenbaum, E.A., 1979. Knowledge engineering for medical decision making: a review of computer-based clinical decision aids. Proc. IEEE 67 (9), 1207–1224. https://doi.org/10.1109/PROC.1979.11436.

Shvets, A.A., Rakhlin, A., Kalinin, A.A., Iglovikov, V.I., 2018. Automatic instrument segmentation in robot-assisted surgery using deep learning. In: 2018 17th IEEE International Conference on Machine Learning and Applications (ICMLA), pp. 624–628.

Sidey-Gibbons, J.A.M., Sidey-Gibbons, C.J., 2019. Machine learning in medicine: a practical introduction. BMC Med. Res. Methodol. 19 (1), 64. https://doi.org/10.1186/s12874-019-0681-4.

Simonyan, K., Zisserman, A., 2015. Very deep convolutional networks for large-scale image recognition. In: 3rd International Conference on Learning Representations.

Snyderman, R., Weil, A.T., 2002. Integrative medicine: bringing medicine back to its roots. Arch. Intern. Med. 162 (4), 395–397. https://doi.org/10.1001/archinte.162.4.395.

Son, L.H., Thong, N.T., 2015. Intuitionistic fuzzy recommender systems: an effective tool for medical diagnosis. Knowl. Based Syst. 74, 133–150. https://doi.org/10.1016/j.knosys.2014.11.012.

Sorokin, I., Seleznev, A., Pavlov, M., Fedorov, A., Ignateva, A., 2015. Deep attention recurrent q-network. In: Deep Reinforcement Learning Workshop. NeurIPS.

Specht, D.F., et al., 1991. A general regression neural network. IEEE Trans. Neural Netw. 2 (6), 568–576. https://doi.org/10.1109/72.97934.

Stanford Institute for Human-Centered Artificial Intelligence (HAI), 2021. COVID-19 and AI: a virtual conference. https://hai.stanford.edu/events/covid-19-and-ai-virtual-conference. (Accessed 17 March 2021).

Stark, B., Knahl, C., Aydin, M., Elish, K., 2019. A literature review on medicine recommender systems. Int. J. Adv. Comput. Sci. Appl. 10 (8), 6–13. https://doi.org/10.14569/IJACSA.2019.0100802.

Stewart, A., Diaz-Aviles, E., Nanopoulos, A., 2011. Self-supervised detection of disease reporting events in outbreak reports. In: 2011 IEEE International Conference on Information Reuse Integration, pp. 416–421.

Su, X., Khoshgoftaar, T.M., 2009. A survey of collaborative filtering techniques. Adv. Artif. Intell. 2009. https://doi.org/10.1155/2009/421425.

Suykens, J.A.K., Vandewalle, J., 1999. Least squares support vector machine classifiers. Neural Process. Lett. 9 (3), 293–300. https://doi.org/10.1023/A:1018628609742.

Svensson-Ranallo, P.A., Adam, T.J., Sainfort, F., 2011. A framework and standardized methodology for developing minimum clinical datasets. AMIA Summits Trans. Sci. Proc. 2011, 54.

Szegedy, C., Liu, W., Jia, Y., Sermanet, P., Reed, S., Anguelov, D., Erhan, D., Vanhoucke, V., Rabinovich, A., 2015. Going deeper with convolutions. In: Proceedings of the IEEE Conference on Computer Vision and Pattern Recognition, pp. 1–9.

Szegedy, C., Ioffe, S., Vanhoucke, V., Alemi, A.A., 2017. Inception-v4, inception-ResNet and the impact of residual connections on learning. In: Thirty-First AAAI Conference on Artificial Intelligence, pp. 4278–4284.

Tachibana, R., Näppi, J.J., Hironaka, T., Yoshida, H., 2020. Self-supervised generative adversarial network for electronic cleansing in dual-energy CT colonography. In: Medical Imaging 2020: Imaging Informatics for Healthcare, Research, and Applications, vol. 11318, p. 113181E, https://doi.org/10.1117/12.2549234.

Tajbakhsh, N., Shin, J.Y., Gurudu, S.R., Hurst, R.T., Kendall, C.B., Gotway, M.B., Liang, J., 2016. Convolutional neural networks for medical image analysis: full training or fine tuning? IEEE Trans. Med. Imaging 35 (5), 1299–1312. https://doi.org/10.1109/TMI.2016.2535302.

Tang, P.C., Ash, J.S., Bates, D.W., Overhage, J.M., Sands, D.Z., 2006. Personal health records: definitions, benefits, and strategies for overcoming barriers to adoption. J. Am. Med. Inform. Assoc. 13 (2), 121–126.

Taylor, R.H., Menciassi, A., Fichtinger, G., Fiorini, P., Dario, P., 2016. Medical robotics and computer-integrated surgery. In: Springer Handbook of Robotics, Springer, pp. 1657–1684.

Taylor, R.A., Moore, C.L., Cheung, K.-H., Brandt, C., 2018. Predicting urinary tract infections in the emergency department with machine learning. PLoS One 13 (3), e0194085. https://doi.org/10.1371/journal.pone.0194085.

Thakkar, M., Davis, D.C., 2006. Risks, Barriers, and Benefits of EHR Systems: A Comparative Study Based on Size of Hospital. In: Perspectives in Health Information Management/AHIMA, American Health Information Management Association, 3.

Anon., 2021. The Cancer Genome Atlas Program. (website). https://www.cancer.gov/about-nci/organization/ccg/research/structural-genomics/tcga. (Accessed 16 March 2021).

Thong, N.T., et al., 2015. HIFCF: an effective hybrid model between picture fuzzy clustering and intuitionistic fuzzy recommender systems for medical diagnosis. Expert Syst. Appl. 42 (7), 3682–3701. https://doi.org/10.1016/j.eswa.2014.12.042.

Tibshirani, R., 1996. Regression shrinkage and selection via the lasso. J. R. Stat. Soc. B (Methodol.) 58 (1), 267–288. https://doi.org/10.1111/j.2517-6161.1996.tb02080.x.

Torrey, L., Shavlik, J., 2010. Transfer learning. In: Handbook of Research on Machine Learning Applications and Trends: Algorithms, Methods, and Techniques, IGI global, pp. 242–264.

Tschandl, P., Sinz, C., Kittler, H., 2019. Domain-specific classification-pretrained fully convolutional network encoders for skin lesion segmentation. Comput. Biol. Med. 104, 111–116.

Tu, Z., Bai, X., 2009. Auto-context and its application to high-level vision tasks and 3D brain image segmentation. IEEE Trans. Pattern Anal. Mach. Intell. 32 (10), 1744–1757.

Übeyli, E.D., 2010. Recurrent neural networks employing Lyapunov exponents for analysis of ECG signals. Expert Syst. Appl. 37 (2), 1192–1199. https://doi.org/10.1016/j.eswa.2009.06.022.

Vaicenavicius, J., Widmann, D., Andersson, C., Lindsten, F., Roll, J., Schön, T.B., 2019. Evaluating model calibration in classification. In: Proceedings of the 22nd International Conference on Artificial Intelligence and Statistics (AISTATS), vol. 89.

Valdez, A.C., Ziefle, M., Verbert, K., Felfernig, A., Holzinger, A., 2016. Recommender systems for health informatics: state-of-the-art and future perspectives. In: Machine Learning for Health Informatics, Springer, pp. 391–414.

van Merode, G.G., Groothuis, S., Hasman, A., 2004. Enterprise resource planning for hospitals. Int. J. Med. Inform. 73 (6), 493–501. https://doi.org/10.1016/j.ijmedinf.2004.02.007.

Vapnik, V., 2013. The Nature of Statistical Learning Theory. Springer Science & Business Media.

Vincent, P., Larochelle, H., Lajoie, I., Bengio, Y., Manzagol, P.-A., Bottou, L., 2010. Stacked denoising autoencoders: learning useful representations in a deep network with a local denoising criterion. J. Mach. Learn. Res. 11 (12), 3371–3408.

Virgolin, M., Alderliesten, T., Witteveen, C., Bosman, P.A.N., 2017. Scalable genetic programming by gene-pool optimal mixing and input-space entropy-based building-block learning. In: Proceedings of the Genetic and Evolutionary Computation Conference, pp. 1041–1048.

Virgolin, M., Wang, Z., Alderliesten, T., Bosman, P.A.N., 2020. Machine learning for automatic construction of pediatric abdominal phantoms for radiation dose reconstruction. In: Medical Imaging 2020: Imaging Informatics for Healthcare, Research, and Applications, vol. 11318, p. 1131815.

Vogelzang, M., Zijlstra, F., Nijsten, M.W.N., 2005. Design and implementation of GRIP: a computerized glucose control system at a surgical intensive care unit. BMC Med. Inform. Decis. Mak. 5 (1), 38. https://doi.org/10.1186/1472-6947-5-38.

Wahle, F., Kowatsch, T., Fleisch, E., Rufer, M., Weidt, S., 2016. Mobile sensing and support for people with depression: a pilot trial in the wild. JMIR mHealth uHealth 4 (3), e111. https://doi.org/10.2196/mhealth.5960.

Wang, Z., Fey, A.M., 2018. Deep learning with convolutional neural network for objective skill evaluation in robot-assisted surgery. Int. J. Comput. Assist. Radiol. Surg. 13 (12), 1959–1970. https://doi.org/10.1007/s11548-018-1860-1.

Wang, Z., Qu, Y., Chen, L., Shen, J., Zhang, W., Zhang, S., Gao, Y., Gu, G., Chen, K., Yu, Y., 2018. Label-aware double transfer learning for cross-specialty medical named entity recognition. In: Proceedings of the 2018 Conference of the North American Chapter of the Association for Computational Linguistics: Human Language Technologies, vol. 1, pp. 1–15.

Watkins, C.J.C.H., Dayan, P., 1992. Q-learning. Mach. Learn. 8 (3–4), 279–292.

Weigend, A.S., Rumelhart, D.E., Huberman, B.A., 1991. Back-propagation, weight-elimination and time series prediction. Connectionist Models, 105–116. https://doi.org/10.1016/b978-1-4832-1448-1.50016-0.

Weintraub, W.S., Fahed, A.C., Rumsfeld, J.S., 2018. Translational medicine in the era of big data and machine learning. Circ. Res. 123 (11), 1202–1204. https://doi.org/10.1161/CIRCRESAHA.118.313944.

Weng, W.-H., Gao, M., He, Z., Yan, S., Szolovits, P., 2017. Representation and reinforcement learning for personalized glycemic control in septic patients. In: 31st Conference on Neural Information Processing Systems (NIPS 2017).

Wiens, J., Guttag, J., Horvitz, E., 2014. A study in transfer learning: leveraging data from multiple hospitals to enhance hospital-specific predictions. J. Am. Med. Inf. Assoc. 21 (4), 699–706. https://doi.org/10.1136/amiajnl-2013-002162.

Wiesner, M., Pfeifer, D., 2014. Health recommender systems: concepts, requirements, technical basics and challenges. Int. J. Environ. Res. Public Health 11 (3), 2580–2607. https://doi.org/10.3390/ijerph110302580.

World Health Organization, 2016. Diagnostic Errors. World Health Organization.

Xiao, Y., Wu, J., Lin, Z., Zhao, X., 2018. A deep learning-based multi-model ensemble method for cancer prediction. Comput. Methods Programs Biomed. 153, 1–9. https://doi.org/10.1016/j.cmpb.2017.09.005.

Xu, X.G., 2014. An exponential growth of computational phantom research in radiation protection, imaging, and radiotherapy: a review of the fifty-year history. Phys. Med. Biol. 59 (18), R233.

Yampolskiy, R.V., 2016. Artificial intelligence safety and cybersecurity: a timeline of AI failures. CoRR abs/1610.07997.

Yang, Y., Yan, L.-F., Zhang, X., Han, Y., Nan, H.-Y., Hu, Y.-C., Hu, B., Yan, S.-L., Zhang, J., Cheng, D.-L., et al., 2018. Glioma grading on conventional MR images: a deep learning study with transfer learning. Front. Neurosci. 12, 804. https://doi.org/10.3389/fnins.2018.00804.

Yom-Tov, E., Feraru, G., Kozdoba, M., Mannor, S., Tennenholtz, M., Hochberg, I., 2017. Encouraging physical activity in patients with diabetes: intervention using a reinforcement learning system. J. Med. Internet Res. 19 (10), e338. https://doi.org/10.2196/jmir.7994.

Yu, C., Dong, Y., Liu, J., Ren, G., 2019a. Incorporating causal factors into reinforcement learning for dynamic treatment regimes in HIV. BMC Med. Inform. Decis. Mak. 19 (2), 19–29. https://doi.org/10.1186/s12911-019-0755-6.

Yu, C., Liu, J., Nemati, S., 2019b. Reinforcement learning in healthcare: a survey. CoRR https://dblp.org/rec/journals/corr/abs-1908-08796.html?view=bibtex.

Yu, C., Liu, J., Zhao, H., 2019c. Inverse reinforcement learning for intelligent mechanical ventilation and sedative dosing in intensive care units. BMC Med. Inform. Decis. Mak. 19 (2), 57. https://doi.org/10.1186/s12911-019-0763-6.

Zhang, J., Cao, P., Gross, D.P., Zaiane, O.R., 2013. On the application of multi-class classification in physical therapy recommendation. Health Inform. Sci. Syst. 1 (1), 15. https://doi.org/10.1186/2047-2501-1-15.

Zhang, Q., Zhang, G., Lu, J., Wu, D., 2015. A framework of hybrid recommender system for personalized clinical prescription. In: 2015 10th International Conference on Intelligent Systems and Knowledge Engineering (ISKE), pp. 189–195.

Zhang, J., Xie, Y., Xia, Y., Shen, C., 2019. Attention residual learning for skin lesion classification. IEEE Trans. Med. Imaging 38 (9), 2092–2103.

Zhao, C., Li, G.-Z., Wang, C., Niu, J., 2015. Advances in patient classification for traditional Chinese medicine: a machine learning perspective. Evid. Based Complement. Alternat. Med. eCAM 2015. https://doi.org/10.1155/2015/376716.

Zhu, W., Xie, L., Han, J., Guo, X., 2020. The application of deep learning in cancer prognosis prediction. Cancers 12 (3), 603. https://doi.org/10.3390/cancers12030603.

# Geolocation-aware IoT and cloud-fog-based solutions for healthcare

# 2

**Jaydeep Das**

*Advanced Technology Development Center, Indian Institute of Technology Kharagpur, West Bengal, India*

## Chapter outline

## 1 Introduction

In the modern age, health has become a priority along with food, clothes, shelter, and other necessities. Health awareness is increasing day by day. Health monitoring, sample collection, diagnosis, and disease detection are regular practices in the healthcare field. Advanced internet technology such as the IoT and sensor networks are used to monitor and collect patient health data. Several smartphone applications, including Apple HealthKit, Google Fit, and Samsung Health, collect data from sensor-based devices such as Apple Watch, SmartBand, etc. They collect health data like blood pressure, pulse, body temperature, and oxygen saturation levels in the blood, and send this data via Bluetooth. Smartphones are power-hungry because several build-in applications are running with other

Machine Learning, Big Data, and IoT for Medical Informatics. https://doi.org/10.1016/B978-0-12-821777-1.00017-3

applications. They collect data and send it to nearby servers. Initially, the collected data are analyzed in the distant cloud server. In this case, the communication delay represents a major challenge (Doukas and Maglogiannis, 2012; Hassanalieragh et al., 2015) for healthcare and similar real-time applications.

However, fog computing can overcome these communication delays, as the fog nodes reside near the health applications and IoT devices (Gia et al., 2015; Negash et al., 2018). In the healthcare system, accurate and real-time results are required. Fog computing challenges related to healthcare applications are described in Mutlag et al. (2019). Along with faster results, the accuracy of the result is also a major concern. A deep learning technique was used to classify data and predict results with high accuracy (Faust et al., 2018). However, complex methods of deep learning and neural networks again lead to a time-consuming process. A personalized healthcare framework in an integrated cloud-fog-edge computing environment is proposed in Mukherjee et al. (2021) and Ghosh et al. (2020b). Tuli et al. (2020) proposed a deep learning-based edge resource-enabled computing platform to get accurate results in minimum response time for health-related applications, such as in heart disease monitoring. Location-based services in a cloud-fog integrated environment are described in Ghosh et al. (2020a). Das et al. (2016) elaborates different location-based geospatial query processing in a cloud environment and cloud-fog domain (Das et al., 2020).

In an emergency, patients need to be admitted to a nearby hospital or medical center after the health data have been analyzed by medical personnel. The nearest pharmacy may need to be located to deliver medicine and other medical equipment. Rapid delivery can be crucial for the patient, and the patient's geolocation is an important aspect in identifying the nearest hospital or healthcare center to the patient's current location. The nearest hospital or healthcare center or pharmacy can be determined using overlay analysis. The shortest path analysis can then be used to reach the hospital or healthcare center.

In this chapter, a geolocation-based IoT-fog-cloud-based solution for healthcare is proposed. Health data are collected through the IoT devices and analyzed through the fog node cluster and cloud server. Based on the data analysis and review by health personnel, and according to the geolocation of the patient, the patient can be referred to the appropriate medical facility.

The *key contributions* of this chapter are:

- Proposing an IoT-fog-cloud-based architecture where healthcare data processing is done along with geolocation data of the patient.
- Identifying the nearby medical facilities using a geospatial buffer creation mechanism.
- Obtaining the shortest path to reach medical centers or facilities from the patient with geospatial analysis.
- Comparing the delay and power consumption of the proposed IoT-fog-cloud-based framework with the IoT-cloud framework.

The rest of this chapter is organized as follows: Section 2 presents the state-of-the-art healthcare systems in the IoT-fog-cloud environment. Section 3 describes the proposed IoT-fog-cloud-based healthcare solution framework. It also elaborates on the geospatial analysis to facilitate medical services to patients depending upon their geolocation. The performance evaluation of the proposed healthcare solution and comparison with the cloud-only healthcare solution are given in Section 4. The last section concludes the chapter with future directions.

## 2 Related work

Healthcare-related data processing using cloud computing (Hassanalieragh et al., 2015; Mahmud et al., 2016) and fog computing (Mutlag et al., 2019; Rahmani et al., 2018) is a current emerging research field. To obtain more efficient results in terms of energy and latency researchers have used both environments together (Abdelmoneem et al., 2019; Tuli et al., 2020). Existing health monitoring work can be classified into three categories: (1) cloud computing-based health monitoring systems, (2) fog computing-based health monitoring systems, and (3) cloud-fog computing merged health monitoring systems.

### 2.1 Health monitoring system with cloud computing

Hassanalieragh et al. (2015) focused on clinical examination reports and trying to predict different kinds of diseases. Wearable sensors were used to collect the patient's health data, such as body temperature, blood pressure, respiratory rate, etc. The collected data were transferred to the remote healthcare center through a concentrator. The cloud was used for long-term data storage, data analysis, and data visualization. A cloud-based data analysis framework was developed in Mahmud et al. (2016). They collected population-wise socioeconomic data and health data, and tried to predict the health shock. A fuzzy-based classifier was used to predict the health-shock level of rural and tribal areas. The cloud was used for data capturing, data storing, indexing, and visualizing purposes. Zhang et al. (2015) described a smart health system in which medical data was integrated between public medical facilities and the patient's health devices. A large amount of heterogeneous data storage and data analysis has been carried out on the cloud platform. Another cloud-based work was proposed in Gupta et al. (2017). The cloud was used to store users' health data like heart rate, calories burned, walking speed, and distance traveled. The data were transferred from IoT devices to the cloud through XML. XML ensured that data collection was fast, secure, and reliable. The proposed model triggered an alert message to the medical person if any abnormality was found in the person's collected data. A machine learning classifier was used in Muhammad et al. (2017) to improve the accuracy of a voice pathology monitoring system. Voice signals were captured through the IoT devices and transmitted to the cloud by watermarking, enabling the secure transmission of the signal. The doctor identified the patient's data and diagnosed it. The doctor provided feedback after analyzing the patient's voice.

### 2.2 Health monitoring system with fog computing

Rahmani et al. (2018) and Negash et al. (2018) elaborated on the methods of IoT-based smart e-healthcare systems in which fog computing and e-health gateways (UT-GATE) were used. This gateway was closer to the sensors and received local health data from the patient. They claimed the e-health systems show better patient mobility, scalability, interoperability, reliability, and energy efficiency. The nRF protocol was used in an IoT-based health monitoring system (Gia et al., 2017), for greater energy efficiency of the sensor nodes. These sensor nodes collected ECG, respiration rate, and body temperature data from patients, and forwarded them to the gateway using wireless technology. Real-time alerts were provided after automated decisions were made by the monitoring system. Gia et al. (2015) presented a fog-based IoT-enabled health monitoring system. ECG signal feature extraction was performed at the edge devices as a case study. For real-time notification, they extracted heart rate, P and T waves, and other features from the ECG signals. They performed all these within an appropriate bandwidth utilization and service delivery.

## 2.3 Health monitoring system with cloud-fog computing

Fog computing refers to an intermediate layer between the IoT devices and the cloud server (Chakraborty et al., 2016; Abdelmoneem et al., 2019). IoT devices collect health data from patients, process some data within the fog devices for emergency purposes, and perform quick responses with alarm triggering. Gu et al. (2019) and Ahmad et al. (2016) used a cloud-fog environment for minimizing data leakage. They worked on the privacy of health data, reducing the transfer of data from IoT devices to the distant cloud server. Support for patients with diabetes by analyzing glucose level data with energy efficiency was carried out in Devarajan et al. (2019). For greater accuracy, they used the J48graft classifier. A telehealth application was proposed in Dubey et al. (2015). The fog device analyzes the data series received from the IoT devices, trying to fit a specific pattern. If new patterns are received, they are forwarded to the cloud for further action. Diagnosis of heart disease using deep learning methods in the IoT-fog computing environment was carried out in Tuli et al. (2020). They showed that the proposed method was delay-aware and energy-efficient. A summary of the related works discussed here is presented in Table 1.

From this literature survey, it can be observed that geolocation has not been dealt with in any of the cases. Geolocation has a vital role in the healthcare system. In emergency cases, the patient's transfer to a nearby hospital or healthcare center can be urgently needed.

**Table 1** Comparison of existing schemes for healthcare systems.

| | Features | | | | |
|---|---|---|---|---|---|
| **Existing work** | **Cloud used** | **Fog used** | **Geolocation analysis** | **Power calculated** | **Delay calculated** |
| Muhammad et al. (2017), Hassanalieragh et al. (2015), Mahmud et al. (2016), Zhang et al. (2015), Gupta et al. (2017) | ✓ | X | X | X | X |
| Mukherjee and De (2014) | ✓ | X | X | ✓ | X |
| Rahmani et al. (2018), Negash et al. (2018), Mutlag et al. (2019), Gia et al. (2015) | X | ✓ | X | X | X |
| Gia et al. (2017) | X | ✓ | X | ✓ | X |
| Gu et al. (2019), Devarajan et al. (2019), Ahmad et al. (2016), Dubey et al. (2015), Muhammed et al. (2018) | ✓ | ✓ | X | X | X |
| Chakraborty et al. (2016), Abdelmoneem et al. (2019) | ✓ | ✓ | X | X | ✓ |
| Tuli et al. (2020) | ✓ | ✓ | X | ✓ | ✓ |
| Proposed work | ✓ | ✓ | ✓ | ✓ | ✓ |

# 3 Proposed framework

In this section, Fig. 1 elaborates the hierarchical structure of cloud servers, fog devices, and IoT devices for health data collection, communication, health data analysis, and recommendations from medical professionals. The workflow of the proposed model is depicted in Fig. 2. Health data are collected through IoT and sensor devices and sent to the nearest fog devices. If the patient is in a moving vehicle, then roadside units can serve as fog devices, as well as the router and switches. Fog devices perform the primary health data analysis as it has low computation power needs. Thus $n$ number of fog devices can be engaged for $m$ parameters of the health data analysis where $n \leq m$. If these aggregated parametric data are within the normal range, then the parameter values are considered to be normal. If the parametric data are not within the normal range, then the results are forwarded to the cloud server and medical personnel are consulted. According to the severity of the reports, the medical personnel will contact the nearest medical center or hospital for further treatment.

Moreover, the geospatial data of the region of interest are analyzed and the geolocation of the patients, hospitals, other healthcare centers, pharmacies, diagnosis centers, etc., are pointed out. It determines the nearby healthcare facilities and obtains the shortest path to reach them. The geolocation-based analysis is done in the cloud server, and all location information is sent to the medical center. After getting the doctor's consult, an ambulance can be sent to the patient's geolocation to bring the

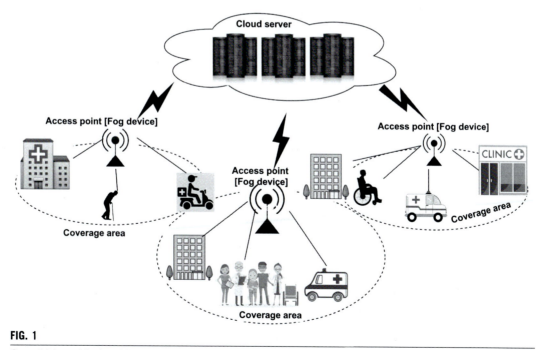

**FIG. 1**

Overall hierarchical architecture.

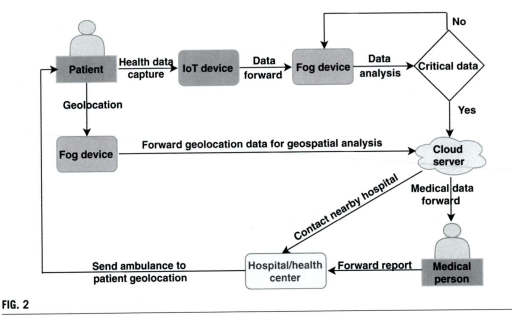

**FIG. 2**

Workflow of proposed model.

patient to the healthcare center for further treatment. If this is not possible, then care can be provided to the patient from the healthcare center by sending medication or a medical team.

## 3.1 Health data analysis

Health data are collected through smart bands worn by the patients. Health data include heart rate, blood pressure, body temperature, and other parameters generated every $n$ minutes. CSV files are generated in different fog nodes for different health parameters. These files are related to individual health data, and each health parameter has an upper bound and lower bound value or a range of values. If it is identified that the collected health data parameters are abnormal or out of the normal range, then an alert will be triggered and the collected health data will be sent to the cloud for further analysis. In the cloud, all historical health data of the patient are present. A medical practitioner or doctor can analyze this collected health data. If anything abnormal or any emergency is identified, then the nearest medical center or hospital is then contacted and a medical team or an ambulance is sent for the patient by the shortest path.

## 3.2 Geospatial analysis for medical facility

Geolocation is an important parameter to obtain the current position of the patient, pharmacies, hospitals, diagnosis centers, etc. It has two parts. One is latitude (i.e., Lat) and another is longitude (i.e., Lon). The Lat/Lon identifies any geographical location on the earth. However, a patient can move from one location to another location by ambulance, car, or other vehicle. If the patient is stationary, that may be at their home, hospital, or any other place for a long time duration. Concern arises if the patient is not in the hospital or a healthcare center, and needs to be moved to a nearby hospital or healthcare center if the condition is critical. For such an emergency, the following two geospatial analyses must be processed:

- Find the nearest hospital or healthcare center.
- Determine the shortest path to reach the nearest hospital or healthcare center.

### 3.2.1 Overlay analysis to obtain nearest medical facilities

In GIS, there are many layers present in the cartography of any area map. Here, Fig. 3 considers five layers, that is, land use land cover (LULC), health, road, rail, and medical shops of area X. The LULC layer describes the overall land structure of area X. The health layer includes hospitals, medical centers,

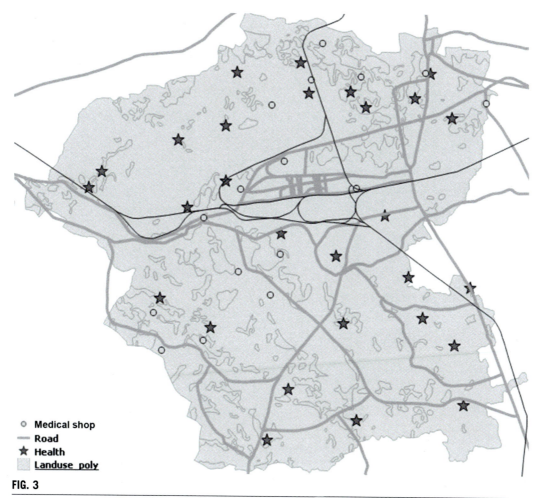

○ Medical shop
— Road
★ Health
  Landuse_poly

**FIG. 3**

Map of area X with five layers.

public health centers (PHCs), block-level public health centers (BPHCs), which are pointed out as a red-colored star. The road layer contains high roads and local roads, which are pointed out as gray-colored lines. Rail is the rail track going through the area X. Black lines indicate these tracks. Medical shops are indicated by green dots.

A buffer of 1 km around the health points (see Fig. 4) has been created. From Fig. 4, it is easily understood, within 1 km, how much area is covered by each medical center. Also, this figure identifies the medical shops within 1 km of the medical centers. Likewise, this can create a buffer around the patient's current geolocation of $x$ kilometer to identify the nearest medical centers and medical shops. The OGC compliant web processing service helps to create a buffer on the fly over the spatial dataset. In that case, the BufferFeatureCollection service is required to create the buffer over the geospatial dataset.

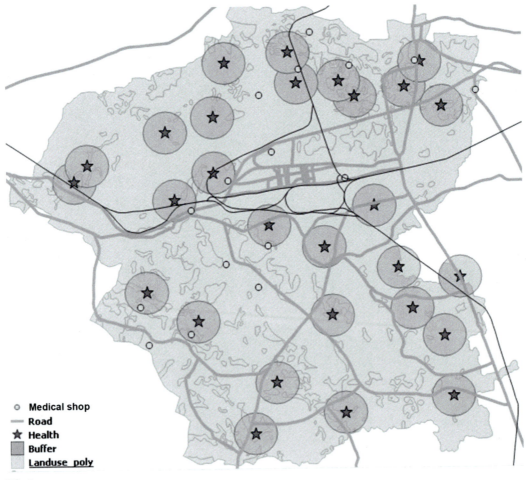

- ○ Medical shop
- — Road
- ★ Health
- ▨ Buffer
- Landuse_poly

**FIG. 4**

Buffer of 1 km for healthcare centers in area X.

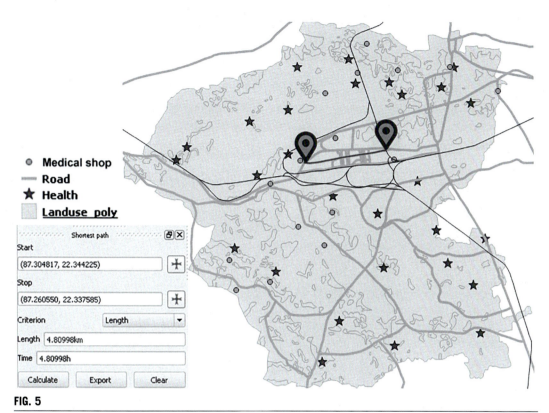

**FIG. 5**

Shortest path determination in area X.

### 3.2.2 Shortest path to reach nearest medical centers

Network analysis in GIS (Cadieux et al., 2020) does the shortest path determination. Here, the road is considered as a network. If the source location is not on the path, then it checks the nearest point that is on the path. From that point, it calculates the path to the nearest point of the destination that is on the road network. Dijkstra's algorithm is used to determine the shortest path between two points (i.e., the patient's current location and nearest healthcare center). Also, it determines the distance between the two points. Our shortest path calculation is portrayed in Fig. 5. Two points (source and destination) of area X are represented with a GPS logo, and the red line shows the shortest path.

## 3.3 Delay and power consumption calculation

Here, delays have been measured (Das et al., 2019, 2020) in the overall process. Total delay is the summation of communication ($\mathcal{D}_{comm}$), propagation ($\mathcal{D}_{prop}$), data processing ($\mathcal{D}_{proc}$), and queueing ($\mathcal{D}_{queu}$) delay:

$$\text{Delay} \quad \mathcal{D} = \sum (\mathcal{D}_{comm} + \mathcal{D}_{prop} + \mathcal{D}_{proc} + \mathcal{D}_{queu}) \tag{1}$$

$$\mathcal{D}_{comm} = (1 + \mathcal{F}) * (d/\mathcal{R}) \tag{2}$$

where $\mathcal{F}$ is failure rate, $d$ is data amount to transmit, and $\mathcal{R}$ is data transmission rate.

Propagation delay $\mathcal{D}_{prop}$ is the time taken for the data to be transmitted from sender node to receiver node:

$$\mathcal{D}_{prop} = d_{sr}/\mathcal{S}_{prop} \tag{3}$$

where $d_{sr}$ is distance between data sender node and data receiver node and $\mathcal{S}_{prop}$ is propagation speed.

Processing delay $\mathcal{D}_{proc}$ is time taken to process the data in a node:

$$\mathcal{D}_{proc} = \mathcal{A}_{proc}/\mathcal{S}_{proc} \tag{4}$$

where $\mathcal{A}_{proc}$ is amount of data processed and $\mathcal{S}_{proc}$ is speed of data processing.

In our case, communications occur between the IoT device and the fog device, fog device and cloud server (if the health data are critical).

So, here the proposed system communication delay is $\mathcal{D}_{sys_{comm}} = \mathcal{D}_{if_{comm}} + \mathcal{D}_{fc_{comm}}$, where $\mathcal{D}_{if_{comm}}$ is IoT to fog and $\mathcal{D}_{if_{comm}}$ is fog to cloud communication delay.

The proposed system's propagation delay $\mathcal{D}_{sys_{prop}} = \mathcal{D}_{if_{prop}} + \mathcal{D}_{fc_{prop}}$, where $\mathcal{D}_{if_{prop}}$ is IoT to fog, and $\mathcal{D}_{if_{prop}}$ is fog to cloud propagation delay.

The proposed system's processing delay $\mathcal{D}_{sys_{proc}} = \mathcal{D}_{f_{proc}} + \mathcal{D}_{c_{proc}}$, where $\mathcal{D}_{f_{proc}}$ and $\mathcal{D}_{c_{proc}}$ are processing delay in fog node and cloud server, respectively.

The proposed system's queueing delay is $\mathcal{D}_{sys_{queu}}$.

The system's overall delay is

$$\mathcal{D}_{sys} = (\mathcal{D}_{sys_{comm}} + \mathcal{D}_{sys_{prop}} + \mathcal{D}_{sys_{proc}} + \mathcal{D}_{sys_{queu}}) \tag{5}$$

The overall power consumption of smartphones has been calculated. During communication with fog nodes, smartphones are in active state $\mathcal{E}_{active}$. The rest of the time smartphones are in idle state $\mathcal{E}_{idle}$.

Power consumption during the communication stage is

$$\mathcal{P}_{sys_{comm}} = \mathcal{E}_{active} * \mathcal{D}_{sys_{comm}} \tag{6}$$

Power consumption during propagation is

$$\mathcal{P}_{sys_{prop}} = \mathcal{E}_{idle} * \mathcal{D}_{sys_{prop}} \tag{7}$$

Power consumption during data processing is

$$\mathcal{P}_{sys_{proc}} = \mathcal{E}_{idle} * \mathcal{D}_{sys_{proc}} \tag{8}$$

Power consumption at queueing stage is

$$\mathcal{P}_{sys_{queu}} = \mathcal{E}_{idle} * \mathcal{D}_{sys_{queu}} \tag{9}$$

So, the overall power consumption is

$$\mathcal{P}_{sys} = (\mathcal{P}_{sys_{comm}} + \mathcal{P}_{sys_{prop}} + \mathcal{P}_{sys_{proc}} + \mathcal{P}_{sys_{queu}}) \tag{10}$$

A comparison of the device delay and power consumption in our proposed framework with the existing cloud-only framework is described in Section 4.

# 4 Performance evaluation

All experiments have been done using the experimental setup listed in Table 2. The GOQii[a] health fitness band was used as an IoT device for tracking the heartbeat, blood pressure, and temperature of the body. These data are stored in the smartphones through the app as .csv files. A smartphone with 2 GB RAM and 8 GB internal memory and three Raspberry Pi 3 with B+ models were used for experiment purposes. The smartphone and Raspberry Pi act as fog devices. Virtual machine (VM) of the Google Cloud Platform (GCP) was used with 3.75 GB RAM, 250 GB storage, and a Windows server. The experiment setup with medical data flow is shown in Fig. 6.

The normal range of human health data is as follows:

Body temperature: 96–98.6°F

**Table 2** **Experimental setup of proposed healthcare system.**

| Device | Details |
|---|---|
| VM in GCP | 3.75 GB RAM, 250 GB storage and Windows server 2012 OS |
| Raspberry Pi 3B+ | 1 GB LPDDR2 SDRAM, 32GB SD card support, ARM Cortex −A53 1.4 GHz 64-bit quadcore and Raspbian Stretch OS |
| Smartphone | 2 GB RAM, 8 GB internal memory, 64-bit 1.2 GHz Qualcomm Snapdragon 410 Quad Core with Android 6.0.1 |
| Smartband | GOQii, body temperature, heart rate, $SpO_2$ tracker |

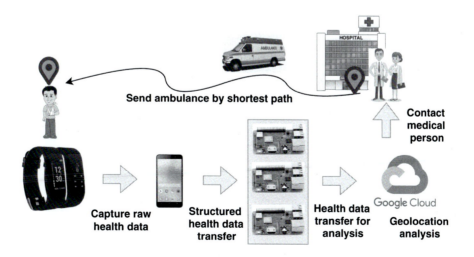

**Send ambulance by shortest path**

**Capture raw health data**　**Structured health data transfer**　**Health data transfer for analysis**　**Geolocation analysis**　**Contact medical person**

**FIG. 6**

Experimental setup for health data transmission.

[a]See https://goqii.com/in-en.

Blood pressure: 60–80 mmHg (diastolic) and 120–140 mmHg (systolic)
Heart rate: 55–80 bpm

In our experiment, hypertension data from research students and faculty members of different age groups were collected. The pictorial view of the hypertension data analysis is shown in Fig. 7. Hypertension data from 30 research students and 10 faculty members were collected. Among the participants, 10 research students were female and 20 were male. Of the faculty member participants, 4 were female and 6 were male (refer to Fig. 7A). The number of students with hypertension was 10, and the number

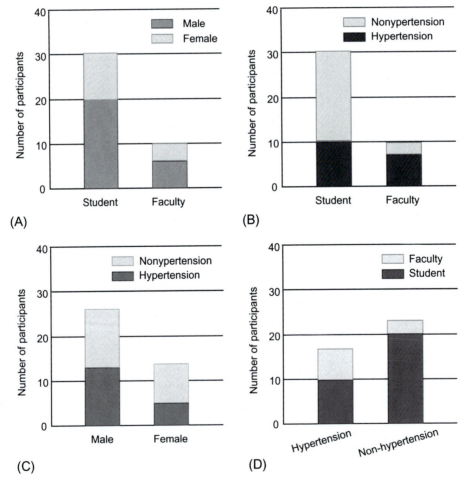

**FIG. 7**

Analysis of hypertension data.

of faculty members was 7 (refer to Fig. 7B). A total of 12 males and 5 females were suffering from hypertension (refer to Fig. 7C). In total, 10 students and 7 faculty members were suffering from hypertension, whereas 20 students and 3 faculty members were free from it (refer to Fig. 7D).

For geospatial analysis, QGIS 2.18.28 was used, which was installed in the GCP VM. All geospatial datasets of area X were kept in the GCP VM. LULC, road, rail, medical center, and medical facility datasets were used for analysis. Five layers were overlaid in the QGIS and integrated, as it is easier to determine the user's interest or apply any algorithms related to the multiple layers. The shortest path creation was carried out using the Dijkstra algorithm. For buffer creation, a built-in function was used for point vector data, as the health centers are considered to be points. The buffer of these health centers is a circle. In the experiment, a buffer around a 1 km radius was considered. The results of buffer creation and the shortest path determination are shown in Figs. 4 and 5.

Delay and power consumption calculations were carried out with varying health data amounts in megabits. Fig. 8 shows that the delay in the fog-cloud environment is much lower than in the only-cloud environment. In the only-cloud domain, all data are processed in the remote cloud server. In our proposed fog-cloud integrated environment, small amounts of data are processed in nearby fog devices. These data are not sent to the remotely located cloud server, which reduces the delay in the overall process. Only the larger amounts of data are processed in the cloud server.

Similarly, different amounts of health data were transmitted to check the user device power consumption. Fig. 9 shows the power consumption of the user devices is much lower in the fog-cloud environment than in the only-cloud environment for health data transmission. A better result is achieved when the data size is increased.

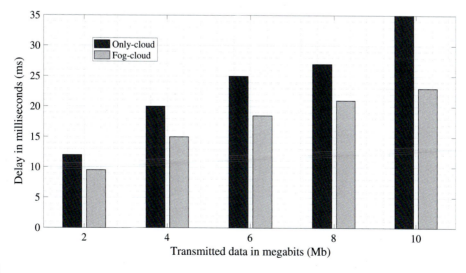

**FIG. 8**

Delay in only-cloud and proposed fog-cloud for health data transmission.

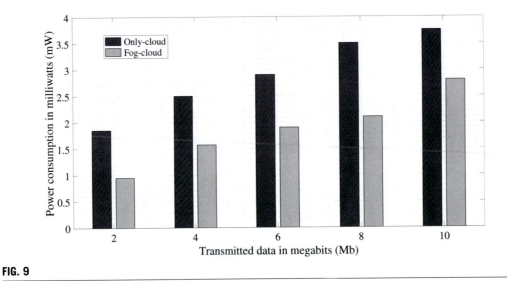

**FIG. 9**

Power consumption of smartphone in only-cloud and proposed fog-cloud for health data transmission.

## 5 Conclusion and future work

In this chapter, geolocation-based healthcare solutions with the support of IoT, cloud, and fog computing are discussed. The health data collection is carried out by IoT devices. Primary analysis is handled in the fog devices. If a critical indication arises in the primary analysis, the system moves to more detailed analysis. Further analysis is done within the cloud server with the patient's historical data analysis by the medical practitioner. In critical situations, an ambulance or medical team can be sent to the patient's geolocation using the shortest route. This chapter illustrates how geospatial analysis can help to find medical necessities in nearby locations and how to reach the medical center or hospital using the shortest path. Moreover, it is observed that the proposed framework outperforms an only-cloud platform with 25%–27% less delay, and 27%–29% less power consumption of smartphones or IoT devices.

In the future, machine learning techniques can be applied for better medical data analysis and health data classification. In this chapter, only hypertension data of patients were considered. Other diseases like diabetes, cancer, hepatitis, etc. can be taken into consideration in future healthcare research with the proposed hierarchical computing environments. Also, incorporating blockchain technology could make the medical data transfer more secure and trustworthy. Patients' data could be generated from the secured devices, and the generated data treated as transactions on the blockchain. The patient health information could then be validated with a smart contract. No third person could change the patient data while it is transferred from the local database to the hospital database. If any health data were to be tampered with during the data transmission, it could easily be identified.

# References

Abdelmoneem, R.M., Benslimane, A., Shaaban, E., Abdelhamid, S., Ghoneim, S., 2019. A cloud-fog based architecture for IoT applications dedicated to healthcare. In: ICC 2019—2019 IEEE International Conference on Communications (ICC), May, IEEE, pp. 1–6.

Ahmad, M., Amin, M.B., Hussain, S., Kang, B.H., Cheong, T., Lee, S., 2016. Health fog: a novel framework for health and wellness applications. J. Supercomput. 72 (10), 3677–3695.

Cadieux, N., Kalacska, M., Coomes, O.T., Tanaka, M., Takasaki, Y., 2020. A python algorithm for shortest-path river network distance calculations considering river flow direction. Data 5 (1), 8.

Chakraborty, S., Bhowmick, S., Talaga, P., Agrawal, D.P., 2016. Fog networks in healthcare application. In: 2016 IEEE 13th International Conference on Mobile Ad Hoc and Sensor Systems (MASS), October, IEEE, pp. 386–387.

Das, J., Dasgupta, A., Ghosh, S.K., Buyya, R., 2016. A geospatial orchestration framework on cloud for processing user queries. In: 2016 IEEE International Conference on Cloud Computing in Emerging Markets (CCEM), October, IEEE, pp. 1–8.

Das, J., Mukherjee, A., Ghosh, S.K., Buyya, R., 2019. Geo-Cloudlet: time and power efficient geospatial query resolution using Cloudlet. In: 2019 11th International Conference on Advanced Computing (ICoAC), December, IEEE, pp. 180–187.

Das, J., Mukherjee, A., Ghosh, S.K., Buyya, R., 2020. Spatio-Fog: a green and timeliness-oriented fog computing model for geospatial query resolution. Simul. Model. Practice Theory 100, 102043.

Devarajan, M., Subramaniyaswamy, V., Vijayakumar, V., Ravi, L., 2019. Fog-assisted personalized healthcare-support system for remote patients with diabetes. J. Ambient Intell. Humaniz. Comput. 10 (10), 3747–3760.

Doukas, C., Maglogiannis, I., 2012. Bringing IoT and cloud computing towards pervasive healthcare. In: 2012 Sixth International Conference on Innovative Mobile and Internet Services in Ubiquitous Computing, July, IEEE, pp. 922–926.

Dubey, H., Yang, J., Constant, N., Amiri, A.M., Yang, Q., Makodiya, K., 2015. Fog data: enhancing telehealth big data through fog computing. In: Inproceedings of the ASE Bigdata & Socialinformatics 2015, pp. 1–6.

Faust, O., Hagiwara, Y., Hong, T., Lih, O., Acharya, U., 2018. Deep learning for healthcare applications based on physiological signals: a review. Comput. Methods Programs Biomed. 161, 1–13.

Ghosh, S., Das, J., Ghosh, S.K., 2020a. Locator: a cloud-fog-enabled framework for facilitating efficient location based services. In: 2020 International Conference on COMmunication Systems & NETworkS (COMSNETS), January, IEEE, pp. 87–92.

Ghosh, S., Das, J., Ghosh, S.K., Buyya, R., 2020b. CLAWER: context-aware cloud-fog based workflow management framework for health emergency services. In: 2020 20th IEEE/ACM International Symposium on Cluster, Cloud and Internet Computing (CCGRID), May, IEEE, pp. 810–817.

Gia, T.N., Jiang, M., Rahmani, A.M., Westerlund, T., Liljeberg, P., Tenhunen, H., 2015. Fog computing in healthcare internet of things: a case study on ECG feature extraction. In: 2015 IEEE International Conference on Computer and Information Technology; Ubiquitous Computing and Communications; Dependable, Autonomic and Secure Computing; Pervasive Intelligence and Computing, October, IEEE, pp. 356–363.

Gia, T.N., Jiang, M., Sarker, V.K., Rahmani, A.M., Westerlund, T., Liljeberg, P., Tenhunen, H., 2017. Low-cost fog-assisted health-care IoT system with energy-efficient sensor nodes. In: 2017 13th International Wireless Communications and Mobile Computing Conference (IWCMC), May, IEEE, pp. 1765–1770.

Gu, J., Huang, R., Jiang, L., Qiao, G., Du, X., Guizani, M., 2019. A fog computing solution for context-based privacy leakage detection for android healthcare devices. Sensors 19 (5), 1184.

Gupta, P.K., Maharaj, B.T., Malekian, R., 2017. A novel and secure IoT based cloud centric architecture to perform predictive analysis of users activities in sustainable health centres. Multimed. Tools Appl. 76 (18), 18489–18512.

Hassanalieragh, M., Page, A., Soyata, T., Sharma, G., Aktas, M., Mateos, G., Kantarci, B., Andreescu, S., 2015. Health monitoring and management using internet-of-things (IoT) sensing with cloud-based processing: opportunities and challenges. In: 2015 IEEE International Conference on Services Computing, June, IEEE, pp. 285–292.

Mahmud, S., Iqbal, R., Doctor, F., 2016. Cloud enabled data analytics and visualization framework for health-shocks prediction. Future Gener. Comput. Syst. 65, 169–181.

Muhammad, G., Rahman, S.M.M., Alelaiwi, A., Alamri, A., 2017. Smart health solution integrating IoT and cloud: a case study of voice pathology monitoring. IEEE Commun. Mag. 55 (1), 69–73.

Muhammed, T., Mehmood, R., Albeshri, A., Katib, I., 2018. Ubehealth: a personalized ubiquitous cloud and edge-enabled networked healthcare system for smart cities. IEEE Access 6, 32258–32285.

Mukherjee, A., De, D., 2014. Femtocell based green health monitoring strategy. In: 2014 XXXIth URSI General Assembly and Scientific Symposium (URSI GASS), August, IEEE, pp. 1–4.

Mukherjee, A., Ghosh, S., Behere, A., Ghosh, S., Buyya, R., 2021. Internet of Health Things (IoHT) for personalized health care using integrated edge-fog-cloud network. J. Ambient Intell. Humaniz. Comput. 12, 943–959. https://doi.org/10.1007/s12652-020-02113-9.

Mutlag, A.A., Ghani, M.K.A., Arunkumar, N.A., Mohammed, M.A., Mohd, O., 2019. Enabling technologies for fog computing in healthcare IoT systems. Future Gener. Comput. Syst. 90, 62–78.

Negash, B., Gia, T.N., Anzanpour, A., Azimi, I., Jiang, M., Westerlund, T., Rahmani, A.M., Liljeberg, P., Tenhunen, H., 2018. Leveraging fog computing for healthcare IoT. In: Fog Computing in the Internet of Things, Springer, Cham, pp. 145–169.

Rahmani, A.M., Gia, T.N., Negash, B., Anzanpour, A., Azimi, I., Jiang, M., Liljeberg, P., 2018. Exploiting smart e-health gateways at the edge of healthcare Internet-of-Things: a fog computing approach. Future Gener. Comput. Syst. 78, 641–658.

Tuli, S., Basumatary, N., Gill, S.S., Kahani, M., Arya, R.C., Wander, G.S., Buyya, R., 2020. HealthFog: an ensemble deep learning based smart healthcare system for automatic diagnosis of heart diseases in integrated IoT and fog computing environments. Future Gener. Comput. Syst. 104, 187–200.

Zhang, Y., Qiu, M., Tsai, C.W., Hassan, M.M., Alamri, A., 2015. Health-CPS: healthcare cyber-physical system assisted by cloud and big data. IEEE Syst. J. 11 (1), 88–95.

# Machine learning vulnerability in medical imaging

3

**Theodore V. Maliamanis and George A. Papakostas**

*HUman-MAchines INteraction Laboratory (HUMAIN-Lab), Department of Computer Science, International Hellenic University, Kavala, Greece*

## Chapter outline

## 1 Introduction

Having the ability to see inside the human body and visualize what is happening there, without the need for surgical access, has long been a goal of medical science. *Radiology* is the branch of medical science that mainly deals with this field and provides the means for the other medical branches to diagnose more effectively. *X-ray* imaging is a method that captures an image of the inner parts of the human body, such as the lungs and bones. *Computed tomography*, *ultrasound tomography*, and *magnetic resonance* are methods that capture many slices of an organ or body part. There are many other specific techniques (Beutel et al., 2000) based on these methods, such as *coronary angiography* and *scintigraphy*, and still others directly use cameras to take internal images. All these methods represent the result as a single image or a set of images for further analysis.

*Medical image analysis* is the field that deals with the analysis of the images made from these medical imaging methods. In early times this analysis was performed by a radiologist or a specifically trained doctor, but as the medical imaging field evolved, the number of images produced increased. This made diagnosis by a single person more difficult or even impossible. The general idea was to find a way to rapidly classify or detect regions of interest in those images and have the doctor decide only about the "suspicious" ones. Computer vision (CV) seemed to be the key, but in earlier times, when its decision accuracy was poor, it was not reliable enough, especially for healthcare tasks. After CV evolved and began to score recognition rates that approached human recognition accuracy, its use in medical image analysis became feasible. This collaboration seemed very promising, because medical images, due to the manner in which they must be captured, have minimized some problems that other images have.

When all began to seem ideal for CV, security issues appeared. Security attacks on CV systems cast doubt on their credibility. Attacks showed the vulnerabilities in CV systems, regardless of the application field. Machine learning vulnerabilities became a threat to medical imaging too. Research of great interest started that not only concerns the applications of CV in medical imaging but in all of CV's critical applications. To date, this research has brought to light many effective attack proposals and also defensive techniques against them. This hunt has improved CV systems, making them more robust against attacks, but also bringing them closer to human perception.

The contributions of this chapter are:

**(1)** The security issues of machine learning-based medical imaging systems are discussed thoroughly for the first time in the literature.
**(2)** The current status of adversarial attacks and defensive strategies for medical imaging systems is described.
**(3)** The importance of developing more secure CV systems for medical imaging is justified through an in-depth analysis.

Next, terms such as computer vision and adversarial computer vision will be defined and, finally, an attempt will be made to capture the current status of the research specific to the subfield of medical imaging CV.

## 2 Computer vision

Computer vision (CV) or machine vision is the field of artificial intelligence (AI) that deals with image recognition and analysis by a machine. An integral part of a modern CV system is the machine learning (ML) model that is used. ML models are systems that, given an input vector of numbers, can compute an output vector. In order to program this computation, the system can be trained with known input–output sets called *training datasets*. When the training process is over, the model has learned the function between input and output vectors, so that if you feed it with an unknown input vector, it can compute the most appropriate output, according to the dataset that the ML model learned from.

A computer vision system can be divided into several parts (see Fig. 1). After image acquisition, the matrices produced, which are three for a colored image or only one for a grayscale image, are processed to make the image features more distinct, with less noise and ready for analysis. The subfield that is responsible for this process and contains all converting and processing methods is called *image processing*. The next step, which is necessary only in some cases, is to detect the target object or the regions of interest and to drop out everything else in the image. Then values representing some chosen features of the image, which are preselected with "feature selection" methods, are computed from the matrix's values.

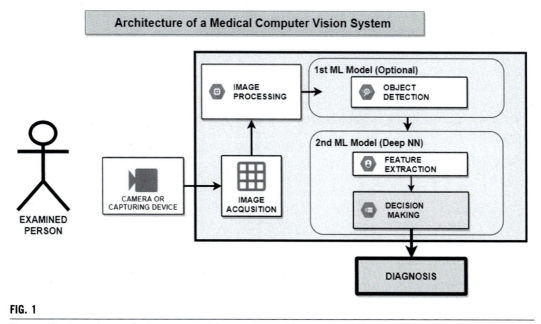

**FIG. 1**

The architecture of a medical computer vision system and its usual workflow.

During training, the ML model divides the hyperplane that is produced by the feature variables into areas that represent the output classes of the specific classification problem. In order to classify the objects from the chosen features, the pretrained ML model is fed with a vector of real numbers representing these feature values and makes a decision as to which area of the hyperplane this vector belongs, classifying the objects that were previously detected in the image, or in some other instances, classifying the entire image. The ability that ML models have of being able to classify "unseen" images, which were not learned during training, is termed the *generalizability* of the model. To rate the accuracy of the model, we test only "unseen" images that were correctly labeled. That is why we usually divide every image dataset into three parts:

- the *training set*, which is used to train the classifier;
- the *validation set*, which is used to validate the training procedure;
- and the *test set*, a smaller set of unused labeled images to test generalizability.

Most of the CV systems have followed this approach; however, the proposal of deep learning (LeCun et al., 2015) introduced new, efficient models. These models are artificial neural networks with many hidden layers. Especially in computer vision, a deep neural network like DCNN (Rawat and Wang, 2017) (Deep Convolutional Neural Network) can undertake some of the most critical processes of a CV system, including feature extraction and decision making (see Fig. 1). Also, the feature selection process that usually took place before the training procedure is now included in the training procedure. Therefore, the features chosen to be extracted cannot be clearly seen and they are imperceptibly included in the first layers of the DCNN, called *convolution filters*. The main advantage of deep ML models is that they can learn from greater datasets, so that they can estimate the output more precisely. Their significantly higher accuracy scores have demonstrated their integrity.

The usual tasks for a CV system are:

- *Classification*, when we want to classify an image of an object. The classes can be only two (healthy or diseased), but can be many more. For instance, the popular ImageNet dataset has 1000 different classes (all the categories of the objects in the dataset).
- *Detection*, when we want to detect several objects in an image.
- *Segmentation*, when we want to find semantic segments and regions of interest in an image.

Other tasks are pose estimation and action recognition, but they have not been applied to medical imaging yet. They may be used later for the development of automated capture of medical images.

The evolution of CV systems has made their use feasible in many fields such as robotics, autonomous vehicles, security systems, cyber-physical systems (CPS), and Internet of Things (IoT) systems. In medical science, except for medical image reconstruction (Hosny et al., 2013; Papakostas et al., 2009), they have been used efficiently in radiology (Rajpurkar et al., 2017); in pathology, especially for cancer detection (Kose and Alzubi, 2020); in dermatology for skin cancer classification (Hosny et al., 2018); and in ophthalmology for retinopathy detection (Wang et al., 2020) and retina biometrics (Badeka et al., 2020). The only problem has seemed to be that sometimes in medical imaging there is a delineation in producing the "ground truth" label that classifies a medical image, because there are instances in which even experts disagree about the classification (Njeh, 2008). Creating a medical image dataset and setting the ground truth labels can be a very sensitive operation, because if the labels are not carefully chosen then the ML system will learn to make wrong decisions.

## 3 Adversarial computer vision

When it seemed that CV systems could understand medical images, and images in general, as efficiently as an expert, some security issues appeared.

Several security issues in healthcare, such as those involving medical files, medical devices, and medical analytics security, are of concern to the scientific community. The use of ML models in healthcare is not related only to CV systems, as these models can also be used for decision making about pharmaceuticals or device evaluation or approval (Finlayson et al., 2019), or about medical data derived from IoT or wearable devices, or filtering and clustering data. Adversarial examples that will be described shortly do not affect only CV systems, but also deep ML models generally. So, the security issues that will be analyzed concern every other ML model use.

The preliminary security issues were found in references about attacks against digital image watermarking (Linnartz et al., 1998), but this did not seem to concern the CV or machine learning field. The first reference to the security of ML was made by Barreno M. et al. in 2008 (Barreno et al., 2008), who also proposed the first taxonomy of attacks on machine learning, basically driven by the research in spam email filtering.

In 2013, Szegedy et al. (Szegedy et al., 2013) had the idea that if we add the appropriate imperceptible perturbation to an image, we can mislead the ML model to make wrong decisions. The appropriate perturbation for a specific image is made by optimizing the input of the ML model, which is the perturbed image, to maximize the prediction error. This first approach means that we know everything about, or rather obtain, the trained ML model that is used in the CV system and the image test set, so we can test the same image adding various kinds of perturbations, which are usually specific noise, finding in this way the minimum perturbation that causes misclassification. This brought a type of the previously mentioned security issues directly to the CV field and then generalized it to the ML field.

Adversarial examples are perturbed images whose purpose is to mislead the ML models (see Fig. 2). In the subfield of CV, these techniques, which include all kinds of attacks using adversarial examples and, in parallel, all the defensive techniques against them, were termed "adversarial computer vision" (adversarial CV). The corresponding term in the more general field of ML was termed "adversarial machine learning" (adversarial ML).

The perturbation, which is usually some kind of noise added to clean images to produce adversarial examples, is not randomly chosen. The main idea that brought up adversarial examples was based on the observation that no CV system can detect positively or classify correctly all the objects of its task for the entire image set given. So, there is a subset of the space of images that causes false decisions in the system, although humans can easily recognize them. This subset of images may be physically perturbed (distortion, deformation, misillumination, misorientation, occlusion) in a way that they significantly influence some of the features that were preselected for extraction and feed them as input to the ML model.

Knowing the trained ML model, we can artificially produce such perturbed images adding noise, randomly or not, to several of them. If we know the features that are selected for extraction in the "feature extraction" phase of the CV systems workflow (see Fig. 1), we can easily choose the appropriate noise to add to an image, so that the applied image feature vector moves to an area of the hyperplane that has been delimited by the ML model to another inappropriate class, resulting in misclassification (see Fig. 3).

It seemed that one needed to obtain the specific pretrained ML model of a CV system, or its parameters and the training dataset, to produce the appropriate adversarial examples. However, based on the observation that adversarial examples made for a specific ML model can surprisingly be efficient for attacking another ML model with other parameters and trained with a dissimilar dataset, we can construct adversarial examples with any ML model in order to attack every other model. This is more effective when we obtain similar ML models or training datasets for producing the adversarial examples, but is still effective in all other instances. This phenomenon is called "attack transferability"

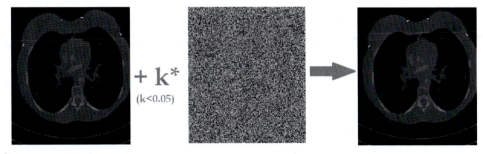

**FIG. 2**

A simple representation of adversarial example production. The adversarial example is shown in the third column, where the parameter $k$ should be optimally minimized while the product effect to the classifier is maximized.

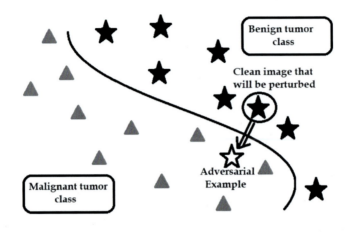

**FIG. 3**

Simplified visualization of the way adversarial examples act in moving from one class area to another, attacking a classifier. Triangles are images that are classified to the malignant tumor class and stars are images that should be classified to the benign tumor class.

(Szegedy et al., 2013; Goodfellow et al., 2014; Papernot et al., 2016a). Therefore the knowledge of the attacked ML model is useful, but it is not the only way to start an attack.

Adding a small, imperceptible-to-humans perturbation, we can artificially produce adversarial examples, but can they be produced accidentally? The answer is yes. These perturbations, such as noise, distortion, deformation, misillumination, misorientation, and occlusion, may be physically applied to an image and if that affects the decision of the ML model, they become accidental adversarial examples. In medical imaging, avoiding or minimizing the previously mentioned perturbations is considered a condition of the utmost importance. Capturing the images is a job that must be done in a predetermined way, and very carefully.

## 4  Methods to produce adversarial examples

There are many methods for generating adversarial examples. Herein, only the methods considered as a base for other variants and those that can have an effective application to medical imaging due to their special characteristics are presented. Before that, it would be useful to be clear that the term *norm*, which will be mentioned often in the following text, is a function from a vector space over the real or complex numbers to the nonnegative real numbers space that satisfies some predefined conditions and has specific properties. Simply, a norm is a way to measure a vector's distance from the zero vector or the distance between two vectors. $L_0$ corresponds to the number of nonzero elements in the vector and cannot be considered as a norm, because it does not satisfy the norm condition. $L_1$ corresponds to the sum of the absolute values of the vector's components. $L_2$ or the Euclidean norm corresponds to the square root of the sum of the squared values of the vector's components, and it finds the shortest distance of the route from the vector to the zeroth vector. L-infinity, $L_\infty$, or max norm corresponds to the maximum of the absolute values of the vector's components. The most popular methods are described as follows.

Fast Gradient Sign Method (FGSM) (Goodfellow et al., 2014) can be considered the base of a family of methods. FGSM generates adversarial examples that are effective in CV systems that use an artificial neural network (ANN), and therefore CNN and DCNN, as they are subsets of the more general ANN set, as a classifier. Given are the values of the parameters $p$ of the model and the cost function $C(p, x,y)$, where $x$ is the input to the model and $y$ the targets associated with $x$, which have been used to train the neural network classifier. The method tries to make the cost function $C(p,x,y)$ linear around the $p$ values, optimizing the $L_\infty$ norm of the constrained perturbation of $\delta$ given in Eq. (1).

$$\delta = \epsilon \cdot \mathrm{sign}(\nabla_x(C(p, x, y))) \tag{1}$$

where $\epsilon$ is a scalar value, sign(.) is the sinus function, and $\nabla_x$ is the gradient of function $C(.)$. FGSM has variants that are based on the gradient of the cost function, such as Fast Gradient-$L_2$ and Fast Gradient-$L_\infty$ (Kurakin et al., 2016a). All the FGSM methods family are executed in one step. FGSM is generally designed for attacks that are not aimed at a specific instance or class, but there are variants that aim at a specific class or the least likely class predicted by the classifier.

Basic Iterative Method (BIM) (Kurakin et al., 2016a) is FGSM based, but it is not a one-step method. First, it applies a $\delta$ perturbation, such as that described in Eq. (1), with a random scalar value of $\epsilon$, and in every following step, it adds another $\delta$ perturbation to the previously perturbed image until it causes misclassification. A variant of BIM worth mentioning, called the "iterative least likely class method" (Kurakin et al., 2016b), is aimed at producing the optimal perturbation so that it makes the classifier misclassify the detected objects or the entire image to the least likely class. Another variant of BIM worth mentioning is projected gradient descent (PGD) (Madry et al., 2017), which is considered the strongest BIM variant. This can make the adversarial examples more effective and disastrous.

L-BFGS (Liu and Nocedal, 1989) is an adversarial example production method so named because, in order to minimize the perturbation's $L_2$ norm, it uses the limited memory quasi-Newton method for large-scale optimization.

Carlini & Wagner (C&A) (Carlini and Wagner, 2016) attacks consist of three methods: the C&A-$L_2$, the C&A-$L_0$, and the C&A-$L_\infty$, each minimizing the $L_2$, the $L_0$, and the $L_\infty$ norm of a cost function. That perturbation cost function is different in each of the three variants of the method. C&A attacks are considered to be among the most efficient attacks in adversarial CV.

Jacobian-based Saliency Map Attack (JSMA) (Papernot et al., 2016b) is a method that iteratively changes the values of just a few pixels. It changes the value of one pixel at a time, keeping the changes for the next iteration when it will alter another pixel. After all iterations, it constructs the adversarial saliency map that measures the effectiveness of every perturbed pixel and, finally, it chooses the regions of the map that are most effective to provoke misclassification. In this way JSMA constructs adversarial examples, affecting only a few regions and not the entire image. This characteristic makes the adversarial examples produced imperceptible and suitable for application in medical imaging.

One Pixel Attack (OPA) (Su et al., 2019) is a method that iteratively alters the values of one pixel of the image at a time, evaluating its effect on the classifier. Consequently, another pixel value is altered but, contrary to the JSMA method iteration, it does not keep the previous pixel altered. If the evaluation of the next one-pixel perturbation shows it has more effect than the previous one, the method decides to substitute the perturbation pixel with the last; otherwise it keeps the previously made one. Completing all the iterations, the method chooses the most effective single-pixel perturbation. This method is designed to generate adversarial examples only from probabilistic ML models, so that it can evaluate every perturbation. The method is not the most effective, but it proves that in some cases only one specific pixel perturbed is enough to change the classification results. Based on this conclusion, we can easily understand how important it is to care about all the conditions of the subject, the background, and the device during image capturing.

Universal Adversarial Perturbation (UAP) (**Moosavi-Dezfooli et al., 2017**) is a family of methods that constructs a single perturbation that is added to all images of the image set. In the previously mentioned methods, a different perturbation is constructed for each image, in a way so as to be optimally effective and imperceptible. With UAP, using a single "universal" perturbation applying it to a set of clean images we can produce a set of adversarial examples. This family of methods is not one of the most effective ones, but its characteristics make it one of the most easily applicable. UAP methods are useful because some of them can directly apply to any physical object. Moreover, the perturbation produced can be materialized, for example a film that can be applied physically on a camera's lens so that the universal perturbation can be applied to any image produced, causing misclassification most of the time.

The first four methods and their variants presented earlier are based on the same idea of maximizing the effect of the adversarial example on the classifier, overminimizing the perturbation cost that makes the perturbation imperceptible. This is made either in one step or iteratively. They differ based on the kind of perturbation they apply, and the cost function of the perturbation used for minimization. The latter three methods are chosen because of their special characteristics and their applicability to medical imaging, as described. Other adversarial example constructions that are worth a reference are STAds (Spatial Transformed Adversarial examples) (Xiao et al., 2018), DeepFool (Moosavi Dezfooli et al., 2016), ZOO Attack (Zeroth Order Optimization Attack) (Chen et al., 2017), Levy-Attack (Srinivasan et al., 2019), UPSET and ANGRI (Sarkar et al., 2017), EAD (Elastic-net attacks) (Chen et al., 2018), and Houdini (Cisse et al., 2017). Many more can be found in the collection of papers in (Carlini, 2019) and many other sources on the internet that are continuously updated.

## 5 Adversarial attacks

An adversarial attack in computer vision can be defined as the application of an adversarial example as input to a CV system, with the purpose of misclassification. We call it misclassification when the CV system classifies an image in a different class than a human does. However, how should it be defined in what class a human classifies an image? How can we decide the "ground truth" class labels corresponding to an image set? Clearly, there is a sense of relativity and therefore the labels of each image must be carefully selected, statistically considering the opinion of a group of specialties and not the classification made by only one expert. In (Carlini, 2019) it is stated that "Ground truth is often ambiguous," which means that, in some instances, especially in medical image analysis, even specialties do not agree on the same classification. If we train an ML model with clumsily chosen labels, it will affect the way the model delimits the classes in the theoretical hyperplane of the feature variables. Choosing a reliable dataset for the training procedure, as for the testing procedure too, affects directly the accuracy of the model's effectiveness and rating. Using a dataset containing adversarial examples, but correctly labeled, can be used to make the ML model more robust to some attacks (Szegedy et al., 2013) and will be analyzed thoroughly later in this chapter.

In the means of attack transferability described earlier, adversarial examples can be used to attack either the same model that they have been created and optimized with, or any other model.

Some adversarial examples can be implemented in the real world, applied physically to objects, but some others can be used only in the cyberworld for perturbing digital images. Some adversarial examples are targeting a specific class or a group of classes, and others are constructed for universal attacks. These ways of using adversarial examples characterize the attacks, so we can taxonomize them.

Many taxonomies have been proposed, but they seem to be influenced by the subject of a specific research subfield. The research, since the first reference to ML security in 2008 (Barreno et al., 2008) and adversarial CV in 2013 (Szegedy et al., 2013), has advanced and new directions taken as the physical implementation of the perturbations appeared (Finlayson et al., 2019; Kurakin et al., 2016a; Elsayed et al., 2018; Eykholt et al., 2018). The latest taxonomy of adversarial CV attacks (Maliamanis and Papakostas, 2020a) that will be presented shortly seems to be more general and updated to the needs of the latest research directions. The taxonomy is based on three axes, the knowledge of the targeted CV system axis, the specificity of the attack axis, and the applicability to the physical objects axis, as is seen in Fig. 4:

- *Knowledge axis.* This consists of three categories of attacks:
  — *White box attacks.* Corresponds to attacks that are constructed having complete knowledge of the type of the ML model, and all its parameters, that the CV system is using, as well as the training method and the training dataset. As previously mentioned, in this

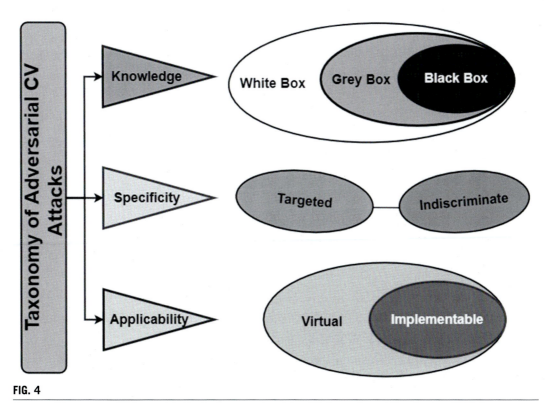

**FIG. 4**

A general taxonomy of adversarial attacks in computer vision (Maliamanis and Papakostas, 2020a).

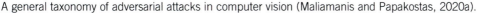

way adversarial examples can be constructed optimally, maximizing their effectiveness. These attacks are the strongest of the three categories.

— *Gray box attacks.* Corresponds to attacks that are constructed having only some knowledge about the classifier. These attacks are usually paired with an attack strategy, depending on the knowledge obtained. These attacks are usually of moderate strength.

— *Black box attacks.* Corresponds to attacks that are constructed without having any knowledge about the classifier. In this case, the attack is made using a classifier and training dataset the attacker already has, hoping that the phenomenon of attack transferability will be effective in the use case. These attacks do not have a constant effectiveness in every case of application, but have the advantage of the universality of use.

- *Specificity axis.* This consists of two categories of attacks:
  - *Targeted attacks.* Corresponds to attacks that try to change the classifier's decision of a single class or a deteriorated group of classes. For example, an attack that intends to change the classification of one disease to another and does not affect the classes of other diseases is a targeted attack.
  - *Indiscriminate attacks.* Corresponds to those attacks that have an effect on all classes without discrimination.

- *Applicability axis.* This consists of two categories of attacks:
  - *Virtual attacks.* Corresponds to attacks that can be found only in digital data forms. These attacks refer to CV systems used on cyber recognition, as digital images, or text recognition from text files.
  - *Implementable attacks.* Corresponds to attacks that can also be materialized in physical form in the real world. These attacks can be applied to physical objects, or in the case of using a universal perturbation on image-capturing devices.

To fully categorize an attack, we need to choose three characterizations, one for each axis of the preceding taxonomy. For example, a black box, indiscriminate, and implementable attack is an attack that was made without any knowledge of the targeted classifier, it affects all of the classes, and it can be materialized in physical forms in order to be applied directly on objects.

There is also research on attack strategies that can pair with a set of attack categories. An interesting attack strategy, called the Oracle Attack Method (Goodfellow et al., 2014), attacks a remote classifier, such as a cloud classifier, monitoring the predictions made by the remote system. In this way it creates a dataset to train a substitute model locally afterwards. The produced local ML model, which resembles the remote one a great deal, can be used for producing adversarial examples. This strategy converts black-box attacks to gray box, obtaining knowledge for the targeted system, concluding in attack efficiency improvement.

# 6 Adversarial defensive methods

Some defensive strategies and methods have been proposed for degrading the effect of adversarial attacks, but among them there is no universal defense capable of making CV systems robust against every attack. Their application to medical CV systems shows no restrictions or differences compared to other CV applications, because, as was mentioned, in medical imaging the conditions may be different but the CV systems used are the same as in other applications.

Lately, the research has been focused on finding the reason for the effectiveness of adversarial attacks against ML models and the reason for the "transfer learning" phenomenon also. These seem to be the keys to designing ML models that are robust against adversarial attacks. An interesting hypothesis, that we support, is that a DCNN, which is the most popular ML model for CV systems, models, among robust features, also nonrobust ones that are imperceptible to humans (Ilyas et al., 2019). Adversarial examples are altering these nonrobust features, which is why they are so effective and imperceptible. The same hypothesis can explain the phenomenon of attack transferability, since altering the nonrobust features of an image can have an effect on another ML model from the targeted one, because it also has modeled some of the same features during training.

Summarizing the main defense proposals, considering the way they act, we concluded on the following categorization:

- *Defensive methods that improve the training process.* Using adversarial examples, correctly labeled, among clean images, to train an ML model with this augmented dataset, is termed "adversarial training." Adversarial training is a very popular defensive method but, besides the fact that it is effective against only the attack methods that are using similar adversarial examples, such as those used for augmenting the training, it drops the accuracy of the model on clean images (Papernot et al., 2016a). This observation can be a clue supporting the hypothesis of nonrobust feature modeling. Another defensive method is the one termed the "distillation method of training" (Papernot et al., 2016c), which uses an additional probabilistic classifier that outputs probabilities of the classes rather than classifying to a "hard" label, in order to provide the "soft" made labels. Subsequently it uses them to train the main ML model. This helps the classifier to classify the adversarial examples more accurately.
- *Defensive methods that improve the image processing step.* Applying on an image a common compression like JPG, which removes the imperceptible high-frequency components from the images, can cause some attacks to become less efficient (Das et al., 2017). Finding the region of interest and cropping the image to it, discarding everything else, using foveation-based mechanisms (Luo et al., 2015), can also reduce the effectiveness of many adversarial attacks.
- *Defensive methods that modify the classifier's architecture.* The observation in (Papernot et al., 2016a) that adversarial training is more effective on deeper DNN classifiers led to the method of increasing the capacity of a DNN. Adding layers to such a model can also be combined with appropriate training (Madry et al., 2017), constructing a classifier that is more robust against attacks. This is an improvement, compared to the single adversarial training, but it is also incapable of constructing a classifier robust to all attacks but instead only to the trained ones. Another method that alters the classifier's architecture is its combination with an autoencoder used before the main classifier with the purpose of "denoising" the input image. This method was termed Deep Contractive Networks (DCNs) (Gu and Rigazio, 2014). They are effective because autoencoders, and especially Contractive Auto-Encoders (CAEs) (Rifai et al., 2011), can optimally compress the input vector, transforming the features to another form that minimizes the correlation between them. In addition, in discarding the contained information that is not useful for the classification process, they discard a major part of the adversarial perturbation applied to an adversarial example.

- *Defensive methods that detect adversarial examples.* These methods are simply trying to detect adversarial examples before forwarding them as inputs to the classifier. The detection idea may be simple, but the execution is difficult. None of the methods that have been proposed can detect all kinds of adversarial attacks (Carlini and Wagner, 2017). If they find an adversarial example, they can denoise it, or substitute it with a clean image, or even discard it. There is a plethora of such detection methods because it has been a favorite problem of researchers from early times. Among others worth referring to are the Convolutional Filter Statistics method (Li and Li, 2017), Feature Squeezing method (Xu et al., 2017), and Magnet method (Meng and Chen, 2017). Although the idea of primary detection is simple, the execution is difficult and the methods are not universally effective. This strategy is of great research interest because, parallel to its evolution, it challenges the attack methods to try to be "invisible."

It is easily concluded but worth mentioning that these methods of adversarial defense can be combined and that is rather necessary when the CV system will be applied to sensitive applications such as healthcare and medical image analysis.

## 7 Adversarial computer vision in medical imaging

The main physical problems that occur during image capture and that affect CV are distortion, deformation, misillumination, misorientation, and occlusion. Specifically to medical images, occlusion is missing, misorientation and misillumination are minimized if the images are captured carefully, and distortion usually is due to lens characteristics that are minimized in modern medical devices. Finally, deformation could be a real problem in some cases, when for instance the image capturing is applying pressure to a body part, but with supervision by specialized personnel it is minimized. The main target during capturing medical images of a body part is to have the same conditions applied to all of them. As mentioned earlier in this chapter, medical images are ideally captured for CV systems and that is the reason why medical CV is one of the most popular applications, with such a large amount of research interest.

From the previous discussion, it is obvious that general adversarial CV attacks can also attack medical images. The same happens to the defensive mechanisms proposed. However, some specific questions arise:

- Do all these attacks have the same efficiency against medical imaging?
- Are some of the defensive mechanisms less and some others more powerful when they apply to medical imaging CV?
- What is the reason for any differentiation?

To answer these, we will analyze some statements that have been studied. In this way we will capture the status of research on the vulnerabilities and, more generally, the differentiations of the adversarial medical CV subfield.

*Some adversarial attack methods have little or no effect on a large part of medical CV.* In (Taghanaki et al., 2018) Taghanaki et al., among others, discovered that the One Pixel Attack (OPA) method did not have any effect on the two-class problem of the classification of chest X-ray images. The OPA attack failed in both ways the attack method was applied, as a black box attack and as a generally much stronger white box attack. This happened because OPA is more effective against RGB color images, where changing a pixel means altering three values, in contrast to the gray-scale images, where it is more difficult to fool a state-of-the-art ML model by altering a single value.

*Medical CV systems are generally more vulnerable to adversarial attacks, compared to others.* As in (Ma et al., 2020) Ma et al. found out that medical DNN models are more powerless against attacks. As they claim, the reasons for this differentiation may be the fact that medical images contain complex biological textures that can be easy targets for effective perturbing. Moreover, most medical classification tasks have deteriorated output classes, which are usually two, more rarely more. The ML models used are designed for large-scale tasks and maybe overparameterized for the simple medical image analysis tasks.

*Adversarial examples of medical images can easily be detected.* As analyzed earlier in this chapter, perturbations applied to images are optimized by the targeted ML model (white box attacks) or another model that transfers the attack. This procedure of optimization, which differs between the method families, chooses to perturb regions of the image that will be more effective, staying as much as possible imperceptible to humans. In (Taghanaki et al., 2018) it is observed that the perturbations applied, especially from strong attacks, can easily be seen by the naked eye, which means that the methods needed to apply more perturbation in order to be effective. This does not keep them from being considered as adversarial examples, because the maximum perceptibility of the perturbation has not ever been defined. The same statement was also supported in (Ma et al., 2020), where it was mentioned that the adversarial features that adversarial perturbation added to medical images are linear, separable from the features that are really needed for the classification, in opposition to the perturbations made to natural images for the general tasks of CV, where the added features are more mixed. This means that sometimes applying a filter that discards the "high- frequency" features can drop a major part of the adversarial perturbation. This supports the fact that the defensive techniques that are more effective for medical ML models are those that detect adversarial examples and those that improve the image-processing step, which were both mentioned earlier in this chapter, as the last two defense categories.

*Medical ML is among the top and easy targets of adversarial attacks.* Healthcare, medicine, and insurance companies are connected industries that care a lot about healthcare data and their security. There are strong financial incentives, due to competition, to adversarially attack medical data and therefore medical images. Moreover, the healthcare infrastructure, especially computers and medical devices that manipulate medical data, is rather slowly updated, a fact that makes medical data easy to attack (Finlayson et al., 2019). The protocols used for encapsulating images and other medical data are not so safe anymore. The DICOM standard (Mildenberger et al., 2002), which packs medical images together with other patient's data, has been broadly used for over 20 years.

*Attack transferability is increased when we use pretrained ML models for medical image analysis tasks.* Using a pretrained model, and consequently "transfer learning" (Weiss et al., 2016) techniques, to additionally train the model with a more specialized training set makes the classifier more effective and increases its accuracy, as compared to a model that is only trained with the second training set. Most of the pretrained CV ML models that can be found are trained on the same, very popular, ImageNet dataset. The observation made by S.C. Wetstein et al. (Wetstein et al., 2020) was that these two-phase trained models in medical image analysis tasks are more vulnerable to black box or gray box attacks optimized with substitute ML models that were also pretrained to the same dataset, compared to the same two-phase models that in the second phase of additional "transfer learning" were trained for more general tasks. As they assume, this is because the pretrained ML model's decision boundaries are more similar, due to the initialization over the same general dataset, than those randomly initialized.

In the preceding discussion, there are many assumptions made explaining the reasons for every statement. This happens because most of the ML models, especially DCNNs, act as black boxes. No one can tell what exactly is happening in every step of the procedure or what features of the images are modeled during training to set the boundaries of the classes for the classification task. As it is usually termed, the "interpretability" of these models is close to zeroth, but the same applies to the human neural networks. After all, artificial NNs aspire to imitate the architecture of human NNs. As these models act this way, the only thing you can surely tell is their result. That is why researchers are trying to use experimental results to make assumptions, and not proofs, about their reasons.

## 8 Adversarial examples: How to generate?

It is not easy to find ready-made medical adversarial examples, except for some samples in paper-related codes, for experimenting with this specific topic. Additionally, the search for "synthetic medical images" is not equivalent to the "medical imaging adversarial examples" search, because the first are mainly used for data augmentation of small datasets, which means that they are not constructed to mislead ML models but the opposite.

The only certain way to experiment with the topic is to generate adversarial examples before using them. First of all, the researcher should find an appropriate, for the experimental concerns, clean image dataset (Kaggle, 2021; OpenNeuro, 2021; The Medical Image Bank of Valencia, 2021). Using one of the adversarial example generating methods described earlier, the researcher can process a part of the dataset if the purpose is testing or alter the whole dataset for experimenting in adversarial training, ML models, or adversarial attack methods evaluation.

The most widespread coding language used for ML tasks is Python, less common is C++, and Matlab is rarely used for some tasks. The most code examples, experiments, and documentation can be found in Python, using several libraries and APIs appropriate for ML (Tensorflow, 2021; Keras, 2021; Scikit-learn, 2021; Pytorch, 2021) and adversarial attacks (Goodfellow et al., 2016; Nicolae et al., 2018; SecML, 2021; Corona et al., 2016).

## 9 Conclusion

Machine learning methods in medical imaging represent a trending field. Adversarial computer vision attacks touch, with some small differentiations in the general tasks, the medical image analysis field.

The latest research is focused on finding new vulnerabilities (Maliamanis and Papakostas, 2020b) and, in parallel, ways to make ML models robust against all kinds of adversarial attacks. Understanding the way these attacks act effectively and investigating the reason why their effectiveness varies from general to more specialized tasks, such as medical image analysis, can help the scientific community to find a universal solution to ML security vulnerabilities. The application of adversarial attacks and defensive techniques to medical machine learning has revealed some small efficiency variations and differentiations that can be very useful for researchers in understanding and supporting or discarding many assumptions.

An obstacle is that the most effective ML models have low interpretability, due to their architecture. Changing the architecture of the models, making them more interpretable, can bring a universal solution to the adversarial CV problem, but can also improve the classification accuracy. Moreover, other security techniques, such as medical file encryption and medical image watermarking, can be applied to secure the files and make attack application harder.

The fact is that the AI field is still far from being equal to human perception, but the goal is to set the ML models capable of an effective and secure manipulation of smaller deteriorated tasks. Even if AI ever touches or outperforms human classification accuracy regarding all clean and adversarial perturbated images, there awaits another problem to be solved, the "hard problem of consciousness" (Chalmers, 1995).

## Acknowledgment

This work was supported by the MPhil program "Advanced Technologies in Informatics and Computers," hosted by the Department of Computer Science, International Hellenic University, Greece.

## References

Badeka, E., Papadopoulou, C.I., Papakostas, G.A., 2020. Evaluation of LBP variants in retinal blood vessels segmentation using machine learning. In: 4th International Conference on Intelligent Systems and Computer Vision (ISCV 2020), 9-11 June, Fez, Morocco.

Barreno, M., Nelson, B.A., Joseph, A.D., Tygar, D., 2008. The Security of Machine Learning., https://doi.org/10.21236/ada519143.

Beutel, J., Kundel, H.L., Van Metter, R.L., 2000. Handbook of Medical Imaging. SPIE.

Carlini, N., 2019. A Complete List of all (arxiv) Adversarial Example Papers. https://nicholas.carlini.com/writing/2019/all-adversarial-example-papers.html.

Carlini, N., Wagner, D., 2016. Towards Evaluating the Robustness of Neural Networks. arXiv: 1608.04644,.

Carlini, N., Wagner, D., 2017. Adversarial examples are not easily detected: bypassing ten detection methods. In: Proceedings of the 10th ACM Workshop on Artificial Intelligence and Security. ACM, pp. 3–14.

Chalmers, D.J., 1995. Facing up to the problem of consciousness. J. Conscious. Stud. 2, 200–219.

Chen, P.-Y., Zhang, H., Sharma, Y., Yi, J., Hsieh, C.-J., 2017. ZOO: zeroth order optimization based black-box attacks to deep neural networks without training substitute models. In: Proceedings of the 10th ACM Workshop on Artificial Intelligence and Security. ACM, New York, NY, USA, pp. 15–26.

Chen, P.-Y., Sharma, Y., Zhang, H., Yi, J., Hsieh, C.-J., 2018. EAD: Elastic-net attacks to deep neural networks via adversarial examples. In: Thirty-second AAAI conference on artificial intelligence, aaai.org.

Cisse, M., Adi, Y., Neverova, N., Keshet, J., 2017. Houdini: Fooling Deep Structured Prediction Models. https://arxiv.org/abs/1707.05373.

Corona, I., Biggio, B., Maiorca, D., 2016. AdversariaLib: an open-source library for the security evaluation of machine learning algorithms under attack. arXiv [cs.CR].

Das, N., Shanbhogue, M., Chen, S.-T., Hohman, F., Chen, L., Kounavis, M.E., Chau, D.H., 2017. Keeping the Bad Guys Out: Protecting and Vaccinating Deep Learning with JPEG Compression. http://arxiv.org/abs/1705.02900.

Elsayed, G., Shankar, S., Cheung, B., Papernot, N., Kurakin, A., Goodfellow, I., Sohl-Dickstein, J., 2018. Adversarial examples that fool both computer vision and time-limited humans. In: Bengio, S., Wallach, H.,

Larochelle, H., Grauman, K., Cesa-Bianchi, N., Garnett, R. (Eds.), Advances in Neural Information Processing Systems. Vol. 31. Curran Associates, Inc, pp. 3910–3920.

Eykholt, K., Evtimov, I., Fernandes, E., Li, B., Rahmati, A., Xiao, C., Prakash, A., Kohno, T., Song, D., 2018. Robust Physical-World Attacks on Deep Learning Visual Classification., https://doi.org/10.1109/cvpr.2018.00175.

Finlayson, S.G., Chung, H.W., Kohane, I.S., Beam, A.L., 2019. Adversarial Attacks Against Medical Deep Learning Systems. arXiv [cs.CR] http://arxiv.org/abs/1804.05296v3.

Goodfellow, I.J., Shlens, J., Szegedy, C., 2014. Explaining and Harnessing Adversarial Examples. https://arxiv.org/abs/1412.6572.

Goodfellow, I., Papernot, N., McDaniel, P., Feinman, R., Faghri, F., Matyasko, A., Hambardzumyan, K., Juang, Y.-L., Kurakin, A., Sheatsley, R., et al., 2016. Cleverhans v0. 1: an adversarial machine learning library. arXiv preprint arXiv:1610.00768 1.

Gu, S., Rigazio, L., 2014. Towards Deep Neural Network Architectures Robust to Adversarial Examples. arXiv preprint arXiv:1412.5068,.

Hosny, K.M., Papakostas, G.A., Koulouriotis, D.E., 2013. Accurate reconstruction of noisy medical images using orthogonal moments. In: 2013 18th International Conference on Digital Signal Processing (DSP), Fira, pp. 1–6, https://doi.org/10.1109/ICDSP.2013.6622675.

Hosny, K.M., Kassem, M.A., Foaud, M.M., 2018. Skin Cancer classification using deep learning and transfer learning. In: 2018 9th Cairo International Biomedical Engineering Conference (CIBEC)., https://doi.org/10.1109/cibec.2018.8641762.

Ilyas, A., Santurkar, S., Tsipras, D., Engstrom, L., Tran, B., Madry, A., 2019. Adversarial Examples Are Not Bugs, They Are Features. http://arxiv.org/abs/1905.02175.

Kaggle, 2021. https://www.kaggle.com/datasets (Accessed 17 March 2021).

Keras, 2021. https://keras.io/about/. (Accessed 17 March 2021).

Kose, U., Alzubi, J., 2020. Deep Learning for Cancer Diagnosis. Springer.

Kurakin, A., Goodfellow, I., Bengio, S., 2016a. Adversarial Machine Learning at Scale. https://arxiv.org/abs/1611.01236.

Kurakin, A., Goodfellow, I., Bengio, S., 2016b. Adversarial Examples in the Physical World. https://arxiv.org/abs/1607.02533.

LeCun, Y., Bengio, Y., Hinton, G., 2015. Deep learning. Nature 521, 436–444.

Li, X., Li, F., 2017. Adversarial examples detection in deep networks with convolutional filter statistics. In: Proceedings of the IEEE International Conference on Computer Vision, pp. 5764–5772. openaccess.thecvf.com.

Linnartz, J.-P.M.G., Jean-Paul, M., van Dijk, M., 1998. Analysis of the Sensitivity Attack against Electronic Watermarks in Images., https://doi.org/10.1007/3-540-49380-8_18.

Liu, D.C., Nocedal, J., 1989. On the limited memory BFGS method for large scale optimization. Math. Program. 45, 503–528.

Luo, Y., Boix, X., Roig, G., Poggio, T., Zhao, Q., 2015. Foveation-based Mechanisms Alleviate Adversarial Examples. http://arxiv.org/abs/1511.06292.

Ma, X., Niu, Y., Gu, L., Wang, Y., Zhao, Y., Bailey, J., Lu, F., 2020. Understanding adversarial attacks on deep learning based medical image analysis systems. Pattern Recogn. https://doi.org/10.1016/j.patcog.2020.107332.

Madry, A., Makelov, A., Schmidt, L., Tsipras, D., Vladu, A., 2017. Towards Deep Learning Models Resistant to Adversarial Attacks. http://arxiv.org/abs/1706.06083.

Maliamanis, T., Papakostas, G.A., 2020a. Adversarial computer vision: a current snapshot. In: Twelfth International Conference on Machine Vision (ICMV 2019)., https://doi.org/10.1117/12.2559582.

Maliamanis, T., Papakostas, G.A., 2020b. DOME-T: Adversarial computer vision attack on deep learning models based on Tchebichef image moments. In: Thirteenth International Conference on Machine Vision (ICMV 2020).

Meng, D., Chen, H., 2017. Magnet: a two-pronged defense against adversarial examples. In: Proceedings of the 2017 ACM SIGSAC Conference on.

Mildenberger, P., Eichelberg, M., Martin, E., 2002. Introduction to the DICOM standard. Eur. Radiol. 12.

Moosavi Dezfooli, S.-M., Fawzi, A., Frossard, P., 2016. DeepFool: A Simple and Accurate Method to Fool Deep Neural Networks., https://doi.org/10.1109/cvpr.2016.282.

Moosavi-Dezfooli, S.-M., Fawzi, A., Fawzi, O., Frossard, P., 2017. Universal Adversarial Perturbations., https://doi.org/10.1109/cvpr.2017.17.

Nicolae, M.-I., Sinn, M., Tran, M.N., Rawat, A., Wistuba, M., Zantedeschi, V., Baracaldo, N., Chen, B., Ludwig, H., Molloy, I.M., Edwards, B., 2018. Adversarial Robustness Toolbox v0.4.0. arXiv [cs.LG].

Njeh, C.F., 2008. Tumor delineation: the weakest link in the search for accuracy in radiotherapy. J. Med. Phys./Assoc. Med. Phys. India 33 (4), 136.

OpenNeuro, 2021, https://openneuro.org/ (Accesed 17 March 2021).

Papakostas, G.A., Mertzios, B.G., Karras, D.A., 2009. Performance of the orthogonal moments in reconstructing biomedical images. In: 2009 16th International Conference on Systems, Signals and Image Processing, Chalkida, pp. 1–4, https://doi.org/10.1109/IWSSIP.2009.5367686.

Papernot, N., McDaniel, P., Goodfellow, I., 2016a. Transferability in Machine Learning: from Phenomena to Black-Box Attacks using Adversarial Samples. https://arxiv.org/abs/1605.07277.

Papernot, N., McDaniel, P., Jha, S., Fredrikson, M., Berkay Celik, Z., Swami, A., 2016b. The Limitations of Deep Learning in Adversarial Settings., https://doi.org/10.1109/eurosp.2016.36.

Papernot, N., McDaniel, P., Wu, X., Jha, S., Swami, A., 2016c. Distillation as a defense to adversarial perturbations against deep neural networks. In: 2016 IEEE Symposium on Security and Privacy (SP). ieeexplore.ieee.org, pp. 582–597.

Pytorch, 2021. https://pytorch.org/ (Accessed 17 March 2021).

Rajpurkar, P., Irvin, J., Zhu, K., Yang, B., Mehta, H., Duan, T., Ding, D., Bagul, A., Langlotz, C., Shpanskaya, K., Lungren, M.P., Ng, A.Y., 2017. CheXNet: Radiologist-Level Pneumonia Detection on Chest X-Rays With Deep Learning. arXiv [cs.CV] http://arxiv.org/abs/1711.05225.

Rawat, W., Wang, Z., 2017. Deep convolutional neural networks for image classification: a comprehensive review. Neural Comput. 29, 2352–2449.

Rifai, S., Vincent, P., Muller, X., Glorot, X., Bengio, Y., 2011. Contractive auto-encoders: explicit invariance during feature extraction. In: Proceedings of the 28th International Conference on International Conference on Machine Learning. pp. 833–840, Omnipress, USA.

Sarkar, S., Bansal, A., Mahbub, U., Chellappa, R., 2017. UPSET and ANGRI : Breaking High Performance Image Classifiers. http://arxiv.org/abs/1707.01159.

Scikit-learn, 2021. https://scikit-learn.org/stable/index.html (Accessed 17 March 2021).

SecML, 2021. https://secml.gitlab.io/. (Accessed 17 March 2021).

Srinivasan, V., Kuruoglu, E.E., Müller, K.-R., Samek, W., Nakajima, S., 2019. Black-Box Decision based Adversarial Attack with Symmetric α-stable Distribution. https://arxiv.org/abs/1904.05586.

Su, J., Vargas, D.V., Sakurai, K., 2019. One Pixel Attack for Fooling Deep Neural Networks., https://doi.org/10.1109/tevc.2019.2890858.

Szegedy, C., Zaremba, W., Sutskever, I., Bruna, J., 2013. Intriguing Properties of Neural Networks. arXiv preprint arXiv,.

Taghanaki, S.A., Das, A., Hamarneh, G., 2018. Vulnerability analysis of chest X-ray image classification against adversarial attacks. In: Understanding and Interpreting Machine Learning in Medical Image Computing Applications, pp. 87–94, https://doi.org/10.1007/978-3-030-02628-8_10.

Tensorflow, 2021. https://www.tensorflow.org/ (Accessed 17 March 2021).

The Medical Image Bank of Valencia, 2021. https://bimcv.cipf.es/ (Accessed 17 March 2021).

Wang, X.-N., Dai, L., Li, S.-T., Kong, H.-Y., Sheng, B., Wu, Q., 2020. Automatic grading system for diabetic retinopathy diagnosis using deep learning artificial intelligence software. Curr. Eye Res., 1–6.

Weiss, K., Khoshgoftaar, T.M., Wang, D., 2016. A survey of transfer learning. J. Big Data. https://link.springer.com/article/10.1186/s40537-016-0043-6.

Wetstein, S.C., González-Gonzalo, C., Bortsova, G., Liefers, B., Dubost, F., Katramados, I., Hogeweg, L., van Ginneken, B., Pluim, J.P.W., de Bruijne, M., Sánchez, C.I., Veta, M., 2020. Adversarial Attack Vulnerability of Medical Image Analysis Systems: Unexplored Factors. arXiv [cs.CR] http://arxiv.org/abs/2006.06356.

Xiao, C., Zhu, J.-Y., Li, B., He, W., Liu, M., Song, D., 2018. Spatially Transformed Adversarial Examples. http://arxiv.org/abs/1801.02612.

Xu, W., Evans, D., Qi, Y., 2017. Feature Squeezing: Detecting Adversarial Examples in Deep Neural Networks. http://arxiv.org/abs/1704.01155.

# Skull stripping and tumor detection using 3D U-Net

**Rahul Gupta, Isha Sharma, and Vijay Kumar**

*National Institute of Technology, Hamirpur, Himachal Pradesh, India*

## Chapter outline

## 1 Introduction

Digital image processing has been adeptly applied in medical science, increasing efficiency in the study of anatomical structure, diagnosis, surgical planning, treatment planning, research, computer integrated surgery, and many other areas. The emerging field of image processing and artificial intelligence has gained much recent attention in medical research and applications. Among all of the techniques used, MRI (magnetic resonance imaging) stands out. This technology makes use of a strong magnetic field and radio waves in order to obtain detailed images of various body organs and tissues (Rutegard et al., 2017; Smith-Bindman et al., 2012). It has high anatomical resolution and hence provides more detailed information on the anatomical structure. This is considered to be a crucial field of research, as it is necessary to reduce the need for human intervention in the preliminary step of image processing, i.e., skull stripping, or brain extraction, in which nonbrain tissues are separated from brain tissues,

Machine Learning, Big Data, and IoT for Medical Informatics. https://doi.org/10.1016/B978-0-12-821777-1.00014-8

in order to decrease the variance and delay due to the time-consuming process of manual processing, which obstructs analysis and large-scale diagnosis and treatment. MRI is usually preferred over other techniques, as it can create efficient contrast in both the interior and exterior brain tissues, and thus it enhances the automated skull stripping process.

Medical image processing and research is a critical part of study and prognosis using magnetic resonance imaging (MRI). It is used in the study of the brain's anatomical structure, in which image segmentation has become a vital part of neurosurgical medical research, as a highly weighted step in the process of extracting features from the image. It is easier to perform analysis of skull-stripped images; therefore an accurate and unbiased skull segmentation method has become a much-valued technique. The tissues of the brain have various important features that are used in brain segmentation. However, detecting the border of the brain can become challenging due to low contrast and artifacts, and the segmentation can easily be corrupted due to noise, bias-field effects, or partial volume effects, possibly resulting in misleading outputs that can lead to faulty observations and diagnosis. This challenge becomes more severe in the case of deformities in brain tissues, sometimes due to the presence of diseases such as tumors, Alzheimer's disease, etc. As a result, this step is considered to be one of the challenging tasks in image processing.

Various approaches have been developed for brain tissue extraction purposes, but no one method is suitable for all types of images. There are several classical approaches that, according to Liu et al. (2014), can be categorized as region-based, boundary-based, atlas-based, and hybrid-based approaches. Also, there are many approaches based on neural networks or deep learning (Lin et al., 2016), which can easily handle bulky datasets and can justifiably derive useful information from them.

Automatic brain tumor detection is another challenging step, due to the variability of shapes and sizes, variable positions, and intensities (Rehman et al., 2020). Brain tumors are of two main types, primary and secondary, where primary tumors are noncancerous while secondary are cancerous. Due to the complexity of this task, various techniques have been developed in the past making use of the different existing imaging techniques, such as CT, PET, MRI, and multimodal imaging techniques. These provide information by using the various tissue features present in the brain. In our work we have specifically focused on the MRI imaging technique, for which there have been various methods developed for tumor detection, including thresholding methods (Singh and Magudeeswaran, 2017), region growing methods (Deng et al., 2010), edge-based methods (Aslam et al., 2015), fuzzy clustering techniques, morphological-based methods, atlas-based methods, and neural network-based methods. Apart from all the previous methods, there are still many challenges in tumor detection techniques, due to artifacts and noise interruptions. It is crucial to be able to detect tumors accurately, as the entire process of diagnosis and treatment can collapse with inefficient automatic skull stripping and tumor detection techniques. In our methodology, an effective approach has been demonstrated that can efficiently minimize these challenges by implementing a 3D U-Net approach for performing neural-based automatic skull stripping, along with supporting detection of the presence of lower-grade gliomas from the MRI dataset.

## 1.1 Previous work

The segmentation of brain tissues is an initial but critical step in the field of medical image processing for accurate diagnosis and surgery estimations. There are numerous generally available datasets that can be used in different skull-stripping algorithms, such as the Alzheimer's Disease Neuroimaging Initiative (ADNI) dataset ( Jack et al., 2008), which has been developed in many steps. Some of the major datasets available are: (1) ADNI1 (2004–2009), ADNI2 (2010–2016), and ADNI3; (2) Open Access Series of Imaging Studies (OASIS) dataset (Marcus et al., 2007); (3) LPBA40, which shows digital brain atlases (Shattuck et al., 2008); (4) Internet Brain Segmentation Repository (IBSR) (IBSR, 2020), which shows manually delineated results with MRI data; (5) National Alliance for Medical Image Computing (NAMIC), which consists of T2W images with skull-stripped data; and (6) Neuro-feedback Skull-stripped (NFBS) database (NFBS, 2020), which is publicly available having a total of 125 MRI images with 48:77 skull-stripped datasets for men and women, respectively.

There are basically three types of MRI brain images: T1-weighted, T2-weighted, and PD-weighted images, which focus on different contrast characteristics of brain tissues (Akkus et al., 2017). Various steps are required before images of the brain can be processed, among which is segmentation, considered to be a crucial stage in image processing, as previously mentioned. A great deal of work has been proposed in this field of segmentation, which can typically be classified into two major types of approaches: classical approaches and neural network-based approaches.

In the field of classical skull-stripping approaches, *morphology-based methods* have been applied (Brummer et al., 1993), wherein histogram thresholding was used prior to applying morphology filters. Atkins and Mackiewich (1998) developed a multistage model. Various methods based on histogram analysis for skull segmentation were proposed by Shan et al. (2002) and Galdames et al. (2012). Another approach, called the Brain Extraction Approach (BEA), was proposed by Somasundaram and Kalaiselvi (2010, 2011); it works by adjustment of the deformable model until the expected borders are reached. The Brain Surface Extraction (BSE) approach was proposed by Shattuck et al. (2001).

*Atlas-based methods* are based on prior knowledge from reference images (Cabezas et al., 2011). Leung et al. (2011) proposed a multiple atlas propagation and segmentation technique (MAPS); this method generates multiple segmentations using library templates and an algorithm called simultaneous truth and performance level estimation (STAPLE). The BEaST (brain extraction based on nonlocal segmentation technique) method was developed by Manjon et al. (2014), using a sum of squared differences in order to observe the brain mask. A new multiatlas brain segmentation (MABS) method was proposed by Del Re et al. (2016). Unlike atlas-based algorithms, MABS uses weights for the atlases according to their similarity to the target image.

*Region growing methods* are based on pixels merging with their neighbors according to their similarity criteria. Based on this methodology, Justice et al. (1997) have presented a 3D SRG (seeded region growing) method for brain MRI segmentation. Park and Lee (2009) have presented a 2-dimensional (2D) RG for brain T1W MRIs, where seed and nonseed regions are generated using masks developed by morphological operations; however, this approach was limited for coronal orientation of brain MRIs. This limitation was handled by Roura et al. (2014) using both axial views and low-quality brain images, with a multispectral adaptive region growing algorithm (MARGA) for skull stripping. A level set approach by Wang et al. (2010) based on local Gaussian distribution fitting energy for brain extraction in MRI has given more accurate results when used in a region-based methodological approach. A drawback faced by region-based algorithms is oversegmentation of the brain tissue, which can be handled by various other methods such as hybrid models or neural network models.

In *hybrid models* combinations of various methods are used, according to the pros and cons of various already-proposed methodologies and imaging techniques, in order to generate the best combination of techniques for fully automating the segmentation process with better analysis and performance. A popular combination of an atlas-based active contour skull stripping algorithm with a level setting-based algorithm was devised by Bauer et al. (2012a, 2012b). BEMA, another Brain Extraction Meta Algorithm, used a combination of quad extractors along with a registration process to generate more accurate results (Rex et al., 2004). MRI brain segmentation framework was developed in two stages. Initially, all nonbrain tissues were removed and then applied automatic gravitational search algorithm to pull out brain tissues from skull stripped images (Kumar et al., 2014).

Currently, the deep learning-based approach also makes use of numerous techniques. They are easily deployable and deep learning has proved to be an accurate and unbiased approach for extracting brain masks. In Kleesiek et al. (2016) a fully neural network-based technique for skull stripping was devised, which has shown better performance than the previous classical techniques. A deep-learning technique based on the U-Net architecture was developed to attain volumetric segmentations from a sparse annotation; a DeepMedic was trained over a smaller amount of data using BRATS 2016 and was able to show outstanding results in terms of Dice. It is sustainable for datasets that require no minimal preprocessing, like BRATS 2015 and 2016. The question as to whether a model will perform in the same manner when trained on one dataset and tested on another was analyzed. Yet another method was reported by Lu et al. (2019), in which a 3D CNN architecture of three levels was used where each level is followed by pooling process along with usage of ConvNet1 and ConvNet2 models, yielding large parameters, followed by tuning of parameters in order to maintain balance between computational time and efficiency.

Tumor detection is best when achieved in the early phases of tumor building, as it can be diagnosed and treated accordingly. In this field of research and study, MRI images have shown better outputs as compared to CT scans or ultrasound. Automated tumor detection is very challenging; better outcomes are obtained with the use of convolution neural networks. In Xu et al. (2015) the methodology made use of ImageNet for extracting features and showed 97.5% accuracy in classification and 84% accuracy in segmentation. In Pan et al. (2015) multiphase MRI images for tumor grading were analyzed and a comparative study was done between deep-learning structures and base neural networks; based on the sensitivity and specificity of the CNN, the performance of the structure was improved by 18% compared to the neural networks. In a study by Siar and Teshnehlab (2019), feature extraction along with a CNN was deployed after preprocessing of images, which showed 98.67% accuracy with the Softmax classifier, 97.34% with the radial basis function (RBF) classifier, and 94.24% with the decision tree (DT) classifier.

## 2  Overview of U-net architecture

U-Net is basically a 2D convolution neural network introduced by Ronneberger et al. (2015). This network consists of normal convolutional layers and max-pooling layers followed by an equal number of up-convolutional layers. These convolutional and up-convolutional layers in the network are connected by skip connections.

### 2.1  3D U-net

The 3D U-Net architecture was constructed by Cicek et al. (2016) for 3D images. In this architecture 3D kernels are used, unlike in the 2D U-Net. When tested, this architecture has been shown to train and generate prediction results for an entire voluminous image. The large memory requirement for analyzing a 3D image is a major drawback for conventional techniques, which can be easily dealt with using

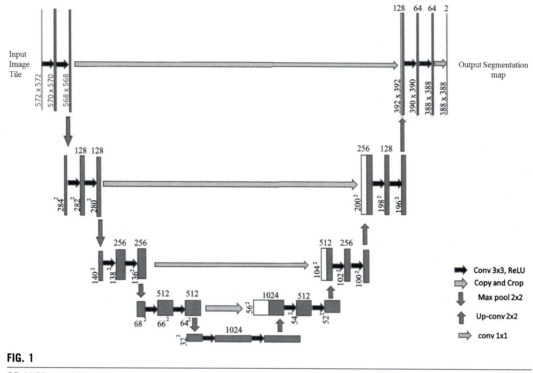

**FIG. 1**

3D U-Net architecture.

this architecture. The analysis path uses max pooling and performs two convolutions per max-pooling operation of kernel size 3 × 3 and with stride 1. Padding is performed on the data so that the output size comes out to be equal to the input. The U-Net architecture is especially well-suited for image segmentation. This network is a fully convolutional network, and the original reason that this architecture was developed was for use in biomedical image segmentation. The architecture is U-shaped, which is why it is called U-Net. In this architecture, the left part is called the contraction path or encoder path, whereas the right part is called the expansion path or decoder path. We can also modify the various parameters of the architecture based on the problem statement and dataset. The contraction path is used to pull out the global features. This consists of the convolution block and max pooling. The convolution block comprises the batch normalization (Ioffe and Szegedy, 2015), convolution, and an activation function called the rectified linear unit (ReLU). This architecture as shown in Fig. 1 and uses padding and maximum pooling as shown in Fig. 3.

### 2.1.1 Batch normalization

Normalization is used to convert various data values in common scale types of values; by using batch normalization, the neural network becomes faster and more stable.

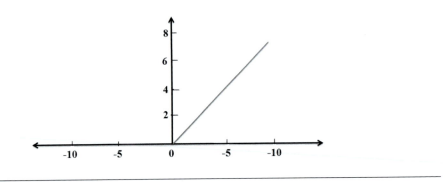

**FIG. 2**

ReLU activation function.

### 2.1.2 Activation function

Activation functions are types of mathematical expressions used to find the output of a neural network. There are various types of activation functions, including ReLU, Leaky ReLU, Sigmoid, and so on. ReLU is one of the linear functions that gives a positive output for positive input values, else zero. This activation function is used to reduce the vanishing gradient problem, and it is used in our model also (Fig. 2).

$$R(z) = \max(0, z)$$

### 2.1.3 Pooling

The main idea for the use of pooling is to reduce the dimension of the matrix and accept some features based on some assumptions, similar to a filter applied to the feature map. Various pooling techniques are used, such as max pooling, min pooling, mean pooling, and so on. In this U-Net architecture, max pooling is used, of size $2 \times 2$ pixels. This $2 \times 2$ size of the pooling matrix is placed on the pixels of the image and the max pixel is pulled out from that image in $2 \times 2$ matrixes, as shown in Fig. 3.

### 2.1.4 Padding

Padding can be defined as "a measure of pixels to be added to an image when it is being prepared by the kernel of a CNN." For this U-Net architecture, padding is defined as "same": i.e., the output image is to have the same dimensions as the input image.

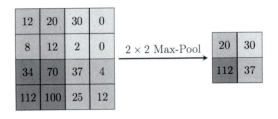

**FIG. 3**

$2 \times 2$ Max pooling.

### 2.1.5 Optimizer

Optimizers perform the adjustment of the learning rate for individual parameters. There are various algorithms for optimizing stochastic gradient descent (SGD) in neural networks, such as Momentum, Adagrad, Adadelta, RMSprop, and Adam. Adagrad is the foremost optimizer, which optimizes the image on a greater level by adding up the gradient history. Hence this makes it suitable for use with small datasets. RMSprop scales its learning rate by finding the mean of the recent gradients of the parameters. Adam is one of the most recently introduced optimizers; it uses first- and second-order momentum to scale the learning rate for each parameter.

## 3  Materials and methods

### 3.1  Dataset

The dataset used contains brain MR images together with manual FLAIR abnormality segmentation masks. The images were obtained from The Cancer Imaging Archive (TCIA). They correspond to 110 patients included in The Cancer Genome Atlas (TCGA) lower-grade glioma collection with at least fluid-attenuated inversion recovery (FLAIR) sequence and genomic cluster data available. This model was trained on 2828 MRIs with parameters as follows: number of epochs 50, batch size 32, and learning rate 0.0001. The performance of the 3D U-Net was evaluated on a dataset "LGG Segmentation Dataset" that is publicly available (LGG, 2019); the results were obtained by this model for 373 MRIs. Here, the input size of each scan was $256 \times 256 \times 3$. In this dimension, $256 \times 256$ defines the length and width, respectively, whereas 3 defines the depth of scan, or RGB image.

### 3.2  Implementation

The implementation of this model was carried out as follows:

Step 1: Image Acquisition.
   Initially, images were collected from the dataset of both types of normal MRI and their respective mask images.
Step 2: Data Visualization.
   After collecting the data, the MRI was visualized with the help of the collected dataset. For this, we imported the cv2 library and converted the BGR images to RGB images.
Step 3: Train and Test Dataset.
   Then the dataset was split for the training and testing of the model. For the training, 2828 MRI sets were used, and for testing the model, 393 MRI sets were collected.
Step 4: Data Generation and Data Augmentation.
   With this step, we generated image and mask at the same time and used the same seed for image data generation and mask generation to ensure the transformation of the images.
Step 5: Define U-Net Architecture.
   In this step, the architecture of U-Net was defined with the ReLU and sigmoid activation function. Normalization, padding, and strides were also used to prepare the model. With this, the total parameters were 31,043,521 (trainable parameters are 31,037,633 and nontrainable parameters are 5888).

Step 6: Train the Model.

The model was trained with 50 epochs, batch size of 32, and learning rate of 0.0001. The Adam optimizer was also used to compile the model. From this, we obtained train and test evaluation metrics.

Step 7: Test the Model.

After training the model, the model was tested on 393 images and achieved better accuracy, Dice coefficient, and IoU than existing methods. Some original and predicted results as obtained by the model are shown in Fig. 5.

# 4 Results

## 4.1 Experimental result

Various implementations of skull segmentation have been done using non-deep learning methods, such as Brain Surface Extractor (BSE) and Robust Brain Extraction (ROBEX) (Iglesias et al., 2011), and also deep learning-based methods, such as Kleesiek's method (Kleesiek et al., 2016). The BSE algorithm works by filtering the image, detecting the edges, performing a morphological operation, followed by surface cleanup to identify the brain. ROBEX is an automatic whole-brain extraction tool for T1-weighted MRI data; it aims for robust skull-stripping across datasets with no parameter settings..

### 4.1.1 Dice coefficient

The Dice coefficient can be defined as "the ratio of twice the intersection of the pixels of both images to the sum of all pixels of both the images."

$$\text{Dice coefficient} = \frac{2|IP_1 \cap IP_2|}{|IP_1| + |IP_2|}$$

where $IP_1$ and $IP_2$ are the image pixels of image 1 and image 2, respectively.

This can also be defined in terms of a confusion matrix:

$$\text{Dice coefficient} = \frac{2TP}{2TP + FP + FN}$$

### 4.1.2 Accuracy

The accuracy is the ratio of truly predicted data points out of all data points. It can also be defined as the ratio of the sum of true positive, true negative to the sum of true positive, true negative, false positive, and false negative.

$$\text{Accuracy} = \frac{TP + TN}{TP + TN + FP + FN}$$

### 4.1.3 Intersection over Union (IoU)

Intersection over Union is the ratio of the intersection of pixels of images to the union of all the pixels of all the images. It is also called the Jaccard Index. This metric is used for image segmentation and object detection. If $IoU\ score \geq 0.5$ then that score is considered a good score.

**Table 1 Quantitative analysis for the MRI dataset.**

| Epochs | Accuracy | IoU | Dice Coefficient | Val_Accuracy | Val_IoU | Val_Dice coefficient |
|---|---|---|---|---|---|---|
| 1 | 0.9176 | 0.0509 | 0.0957 | 0.9890 | 0.0119 | 0.0233 |
| 5 | 0.9810 | 0.1417 | 0.2439 | 0.9886 | 0.1017 | 0.1818 |
| 10 | 0.9956 | 0.4474 | 0.6104 | 0.9958 | 0.4697 | 0.6331 |
| 15 | 0.9960 | 0.5726 | 0.7205 | 0.9946 | 0.3850 | 0.5497 |
| 20 | 0.9969 | 0.6941 | 0.8155 | 0.9972 | 0.7014 | 0.8128 |
| 25 | 0.9972 | 0.7296 | 0.8393 | 0.9970 | 0.7118 | 0.8294 |
| 30 | 0.9973 | 0.7421 | 0.8446 | 0.9969 | 0.7079 | 0.8207 |
| 35 | 0.9974 | 0.7639 | 0.8625 | 0.9972 | 0.7385 | 0.8456 |
| 40 | 0.9972 | 0.7447 | 0.8482 | 0.9958 | 0.5870 | 0.7248 |
| 45 | 0.9974 | 0.7677 | 0.8652 | 0.9975 | 0.7620 | 0.8547 |
| 50 | 0.9975 | 0.7849 | 0.8753 | 0.9976 | 0.8007 | 0.8882 |

**Table 2 Result of MRI dataset.**

| Accuracy | IoU | Dice coefficient |
|---|---|---|
| 0.9978 | 0.7903 | 0.8819 |

$$IoU = \frac{Area\ of\ Intersection}{Area\ of\ Union}$$

This model was trained on 2828 MRIs with parameters as follows: number of epochs 50, batch size 32, and learning rate 0.0001; some of the results are shown in Table 1.

The results obtained by this model for the 373 MRIs tested using the U-Net architecture are depicted in Table 2.

## 4.2 Quantitative result

Using the Table 1 data, we can summarize in graphs, as shown in Fig. 4. Both types of data are plotted on the graph: i.e., training data is shown in red and test data is shown in blue. A graph of the entire metrics as well as a loss graph are also plotted.

## 4.3 Qualitative result

The model was tested on 373 MRIs with an accuracy of 0.9978. We can see the results of the images with their respective masks which were tested on the proposed model and lower-grade gliomas, using shape features which were automatically extracted by the proposed model as shown in Fig. 5.

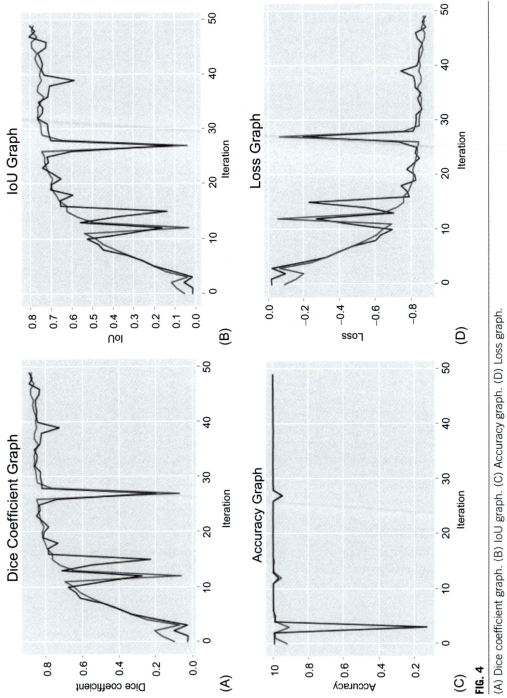

**FIG. 4**

(A) Dice coefficient graph. (B) IoU graph. (C) Accuracy graph. (D) Loss graph.

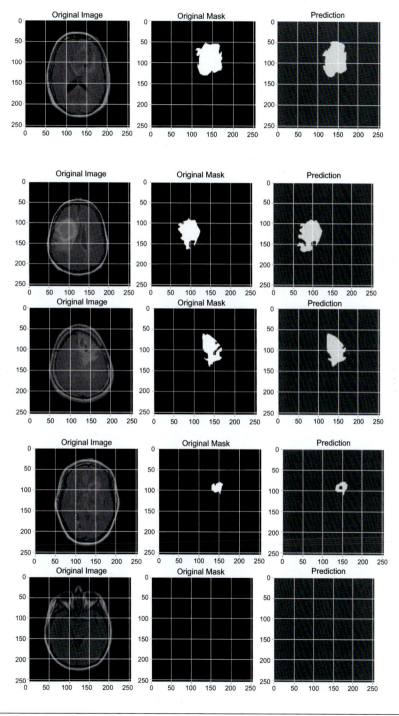

**FIG. 5**

Lower-grade gliomas predicted with respect to their original image and original mask with the use of 3D U-Net architecture.

## 5 Conclusion

We have implemented a 3D U-Net to segment the brain and for extraction of lower-grade gliomas from the stripped tissues. This method is capable of performing automatic skull stripping and extraction of lower-grade gliomas from the MRI dataset of the human brain that was used. When trained appropriately, this model has shown effective results according to the Dice coefficient, IoU metrics, etc., as has been demonstrated. Also, this model can be beneficial in making clear estimations of tumor stages because of the model's well-defined architecture. We believe that the implemented technique will be useful for very large-scale case studies and treatment. In future, this approach can be modified for detection of other types of brain tumors by analysis of other features without being affected by issues of inhomogeneity.

## References

Akkus, Z., Galimzianova, A., Hoogi, A., Rubin, D.L., Erickson, B.J., 2017. Deep learning for brain MRI segmentation: state of the art and future directions. J. Digit. Imaging 30, 449–459. https://doi.org/10.1007/s10278-017-9983-4. In this issue.

Aslam, A., Khan, E., Beg, M.M.S., 2015. Improved edge detection algorithm for brain tumor segmentation. Procedia Comput. Sci. 58, 430–437.

Atkins, M.S., Mackiewich, B.T., 1998. Fully automatic segmentation of the brain in MRI. IEEE Trans. Med. Imaging 17 (1), 98–107. https://doi.org/10.1109/42.668699.

Bauer, S., Fejes, T., Reyes, M., 2012a. A skull-stripping filter for ITK. Insight J. 96, 70–78.

Bauer, S., Nolte, L.P., Reyes, M., 2012b. Skull-Stripping for Tumor-Bearing Brain Images. arXiv preprint arXiv:1204.0357, p. 97.

Brummer, M.E., Mersereau, R.M., Eisner, R.L., Lewine, R.J., 1993. Automatic detection of brain contours in MRI data sets. IEEE Trans. Med. Imaging 1993 (12), 153–166. https://doi.org/10.1109/42.232244.

Cabezas, M., Oliver, A., Lladó, X., Freixenet, J., Bach Cuadra, M., 2011. A review of atlas-based segmentation for magnetic resonance brain images. Comput. Methods Prog. Biomed. 104 (3), e158–e177.

Cicek, O., Abdulkadir, A., Lienkamp, S.S., Brox, T., Ronneberger, O., 2016. 3D U-net: learning dense volumetric segmentation from sparse annotation. Lect. Notes Comput. Sci, 424–432.

Del Re, E.C., Gao, Y., Eckbo, R., Petryshen, T.L., Blokland, G.A., Seidman, L.J., Konishi, J., Goldstein, J.M., McCarley, R.W., Shenton, M.E., et al., 2016. A new MRI masking technique based on multi-atlas brain segmentation in controls and schizophrenia: a rapid and viable alternative to manual masking. J. Neuroimaging 2016 (26), 28–36.

Deng, W., Xiao, W., Deng, H., Liu, J., 2010. MRI brain tumor segmentation with region growing method based on the gradients and variances along and inside of the boundary curve. In: 2010 3rd International Conference on Biomedical Engineering and Informatics.

Galdames, F.J., Jaillet, F., Perez, C.A., 2012. An accurate skull stripping method based on simplex meshes and histogram analysis for magnetic resonance images. J. Neurosci. Methods 206, 103–119.

IBSR, 2020. Dataset. Available at: https://www.nitrc.org/projects/ibsr. (Accessed 4 June 2020).

Iglesias, J.E., Liu, C.Y., Thompson, P.M., Tu, Z., 2011. Robust brain extraction across datasets and comparison with publicly available methods. IEEE Trans. Med. Imaging 2011 (30), 1617–1634.

Ioffe, S., Szegedy, C., 2015. Batch Normalization: Accelerating Deep Network Training by Reducing Internal Covariate Shift. preprint arXiv:1502.03167.

Jack, C.R., Bernstein, M.A., Fox, N., Thompson, P., Alexander, G., Harvey, D., Borowski, B., Britson, P.J., Whitwell, J.L., Ward, C., et al., 2008. The Alzheimer's disease neuroimaging initiative (ADNI): MRI methods. J. Magn. Reson. Imaging 27, 685–691.

Justice, R., Stokely, E., Strobel, J., Ideker, R., Smith, W., 1997. Medical image segmentation using 3D seeded region growingc. In: SPIE. Vol. 3034.

Kleesiek, J., Urban, G., Hubert, A., Schwarz, D., Maier-Hein, K., Bendszus, M., Biller, A., 2016. Deep MRI brain extraction: A 3D convolutional neural network for skull stripping. NeuroImage 2016 (129), 460–469.

Kumar, V., Chhabra, J.K., Kumar, D., 2014. Automatic MRI brain image segmentation using gravitational search-based clustering technique research developments in computer vision and image processing. Methodol. Appl., 313–326.

Leung, K.K., Barnes, J., Modat, M., Ridgway, G.R., Bartlett, J.W., Fox, N.C., Ourselin, S., 2011. Brain MAPS: an automated, accurate and robust brain extraction technique using a template library. Neuroimage 55 (3), 1091–1108. https://doi.org/10.1016/j.neuroimage.2010.12.067.

LGG, 2019. Dataset. https://www.kaggle.com/mateuszbuda/lgg-mri-segmentation. (Accessed 4 June 2020).

Lin, D., Vasilakos, A.V., Tang, Y., Yao, Y., 2016. Neural networks for computer-aided diagnosis in medicine: a review. Neurocomputing 216, 700–708.

Liu, J., Li, M., Wang, J., Wu, F., Liu, T., Pan, Y., 2014. A survey of MRI-based brain tumor segmentation methods. Tsinghua Sci. Technol. 19 (6), 578–595.

Lu, H., Wang, H., Zhang, Q., Yoon, S.W., Won, D., 2019. A 3D convolutional neural network for volumetric image semantic segmentation. Procedia Manuf. 39, 422–428. https://doi.org/10.1016/j.promfg.2020.01.386.

Manjon, J.V., Eskildsen, S.F., Coupe, P., Romero, J.E., Collins, D.L., Robles, M., 2014. Nonlocal intracranial cavity extraction. Int. J. Biomed. Imaging 2014, 820205. https://doi.org/10.1155/2014/820205.

Marcus, D., Wang, T.H., Parker, J., Csernansky, J.G., Morris, J.C., Buckner, R.L., 2007. Open access series of imaging studies (OASIS): cross-sectional MRI data in young, middle aged, nondemented, and demented older adults. J. Cogn. Neurosci. 19, 1498–1507.

NFBS, 2020. Dataset. Available at: http://preprocessed-connectomes-project.org/NFB_skullstripped. (Accessed September 2020).

Pan, Y., et al., 2015. Brain tumor grading based on neural networks and convolutional neural networks. In: 37th Annual International Conference of the IEEE Engineering in Medicine and Biology Society (EMBC), pp. 699–702.

Park, J.G., Lee, C., 2009. Skull stripping based on region growing for magnetic resonance brain images. NeuroImage 47, 1394–1407. https://doi.org/10.1016/j.neuroimage.2009.04.047.

Rehman, H.Z.U., Hwang, H., Lee, S., 2020. Conventional and deep learning methods for skull stripping in brain MRI. Appl. Sci. 10 (5), 1773.

Rex, D.E., Shattuck, D.W., Woods, R.P., Narr, K.L., Luders, E., Rehm, K., Stolzner, S.E., Rottenberg, D.A., Toga, A.W., 2004. A meta-algorithm for brain extraction in MRI. NeuroImage 23, 625–637.

Ronneberger, O., Fischer, P., Brox, T., 2015. U-Net: convolutional networks for biomedical image segmentation. CoRR. http://arxiv.org/abs/1505.04597.

Roura, E., Oliver, A., Cabezas, M., Vilanova, J.C., Rovira, A., Ramio-Torrenta, L., Llado, X., 2014. MARGA: multispectral adaptive region growing algorithm for brain extraction on axial MRI. Comput. Methods Prog. Biomed. 113, 655–673. https://doi.org/10.1016/j.cmpb.2013.11.015. Appl. Sci. 2020, 10, 1773 27 of 30.

Rutegard, M.K., Batsman, M., Axelsson, J., Brynolfsson, P., Brannstrom, F., Rutegard, J., Singh, J.F., Magudeeswaran, V., 2017. Thresholding based method for segmentation of MRI brain images. In: 2017 International Conference on I-SMAC (IoT in Social, Mobile, Analytics and Cloud) (I-SMAC).

Shan, Z.Y., Yue, G.H., Liu, J.Z., 2002. Automated histogram-based brain segmentation in T1- weighted three-dimensional magnetic resonance head images. NeuroImage 17, 1587–1598.

Shattuck, D.W., Sandor-Leahy, S.R., Schaper, K.A., Rottenberg, D.A., Leahy, R.M., 2001. Magnetic resonance image tissue classification using a partial volume model. NeuroImage 13, 856–876.

Shattuck, D.W., Mirza, M., Adisetiyo, V., Hojatkashani, C., Salamon, G., Narr, K.L., Poldrack, R.A., Bilder, R.M., Toga, A.W., 2008. Construction of a 3D probabilistic atlas of human cortical structures. NeuroImage 39 (3), 1064–1080.

Siar, M., Teshnehlab, M., 2019. Brain tumor detection using deep neural network and machine learning algorithm. In: 2019 9th International Conference on Computer and Knowledge Engineering (ICCKE).

Singh, J.F., Magudeeswaran, V., 2017. Thresholding based method for segmentation of MRI brain images. 2017 International Conference on I-SMAC (IoT in Social, Mobile, Analytics and Cloud) (I-SMAC). IEEE, pp. 280–283.

Smith-Bindman, R., Miglioretti, D.L., Johnson, E., Lee, C., Feigelson, H.S., Flynn, M., Williams, A.E., 2012. Use of diagnostic imaging studies and associated radiation exposure for patients enrolled in large integrated health care systems, 1996-2010. JAMA 307 (22).

Somasundaram, K., Kalaiselvi, T., 2010. Fully automatic brain extraction algorithm for axial T2-weighted magnetic resonance images. Comput. Biol. Med. 2010 (40), 811–822.

Somasundaram, K., Kalaiselvi, T., 2011. Automatic brain extraction methods for T1 magnetic resonance images using region labeling and morphological operations. Comput. Biol. Med. 2011 (41), 716–725. https://doi.org/10.1016/j.compbiomed.2011.06.008.

Wang, L., Chen, Y., Pan, X., Hong, X., Xia, D., 2010. Level set segmentation of brain magnetic resonance images based on local Gaussian distribution fitting energy. J. Neurosci. Methods 2010 (188), 316–325. https://doi.org/10.1016/j.jneumeth.2010.03.004.

Xu, Y., et al., 2015. Deep convolutional activation features for large scale brain tumor histopathology image classification and segmentation. In: IEEE International Conference on Acoustics, Speech and Signal Processing (ICASSP), pp. 947–951.

# Cross color dominant deep autoencoder for quality enhancement of laparoscopic video: A hybrid deep learning and range-domain filtering-based approach

**Apurba Das[a,b] and S.S. Shylaja[a]**

*Department of CSE, PES University, Bangalore, India[a] Computer Vision (IoT), Tata Consultancy Services, Bangalore, India[b]*

## Chapter outline

## 1 Introduction

It has been well accepted (Stoyanov, 2012) that laparoscopic video streams are one of the best modalities for operating surgeons as far as the intraoperative data is concerned. Quality degradation due to multiple artifacts like haze, blood, nonuniform illumination, and specular reflection impacts not only the visibility of the surgeon but also the accuracy of image/video analytics. Haze is directly responsible for reducing the contrast of the surgical video stream. Hence, it is of the utmost importance to dehaze laparoscopic videos in guided surgery to ensure improved visualization of the operative field. Laparoscopic desmoking has been addressed in a few recent works (Kotwal et al., 2016; Baid et al., 2017; Tchakaa et al., 2017) that essentially utilized the idea of the dark channel prior (DCP) dehazing algorithm (He et al., 2011, 2013) for images, as depicted in Eq. (1):

$$I(x) = J(x)t(x) + A(1 - t(x)) \tag{1}$$

where $I$ is the observed intensity, $J$ is the scene radiance, $A$ is the global atmospheric light, and $t$ is the medium transmission describing the light that reaches the camera without suffering from scatter due to dust or water particles in the medium. The goal of any dehazing algorithm is to extract the scene radiance $J$ from a hazy input image $I$.

He et al. (2011) observed that, in outdoor environments, most of the local patches have lowest intensity in at least one color channel. Based on this observation, they proposed the DCP model, which has been considered to be the traditional model for dehazing an image since its publication. Later, the use of a guided filter (He et al., 2013) was proposed to improve the quality of the results. However, there is a basic difference between dehazing an outdoor scene and a laparoscopic video. Essentially, concentration of haze in an outdoor scene is dependent on scene depth whereas in laparoscopy the haze or smoke is a local phenomenon. Rather, it depends on the tip of the thermal cutting instrument. In laparoscopic surgery, the light source does not ensure uniform illumination nor is the organ surface Lambertian (which assures only defused reflection). These constraints violate the assumptions of Eq. (1). Wang et al. (2018) have analyzed the same and proposed a new algorithm considering two specialized properties of laparoscopic dehazing: haze has low contrast and low intrachannel differences. But most of the works until now, to the best of our knowledge, focussed on defogging images and completely ignored the intraframe correspondence in laparoscopic "video." Das et al. (2018a) and Das and Shylaja (2020) have proposed a fast bilateral filter using two different layers of adaptiveness to the filter for dehazing and deraining. In the current work, we exploit the property of intraframe correspondence in laparoscopic videos and dominance of cross color in the domain of organ surgery. This improves not only the clarity of vision but also further image analytics in distinctive detection/segmentation of the object of interest in near real time. The chapter is organized as follows. In Section 2, the fundamental idea of bilateral filtering is described. Next, in Section 3, the novel algorithm of a color dominant deep autoencoder is presented. Section 4 depicts the experimental results of cross color dominant deep autoencoder quality enhancement on laparoscopic video. Finally, our observations and findings are summarized in Section 5.

## 2 Range-domain filtering

Since the bilateral filter concept was proposed by Tomasi and Manduchi (1998), it has been a major area of contribution in the image processing and computer vision community. Consider a high-dimensional image $f: \mathbb{Z}^d \to \mathbb{R}^n$ and a *guide* image $p: \mathbb{Z}^d \to \mathbb{R}^\rho$. Here $d$ is the dimension of the domain, and $n$ and $\rho$ are dimensions of the ranges of the input image $f$ and guide $p$, respectively. The output of the bilateral filter $h: \mathbb{Z}^d \to \mathbb{R}^n$ is given as

$$h_j = \frac{1}{k_j} \sum_{i \in W} \omega(i)\, \phi(p_{j-i} - p_j) f_{j-i}, \tag{2}$$

where

$$k_j = \sum_{i \in W} \omega(i) \, \phi(p_{j-i} - p_j).$$

(3)

Here $\omega : \mathbb{R}^d \to \mathbb{R}$ is the spatial kernel and $\phi : \mathbb{R}^n \to \mathbb{R}$ is the range kernel. If $f$ and $p$ are different, then this filter is a cross-bilateral filter (Eisemann and Durand, 2004; Petschnigg et al., 2004).

The said filter is not only restricted to gray images but also extends the operations to color images with the promise to solve different applications in computer vision, such as dehazing and joint upsampling. Traditional spatial filtering is *domain* filtering, and enforces closeness by nonuniformly weighing neighboring pixel values. On the other hand, *range* filtering averages image values with weights that decay with dissimilarity in intensity. Range filtering is nonlinear and its output changes for every pixel to be filtered. The computations in Eqs. (2), (3) are performed over set $W$, which is a set of neighborhood pixels around the pixel of interest. Various examples of input $f$ are discussed in Nair and Chaudhury (2017). The aforementioned variation of bilateral filters has been tested both for gray and color images and has shown superior enhancement ensuring edge preservation, as depicted in Figs. 1 and 2, respectively.

## 3 Cross color dominant deep autoencoder ($C^2D^2A$) leveraging color spareness and saliency

In the current work, we have leveraged the property of dimension reduction of the autoencoder (Chen and Lai, 2019) to extract the dominant color from the larger color range present in any image. The idea of sparse color occupancy for any group of images depicting the same object or action has been utilized

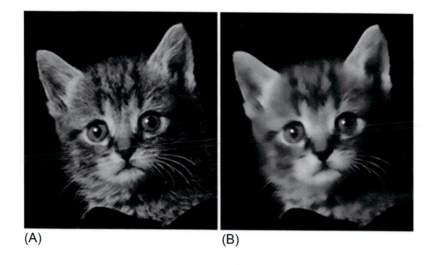

(A)                                    (B)

**FIG. 1**

Bilateral smoothing filter applied on gray image, ensuring edge preservation (Tomasi and Manduchi, 1998).

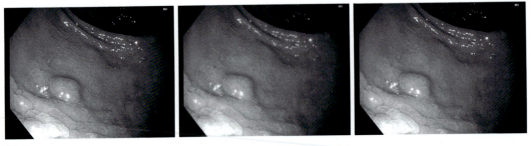

**FIG. 2**

Bilateral smoothing filter applied on color image: Ensuring edge preservation and no phantom color (Tomasi and Manduchi, 1998): The left one is the input laparoscopic image, the middle one is the output of classical smoothening filter making the edges also blurred, and the right most one is the output of bilateral filtering maintaining the edges.

further to create the dominant color map (DCM) offline as a table to be referenced in real time. The offline DCM table has next been used as an LUT for real-time processing, ensuring much faster bilateral filtering with respect to the state of art.

## 3.1 Evolution of DCM through $C^2D^2A$

The principal idea here is to determine dominant/salient colors from a group of homogeneous images (e.g., laparoscopic or endoscopic images; Ye et al., 2015). The dominant colors might be even interpolated colors of the quantized available colors in the image set. The autoencoder architecture, as depicted in Fig. 3, has been employed to determine the salient/dominant color for different groups of homogeneous images at a time with the objective of deriving a DCM (Das and Shylaja, 2021) in a coded and reduced dimension format, offline. This DCM further would be processed during image filtering. The proposed method of DCM derivation has the five following stages:

1. Imagification of weighted histogram as input to the autoencoder ($C^2D^2A$).
2. Unsupervised learning of DCM from large number of images for 1000 epochs.
3. Validating the converged DCM for unseen query image.
4. Hyperparameter tuning and retraining the $C^2D^2A$ if the result of previous stage is unsatisfactory.
5. Freezing the $C^2D^2A$ as offline look-up table (LUT) to be referred for primary path of bilateral image filtering.

In order to improve the speed of the bilateral image filtering, it is important to identify the dominant color from the sparse color occupancy in the entire color gamut. The process of histogram imagification and extracting the DCM are the activities to achieve the aforementioned target. First, the histograms of red, green, and blue color channels are calculated and normalized between 0 and 255, to be represented as the image shown in Fig. 4. The representation has been depicted in Eq. (4).

$$red = countOf(I(:,:,1)), \tag{4a}$$

$$green = countOf(I(:,:,2)), \tag{4b}$$

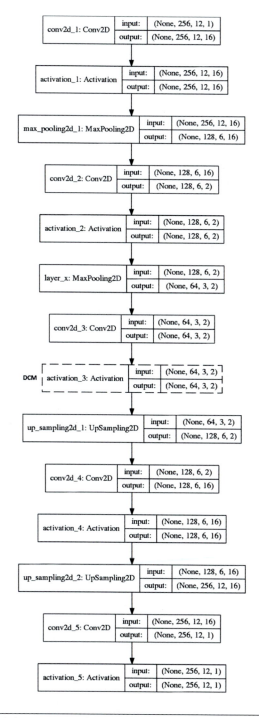

**FIG. 3**

$C^2D^2A$: Cross color dominant deep autoencoder architecture to create the DCM.

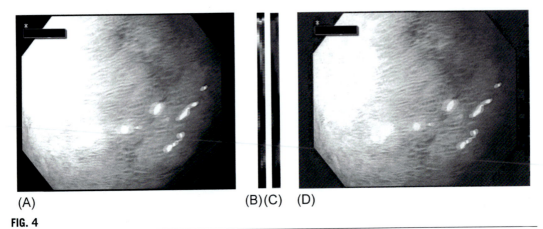

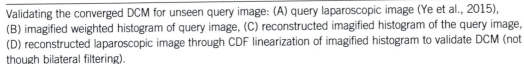

(A)　　　　　　　　　　　　(B)(C)　(D)

**FIG. 4**

Validating the converged DCM for unseen query image: (A) query laparoscopic image (Ye et al., 2015),
(B) imagified weighted histogram of query image, (C) reconstructed imagified histogram of the query image,
(D) reconstructed laparoscopic image through CDF linearization of imagified histogram to validate DCM (not
though bilateral filtering).

$$blue = countOf(I(:,:,3)),$$
(4c)

$$Img_{hist}(:,1:4) = red \times 256 \frac{red(:,:) - min(red)}{max(red) - min(red)} ones(4256),$$
(4d)

$$Img_{hist}(:,5:8) = green \times 256 \frac{green(:,:) - min(green)}{max(green) - min(green)} ones(4256),$$
(4e)

$$Img_{hist}(:,9:12) = blue \times 256 \frac{blue(:,:) - min(blue)}{max(blue) - min(blue)} ones(4256).$$
(4f)

As described in Eq. (4), the color histogram has been imagified and repeated four times as four columns
of $Img_{hist}(:,:)$ to enable the imagified weighted histogram to be consumed by the autoencoder (Fig. 3).
One sample laparoscopic image and its imagified histogram has been shown in Fig. 4. For training the
autoencoder to extract the DCM for laparoscopic/endoscopic images, 1000 laparoscopic images have
been used for training samples. As depicted in the autoencoder architecture, the encoded form has dimension $64 \times 3$, which is the reduced dimension from the original dimension of $256 \times 3$. This dimensionality reduction is exactly 75% and the same could be reconstructed from the DCM as shown in
Fig. 4D; this image was reconstructed by CDF linearization, an idea described by Das (2015). It
can be observed that the specular reflection also was reasonably addressed in the reconstructed frame.
In this case, the number 64 could be treated as the number of clusters having the dominant encoded
color of the selected class images. The same can be interpolated to any other number of clusters.
Fig. 4 also shows that the compromise of color is at the background of the scene, not at the region
of interest. The reconstructed histogram (Fig. 4C) has a similar relative pattern to the input imagified
histogram (Fig. 4B). This is only in the verification stage through CDF linearization.

## 3.2 Inclusion of DCM into principal flow of bilateral filtering

Based on clustering of sparse color space, Durand and Dorsey (2002) and Yang et al. (2009, 2015) have proposed to quantize the range space to approximate the filter using a series of fast spatial convolutions. Motivated by the aforementioned work, Nair and Chaudhury (2017) has proposed an algorithm based on clustering of the sparse color space. There the idea is to perform high-dimensional filtering on a cluster-by-cluster basis. For $K$ number of clusters, where $1 \leq k \leq K$,

$$h_k(i) = \sum_{j \in W} \omega(j)\phi(p_{i-j} - \mu_k)f_{i-j},$$     (5)

$$\alpha_k(i) = \sum_{j \in W} \omega(j)\phi(p_{i-j} - \mu_k).$$     (6)

Here, Eqs. (5), (6) represent the numerator and denominator of Eqs. (2), (3) replacing $p_i$ by the cluster centroids $\mu_k$. The scheme of hybridizing online and offline processing has been shown in Fig. 5. As the algorithm to construct the color LUT is working offline and the principal flow of filtering is operated in real time, the performance has been improved significantly, as presented in Das et al. (2018b).

## 4 Experimental results

In the preceding sections, the necessity of dehazing in laparoscopic video has been established along with its challenges in achieving real-time performance, especially for videos. The idea (Das et al.,

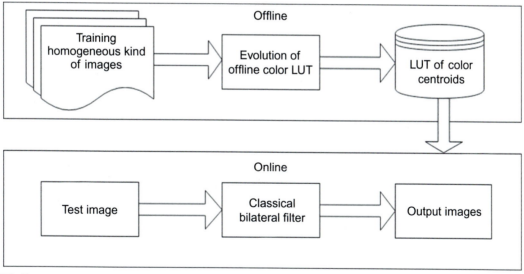

**FIG. 5**

Scheme of hybridization between offline and online processing in proposed fast bilateral filtering: the LUT has been derived from DCM through decoding the same in the reverse path of the autoencoder.

| Table 1 Performance of laparoscopic video (containing 704 frames from video (Ye et al., 2015)) dehazing by $C^2D^2A$-based dynamic bilateral filtering. | | |
|---|---|---|
| **Key-frame (KF) interval** | **Execution time (s)** | **FPS** |
| All | 1359 | 0.5 |
| 3 | 525 | 1.3 |
| 5 | 395 | 1.8 |
| 10 | 200 | 3.5 |
| 15 | 161 | 4.4 |
| Dynamic (avg. = 22.5) | 147 | 4.8 |

2018a) of key-frame identification, estimation of atmospheric and transmission parameters from key frames, and applying the aforementioned onto subsequent frames without further estimation computation would ensure fast processing, as shown in Table 1. The flow chart has been presented in Fig. 6. Both manual key-frame selection and dynamic automated key-frame detection have been employed to present the results. Finally, the laparoscopic video enhancement has been depicted through two sample frames in Fig. 7. Here, $C^2D^2A$-based dynamic bilateral filtering is applied on laparoscopic video (Ye et al., 2015). It is clearly observed that the enhancement of dominant colors ensures significant emphasis on the regions of veins and arteries. It is also observed that the unwanted noise could be

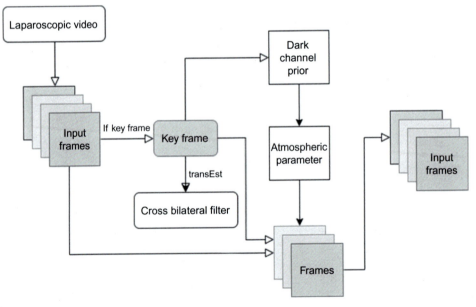

**FIG. 6**

Flow diagram representing key-frame-based dynamic $C^2D^2A$ dehazing.

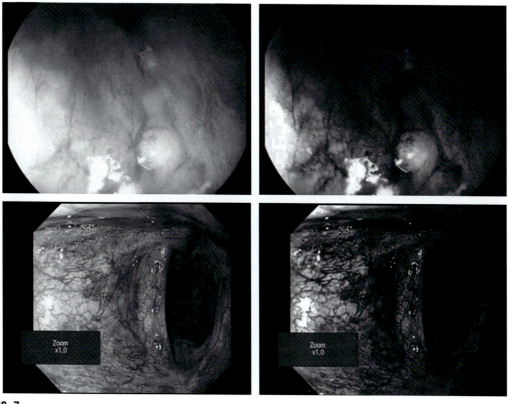

**FIG. 7**

$C^2D^2A$-based dynamic bilateral filtering on laparoscopic video (Ye et al., 2015). *Left column*: Two sample frames as inputs; *right column*: corresponding outputs.

cleaned without disturbing the detailing, edges, and thin lines in the video frame. This confirms the effectiveness of the proposed algorithm both in terms of quality of enhancement and performance.

## 5  Conclusion

For minimally invasive surgeries like laparoscopy and invasive medical procedures like endoscopy, the laparoscopic/endoscopic videos are well-accepted best modalities for analysis and inference. The quality of the aforementioned videos is largely deteriorated by haze, blood, etc., which in turn makes the quality of acquisition unacceptable. The current work focuses on efficient dehazing of laparoscopic/endoscopic videos addressing both quality and performance requirements. In the current chapter, we have discussed an algorithm of cross color dominant deep autoencoder ($C^2D^2A$)-based bilateral filtering, which enabled the method of video quality enhancement to achieve the aforementioned performance objective, too. We have presented promising results on the target modality of videos, showing the strength of a hybrid model of deep learning and bilateral filtering in medical video enhancement.

## Acknowledgments

The authors would like to acknowledge Ms. Pallavi Saha, Mr. Shashidhar Pai, and Ms. Shormi Roy for their support in data annotation and cleaning.

## References

Baid, A., Kotwal, A., Bhalodia, R., Merchant, S.N., Awate, S.P., 2017. Joint desmoking, specularity removal, and denoising of laparoscopy images via graphical models and Bayesian inference. In: IEEE International Symposium on Biomedical Imaging (ISBI), pp. 732–736.

Chen, R., Lai, E.M.K., 2019. Convolutional autoencoder for single image dehazing. In: 2019 IEEE International Conference on Image Processing (ICIP), pp. 4464–4468, https://doi.org/10.1109/ICIP.2019.8803478.

Das, A., 2015. Guide to Signals and Patterns in Image Processing. Springer.

Das, A., Shylaja, S.S., 2020. Video deraining for mutual motion by fast bilateral filtering on spatiotemporal features. Int. J. Innov. Technol. Explor. Eng. 9 (3), 1772–1782.

Das, A., Shylaja, S.S., 2021. Efficient quality enhancement of gastrointestinal endoscopic video by a novel method of color salient bilateral filtering. Multimed. Tools Appl. 80, 6235–6245. In this issue.

Das, A., Pai, S., Shylaja, S.S., 2018a. D2ehazing: real-time dehazing in traffic video analytics by fast dynamic bilateral filtering. In: Proceedings of Computer Vision and Image Processing, pp. 127–137.

Das, A., Shenoy, V.S., Vinay, T., Shylaja, S.S., 2018b. A faster high-dimensional bilateral image filtering by efficient utilization of color sparsness offline. In: IEEE Applied Signal Processing Conference (ASPCON), pp. 49–53.

Durand, F., Dorsey, J., 2002. Fast bilateral filtering for the display of high-dynamic-range images. ACM Trans. Graph. 21, 257–266.

Eisemann, E., Durand, F., 2004. Flash photography enhancement via intrinsic re-lighting. In: ACM Transactions on Graphics (Proc. SIGGRAPH 04), pp. 673–678.

He, K., Sun, J., Tang, X., 2011. Single image haze removal using dark channel prior. IEEE Trans. Pattern Anal. Mach. Intell. 33 (12), 2341–2353.

He, K., Sun, J., Tang, X., 2013. Guided image filtering. IEEE Trans. Pattern Anal. 35 (6), 1397–1409.

Kotwal, A., Bhalodia, R., Awate, S.P., 2016. Joint desmoking and denoising of laparoscopy images. In: IEEE International Symposium on Biomedical Imaging (ISBI), pp. 1050–1054.

Nair, P., Chaudhury, K.N., 2017. Fast high-dimensional filtering using clustering. In: International Conference of Image Processing (Accepted).

Petschnigg, G., Szeliski, R., Agrawala, M., Cohen, M., Hoppe, H., Toyama, K., 2004. Digital photography with flash and no-flash image pairs. In: ACM Transactions on Graphics (Proc. SIGGRAPH 04), pp. 664–672.

Stoyanov, D., 2012. Surgical vision. Ann. Biomed. Eng. 40 (2), 332–345.

Tchakaa, K., Pawara, V.M., Stoyanova, D., 2017. Chromaticity based smoke removal in endoscopic images. In: Proceedings of SPIE, p. 101331M-1.

Tomasi, C., Manduchi, R., 1998. Bilateral filtering for gray and color images. In: International Conference on Computer Vision, pp. 839–846.

Wang, C., Cheikh, F.A., Kaaniche, M., Elle, O.J., 2018. A smoke removal method for laparoscopic images. CoRR abs/1803.08410.

Yang, Q., Tan, K.H., Ahuja, N., 2009. Real-time O(1) bilateral filtering. In: IEEE Conference on Computer Vision and Pattern Recognition, 2009. CVPR 2009, pp. 557–564.

Yang, Q., Tan, K.H., Ahuja, N., 2015. Constant time median and bilateral filtering. Int. J. Comput. Vis. 112, 307–318.

Ye, M., Giannarou, S., Meining, A., Yang, G.Z., 2015. Online tracking and retargeting with applications to optical biopsy in gastrointestinal endoscopic examinations. Med. Image Anal. 112 (3), 307–318.

# Estimating the respiratory rate from ECG and PPG using machine learning techniques

6

**Wenhan Tan and Anup Das**

*Electrical and Computer Engineering, Drexel University, Philadelphia, PA, United States*

## Chapter outline

## 1 Introduction

### 1.1 Motivation

Respiratory rate (RR) is a known factor in many conditions causing physiological deterioration in patients. Its measurement accuracy is of substantial importance for many medical uses, including mobile health, home monitoring applications, and hospitals. Most hospitals and personal clinics use pulse oximetry to continuously measure heart rate (HR) and peripheral blood oxygen saturation (SpO2), but the measurement of RR relies on the use of other equipment, for instance capnometry or measurement of gas flow. Therefore, it is necessary to improve RR estimation from the electrocardiogram (ECG), the photoplethysmogram (PPG) collected from pulse oximeters, and other signals that are related to RR.

Mobile healthcare, or smart devices that monitor patients, has received much attention recently. Most patients during the day will not tolerate wearing sensors constantly, since these devices are uncomfortable over a long duration. They would rather use pulse oximeters and other devices that are easily accessed and simple for patients to use. However, pulse oximeters provide no information about RR and it is significantly challenging to improve RR estimation methods, primarily because of movement artifacts.

Recent technologies are calling for inclusion of RR estimation from the PPG and the ECG. This is influenced by the large number of health trackers and other fitness devices. Their aim is to maintain and report the fitness status of the mostly healthy people who wear them. This is different from hospital and clinic needs, as a long-term and costly validation is required to be able to use any new technology in hospitals and clinics. The majority of current smart devices include a small version of accelerometers for tracking "fitness data" and the state-of-the-art generation includes sensors such as pulse oximeters (e.g., Apple Watch from Apple, Inc., United States) and bioimpedance sensors (e.g., UP3 from Jawbone, United States). If a better means of estimating RR existed, then it could be used on these devices, increasing the amount of physiological data they can provide.

## 1.2 Background

The ECG is a measure of the electrical activity of the heartbeat: each beat causes an electrical impulse to travel through the heart and body. The most prominent feature is known as the QRS complex, which represents the main pumping duration of the heart. The QRS complex is shown in Fig. 1.

The PPG works a little bit differently from the ECG. It measures the change in light absorption under human skin. The change appears each time the heart beats. The amplitude of this signal is directly related to pulse pressure from blood pumping, as shown in Fig. 2.

The ECG and the PPG are both related to heartbeat, as shown in Fig. 3, but the goal of this work is to estimate respiratory rate (RR) from these two signals. The ECG and the PPG have the same peak time showing each heartbeat. Fig. 3 depicts a MATLAB generated plot using the publicly available BIDMC dataset.

The goal of this work is to test whether machine learning-based RR estimation from the ECG and the PPG could be a part of the signal processing or eventually replace the signal processing in wearable devices. The proposed method will be evaluated on both the ECG and the PPG and eventually compared with existing methods that rely on signal processing entirely.

*Contributions*: The following are our key contributions:

- data preprocessing including extracting respiratory rate signal by filtering;
- classifying extracted respiratory rate signals by window size of 32 s using neural network and support vector machine;
- exploring hyperparameters to improve model accuracy;
- evaluating 53 subjects by comparing number of classes and model accuracy.

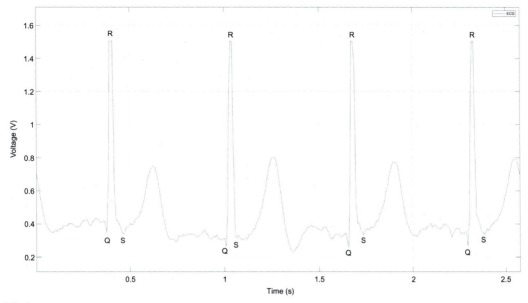

**FIG. 1**

The QRS complex. Each letter indicates a different place of the signal. The *R* peak is the largest amplitude of electrical activity and used most in measurements of heart rate. Generated by MATLAB. More details refer to Soehn (2017).

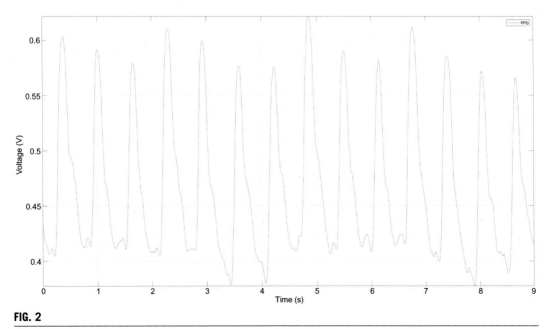

**FIG. 2**

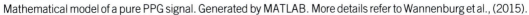

Mathematical model of a pure PPG signal. Generated by MATLAB. More details refer to Wannenburg et al., (2015).

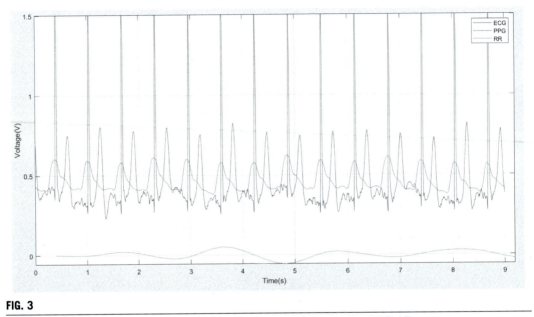

**FIG. 3**

Plot of the ECG, the PPG, and RR signal over a period of 9 s. Generated by MATLAB.

## 2 Related work

Current methods for estimating RR from the ECG and the PPG are often used on windows of time-series data. RR is produced from each window during estimation. There are usually three main steps of estimation, as illustrated in Fig. 4.

The first step is extracting the respiratory component from the raw signal. There are many ways to perform extraction and they often rely on the extraction of features from the raw signal, such as the pulse width, peak-trough detection in the time domain. Techniques such as digital filters, Fourier transforms, and joint time-frequency analysis have all been used.

The second step is to estimate respiratory rate from the extracted respiratory signal. This part of the entire RR estimation is all about signal processing. Over 100 algorithms have been proposed to estimate RR (Charlton et al., 2016) and they have been rarely compared systematically to decide which algorithm performs the best (Charlton et al., 2016). For example, the PPG signal has been analyzed using a short-time Fourier transform using a moving window of a certain time duration. The maximum frequency in the range of respiratory frequency is noted as RR (Pimentel et al., 2017).

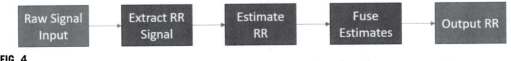

**FIG. 4**

Steps of traditional RR estimation. Generated by PowerPoint.

A more recent algorithm was proposed in 2014 (Garde et al., 2014), which is based on the time-varying correntropy spectral density function (CSD) being applied on the PPG. CSD is a similarity measure of time-varying structure and the statistical characteristics of a signal. This algorithm first detects the heart rate by looking for the maximum frequency peak and then extracts the RR signal with a cutoff frequency of 0.1 Hz (Garde et al., 2014).

One of the most recently proposed algorithms describes a method that estimates RR from PPG data collected from pulse oximetry using three respiratory-induced variations (RIIV, RIAV, RIFV). RIIV is the respiratory-induced intensity variation, the time series of amplitudes of PPG peaks (Pimentel et al., 2017). RIAV is the respiratory-induced amplitude variation, the peaks of the PPG (Pimentel et al., 2017). RIFV is the respiratory-induced frequency variation, the change in the value of the instantaneous HR during the respiratory cycle (Pimentel et al., 2017).

The last step is the fusion of estimated RR. Its purpose is to combine different estimated RR results and generate a single output. The proposed "smart fusion" method analyzes the frequency from each of the respiratory-induced variations. Then the "smart fusion" method takes their mean and combines the results. Artifacts and low-quality estimations are discarded in the end. This has been demonstrated to be the most effective algorithm of fusing RR by Pimentel et al. (2017).

In Chon et al. (2009), an algorithm based on best time and frequency resolution uses variable-frequency complex demodulation (VFCDM) to increase the accuracy of respiratory rate estimation from PPG. Both CWT and AR methods have been shown to output good estimates of respiratory rate in the normal range (12–26 breaths/min). The VFCDM method was tested on 15 different subjects for breathing frequencies between 0.2 and 0.6 Hz (12–36 breaths/min) and compared with the continuous wavelet transform (CWT) and autoregressive (AR) methods. The VFCDM has significantly lower median error among them.

In Karlen et al. (2011), a way of extracting respiratory sinus arrhythmia (RSA) from the PPG-derived heart rate variability (HRV) was introduced. The method was tested on data from 299 children and 13 adults undergoing general anesthesia. The research compared the RSA from both ECG and PPG, with reference RR from a capnograph. The results show that RSA on PPG is possible and slightly better than that on ECG.

In Karlen et al. (2013), a new method of estimating respiratory rate from PPG in real time was introduced. The method contains three respiratory-induced variations (frequency, amplitude, and intensity) extracted from PPG and uses fast Fourier transforms. Then the proposed smart fusion is used to combine the three results using a transparent mean calculation. The algorithm was tested on data from 29 children and 13 adults. The results show that combining the three respiratory-induced variations improves estimation by lowering the mean square error. The algorithm is also applied in a mobile pulse oximeter to diagnose severe childhood pneumonia in remote areas.

In Pimentel et al., an algorithm using autoregressive models was proposed. It uses multiple autoregressive models of different orders for determining the dominant respiratory frequency in the three respiratory-induced variations (frequency, amplitude, and intensity) from PPG. The method was tested on two different datasets that contain 95 8-min PPG datasets from both children and adults. The results are then compared with existing methods using two window sizes (32 and 64 s). It achieves comparable accuracy to existing methods and provides RR estimates from a larger window size.

In Hernando et al. (2019), two PPG signals were compared, one from the finger and the other from the forehead. Both were recorded from 35 subjects during a controlled experiment that required a constant rate from 0.1 Hz to 0.6 Hz in 0.1-Hz steps. Four PPG-derived respiratory (PDR) signals were extracted from both PPG locations and were used to estimate respiratory rate. Different combinations of PDR signals have been analyzed. The results show that when (i) using finger PPG; (ii) respiratory rate is less than 0.4 Hz; and (iii) the RIIV signal is not considered, the accuracy is better: 85 success rates at 0.1 and 0.2 Hz, 90% at 0.3 Hz, and above 75% at 0.4 and 0.5 Hz.

Recently, machine-learning techniques have also been used for ECG RR detection and classification. In Das et al. (2018a), a novel method of heart-rate estimation from electrocardiogram (ECG) data was designed and implemented. The approach was to use a spiking neural network, specifically a liquid state machine, and an unsupervised readout based on fuzzy $c$-means consisting of spiking responses, selected by using particle swarm optimization. The results showed high accuracy and low energy consumption in heart-rate estimation for wearable devices. This work also contributes to neuromorphic algorithms and applications.

In Das et al. (2018b), a different machine-learning algorithm was proposed to classify cardiac arrhythmia. It is based on a representation using time-frequency joint distribution of ECG data from the MIT-BIH arrhythmia database. The proposed algorithm is a multilayer perceptron used on wearable health devices. The results show that the approach has an average accuracy of 95.7% and significant improvement with respect to existing ECG signal classification techniques.

In Messinger et al. (2019), an artificial neural network is introduced to predict the pediatric-automated asthma respiratory score (pARS). A manual pediatric asthma score (PAS) is used as clinical care standard data for comparison. Total PAS distribution is not a straight horizontal line. Most data fall between PAS values of 6 to 9. First, vital sign data including heart rate, respiratory rate, and pulse oximetry are merged with the manual pediatric asthma score for children of ages between 2 and 18. Children are selected if they are admitted to the pediatric intensive care unit (PICU) for status asthmaticus. The merged signals are split into train and test sets for the artificial neural network (ANN). The ANN is trying to predict a respiratory score that would further be compared to two other approaches via a 10-fold cross-validation method. The two approaches are a normal and a Poisson distribution used as a reference to compare with the purposed machine-learning regression results. The results show that pARS has the smallest mean absolute error (MAE) overall. The normal and Poisson yield a slightly higher MAE for extreme PAS values, including 5, 6, 7, and 13.

In Zeiberg et al. (2019), a developed machine-learning algorithm is introduced to predict acute respiratory distress syndrome (ARDS). The datasets used were extracted from electronic health record (EHR) data during data preprocessing. One extracted dataset from 2016 was used for training and the other dataset from 2017 was used for testing. The proposed training method uses fivefold cross validation and eventually generated 984 features with L2-logistic regression for testing. The results showed an overall AUC value of 0.81. With a threshold based on the 85th percentile of risk, the results showed a sensitivity of 56% and specificity of 86%, and a positive predictive value of 9%.

In Sauthier et al. (2020), a random forest machine-learning algorithm was introduced to predict prolonged acute hypoxemic respiratory failure in influenza-infected critically ill children. Most acute respiratory distress syndrome (ARDS) predictive models use logistic regression, but it is limited in exploiting nonlinear features. Random forest, on the other hand, does not easily overfit and has shown better results for some clinical cohorts. In the results, respiratory, $FiO_2$, and pH are the most important features and the random forest algorithm generated an AUC value of 0.93.

In Bashar et al. (2019), a decision tree regression algorithm was introduced to extract heart rate from the PPG signal. The PPG signal was first collected from wearable devices and then split into noisy and nonnoisy data using the $k$-means clustering method, an unsupervised machine-learning algorithm. A decision tree algorithm was then implemented on the nonnoisy data to compute heart rate. The metric being used here was root mean square error and average error. The results showed that fewer model features produce the same absolute error rate as all model features do. This demonstrates the potential of calculating heart rate on wearable devices by applying unsupervised machine-learning algorithms.

Recently, in Mian Qaisar and Subasi (2020), a cloud-purposed ECG acquisition and machine-learning techniques were introduced to collect only significant data for cloud monitoring purposes. The motivation was that wearable devices are meant to be small and should not require massive computing processes, which also cost battery life. The database used was the MIT-BIH Arrhythmia and the acquisition frequency was 360 Hz. The collected ECG signal was first filtered using several embedded processing techniques, including event-driven analog-to-digital converters (EDADCs), adaptive rate resampling, etc. The resampled and filtered ECG signals were then used in cloud-based processing, including feature extraction and machine-learning detection of cardiac arrhythmia. The feature extraction method used was the autoregressive Burg method and the machine-learning algorithms used were SVM, k-NN, ANN, random forest, and rotation forest. All classification-based results showed an accuracy between 90% and 96% and an AUC value between 0.97 and 0.997. These results indicate the power and future of medical and health monitoring functions on wearable devices.

# 3  Methods

## 3.1  Data

All datasets used in this work are from a publicly available database called BIDMC PPG and the Respiration dataset downloaded from the PhysioNet website: https://physionet.org/content/bidmc/1.0.0/ (Pimentel et al., 2018). This dataset contains signals from the much larger MIMIC II matched waveform database, along with manual breath annotations made from two annotators, using the impedance respiratory signal (Goldberger et al., 2000). The data was collected from critically ill patients at the Beth Israel Deaconess Medical Center (Boston, MA, United States) during hospital care. There are a total of 53 recordings of 53 patients within the dataset and each one is 8 min in duration. Each recording includes the ECG and the PPG sampled at 125 Hz and other physiological parameters such as the heart rate (HR) and respiratory rate (RR) sampled at 1 Hz. They also contain fixed parameters, such as age and gender for each patient.

## 3.2  Steps

The proposed algorithms in this work replace the estimation of RR and fusion of RR with machine learning, as shown in Fig. 5. The reason for keeping extraction of the RR signal is to eliminate unnecessary noise and frequency components from the raw signal.

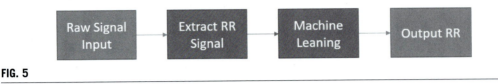

**FIG. 5**

Steps of proposed algorithms. Generated by PowerPoint.

### 3.3 RR signal extraction

As described in Pimentel et al. (2017), the first fundamental stage of the RR algorithms is extraction, in which a time series dominated by respiratory modulation is extracted from the original signal (Pimentel et al., 2017). As illustrated in Fig. 3, the RR signal is extracted from the ECG (blue plot; dark gray in print versions) and the PPG (orange plot; medium gray in print versions) as well as RR (yellow plot; light gray in print versions) signals.

The algorithms of RR signal extraction, as mentioned previously, have more than 100 types. They have been split into one of two main methods: filter-based extraction and feature-based extraction, as shown in Fig. 6. The algorithm used in this work is feature-based extraction: extracting a component, such as pulse wave amplitude, from each cardiac cycle. Feature-based extraction has six components, as shown in Fig. 6: elimination of very high frequencies (EHF), beat detection with R-spike detection (RDt), fiducial point identification (FPt), extraction of feature measurements (FMe), resampling at a regular sampling frequency (RS), and elimination of very low frequencies (ELF).

### 3.4 Machine learning

A neural network (NN) and support vector machine (SVM) were used in the work. They were both tested on the ECG and the PPG.

*Features.* The extracted RR signals are used to estimate RR with a moving window of 32 s. The signal data from each window of 32 s becomes the input data for future machine learning. Each recording is about 8 min long and produces around 14 windows. The total number of windows over 53 recordings are exactly 740, as shown in Fig. 7, and these windows become features of this work. The reason is that wearable devices are not as powerful as hospital and clinic applications, and it is necessary to reduce the amount of hardware power and energy by treating the entire collection of windows as features.

*Classes.* The RR results estimated from one of the traditional estimation algorithms are used to label the class of each window. The traditional estimation algorithm chosen for this work is a frequency-domain technique called autoregressive spectral analysis, using the median spectrum for orders 2–20 (ARM). Then it is fused using a modulation-fusion technique called Smart Fusion (SFU). Table 1 introduces different respiratory rates among different age ranges. However, 30 breaths per minute falls into the first three rows of Table 1, so the number of classes is not settled in this work, as shown in Table 2.

## 4 Experimental results

As shown in Figs. 8 and 9, the proposed RR estimation algorithm on ECG generally has a higher accuracy than that on PPG. The traditional results also demonstrate that estimation on ECG has a higher

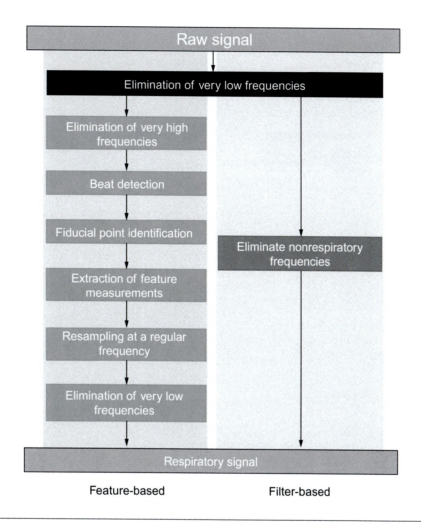

**FIG. 6**

Two main methods of RR signal extraction algorithms. Left column shows feature-based and right column shows filter-based extraction. Generated by PowerPoint. More details refer to Pimentel et al., (2017).

accuracy than that on PPG on average. For both types of signals, the accuracy drops significantly once the number of classes increases. For the neural network (NN), the accuracy is below 80% when there are more than five classes. For support vector machine (SVM), the accuracy is below 70% once there are more than four classes. In addition, NN outperforms SVM in general.

# 5 Discussion and conclusion

The goal of this work was to demonstrate the usefulness of machine learning in RR estimation and its potential for further study in wearable devices, and this goal has been achieved. The accuracy of RR estimation from ECG is above 80% when there are five classes. Five classes

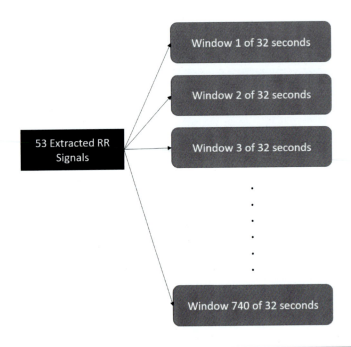

**FIG. 7**

Extracted RR signals from 53 records split into a total of 740 time-series windows. Each window is 32 s. Generated by PowerPoint.

| Table 1 Normal respiratory rate ranges among different age ranges. Generated by PowerPoint. | |
| --- | --- |
| **Age range** | **Normal respiratory rate** |
| 0–12 months | 30–60 per minute |
| 1–3 years | 24–40 per minute |
| 4–5 years | 22–34 per minute |
| 6–12 years | 18–30 per minute |
| 13–18+ years | 12–16 per minute |

for RR estimation is probably enough to monitor a patient or healthy person's "fitness" status. Estimation from the ECG has a higher accuracy than that from the PPG, so treating the ECG as input data is preferred. The accuracy of this work has room to increase, and there are many other features that can be generated, such as spectra from the short-time Fourier transform (STFT), as well as other signal feature generation algorithms. In addition, deep learning is an effective method of replacing traditional machine-learning algorithms and probably can provide better

**Table 2** Number of classes and their corresponding RR ranges. Generated by PowerPoint.

| | 2 Classes | 3 Classes | 4 Classes | 5 Classes | 6 Classes | 7 Classes | 8 Classes | 9 Classes |
|---|---|---|---|---|---|---|---|---|
| Class 1 | RR < 30 | RR < 30 | RR < 25 | RR < 25 | RR < 20 | RR < 15 | RR < 10 | RR < 10 |
| Class 2 | 30 < RR | 20 < RR < 35 | 25 < RR < 30 | 25 < RR < 30 | 20 < RR < 25 | 15 < RR < 20 | 10 < RR < 15 | 10 < RR < 15 |
| Class 3 | | 35 < RR | 30 < RR < 35 | 30 < RR < 35 | 25 < RR < 30 | 20 < RR < 25 | 15 < RR < 20 | 15 < RR < 20 |
| Class 4 | | | 35 < RR | 35 < RR < 40 | 30 < RR < 35 | 25 < RR < 30 | 20 < RR < 25 | 20 < RR < 25 |
| Class 5 | | | | 40 < RR | 35 < RR < 40 | 30 < RR < 35 | 25 < RR < 30 | 25 < RR < 30 |
| Class 6 | | | | | 40 < RR | 35 < RR < 40 | 30 < RR < 35 | 30 < RR < 35 |
| Class 7 | | | | | | 40 < RR | 35 < RR < 40 | 35 < RR < 40 |
| Class 8 | | | | | | | 40 < RR | 40 < RR < 45 |
| Class 9 | | | | | | | | 45 < RR |

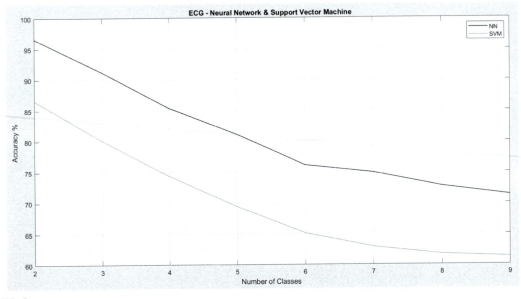

**FIG. 8**

Plot of number of classes vs. accuracy on ECG using NN and SVM. Generated by MATLAB.

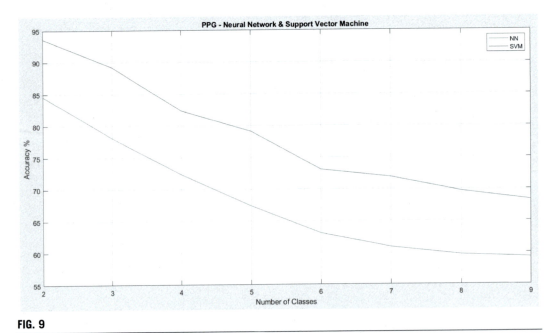

**FIG. 9**

Plot of number of classes vs. accuracy on PPG using NN and SVM. Generated by MATLAB.

results. In the future, there is a need to explore other machine intelligence techniques, such as random forest and the echo state network, to improve the accuracy. However, most wearable devices are tiny and do not have the power or processing speed to generate features while trying to conserve their battery life. Thus finding the balance between the complexity of RR estimation algorithms and the amount of energy being distributed to this from wearable devices is important.

## Acknowledgments

This work is supported by the National Science Foundation Award CCF-1937419 (RTML: Small: Design of System Software to Facilitate Real-Time Neuromorphic Computing). We would like to thank Dr. Andrew R. Cohen from the Electrical and Computer Engineering Department at Drexel University for his guidance in machine learning and pattern recognition.

## References

Bashar, S.S., Miah, M.S., Karim, A.H.M.Z., Al Mahmud, M.A., 2019. Extraction of heart rate from PPG signal: a machine learning approach using decision tree regression algorithm. In: 2019 4th International Conference on Electrical Information and Communication Technology (EICT), Khulna, Bangladesh, pp. 1–6, https://doi.org/10.1109/EICT48899.2019.9068845.

Charlton, P.H., et al., 2016. An assessment of algorithms to estimate respiratory rate from the electrocardiogram and photoplethysmogram. Physiol. Meas. 37 (4), 610.

Chon, K.H., Dash, S., Ju, K., 2009. Estimation of respiratory rate from photoplethysmogram data using time–frequency spectral estimation. IEEE Trans. Biomed. Eng. 56 (8), 2054–2063. https://doi.org/10.1109/TBME.2009.2019766.

Das, A., et al., 2018a. Unsupervised heart-rate estimation in wearables with liquid states and a probabilistic readout. Neural Netw. 99, 134–147.

Das, A., Catthoor, F., Schaafsma, S., 2018b. Heartbeat classification in wearables using multi-layer perceptron and time-frequency joint distribution of ECG. In: 2018 IEEE/ACM International Conference on Connected Health: Applications, Systems and Engineering Technologies (CHASE), Washington, DC, USA, pp. 69–74, https://doi.org/10.1145/3278576.3278598.

Garde, A., et al., 2014. Estimating respiratory and heart rates from the correntropy spectral density of the photoplethysmogram. PLoS One 9 (1), e86427.

Goldberger, A., et al., 2000. PhysioBank, PhysioToolkit, and PhysioNet: components of a new research resource for complex physiologic signals. Circulation 101 (23), e215–e220.

Hernando, A., et al., 2019. Finger and forehead PPG signal comparison for respiratory rate estimation. Physiol. Meas. 40, 095007.

Karlen, W., Brouse, C.J., Cooke, E., Ansermino, J.M., Dumont, G.A., 2011. Respiratory rate estimation using respiratory sinus arrhythmia from photoplethysmography. In: 2011 Annual International Conference of the IEEE Engineering in Medicine and Biology Society, Boston, MA, pp. 1201–1204, https://doi.org/10.1109/IEMBS.2011.6090282.

Karlen, W., Raman, S., Ansermino, J.M., Dumont, G.A., 2013. Multiparameter respiratory rate estimation from the photoplethysmogram. IEEE Trans. Biomed. Eng. 60 (7), 1946–1953. https://doi.org/10.1109/TBME.2013.2246160.

Messinger, A.I., Bui, N., Wagner, B.D., Szefler, S.J., Vu, T., Deterding, R.R., 2019. Novel pediatric-automated respiratory score using physiologic data and machine learning in asthma. Pediatr. Pulmonol. 54, 1149–1155.

Mian Qaisar, S., Subasi, A., 2020. Cloud-based ECG monitoring using event-driven ECG acquisition and machine learning techniques. Phys. Eng. Sci. Med. 43 (2), 623–634. https://doi.org/10.1007/s13246-020-00863-6.

Pimentel, M.A.F., et al., 2017. Toward a robust estimation of respiratory rate from pulse oximeters. IEEE Trans. Biomed. Eng. 64 (8), 1914–1923. http://ieeexplore.ieee.org/stamp/stamp.jsp?tp=&arnumber=7748483&isnumber=7981410.

Pimentel, M.A.F., et al., 2018. BIDMC PPG and Respiration Dataset. Version: 1.0.0, PhysioNet. https://physionet.org/content/bidmc/1.0.0/.

Sauthier, M.S., et al., 2020. Machine learning predicts prolonged acute hypoxemic respiratory failure in pediatric severe influenza. Crit. Care Explor. 2 (8), e0175. https://doi.org/10.1097/CCE.0000000000000175.

Soehn, A., 2017. Measuring the Heart—How Do ECG and PPG Work. https://imotions.com/blog/measuring-the-heart-how-does-ecg-and-ppg-work/.

Wannenburg, J., Malekian, R., 2015. Body sensor network for mobile health monitoring, a diagnosis and anticipating system. IEEE Sensors J. 15, 6839–6852. https://doi.org/10.1109/JSEN.2015.2464773.

Zeiberg, D., Prahlad, T., Nallamothu, B.K., Iwashyna, T.J., Wiens, J., et al., 2019. Machine learning for patient risk stratification for acute respiratory distress syndrome. PLoS One 14 (3). https://doi.org/10.1371/journal.pone.0214465, e0214465.

# Machine learning-enabled Internet of Things for medical informatics

**Ali Nauman[a], Yazdan Ahmad Qadri[a], Rashid Ali[b], and Sung Won Kim[a]**

*Department of Information and Communication Engineering, Yeungnam University, Gyeongsan, Republic of Korea[a]*
*School of Intelligent Mechatronics Engineering, Sejong University, Seoul, Republic of Korea[b]*

## Chapter outline

## 1 Introduction

The diminishing divide between the physical world and cyberspace is ushering in a new phase of Internet of Things (IoT). The emergence of IoT in the recent years envisages to cover the gaps in the network models of the cyber and physical world and leads to a paradigm shift of human-machine interaction. The IEEE defines IoT as "a network of items, each of which is embedded with sensors and these sensors are connected to the internet" (Qadri et al., 2020).

The amalgamation of IoT in the healthcare sector is referred to as Medicine 4.0, also known as Health 2.0. Medicine 4.0 is driving an exponential adoption of diagnostic tools in the healthcare sector.

The applications of Medicine 4.0 vastly lie in ubiquitous monitoring of the patients, which assist in the prior detection of disease and the implementation of a proactive treatment plan. The applications of IoT in the medical field such as ubiquitous monitoring encompass the definition of healthcare Internet of Things (H-IoT). The principal enabling technology for IoT is wireless sensor networks and for H-IoT is body sensor networks (BSNs). The BSNs are a network of sensors deployed in and on the human body (Yang et al., 2017).

With the advances in wireless body area networks (WBSNs), the H-IoT is continuously evolving. The primary features of WBAN-based H-IoT are (1) miniature sensors, (2) data security, (3) fault tolerance, (4) quality of service (QoS), (5) quality of experience, (6) interoperability, (7) real-time processing, and (8) mobility support (Filipe et al., 2015).

Machine learning (ML) is a subset of artificial intelligence (AI) that provides statistical tools, algorithms, and schemes for machines to learn from data. In ML techniques, machines take actions in particular states using the knowledge from their training on structured/unstructured data sets. ML predicts future data or patterns based on observations and experiences. ML is a key enabling means for IoT, which provides information inference, data processing, and intelligence for IoT devices to enhance network performance (Samie et al., 2019).

ML techniques are becoming interestingly important in many communication systems. The innovative ML technologies improve the overall performance at multiple layers of the H-IoT protocol stack, which optimizes the entire system. At the application layer, ML is used for signal processing, security, and error correction. ML techniques predict network traffic, link quality evaluation, and resource allocation at data link layer. At the network layer, ML techniques aid in optimizing routing protocols. ML also optimizes resource management and data processing at higher layers.

## 1.1 Healthcare Internet of Things

The H-IoT is one of the major subset of IoT application. The IoT application deployed in the healthcare sector is known as H-IoT. The H-IoT systems follow a similar three-layer network architecture as of traditional IoT network. However, the difference lies in their underlying technologies that are summarized in Table 1.

**Table 1 Comparison between generic IoT and healthcare IoT.**

| Sr. no. | Generic IoT | Healthcare IoT |
|---------|-------------|----------------|
| 1 | Large-scale geographical deployment | Deployed in or around the human body |
| 2 | Renewable energy is wind and solar | Sensors can harvest energy from human body |
| 3 | Environment monitoring | Human patient monitoring |
| 4 | Application-dependent size | Miniature in size |
| 5 | Mostly stationary sensor nodes | Essentially mobile associated with human body |
| 6 | Easy deployment | Mostly require invasive procedure in case of implant |
| 7 | Data are not necessarily preserved | Data related to patient must be preserved |

### 1.1.1 H-IoT architecture

The abrupt increase in the usage of wearable devices and fitness trackers over the past few years indicates the exponential increase of these devices and the implants in the future (Statista Research Department, 2016). The integration of smart health monitoring systems with IoT infrastructure has motivated the development of the IoT networks for the healthcare system known as IoThNet. The enormous potential of these systems to track the health conditions of the patient's vital organs for better diagnosis and medical care has raised the need for the development of standardized architecture. A standard architecture would be the key enabler for H-IoT systems. The IEEE standardization working group is established for point-of-service healthcare devices, which define the communication protocol stack for H-IoT, and it is key parameter indicators (KPIs) (IEEE Standard Association, 2018).

### 1.1.2 Three-tier H-IoT architecture

The traditional IoT encompasses three basic elements that are hardware sensors, communication enabling technologies, and servers for data processing. These elements form a three-layered H-IoT architecture: (1) things layer, (2) communication layer, and (3) processing layer as depicted in Nauman et al. (2020) (Fig. 1).

*Things layer*: The first layer of H-IoT architecture is known as things layer. Literature refers this layer as perception, sensor, or device layer. This layer consists of hardware sensors or actuators as things. The hardware sensors record various indices of the H-IoT system based on the application, while the actuator is a feedback system which takes input from user after processing. Sensors transmit the acquired data on uplink transmission, while actuators have downlink transmissions as well for user feedback or instructions. The major objective of this layer is to connect things in the H-IoT network. The things sense and acquire data from the physical world and transmit the data to processing servers via gateways.

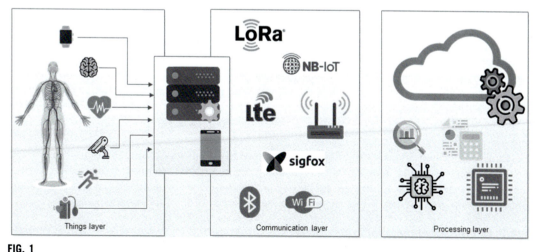

**FIG. 1**

Three-tier H-IoT architecture.

*Communication layer*: The things layer is connected to the processing layer via the communication layer. It is the middle layer, also known as the transmission layer. The layer is virtually divided into two sublayers that are access layer and the core network. The main objective of the access layer is to connect things and applications through gateway or interfaces using communication protocols. The core sublayer determines the optimum route for data transmission. The low-power wireless communication protocols utilized in this layer are Bluetooth Low Energy, Zigbee, Radio Frequency Identification, and Wi-Fi.

*Processing layer*: The acquired data at the thing layer are processed at the processing layer. The processing layer analyzes the data for extracting useful information that is termed as features using local servers or remote cloud processors. The amount of data generated at things layer is substantial, so the cloud-based solutions for processing are more flexible. However, transmitting all the acquired data to cloud incurs significant delay, which can be reduced using local processing units known as *edge node*. Sometimes an additional distributed computing layer is included, which is known as *fog layer*. The additional fog layer reduces latency, improves processing, enhances security, and supports interoperability.

# 2 Applications and challenges of H-IoT
## 2.1 Applications of H-IoT

The H-IoT systems vary depending upon the application and QoS requirements. Few of the major H-IoT applications are classified as follows:

- fitness tracking;
- neurological disorders;
- cardiovascular disorders; and
- ambient-assisted living.

### 2.1.1 Fitness tracking
Fitness tracking is one of the major applications of H-IoT using electronic wearable devices, which include smart wrist bands and smart clothing (Haghi et al., 2017). The fitness band monitors and records motions and pulse rate, while the smart clothing monitors cardiac activity. The collected data are transmitted to cloud servers using enabling technologies to determine the status of health of the user. The sensor layer is the input interface between the cloud/local server and the application layer (user) in a three-layer architecture. The locally preprocessed data are sent to the cloud database server for storage. The cloud database can be remotely accessed by the doctor or user for monitoring or tracking. The sensors mostly used in fitness tracking include pulse sensors, temperature sensors, and accelerometers. All the sensors are attached to the commonly available fabric that emulates a smart fabric (Kansara et al., 2018). Fig. 2 summarizes the overview of the fitness tracking system.

### 2.1.2 Neurological disorders
The detection and diagnosis of neurological disorders, such as Parkinson's disorder (PD), epilepsy, and Alzheimer's disease, are one of the major application areas of H-IoT systems. The electrical activities of the brain are called as electroencephalogram (EEG). The EEG data are used for neurological

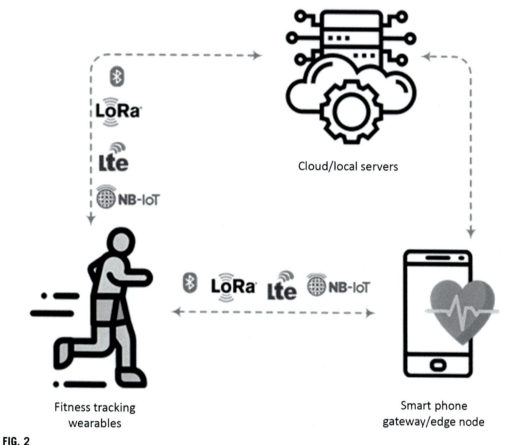

**FIG. 2**

An overview of fitness tracking system.

disorder diagnostics. The EEG is considered to be the standard tool for neurological disorder diagnosis. The H-IoT systems are utilized to monitor the body temperature, body movements, and audio for epileptic seizure detection (Jagtap and Bhosale, 2018). EEG is used for the detection of epilepsy by mounting sensors on a headband that is connected to an edge node, which also acts as an intermediary node. The gateway processes the data and generates as emergency alert to alert the custodian. The gateway transmits the data to the cloud server for long-term storage and precision analysis by healthcare professionals (Lin et al., 2018).

The major symptoms of PD are tremors. Accelerometer and gyroscope are used to quantify tremors. Sensors are used to record the body movements, and treatment for the patient is determined from the generated and recorded data. The data are preprocessed at the device level and transmitted to the diagnostic level via a gateway. The diagnostic level has an interface, for example, mobile application (Vijay et al., 2018). Freezing of gait is one of the symptoms of PD, and inertial sensors within a smartwatch are used to track vital signs of the body movements. The diagnostics follow the same three-tier

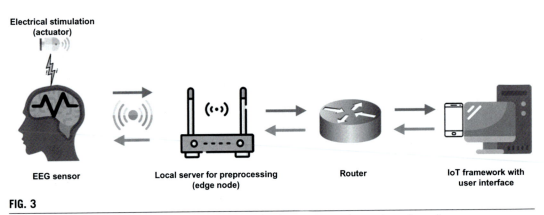

**Electrical stimulation (actuator)**

EEG sensor      Local server for preprocessing (edge node)      Router      IoT framework with user interface

**FIG. 3**

The architectural framework for real-time sensing and seizure suppression systems for epilepsy.

architecture that constitutes smartwatch as a device layer, smartphone as a gateway, and cloud servers as processing layer (Šatala et al., 2018). An overview of the architectural framework for seizure suppression system for epilepsy is shown in Fig. 3.

### 2.1.3 Cardio vascular disorders

Cardiovascular diseases (CVDs) are the types of diseases that affect blood vessels and heart. The most common CVDs include high blood pressure, hypertension, and cerebrovascular diseases, which are referred to as stroke or heart attack. Some of the reasons for heart attack are hypertension, triglyceride levels in the blood, elevated cholesterol, smoking, diabetes, sedentary lifestyle, and obesity. The detection and diagnosis are performed by analyzing the electrical activity of the heart known as electro-cardiogram (ECG). The monitoring and analysis of ECG by IoT-based systems are used for the detection and prevention of CVDs. Most of the H-IoT architectures for CVDs follow the same three-tier architecture as shown in Fig. 1. Usually, heart rate and body temperature sensors are used to predict and prevent CVDs.

### 2.1.4 Ambient-assisted living

The world population is facing a global phenomenon known as population aging. It is predicted that 10% of the population of the Organization for Economic Cooperation and Development (OECD) countries will be more than 80 years old. This will surge the dependency on healthcare facilities exponentially. IoT-based assisted ambient living (AAL) can assist the remote behavior monitoring, emergency detection, and alert generation such as pollution-level alerts (Wan et al., 2017). Wan et al. (2017) summarized the four-layered H-IoT-based AAL architecture as shown in Fig. 4. The sensing layer constitutes the sensors and trackers. The networking layer is composed of communication enabling technologies like Internet, wide area networks (WAN), and personal area networks (PAN). The third layer is the data processing system in the architecture with faculties for multiple approaches. The fourth layer is the application layer, which provides the interface to users for AAL support systems.

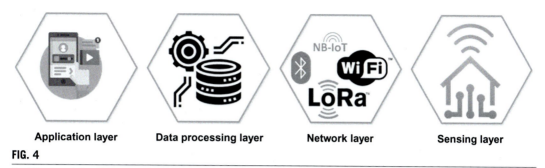

|  Application layer | Data processing layer | Network layer | Sensing layer |

**FIG. 4**

Architecture of ambient-assisted living systems with IoT (Wan et al., 2017).

## 2.2 Challenges of H-IoT system

The KPIs evaluate the performance of H-IoT systems is classified into two categories, as shown in Fig. 5. These categories also determine the challenges that H-IoT system faces are as follows:

- QoS improvement and
- Scalability challenges.

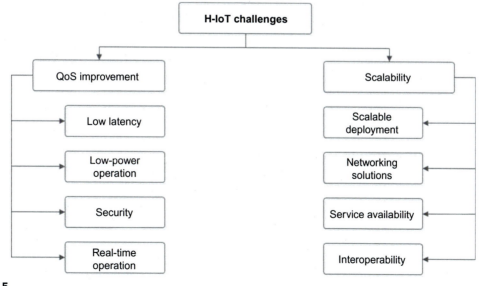

**FIG. 5**

H-IoT challenges.

### 2.2.1 QoS improvement

The QoS improvements required for the H-IoT system include low latency, low-power operation, security, and real-time operations. These requirements are explained as follows:

1. *Low latency*: The time-critical nature of the H-IoT application requires minimum latency. The total end-to-end delay is the sum of transmission delay and processing delay. The transmission delay is reduced by selecting the enabling communication technology with wide bandwidth availability. The processing delay is minimized by utilizing ML-based approaches, fog/edge computing, and cloud computing. The combination of ML, fog/edge, and cloud computing would significantly improve the system performance (Kumar et al., 2018).
2. *Low-power operation*: The miniature of IoT and wearable devices require minimum power consumption so that the devices should be recharged after a long period of time. The wearable devices can be recharged; however, implants require a battery that can sustain a battery time lasting for years. Therefore, novel and innovation solutions are required for the development of batteries that are long lasting and safe for use within the body (She et al., 2019). In addition, lightweight operating systems (OS) are required to operate with low-power consumption. Moreover, efficient resource management can enhance energy conservation. The efficient utilization of limited power, memory, and processing capability can lead toward the optimum working of H-IoT sensors. ML-enabled energy harvesting algorithms are one of the most suitable solutions to optimize the H-IoT systems (Ortiz et al., 2016). ML algorithms can easily optimize the OS, resource management, and overall performance of the system.
3. *Security*: The confidentiality of the patient's data is of paramount importance in H-IoT systems. The manipulation in the user's data or communication link has serious safety implications. The cryptographic techniques enable secure data access for only authorized users. However, unorthodox methods compromise the patient's private data. Intelligent security techniques are required to mitigate new attacks. AI provides effective and efficient solutions. However, resource-constrained H-IoT sensors to require lightweight algorithms, so it is imperative to devise efficient ML algorithms (Al-Garadi et al., 2018).
4. *Real-time operations*: The vast application area of H-IoT includes real-time patient monitoring and teleoperations. Therefore, the substantial amount of H-IoT data should be processed in real time with minimum latency. Extracting useful information refers as *features* from the data with minimum processing is another challenge. Deep learning (DL) algorithms augment the performance to analyze, process, and extract features with minimum latency and processing.

### 2.2.2 Scalability challenges

The deployment of the H-IoT system over a large scale in a smart city requires the system to be highly scalable. There are number of factors responsible for scalable H-IoT systems.

1. *Scalable deployment*: A smart city requires large-scale deployment of H-IoT devices. The same trend is observed with the exponential increase in wearable devices from 80 million in 2015 to 200 million in 2019, which indicates the potential of H-IoT systems (Seneviratne et al., 2017). The scalable and interoperable platforms and underlying communication technologies can enable large-scale deployment of H-IoT devices. Therefore, the standardization of communication technology for heterogeneous wearable and implantable sensors is of great importance.

In addition, the network resources should be scalable to support large-scale deployment of H-IoT devices. Innovative multiplexing and multiple access solutions for efficient use of the electromagnetic spectrum is in need. The 5G network is expected to support large-scale deployment of IoT devices with an increase in network capacity, while providing 10-fold improvement in energy efficiency. The terahertz (THz) communication is one of the potential solutions for the scarced network spectrum (Chen et al., 2019).

2. *Network solutions*: The large-scale deployment of H-IoT devices requires efficient network mechanisms. The network should be capable to support massive channel access mechanism in an ultradense environment. The miniature form factor renders the H-IoT devices resource constrained, whereas the channel access mechanism is power-consuming process. Therefore, it is of immense importance to design an intelligent, fast, and low-power consumption channel access mechanism. In this regard, ML provides efficient and promising results. Specifically, reinforcement learning (RL) techniques in ML provide lightweight and distributed algorithms to enhance current standards such as IEEE 802.15.4 and IEEE 802.15.6. In addition, ML techniques can predict traffic patterns in the network and allocate network resources accordingly to meet QoS requirements.

3. *Service availability*: The H-IoT devices and medical implants are placed on the human body, which is in constant mobility. Due to mobility, the network performance degrades. Hence, service availability and localization are major challenges in mobility. The service must be available in spite of the human mobility. The Internet Protocol version 6 (IPv6) provides an effective solution for network service availability with minimum handover time between different networks. ML algorithms learn the mobility patterns of the network to provide a potential solution for the dynamic network.

4. *Interoperability*: The H-IoT systems are envisioned to be deployed over a large scale from many original equipment manufacturer (OEM). The data generated from different OEMs vary significantly in format. The interoperability requires data handling, network management, and security. The regulatory authorized needs to put forward an unified standard and data format for heterogeneous devices connected over the Internet.

## 3 Machine learning

AI enables machines to mimic the human brain-like intelligence. The capabilities of AI include natural language processing, knowledge-based decisions, and perception. ML is the subset of AI (Sianaki et al., 2019). ML is the general technique of AI that can learn directly from structured and unstructured data provided by the information technology without any explicit programming. The ML techniques that can learn from labeled and unlabeled data sets for prediction are termed as supervised and unsupervised learning. The ML techniques enable the machines to learn themselves without any prior knowledge related to data set by interacting with the environment itself just like humans. Such ML techniques are termed as reinforcement learning (RL). Fig. 6 shows the relationship between AI, ML, and DL. Therefore, it classifies the ML into three categories that are supervised, unsupervised, and RL. Few examples of ML algorithms are K-means, Naïve Bayes, and support vector machine (SVM).

There are few techniques which learn from most of the unlabeled data; however, they also use a small amount of labeled data. Such techniques are known as semisupervised learning. DL is a subclass of ML with a multilayered system to perform higher capabilities. DL techniques include deep belief

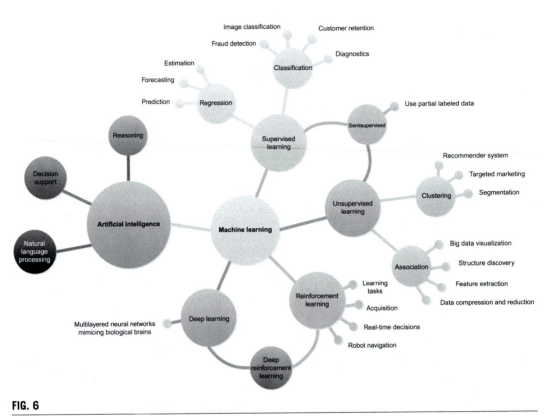

**FIG. 6**

Relationship between artificial intelligence, machine learning, and deep learning.

networks and neural networks (NNs). The association of DL and RL exploits the advantage of both techniques, which promote high-performance algorithms such as deep Q-networks (DQNs).

AI is advancing and revolutionizing all technological and scientific areas, including IoT. ML is also transforming H-IoT applications. The use of ML significantly improves the diagnosis of complex medical disorders. The applications of ML in the field of personalized medical care are categorized into three major categories as follows:

- diagnostics;
- patient monitoring and alarm systems; and
- assistive systems.

For the sake of better understanding, this chapter classifies the applications of ML in H-IoT into two categories that are

- application level and
- network level

The advancements of H-IoT at the application level include improvements in diagnostics, personalized assistive, and monitoring systems. Whereas, the network-level advancements of H-IoT include the improvement in network latency, data processing, real-time operations, and network security.

## 3.1 Machine learning advancements at the application level of H-IoT

This section includes the recent ML algorithms to improve the H-IoT at the application level. Walinjkar and Woods (2017) propose a prediction algorithm to predict arrhythmias. The algorithm utilizes k-nearest neighbors (kNN) for 97% detection accuracy of arrhythmias of the heart in real time. The ECG and temperature data collected from a personalized wearable device are compared with thresholds to generate alarms. The data can be further processed using the proposed algorithm to predict arrhythmias. H-IoT has been exploited for limb rehabilitation after stroke. The data collected from sensors embedded in wrist wearable devices are processed with ML-based classification complexity estimating algorithms and principal component analysis (PCA), which helps in the detection of surface electromyography with 97% accuracy. The results can be utilized by robotic hands (Yang et al., 2018).

ML has been used for detection of patients falling by ML-based video analyzer from a video feed in a smart home. The system yields an accuracy of 99% detection and generating timely alerts (Hsu et al., 2017). To enhance the personal assistive system with the risk assessments feature, ML can be implemented. The system with gyroscope a data analyzer from wrist band with ML algorithms using kNN giving an accuracy of 82.2% (Ramachandran et al., 2018). The intelligent analysis of sleep patterns can improve health. The DL approach which utilizes long short-term memory (LSTM) to analyze the multimodal inputs that are electrooculogram, ECG, and EEG. The LSTM is an efficient DL approach in learning patterns of temporal data. The patterns are then clustered as normal and abnormal using k-medoid algorithms. The classification of eye movement and sleep postures is also used to classify sleep patterns. The prepossessed data using PCA are further analyzed using SVM to classify data into clusters (Matar et al., 2016).

Real-time disease detection is one of the major research areas in the field of H-IoT, of which breast cancer detection is being explored extensively. The ML-based body fluid analysis using implants or wearable devices at the point of care (PoC) can help real-time breast cancer detection (Firouzi et al., 2018). Diabetes is one of the chronic deceases, causing deaths up to more than 2 million over the globe. The personalized diabetic data analysis could improve the early detection and prevention of deaths. The ML-based classifier estimates the medical condition from the data and compares the data with patients historical record in order to check if the vitals are breached (Asthana et al., 2017). A generative adversarial network is an unsupervised learning algorithm that could improve the classification process (Yang et al., 2019).

## 3.2 Machine learning advancements at network level of H-IoT

This section provides the recent work on ML, which improves communication in H-IoT networks. One of the important issues in the H-IoT network is related to security and privacy. The issue becomes more serious when the private personalized data are transmitted to the cloud for processing. It is of vital importance that the network should be protected from all breaches. In addition, manipulation of the data has severe and fatal implications. ML is an efficient tool for improving the security of the H-IoT systems. DL algorithm incorporating LSTM for encoding and decoding the data can be used for preserving the privacy of AAL systems. Only authorized individuals can access the data based on the permission level. The LSTM identifies different types of data and permission levels. Any manipulation of data or malicious entity to access the data can be located promptly by the LSTM system (Psychoula et al., 2018).

The life expectancy of the H-IoT device is of critical importance. The H-IoT devices transmit all the acquired data to the processing unit over energy-limited resources. The ML-based approach utilizing the SVM optimizes the system by preprocessing the data and classifies the data onboard. This approach could significantly increase the battery lifetime from 13 to 997 days (Fafoutis et al., 2018).

The selection of frequency channels is of critical importance, as massive H-IoT devices are expected to be deployed in the future. In a dense-deployed environment, channel selection with minimum latency and high fault tolerance. The RL-based channel selection termed as RL channel assignment algorithm (RL-CAA) meets the QoS requirements of H-IoT. It uses the history of the amount of traffic on the channel to learn traffic patterns on different channels (Ahmed et al., 2016).

The routing is one of the crucial network parameters to optimize network performance. Optimal routing decision also optimizes the latency, energy, and network lifetime. Q-learning is a type of RL for real-time operations, such as finding the optimal route between source and destination (Kiani, 2017). Furthermore, clustering can improve the energy efficiency by reducing the traffic load from the nodes and route to the node which can handle maximum traffic load.

The redundant or less priority data aggregation leads to an increase in resource consumption. ML-based data aggregation utilizing SVM classifier to aggregate the data based on data type and priority. This approach increases the efficiency in keeping the load balanced and energy conservation. This could also help in designing the routing algorithms for their critical routing selection decision to enable prioritized routing (Praveen Kumar et al., 2019).

## 4 Future research directions

The current consumer market reflects the diversity of applications of H-IoT technology. The health tracking systems offered by the numerous OEMs reflects this trend. The development of technologies such as 5G networks, AI, and smart materials is inspiring new areas of applications. Research and development in the H-IoT field are increasingly becoming a cross-domain exercise. Therefore, future research opportunities encompass a multitude of technological areas. ML supports a large number of applications in the H-IoT domain, and more possible applications are being found. The future of ML in H-IoT falls into two groups. The first being the novel applications of H-IoT that is supported by ML. The second being the new ways in which ML can enhance the network-level performance of an H-IoT system.

### 4.1 Novel applications of ML in H-IoT

The development of the AI, especially novel ML algorithms, is spearheading new application areas of H-IoT. In many upcoming technologies such as the Internet of Nano Things (IoNT), ML is playing an essential role in optimizing the performance and development of efficient and autonomous IoT monitoring systems.

### 4.1.1 Real-time monitoring and treatment

The primary purpose that the IoT devices perform is monitoring. However, in the case of healthcare applications, monitoring the patient's health is equipped with a response system. In addition to the generation of an alarm and alerting the healthcare support staff, the autonomous system can administer a "first aid." Multiple-use cases can be explored such as:

- *Autonomous blood sugar regulation system*: These system monitors and predicts the usage of glucose or blood sugar. ML algorithms can be trained to identify the optimum level of blood sugar and thus automatically administer a suitable level of glucose via an implant.
- *Precision medicine systems*: The overdose of prescription drugs is a significant problem in the healthcare industry. Sometimes, the doctors prescribe a dosage higher than the required amount. Therefore, to optimize the administration of drugs, an ML-based precision drug administration module can be implemented. The levels of various chemicals in the bloodstream are continuously monitored, and the user is alerted about the exact amount of the drug dosage. This ML-based system controls the overdose of medicines by training from the standard blood composition. If an anomaly is detected, the drug usage is regulated accordingly.
- *Prediction of neurological and cardiological events*: The prevalence of cardiological and neurological disorders, like stroke and epilepsy, highlights the importance of H-IoT in health monitoring. The occurrence of stroke and epileptical seizure is possible to predict from the events on the ECG and EEG, respectively. AI-based algorithms can identify the events or changes on the wave forms that precede a seizure or a stroke. In addition, countermeasures and alerts can be generated before the event occurs. Multiple countermeasures are defined for a stroke or seizure that can be implemented to mitigate the fatal risks of these two disorders.

### 4.1.2 Training for professionals

The healthcare professionals can improve their skills by using AI-based training modules that can test the knowledge and effectiveness of the medical students by generating random scenarios. These scenarios are based on real-life cases using which the algorithm is trained.

### 4.1.3 Advanced prosthetics

A large part of the world population faces some form of physical disability, and many among those depends on others for necessary activities. Therefore, ML-based prosthetics work by analyzing the signals in the central nervous system. The analysis can allow a robotic prosthetic package to obey the command of the user.

## 4.2 Research opportunities in network management

The H-IoT systems, like their generic IoT counterparts, are resource constrained. Therefore, for the processing of the packets, access management, channel access, and routing should be optimized. The optimization can occur at various levels of the network management system.

### 4.2.1 Channel access

RL algorithms are allowing the use of AI systems in channel access, which has to abide by a strict rule in terms of time delay and reliability. The RL algorithms can form policy and evaluate it to optimize the access to an already limited available channel bandwidth. The random access management can also be improved by utilizing ML algorithms to assign priorities to nodes and data types.

### 4.2.2 Dynamic data management

The continuous streams of data generated by the sensors are mostly composed of redundant data. Therefore, network resources are unnecessarily burdened. The lightweight and efficient ML algorithms can remove the redundancies in the data and prioritize the events that are urgent. The precious channel bandwidth can be preserved using this approach.

### 4.2.3 Fully autonomous operation

In an attempt to optimize network management, AI algorithms can be utilized. The use of lightweight ML algorithms is supported by the resource-constrained IoT nodes and network gateways. The split-second decisions can be made autonomously by ML algorithms that learn the traffic patterns and traffic load. The routing algorithms can be improved by predicting the future requirements of nodes based on the past experiences of the nodes.

### 4.2.4 Security

The security of patient data is a critical part of the H-IoT system. Multiple approaches to protect the privacy and the patient data are in use. However, the use of ML-based algorithms is also being popularized, such as in the case of intrusion detection systems (IDS). The ML algorithms learn the traffic features and patterns to identify a baseline upon which classification algorithms are applied. This approach is extended to other attack types, and the suitable ML algorithm is required for such instances. A randomized controlled behavior can be implemented for controlling the access of the nodes to enhance the system performance by utilizing ML algorithms.

## 5 Conclusion

The emergence of the IoT with the interaction of physical and cyberspace evolves a new paradigm for healthcare application, which is referred as healthcare IoT (H-IoT). The exponential increase in H-IoT devices around the globe augments the need for efficient and intelligent H-IoT enabling technologies. As a subset of AI, ML provides statistical tools, algorithms, and schemes for the machine to mimic the human brain-like intelligence. ML improves H-IoT application in diagnostics, assistive systems, and patient monitoring systems. While ML enhances the H-IoT network by reducing latency, improving data delivery rate and life expectancy of H-IoT devices, security, routing, and data classification. The future advancements in H-IoT systems are intelligent prosthetics, precision medicine, neurological and cardiological disorders prediction, and intelligent self-sustaining network.

# References

Ahmed, T., Ahmed, F., Le Moullec, Y., 2016. Optimization of channel allocation in wireless body area networks by means of reinforcement learning. In: 2016 IEEE Asia Pacific Conference on Wireless and Mobile (APWi-Mob), pp. 120–123.

Al-Garadi, M.A., Mohamed, A., Al-Ali, A.K., Du, X., Guizani, M., 2018. A survey of machine and deep learning methods for internet of things (IoT) security. CoRR abs/1807.11023. http://arxiv.org/abs/1807.11023.

Asthana, S., Megahed, A., Strong, R., 2017. A recommendation system for proactive health monitoring using IoT and wearable technologies. In: 2017 IEEE International Conference on AI Mobile Services (AIMS), pp. 14–21.

Chen, Z., Ma, X., Zhang, B., Zhang, Y., Niu, Z., Kuang, N., Chen, W., Li, L., Li, S., 2019. A survey on terahertz communications. China Commun. 16 (2), 1–35.

Fafoutis, X., Marchegiani, L., Elsts, A., Pope, J., Piechocki, R., Craddock, I., 2018. Extending the battery lifetime of wearable sensors with embedded machine learning. In: 2018 IEEE 4th World Forum on Internet of Things (WF-IoT), pp. 269–274.

Filipe, L., Fdez-Riverola, F., Costa, N., Pereira, A., 2015. Wireless body area networks for healthcare applications: protocol stack review. Int. J. Distrib. Sens. Netw. 11 (10), 213705.

Firouzi, F., Farahani, B., Ibrahim, M., Chakrabarty, K., 2018. Keynote paper: from EDA to IoT eHealth: promises, challenges, and solutions. IEEE Trans. Comput. Aided Des. Integr. Circuits Syst. 37 (12), 2965–2978.

Haghi, M., Thurow, K., Stoll, R., 2017. Wearable devices in medical internet of things: scientific research and commercially available devices. Healthcare Inf. Res. 23 (1), 4. https://doi.org/10.4258/hir.2017.23.1.4.

Hsu, C.C., Wang, M.Y., Shen, H.C.H., Chiang, R.H., Wen, C.H.P., 2017. FallCare+: an IoT surveillance system for fall detection. In: 2017 International Conference on Applied System Innovation (ICASI), pp. 921–922.

IEEE Standard Association, 2018. IEEE approved draft standard for service-oriented medical device exchange architecture & protocol binding. IEEE Standard 11073-20701-2018. IEEE Engineering in Medicine & Biology Society.

Jagtap, P.T., Bhosale, N.P., 2018. IoT based epilepsy monitoring using accelerometer sensor. In: 2018 International Conference on Information, Communication, Engineering and Technology (ICICET), pp. 1–3.

Kansara, R., Bhojani, P., Chauhan, J., 2018. Designing smart wearable to measure health parameters. In: 2018 International Conference on Smart City and Emerging Technology (ICSCET), pp. 1–5.

Kiani, F., 2017. Reinforcement learning based routing protocol for wireless body sensor networks. In: 2017 IEEE 7th International Symposium on Cloud and Service Computing (SC2), pp. 71–78.

Kumar, P.M., Lokesh, S., Varatharajan, R., Chandra Babu, G., Parthasarathy, P., 2018. Cloud and IoT based disease prediction and diagnosis system for healthcare using Fuzzy neural classifier. Future Gener. Comput. Syst. 86, 527–534. https://doi.org/10.1016/j.future.2018.04.036.

Lin, S., Istiqomah, Wang, L., Lin, C., Chiueh, H., 2018. An ultra-low power smart headband for real-time epileptic seizure detection. IEEE J. Transl. Eng. Health Med. 6, 1–10.

Matar, G., Lina, J., Carrier, J., Riley, A., Kaddoum, G., 2016. Internet of Things in sleep monitoring: an application for posture recognition using supervised learning. In: 2016 IEEE 18th International Conference on e-Health Networking, Applications and Services (Healthcom), pp. 1–6.

Nauman, A., Qadri, Y.A., Amjad, M., Zikria, Y.B., Afzal, M.K., Kim, S.W., 2020. Multimedia internet of things: a comprehensive survey. IEEE Access 8, 8202–8250.

Ortiz, A., Al-Shatri, H., Li, X., Weber, T., Klein, A., 2016. Reinforcement learning for energy harvesting point-to-point communications. In: 2016 IEEE International Conference on Communications (ICC), pp. 1–6.

Praveen Kumar, D., Amgoth, T., Annavarapu, C.S.R., 2019. Machine learning algorithms for wireless sensor networks: a survey. Inf. Fusion 49, 1–25. https://doi.org/10.1016/j.inffus.2018.09.013.

Psychoula, I., Merdivan, E., Singh, D., Chen, L., Chen, F., Hanke, S., Kropf, J., Holzinger, A., Geist, M., 2018. A deep learning approach for privacy preservation in assisted living. In: 2018 IEEE International Conference on Pervasive Computing and Communications Workshops (PerCom Workshops), pp. 710–715.

Qadri, Y.A., Nauman, A., Zikria, Y.B., Vasilakos, A.V., Kim, S.W., 2020. The future of healthcare internet of things: a survey of emerging technologies. IEEE Commun. Surv. Tutor. 22 (2), 1121–1167.

Ramachandran, A., Adarsh, R., Pahwa, P., Anupama, K.R., 2018. Machine learning-based techniques for fall detection in geriatric healthcare systems. In: 2018 9th International Conference on Information Technology in Medicine and Education (ITME), pp. 232–237.

Samie, F., Bauer, L., Henkel, J., 2019. From cloud down to things: an overview of machine learning in internet of things. IEEE Internet Things J. 6 (3), 4921–4934.

Šatala, P., Gašpar, V., Butka, P., 2018. Using IoT devices for movement detection in medical environment—proof of concept. In: 2018 IEEE 16th World Symposium on Applied Machine Intelligence and Informatics (SAMI), pp. 61–66.

Seneviratne, S., Hu, Y., Nguyen, T., Lan, G., Khalifa, S., Thilakarathna, K., Hassan, M., Seneviratne, A., 2017. A survey of wearable devices and challenges. IEEE Commun. Surv. Tutor. 19 (4), 2573–2620.

She, D., Tsang, M., Allen, M., 2019. Biodegradable batteries with immobilized electrolyte for transient MEMS. Biomed. Microdevices 21 (1). https://doi.org/10.1007/s10544-019-0377-x.

Sianaki, O.A., Yousefi, A., Tabesh, A., Mahdavi, M., 2019. Machine learning applications: the past and current research trend in diverse industries. Inventions 4 (1), 8. https://doi.org/10.3390/inventions4010008.

Statista Research Department, 2016. Wearables sales revenue worldwide 2015–2021. Statista. https://www.statista.com/statistics/641865/wearables-sales-by-category-worldwide/.

Vijay, A.K., Sangeetha, K., Shibani, A.A., Pranitha, M.P., 2018. Tremomarker tremor detection for diagnosis in a non-clinical approach using IoT. In: 2018 Fourth International Conference on Biosignals, Images and Instrumentation (ICBSII), pp. 206–212.

Walinjkar, A., Woods, J., 2017. Personalized wearable systems for real-time ECG classification and healthcare interoperability: real-time ECG classification and FHIR interoperability. In: 2017 Internet Technologies and Applications (ITA), pp. 9–14.

Wan, J., Gu, X., Chen, L., Wang, J., 2017. Internet of things for ambient assisted living: challenges and future opportunities. In: 2017 International Conference on Cyber-Enabled Distributed Computing and Knowledge Discovery (CyberC), pp. 354–357.

Yang, N., Wang, Z., Gravina, R., Fortino, G., 2017. A survey of open body sensor networks: applications and challenges. In: 2017 14th IEEE Annual Consumer Communications Networking Conference (CCNC), pp. 65–70.

Yang, G., Deng, J., Pang, G., Zhang, H., Li, J., Deng, B., Pang, Z., Xu, J., Jiang, M., Liljeberg, P., Xie, H., Yang, H., 2018. An IoT-enabled stroke rehabilitation system based on smart wearable armband and machine learning. IEEE J. Transl. Eng. Health Med. 6, 1–10.

Yang, Y., Nan, F., Yang, P., Meng, Q., Xie, Y., Zhang, D., Muhammad, K., 2019. GAN-based semi-supervised learning approach for clinical decision support in health-IoT platform. IEEE Access 7, 8048–8057.

# Edge detection-based segmentation for detecting skin lesions

**Marwa A. Gaheen[a], Enas Ibrahim[a], and Ahmed A. Ewees[a,b]**

*Department of Computer, Damietta University, Damietta, Egypt[a] Department of e-Systems, University of Bisha, Bisha, Saudi Arabia[b]*

## Chapter outline

## 1 Introduction

One of the largest threats to humans is cancer; it is the second leading cause of death globally (Yuan and Lo, 2017). Skin cancer is one of the most common cancers and its incidence has increased in recent years. Skin cancer is the uncontrolled growth of abnormal skin cells. These cancer cells may diffuse from the skin into other organs and tissues if neglected and unchecked (Li et al., 2018), and may even be lethal. Suitable and timely dissection of skin lesions is of major significance to medical personnel in order to provide the right diagnosis and treatment to their patients (Pal and Subashini, 2020).

Machine Learning, Big Data, and IoT for Medical Informatics. https://doi.org/10.1016/B978-0-12-821777-1.00008-2

Dermoscopy is a noninvasive imaging tactic applied to find melanomas and other skin lesions. With the assistance of dermoscopy, the subsurface construction of skin lesions can be examined, and various types of lesions can be identified with efficient visualization (Navarro et al., 2018). However, a dermatologist employs various dermoscopy methods, such as the ABCDE rule, 7-points checklist, CASH, and the Menzies method for skin lesion detection, and these have some issues. In particular, manual detection using dermoscopic imaging is a time-consuming and slow procedure for a dermatologist. Also, the outcomes are not always perfect, since there is low variance between normal and lesion skin. Furthermore, it is very difficult to determine the variation between melanoma and nonmelanoma skin images. Thus many preprocessing stages are needed for these dermoscopic images to obtain exact results. Therefore, in connection with the accuracy and efficiency, there are different computer-aided approaches for detecting skin lesion from dermoscopic images. Another group of algorithms is the region-based group. These methods aid approaches to automated skin lesion detection from dermoscopic images ( Javed et al., 2020).

The basic approach in improving an automatic diagnostic tool for skin lesion analysis includes segmentation, feature extraction, and classification. Among these three tasks, segmentation is crucial, since the accuracy of segmentation directly affects the successive tasks ( Jaisakthi et al., 2018; Ibrahim et al., 2020). However, skin lesion segmentation from the adjacent skin in automatic dermoscopic imaging has been, and continues to be, a challenge. There is a label imbalance issue in dermoscopic images, due to the fact that different skin lesion areas are very small and are represented by very small areas in the dermoscopic images. Consequently, we must concentrate on the recall average of skin lesion regions, since a minimal recall average will lose the smaller skin lesions. In addition, the skin lesions commonly appear in different colors, shapes, sizes, and positions and they may have ambiguous and irregular boundaries and have low variance from the adjacent skin. Also, artifacts and essential cutaneous characteristics like frames, hairs, vessels, air bubbles, and blood can increase the difficulty of automatic segmentation (Ghalejoogh et al., 2020; Agarwal et al., 2017).

Image segmentation is used to locate the boundary between the lesion area and the surrounding skin. Obtaining an accurate segmentation of the lesion is a critical step to provide minimal error rates in the quantification of the shape, size, and border features of the skin lesion. Generally, the segmentation operation aims at partitioning the image into sets of interrelated pixels in a region of interest (ROI) to assist in the detection of spatial transitions among these sets. The segmentation methods can be mainly categorized as: image thresholding, region segmentation, active contour, artificial intelligence, and edge extraction (Li et al., 2018; Jaisakthi et al., 2018; Gaheen et al., 2020). The thresholding tactics work well in conditions where there is a valid contrast between the skin and the lesion, if possible producing bimodal image histograms. The segmentation becomes an issue and cannot be addressed using thresholding if the histogram modes identical to the lesion and the skin overlap (Ghalejoogh et al., 2020). Another group of algorithms is region-based. These methods face challenges in efficient segmentation when the lesion is inhomogeneous or textured. This is most common since the boundary of the lesion includes dermoscopic contrasting structures that can lead to an over image segmentation. Occasionally, a soft skin tone variation crossing from the lesion to the skin causes imprecise segmentation (Agarwal et al., 2017). The active contour method consists of deformable contours that can be set to a variety of forms. The method contains an energy maximization operation built on edge or region-based methods and has been applied in segmenting different medical images (Munir et al., 2018; Riaz et al., 2018).

The process of segmentation of medical images faces various challenges due to the nature of human organs and the captured image. Several attempts and segmentation algorithms have been presented in the literature to address medical image segmentation problems, especially skin lesion segmentation.

This chapter proposes the eJaya algorithm for detecting skin lesions. The Jaya algorithm is a recent algorithm proposed for resolving restricted and unrestricted optimization issues. The mechanism relies on the concept that the solution acquired for a given issue should move toward the best solution and should avoid the worst solution. This mechanism requires only the common control operators and does not order any algorithm control operators (Rao, 2019a; Rao and Saroj, 2018). The elitist general concept has been applied in different evolutionary mechanisms. The concept is to exchange a worse solution for the better solution before carrying out the next iteration. The idea results in faster movement toward a better solution; therefore, the superior individuals are never lost (Kumar and Yadav, 2019; Rao, 2019b; Gaheen et al., 2021). This mechanism has been applied in several studies that have proven its effectiveness in solving optimization issues. In Raut and Mishra (2019), Jaya and eJaya mechanisms together were implemented to resolve a combinatorial, complex, optimization issue of concurrent network reconfiguration accompanied by DG distribution. The obtained outcomes proved that the suggested method is widely effective in enhancing power loss, extreme load capacity, and lower voltage in parallel with other methods.

This chapter is arranged as follows: Section 2 presents some previous works; Section 3 introduces the materials and methods; Section 4 presents the proposed approach; Section 5 discusses the experiment and the results obtained. The last section presents the conclusions and future work.

## 2  Previous works

Yacin Sikkandar et al. (2020) developed an efficient segmentation using a hybrid classification model for diagnosing skin lesions. The suggested model consisted of four phases: preprocessing, segmentation, feature extraction, and classification. A detailed experimental process was applied to investigate the execution of the presented model. The model was evaluated using the ISIC dataset and exhibited superior results. The experimental outcomes proved that the model presented the highest results among the compared algorithms (sensitivity 93.40%, accuracy of 97.91%, and specificity of 98.70%). Xie et al. (2020) proposed an attention mechanism to detect skin lesion borders based on a convolutional neural network (CNN). The CNN was utilized to obtain the feature maps to support the performance of segmentation. The proposed mechanism was divided into three branches. The first was the main branch, which extracts the local details of the lesion. The second was the spatial attention branch, which obtains features at each spatial position. The third branch was used to extract context information. The output of the main branch was fused with the outputs of the other two branches.

Tan et al. (2020) proposed a variant of the particle swarm optimization (PSO) algorithm, called hybrid learning particle swarm optimization (HLPSO), for the purpose of skin lesion segmentation and classification. HLPSO gathered various search mechanisms, including modified firefly algorithm operations, a new spiral research action, probability distributions, crossover, and mutation procedures, to diversify and improve the original PSO algorithm. It was used in synchrony with the $k$-means clustering algorithm to enhance lesion segmentation. A CNN was used to classify the lesion. Several skin lesion datasets were used in the evaluation, and the results showed superior capabilities in lesion segmentation compared with other related models of skin lesion segmentation. Tang et al. (2019) used a separable U-Net in parallel with stochastic weight averaging to segment skin lesions. The separable U-Net depended on a separable convolutional block in which the image was resized and converted to probability maps by separable U-Net and the final mask of the skin lesion was created. Stochastic weight averaging was used in addition to the U-Net to overcome the overfitting problem.

Dalila et al. (2017) proposed an automated system to segment and classify cancerous lesions corresponding to malignant melanoma features. The ant colony optimization (ACO) algorithm was used to detect the lesion contour and both k-nearest neighbor (kNN) and artificial neural network (ANN) were used as classifiers to test the results retrieved by the ACO algorithm. The confusion matrix showed that the algorithm classified correctly 85.22% and 93.60% of the image by kNN and ANN, respectively. Kumar et al. (2020) presented a semantic segmentation system for skin lesion images. They evaluated the system using three datasets (DermoFit, ISIC ISBI 2017, and PH2). The evaluation proved the superiority of the proposed system to the compared approaches. On the other hand, Mahbod et al. (2020) investigated the effect of applying skin lesion masks to classify dermatoscopic images. The proposed method was evaluated using the ISIC 2017 challenge dataset and its results outperformed the compared approaches. All preprocessing phases were executed with MATLAB software (2018a). All tests were conducted on a single computer with an Intel Core i7-8700 3.20 GHz CPU, and 32 GB of RAM.

Several metaheuristic methods are used in image processing (Sahlol et al., 2020; Ewees et al., 2019; Gaheen et al., 2019; Elatawy et al., 2020) to detect skin lesions, including PSO, genetic algorithm (GA), and ACO. Eltayef et al. (2017) presented an automated approach for detecting melanoma borders based on PSO and Markov random field algorithms, to define the edge of the lesion area in the input images. The outcomes proved that the suggested method drew the lesion edges accurately compared to other approaches. Ashour et al. (2018) performed a novel skin lesion detection approach based on the GA for neutrosophic set process optimization to minimize the indefiniteness of the dermoscopy images. The findings showed that the GA achieved the best performance compared to other approaches. In addition, Sengupta et al. (2019) proposed an optimization edge detection mechanism called ACO to improve skin lesion edge detection. The comparison of outcomes proved notable enhancement in skin lesion image quality from improved edge detection using ACO. Another skin lesion segmentation model introduced by Hawas et al. (2020) is called the optimized clustering estimation for neutrosophic graph cut algorithm (OCE-NGC). This model utilized the GA for optimizing the HBCE procedure using its optimum threshold values. The tests were applied on a computer with a 4-core Intel Core i5-5200U 2.7-GHz CPU and 8 GB RAM. The OCE-NGC platform was trained and estimated using the International Skin Imaging Collaboration (ISIC 2016) dataset for segmentation, which includes 900 and 379 dermoscopic photos. The experimental outcomes established the superiority of the suggested OCE-NGC approach compared to the other approaches.

# 3 Materials and methods

This section introduces the methods used in this chapter.

## 3.1 Elitist-Jaya algorithm

The elitist-Jaya algorithm (eJaya) was developed by Rao and Saroj (2017). This algorithm depends on the notion that the solution acquired for a given issue should proceed toward the best solution and should avoid the poorest solution. The method aims to always approach success and avoid failure.

The steps of the algorithm are represented as follows. Let $O(y)$ represent an objective function that will be minimized or maximized. During the $i$ iteration, $d$ (i.e., $q = 1, 2, ..., d$) refers to the number of design factors, and $p$ (i.e., $r = 1, 2, ..., p$) is the population size. Let $Y_{q,r,i}$ represent the value of the $q$th factor for the $r$th selected through the $i$th iteration; thereafter this value is revised as shown in Eq. (1).

$$Y'_{q,r,i} = Y_{q,r,i} + r_1(Y_{q,best,i} - |Y_{q,r,i}|) - r_2(Y_{q,worst,i} - |Y'_{q,r,i}|) \tag{1}$$

where $Y_{q,best,i}$ indicates the value of the $q$th factor for the best solution and $Y_{q,worst,i}$ indicates the value of the $q$th factor for the poorest solution. $Y'_{q,r,i}$ indicates the recent value of $Y_{q,r,i}$ and $r_1$, $r_2$ are numbers that change randomly in a range [0, 1]. The expression $r_1(Y_{q,best,i} - |Y_{q,r,i}|)$ represents that the solution aims to reach the best solution and the expression $- r_2(Y_{q,worst,i} - |Y_{q,r,i}|)$ represents that the solution aims to avoid the poorest solution. $Y'_{q,r,i}$ is agreeable if the function value created by it is the best. Fig. 1 illustrates the flowchart of the eJaya algorithm.

## 3.2 Otsu's method

Otsu's thresholding technique correlates with the linear discriminant standard, which supposes that the image is composed of only object background and foreground, and the diversity and heterogeneity of the background is neglected. Otsu uses the threshold to try to reduce the iterations of the class allocation. It segments the input image into two dark and light regions. The purpose is to find the threshold value with the minimum entropy for the sum of foreground and background. Otsu's method locates the threshold value depending on the statistical details of the image.

$$F_{Ots} = \sum_{i=0}^{K} A_i(\eta_i - \eta_1)^2 \tag{2}$$

$$A_i = \sum_{j=t_i}^{t_{i+1}-1} P_j \tag{3}$$

$$\eta_i = \sum_{j=t_i}^{t_{i+1}-1} i\frac{P_j}{A_j}, \text{where } P_i = \frac{h_i}{N} \tag{4}$$

where $\eta_1$ refers to the medium intensity of $I$ together with $t_0 = 0$ and $t_{K+1} = L$, while $h_i$ and $P_i$ refer to the iteration and probability of the $i$th gray scale, respectively. $N$ is pixels.

## 4 Proposed method

In this section, the proposed segmentation method is presented, which works to segment the affected skin lesion area. The proposed approach consists of two phases: the first is image preprocessing and the second is edge detection. In this method the eJaya algorithm is used to train the Otsu's method for segmenting the edges of the skin lesion area accurately.

## 4.1 Image preprocessing

In this phase, smoothing techniques are utilized toward the purpose of removing the noise that negatively affects the outcome of the segmentation. The input color image is converted to a gray level.

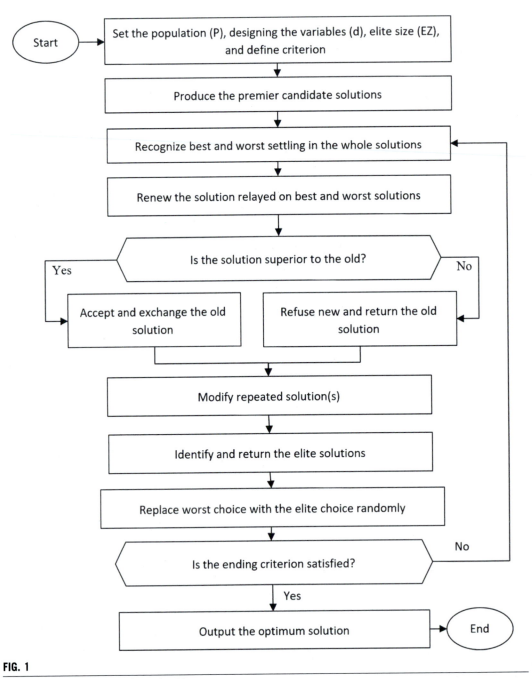

**FIG. 1**
The flowchart of the elitist-Jaya algorithm.

A Gaussian filter is utilized as it has a role in lesion edge detection through overcoming vanished edges, shifted edge position, and phantom edges. Then a morphological closing filter is applied to get rid of the extrinsic and inner noise of the skin lesion area, such as holes and gaps in the contour.

## 4.2 Edge detection

The proposed algorithm utilizes a new approach for segmenting skin lesions by enhancing the quality of the skin image and segmenting the lesion from the skin. The algorithm tries to increase the quality of the segmentation with less error, in order to outperform other ones. The preprocessed image plays an important role in supporting the results of the segmentation procedure. The proposed algorithm depends on training the Otsu's method with the eJaya optimization algorithm to increase the segmentation accuracy, in order to benefit from the advantages of the eJaya in selecting the proper segmentation threshold.

Fig. 2 illustrates the flowchart of the proposed method; the steps of the proposed method can be summarized as follows:

- *Input*: the skin lesion images.
- Resize the images to be on the same size.
- Use a morphological filter to remove the noise.
- Train Otsu's method using eJaya optimization algorithm.
- Segment the image into two levels.
- Binarize the lesion image.
- *Output*: the segmented skin lesion image.

## 5 Experiment and results

This section discusses the experiment and its results.

### 5.1 Dataset

The dataset utilized for training and testing the suggested algorithm was adopted from the HAM10000 dataset, which is a collection of dermatoscopic images representing various classes of skin lesions (Tschandl et al., 2018). The experimental sample consists of a set of 320 images. Fig. 3 shows a sample of these images.

### 5.2 Evaluation metrics

To evaluate the performance of the proposed eJaya segmentation algorithm in segmenting skin lesion images, different well-known evaluation metrics were used, including Accuracy, Precision, and Recall as shown in Eqs. (5)–(7), respectively; the computation time was also used.

$$\text{Accuracy} = \frac{\text{TP} + \text{TN}}{\text{TP} + \text{TN} + \text{FP} + \text{FN}} \tag{5}$$

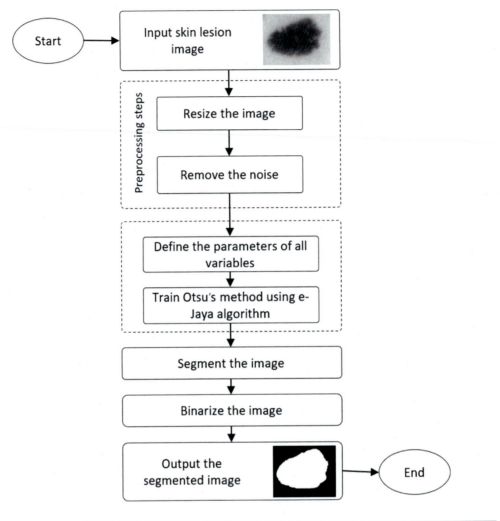

**FIG. 2**

The flowchart of the proposed method.

$$\text{Precision} = \frac{\text{TP}}{\text{TN} + \text{FP}} \qquad (6)$$

$$\text{Recall} = \frac{\text{TP}}{\text{TP} \times \text{FN}} \qquad (7)$$

where TP is the true positive, which refers to the number of classes that segmented correctly. TN is the true negative, which refers to the number of classes that segmented incorrectly. FP is the false positive and FN is the false negative.

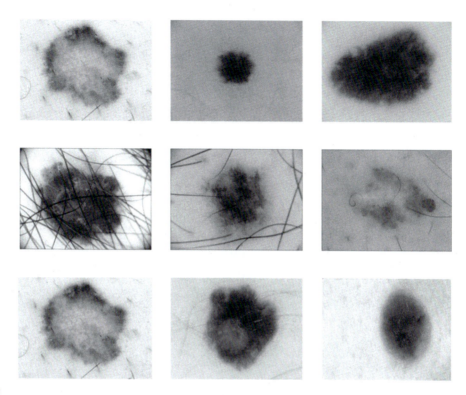

**FIG. 3**

Sample of images from the dataset used.

## 5.3 **Results and discussion**

The proposed segmentation algorithm was compared against the following algorithms: PSO, sine co-sine algorithm (SCA), Grey Wolf Optimizer (GWO), differential evolution (DE), and 2D wavelet algorithm, in terms of accuracy, precision, recall, and time, as displayed in Table 2. The implementation was applied using MATLAB 2014b and run on Windows 10 (64-bit) with a processor Core i7 (2.40 GHz) and 8 GB RAM. The parameter settings of the algorithms are listed in Table 1 and the global parameters are iterations number = 20 and population number = 50. All results, for each algorithm, were calculated using the average of 30 independent runs.

Table 2 and Figs. 4 and 5 show the performance results of all algorithms in segmenting the skin lesion images extracted from the benchmark dataset (i.e., 320 images).

The eJaya algorithm has the highest accuracy rate (0.8229), while the PSO algorithm has (0.8123), followed by the DE algorithm with (0.8108) accuracy rate; then comes the GWO algorithm with (0.7840) accuracy rate, and after that comes the 2D wavelet algorithm with (0.7670) accuracy rate; finally, the SCA algorithm has an accuracy rate of (0.7301). For the precision rate, the eJaya algorithm has the highest rate with (0.8050), while the DE algorithm has (0.8035) precision rate; next is the PSO algorithm with (0.7820) precision rate, followed by the GWO algorithm with (0.7729) precision rate;

**Table 1 Parameter settings of the algorithms.**

| Algorithm | Parameter values |
|-----------|------------------|
| SCA | $a = 2$ |
| PSO | $wDamp = 0.99, w = 1, C1 = 1, C2 = 2$ |
| GWO | $a = [2:0]$ |
| DE | $\beta_{min} = 0.2, pCR = 0.2, \beta_{max} = 0.8$ |
| eJaya | $r = [1, 2]$ |

**Table 2 Average of evaluation metrics obtained by the proposed method and the compared methods.**

| Algorithm | Accuracy | Precision | Recall | Time |
|-----------|----------|-----------|--------|------|
| eJaya | **0.8229** | **0.805** | **0.5297** | 0.0468 |
| PSO | 0.8123 | 0.782 | 0.5117 | **0.0425** |
| SCA | 0.7301 | 0.7293 | 0.5053 | 0.0464 |
| GWO | 0.7840 | 0.7729 | 0.4932 | 0.0471 |
| DE | 0.8108 | 0.8035 | 0.459 | 0.0950 |
| 2D Wavelet | 0.7670 | 0.738 | 0.3845 | 0.3436 |

*The best values are in boldface*

after that comes the 2D wavelet algorithm with (0.738) precision rate, and finally the SCA algorithm has a precision rate of (0.7293).

With regard to the recall rate, the eJaya algorithm has the highest rate with (0.5297). Second is the PSO algorithm with (0.5117) and third is the SCA algorithm with (0.5053); fourth is the GWO algorithm with (0.4932), and fifth is the DE algorithm with (0.4590); finally, the 2D wavelet has a recall rate of (0.3845).

However, in terms of time the PSO algorithm comes first, then the eJaya algorithm; after that is the SCA algorithm, followed by the GWO algorithm, the DE algorithm, and finally the 2D wavelet algorithm.

It can be concluded from Table 1 that the eJaya algorithm outperforms other algorithms in terms of accuracy, precision, and recall. That is due to the major advantage of the eJaya algorithm, which is that it is an algorithmic-specified parameter-minimal algorithm, which avoids the load of tuning of algorithmic-specified parameters.

All of the metaheuristic mechanisms require setting of algorithmic-specified parameters. The tuning of these factors and common control factors like number of iterations, elite size, and population size. The rendering of the metaheuristic tactics is affected by the tuning of these algorithmic-specified parameters and the incorrect setting of the algorithmic-specified parameters leads to trapping in local optima (Ahmed et al., 2017; Penghui et al., 2020; Sahlol et al., 2017). Over and above, the eJaya mechanism has having simple numerical construction and also has a single phase.

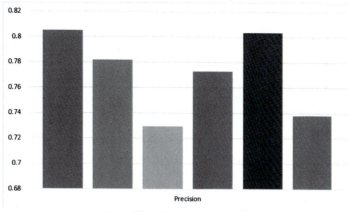

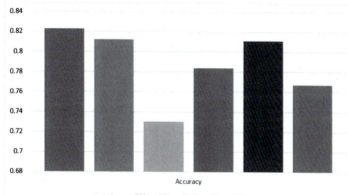

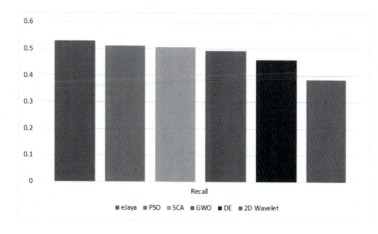

**FIG. 4**

Accuracy, precision, and recall results of all algorithms.

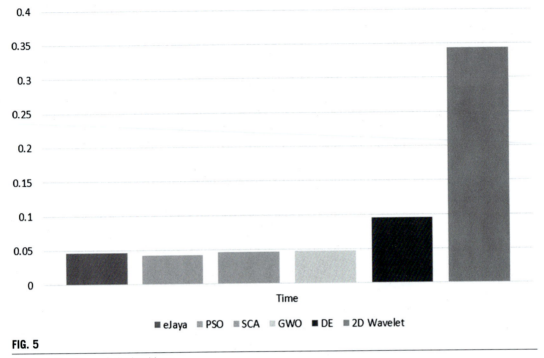

**FIG. 5**

Computation time of all algorithms.

To display the performance of the proposed segmentation method and its positive impact, the results of the segmentation process and the original image are stated for two samples in Fig. 6. This figure displays two samples of the segmented skin lesion images from the HAM10000 dataset using the proposed method and the other segmentation methods. As shown in the figure, the eJaya algorithm has a powerful and positive impact in segmenting the image and detecting the edges of the affected skin cancer area. The produced segmented images are more accurate than those of the other methods, followed by the PSO, whereas the 2D wavelet showed the worst detection results in the images.

## 5.4 Statistical analysis

This section analyzes the performance of the proposed method using the $t$-test statistical test to determine whether there is a significant difference between the eJaya algorithm and the compared methods at a level equal to 5%. The results are recorded in Table 3. This table shows that there are significant differences between the proposed eJaya and the algorithms SCA, GWO, and 2D wavelet with regard to accuracy, precision, and recall measures, whereas the PSO and DE showed similar results to the eJaya algorithm to some extent.

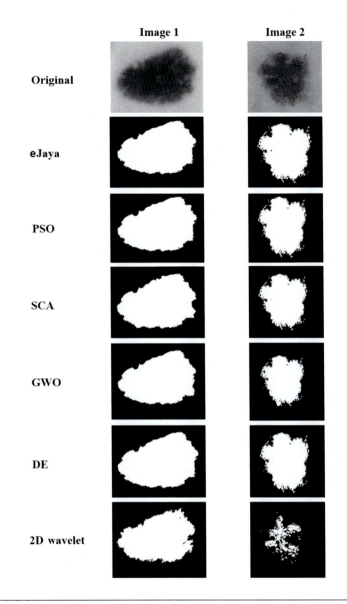

**FIG. 6**

Two samples of the segmented images.

**Table 3 Results of the statistical test.**

| Algorithm | Accuracy | Precision | Recall |
|-----------|----------|-----------|--------|
| PSO | 0.922 | 0.105 | 0.787 |
| SCA | <0.05 | <0.05 | <0.05 |
| GWO | <0.05 | <0.05 | <0.05 |
| DE | 0.851 | 1.673 | <0.05 |
| 2D wavelet | <0.05 | <0.05 | <0.05 |

## 6 Conclusion

This chapter proposed a method for skin lesion segmentation. This method introduces a new model to train Otsu's method based on the elitist-Jaya optimization algorithm. The proposed method consists of two phases: image preprocessing and edge detection. The experimental dataset consists of a set of 320 images. To evaluate the execution of the segmentation method, different evaluation metrics were used, namely accuracy, precision, and recall. The results showed that the suggested method outperformed the other algorithms in all measures, and it showed better segmented images than the compared algorithms. It obtained accuracy equal to 0.82, whereas the PSO was the fastest algorithm in terms of CPU time measure. In future, we will try to extend this work to segment different types of images and fields, such as X-ray images and satellite images. In addition, we plan to use new optimization algorithms and deep learning techniques to detect different types of skin lesions and intend to propose a real-time application to aid decision makers.

## References

Agarwal, A., Issac, A., Dutta, M.K., 2017. A region growing based imaging method for lesion segmentation from dermoscopic images. In: 2017 4th IEEE Uttar Pradesh Section International Conference on Electrical, Computer and Electronics (UPCON), pp. 632–637.

Ahmed, K., Ewees, A.A., Hassanien, A.E., 2017. Prediction and management system for forest fires based on hybrid flower pollination optimization algorithm and adaptive neuro-fuzzy inference system. In: 2017 Eighth International Conference on Intelligent Computing and Information Systems (ICICIS), pp. 299–304.

Ashour, A.S., Hawas, A.R., Guo, Y., Wahba, M.A., 2018. A novel optimized neutrosophic k-means using genetic algorithm for skin lesion detection in dermoscopy images. Signal Image Video Process. 12 (7), 1311–1318.

Dalila, F., Zohra, A., Reda, K., Hocine, C., 2017. Segmentation and classification of melanoma and benign skin lesions. Optik 140, 749–761.

Elatawy, S.M., Hawa, D.M., Ewees, A.A., Saad, A.M., 2020. Recognition system for alphabet Arabic sign language using neutrosophic and fuzzy c-means. Educ. Inf. Technol. 25, 5601–5616. https://doi.org/10.1007/s10639-020-10184-6.

Eltayef, K., Li, Y., Liu, X., 2017. Lesion segmentation in dermoscopy images using particle swarm optimization and Markov random field. In: 2017 IEEE 30th International Symposium on Computer-Based Medical Systems (CBMS), pp. 739–744.

Ewees, A.A., ElLaban, H.A., ElEraky, R.M., 2019. Features selection for facial expression recognition. In: 2019 10th International Conference on Computing, Communication and Networking Technologies (ICCCNT), pp. 1–6.

Gaheen, M.A., Ewees, A.A., Farouk, F., 2019. Face-pose estimation for learning systems. In: 2019 10th International Conference on Computing, Communication and Networking Technologies (ICCCNT), pp. 1–6.

Gaheen, M.A., Ewees, A.A., Eisa, M., 2020. Students head-pose estimation using partially-latent mixture. In: Emerging Trends in Electrical, Communications, and Information Technologies, Springer, pp. 717–729.

Gaheen, M.M., ElEraky, R.M., Ewees, A.A., 2021. Automated students Arabic essay scoring using trained neural network by e-Jaya optimization to support personalized system of instruction. Educ. Inf. Technol. 26, 1165–1181.

Ghalejoogh, G.S., Kordy, H.M., Ebrahimi, F., 2020. A hierarchical structure based on stacking approach for skin lesion classification. Expert Syst. Appl. 145, 113127.

Hawas, A.R., Guo, Y., Du, C., Polat, K., Ashour, A.S., 2020. OCE-NGC: a neutrosophic graph cut algorithm using optimized clustering estimation algorithm for dermoscopic skin lesion segmentation. Appl. Soft Comput. 86, 105931.

Ibrahim, E., Ewees, A.A., Eisa, M., 2020. Proposed method for segmenting skin lesions images. In: Emerging Trends in Electrical, Communications, and Information Technologies, Springer, pp. 13–23.

Jaisakthi, S.M., Mirunalini, P., Aravindan, C., 2018. Automated skin lesion segmentation of dermoscopic images using GrabCut and k-means algorithms. IET Comput. Vis. 12 (8), 1088–1095.

Javed, R., Rahim, M.S.M., Saba, T., Rehman, A., 2020. A comparative study of features selection for skin lesion detection from dermoscopic images. Netw. Model. Anal. Health Inform. Bioinform. 9 (1), 4.

Kumar, V., Yadav, S.M., 2019. Optimization of cropping patterns using elitist-Jaya and elitist-TLBO algorithms. Water Resour. Manag. 33 (5), 1817–1833.

Kumar, A., Hamarneh, G., Drew, M.S., 2020. Illumination-based transformations improve skin lesion segmentation in dermoscopic images. In: 2020 IEEE/CVF Conference on Computer Vision and Pattern Recognition Workshops (CVPRW), pp. 3132–3141.

Li, H., He, X., Zhou, F., Yu, Z., Ni, D., Chen, S., Wang, T., Lei, B., 2018. Dense deconvolutional network for skin lesion segmentation. IEEE J. Biomed. Health Inform. 23 (2), 527–537.

Mahbod, A., Tschandl, P., Langs, G., Ecker, R., Ellinger, I., 2020. The effects of skin lesion segmentation on the performance of dermatoscopic image classification. Comput. Methods Programs Biomed. 197, 105725.

Munir, A., Soomro, S., Lee, C.H., Choi, K.N., 2018. Adaptive active contours based on variable kernel with constant initialisation. IET Image Process. 12 (7), 1117–1123.

Navarro, F., Escudero-Viñolo, M., Bescós, J., 2018. Accurate segmentation and registration of skin lesion images to evaluate lesion change. IEEE J. Biomed. Health Inform. 23 (2), 501–508.

Pal, S., Subashini, M.M., 2020. Skin cancer detection using advanced imaging techniques. In: Smart Computing Paradigms: New Progresses and Challenges, Springer, pp. 229–237.

Penghui, L., Ewees, A.A., Beyaztas, B.H., Qi, C., Salih, S.Q., Al-Ansari, N., Bhagat, S.K., Yaseen, Z.M., Singh, V. P., 2020. Metaheuristic optimization algorithms hybridized with artificial intelligence model for soil temperature prediction: novel model. IEEE Access 8, 51884–51904.

Rao, R.V., 2019a. Applications of Jaya algorithm and its modified versions to different disciplines of engineering and sciences. In: Jaya: An Advanced Optimization Algorithm and Its Engineering Applications, Springer, pp. 291–310.

Rao, R.V., 2019b. Jaya optimization algorithm and its variants. In: Jaya: An Advanced Optimization Algorithm and Its Engineering Applications, Springer, pp. 9–58.

Rao, R.V., Saroj, A., 2017. Constrained economic optimization of shell-and-tube heat exchangers using elitist-Jaya algorithm. Energy 128, 785–800.

Rao, R.V., Saroj, A., 2018. Multi-objective design optimization of heat exchangers using elitist-Jaya algorithm. Energy Syst. 9 (2), 305–341.

Raut, U., Mishra, S., 2019. An improved elitist-Jaya algorithm for simultaneous network reconfiguration and DG allocation in power distribution systems. Renew. Energy Focus 30, 92–106.

Riaz, F., Naeem, S., Nawaz, R., Coimbra, M., 2018. Active contours based segmentation and lesion periphery analysis for characterization of skin lesions in dermoscopy images. IEEE J. Biomed. Health Informatics 23 (2), 489–500.

Sahlol, A.T., Moemen, Y.S., Ewees, A.A., Hassanien, A.E., 2017. Evaluation of cisplatin efficiency as a chemotherapeutic drug based on neural networks optimized by genetic algorithm. In: 2017 12th International Conference on Computer Engineering and Systems (ICCES), pp. 682–685.

Sahlol, A.T., Kollmannsberger, P., Ewees, A.A., 2020. Efficient classification of white blood cell leukemia with improved swarm optimization of deep features. Sci. Rep. 10 (1), 1–11.

Sengupta, S., Mittal, N., Modi, M., 2019. Improved skin lesion edge detection method using ant colony optimization. Skin Res. Technol. 25 (6), 846–856.

Tan, T.Y., Zhang, L., Lim, C.P., 2020. Adaptive melanoma diagnosis using evolving clustering, ensemble and deep neural networks. Knowl. Based Syst. 187, 104807.

Tang, P., Liang, Q., Yan, X., Xiang, S., Sun, W., Zhang, D., Coppola, G., 2019. Efficient skin lesion segmentation using separable-U Net with stochastic weight averaging. Comput. Methods Programs Biomed. 178, 289–301.

Tschandl, P., Rosendahl, C., Kittler, H., 2018. The HAM10000 dataset, a large collection of multi-source dermatoscopic images of common pigmented skin lesions. Sci. Data 5, 180161.

Xie, F., Yang, J., Liu, J., Jiang, Z., Zheng, Y., Wang, Y., 2020. Skin lesion segmentation using high-resolution convolutional neural network. Comput. Methods Programs Biomed. 186, 105241.

Yacin Sikkandar, M.Y., Alrasheadi, B.A., Prakash, N.B., Hemalakshmi, G.R., Mohanarathinam, A., Shankar, K., 2020. Deep learning based an automated skin lesion segmentation and intelligent classification model. J. Ambient. Intell. Human. Comput. https://doi.org/10.1007/s12652-020-02537-3.

Yuan, Y., Lo, Y.-C., 2017. Improving dermoscopic image segmentation with enhanced convolutional-deconvolutional networks. IEEE J. Biomed. Health Inform. 23 (2), 519–526.

CHAPTER

# A review of deep learning approaches in glove-based gesture classification

9

**Emmanuel Ayodele[a], Syed Ali Raza Zaidi[a], Zhiqiang Zhang[a], Jane Scott[b], and Des McLernon[a]**

*School of Electronic and Electrical Engineering, University of Leeds, Leeds, United Kingdom[a] School of Architecture, Planning and Landscape, Newcastle University, Newcastle, United Kingdom[b]*

## Chapter outline

## 1 Introduction

Hand gestures are an important part of nonverbal communication and form an integral part of our interactions with the environment. Notably, sign language is a set of hand gestures that is valuable to millions of disabled people. However, deaf/dumb users experience difficulty in communicating with the outside world as most neither understand nor can use sign language. Gesture recognition and classification platforms can aid in translating the gestures to those who do not understand sign language (Yang et al., 2016). In addition, hand gesture recognition can aid in monitoring the progress of patients who are recovering from stroke and rheumatoid arthritis (Watson, 1993). Healthcare professionals can remotely monitor the performance of several patients using a gesture classification system at a lower cost and time than the traditional method of physically observing the joints in

Machine Learning, Big Data, and IoT for Medical Informatics. https://doi.org/10.1016/B978-0-12-821777-1.00012-4

the hand. Furthermore, hand gesture classification is a vital tool in human-computer interaction. These gestures can be used to control equipment in the workplace and to replace traditional input devices such as a mouse/keyboard in virtual reality applications (Iannizzotto et al., 2001; Conn and Sharma, 2016).

There are two major approaches in the classification of hand gestures. The first approach is the vision-based approach. This involves the use of cameras to acquire the pose and movement of the hand and algorithms to process the recorded images (Kuzmanic and Zanchi, 2007). Although this approach is popular, it is very computationally intensive, as images or videos have to undergo significant pre-processing to segment features such as the image's color, pixel values, and shape of hand (Rautaray and Agrawal, 2015). Furthermore, the current geopolitical climate prevents the widespread application of this approach because users are less inclined to the placement of cameras in their personal space, particularly in applications that require constant monitoring of the hands (Caine et al., 2006). Furthermore, camera-based approaches restrict the movement of the user to within the camera's view. In applications where the user will need to perform their day-to-day activities (e.g., progress monitoring), multiple cameras are required to continuously track the user's movement and will significantly increase the cost of the system.

In contrast, the glove-based approach involves the use of data gloves that record the flexion of the finger joints. This method is less computationally intensive because the glove's sensory data is more easily processed than recorded images. In particular, the sensory data of a glove is simply the intensity of light (fiber-optic sensors), electrical resistance/capacitance (conductive strain sensors), or 3-dimensional positional coordinates (inertial sensors) (5DT, 2020; CyberGlove II, 2020; Lin et al., 2014). This means that researchers can classify the sensory data with little or no preprocessing. Moreover, a data glove allows continuous recording of the hand gestures without restricting the movement of the user. Furthermore, data gloves can be easily constructed with cheap off-the-shelf components such as bend sensors and a textile glove, which acts as a support structure. These advantages motivate a review of data glove-based gesture classification.

Gesture classification is the prediction of the hand gesture from the glove's sensory data. Although for a simple set of gestures such as the opening and closing of the fist, the data can be classified easily because the difference between the two gestures can be visually observed and linearly separated. However, for a more complex set of gestures such as sign language where some gestures are identical, machine learning is required to accurately classify those gestures. In addition, dynamic gestures such as sentences can only be classified with machine learning algorithms.

Therefore, this chapter presents a rigorous review of glove-based gesture classification with machine learning. There have been studies reviewing the application of machine learning in camera-based hand gesture classification (Rautaray and Agrawal, 2015), but to the best of our knowledge, there has been no review of glove-based gesture classification since Watson's 1993 study (Watson, 1993). Therefore, this chapter provides a one-stop destination for researchers interested in glove-based gesture classification. Moreover, we review the application of deep learning in glove-based gesture classification. This is a nascent field with significant work only published within the last 2 years. In addition, we highlight the advantages of deep learning algorithms over classical machine learning algorithms and discuss the limitations that prevent the rapid publication of studies within this field.

This chapter is structured as follows: Section 2 describes data gloves, their design, history, and sensing mechanism; Section 3 discusses gesture taxonomies; Section 4 describes classical machine learning and deep learning algorithms and their applications in glove-based gesture classification; Section 5 discusses the results of this review and postulates ideas for further research; and finally conclusions are presented in Section 6.

## 2 **Data gloves**

A data glove is a wearable device that is worn on a user's hand with the intent of measuring the motion at specified joints in the hand. As shown in Fig. 1, the design of data gloves involves embedding strain or inertial sensors in a textile glove. These sensors are placed near the measured joints for increased accuracy. In addition, processing and power supply are embedded to form an incorporated wearable system.

### 2.1 **Early and commercial data gloves**

The first data glove was developed in 1977 by researchers in MIT (Massachusetts Institute of Technology). It was called the "Sayre Glove" and utilized elementary fiber-optic sensors (Sturman and Zeltzer, 1994). These sensors consisted of tubes that transmitted light between their two ends. The intensity of the light passing through the tubes decreased as the tubes were bent by the flexion at the finger joints. The light intensity was measured by the voltage of a photocell placed at one end

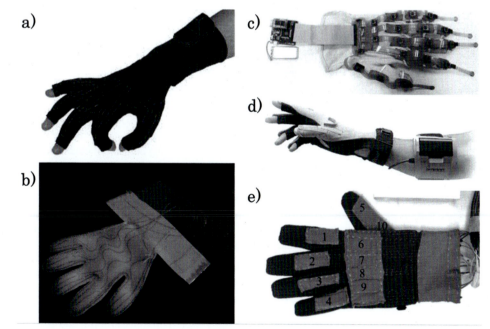

**FIG. 1**

Data gloves: (A) 5DT data glove (5DT, 2020), (B) FBG data glove (da Silva et al., 2011), (C) IMU data glove (Hsiao et al., 2015), (D) Cyberglove II (CyberGlove II, 2020), and (E) a soft sensing glove (Shen et al., 2016).

of the tube. It was observed that there was a strong correlation between the angle of flexion and the voltage of the photocell. Other examples of early data gloves made in the early 1980s include the "Digital Entry Data" and the "Super Glove," which used bend sensors and printed resistive inks respectively (Dipietro et al., 2008).

Recent commercial data gloves include the "Cyberglove," "5DT Data Glove," and "Didjiglove." The Cyberglove developed by Stanford University consists of 18 or 22 piezoresistive sensors. The model with 18 sensors only measures the metacarpophalangeal (MCP) and proximal interphalangeal (PIP) joints, while the model with 22 sensors measures the MCP, PIP, and distal interphalangeal (DIP) joints (CyberGlove II, 2020). In addition, both models measure the abduction, adduction, and wrist movements. The 5DT glove measures movement at the joints using fiber-optic sensors (5DT, 2020). These sensors measure the angle of flexion by its correlation to the weakening of light. It utilizes only one sensor per finger. In particular, the overall flexion at the MP and IP of the thumb is measured by a single sensor, while for other fingers, the overall flexion at the MCP and PIP joints are measured by a single sensor. An upgraded version of the glove uses more sensors to measure abduction and adduction between the fingers. The Didjiglove employs capacitive sensors to measure the flexion at the MCP and PIP joint (Dipietro et al., 2008). The capacitive sensors comprise of two comb-shaped conductive layers that are separated by a dielectric. Although recent data gloves have improved the accuracy of early data gloves, the core design of embedding a strain sensor in a textile glove has been retained. Therefore, it is imperative that we discuss the sensing mechanism of the popular strain sensors used in these data gloves.

## 2.2 Sensing mechanism in data gloves

Data gloves can be categorized based on their sensing mechanism. The three main types of sensors used in data gloves are fiber-optic sensors, conductive strain sensors, and inertial sensors. This section reviews their operating principles, advantages, and disadvantages.

### 2.2.1 Fiber-optic sensors

Fiber-optic sensors measure strain by translating the weakening of the light across its fiber (Lau et al., 2013). They are known for very accurate measurements because of the consistent correlation between the attenuation and the contortion angle of the fiber. However, their main disadvantage is the requirement of a light source, which increases the weight and size of the data glove.

Enhanced configurations of fiber-optic sensors have been utilized in more recent data gloves. Particularly, fiber-Braggs gratings (FBG) sensors were implemented in a data glove to measure the flexion at the interphalangeal joints (da Silva et al., 2011). FBG sensors measure strain by changes in the wavelength of the reflected Bragg signal. However, the FBG sensors are very sensitive to temperature and the equation below illustrates the relationship between changes in the Bragg wavelength and changes in the temperature and strain.

$$\Delta\lambda_B = \lambda_B(1 - \rho_e)\Delta\epsilon + \lambda_B(\alpha_t + \xi_t)\Delta T, \tag{1}$$

where $\Delta\lambda_B$, $\Delta T$, and $\Delta\epsilon$ represent the change in the Bragg wavelength, temperature, and strain respectively. In addition, $\rho_e$, $\xi_t$, and $\alpha_t$ are, respectively, the photoelastic, thermooptic, and thermal expansion coefficients of the fiber core. Despite the high accuracy in measuring joint angles, their use in real-world applications is restricted due to their high sensitivity to temperature changes.

### 2.2.2 Conductive strain sensors

Data gloves have been fabricated by utilizing conductive strain sensors (Chen et al., 2016). These strain sensors are formed from embedding conductive nanomaterials on flexible textile polymers by coating, wet spinning, or knitting. Their sensing mechanism is based on the changes in the relationship between their electrical resistance or capacitance and the strain exerted on them as a result of changes in the flexion of the joints in the hand. This creates a data glove that is textile, accurate, and light weight.

Notably, a conductive strain sensor was formed by coating spandex and silk fibers with graphite flakes with a Mayer rod (Zhang et al., 2016). Another textile strain sensor was developed by coating a Lycra fabric with polypyrrole (Wu et al., 2005). Moreover, multifilament yarns formed from conductive and textile fibers can be knitted to form textile strain sensors (Atalay et al., 2014). Furthermore, conductive strain sensors were created with coaxial fibers comprising of a core-shell structure where a flexible shell wraps the conductive core. They are fabricated by either injecting a textile fiber with conductive nanomaterials or by wet spinning (Tang et al., 2018).

### 2.2.3 Inertial sensors

Inertial sensors in data gloves comprise of gyroscopes and accelerometers that track the position and orientation of the hand joints (Lin et al., 2014; Hsiao et al., 2015). They are more useful in tracking dynamic gestures that require the movement of the wrist rather than other sensors because of the higher degrees of freedom in the wrist compared to the interphalangeal joints. However, they are not as flexible as other sensors and they tend to make the data glove bulky.

## 3 Gesture taxonomies

Gestures are a very important method of communication. For example, a "thumbs up" (G12 in Fig. 2B) can signify approval to the recipient, while a "thumbs down" can signify disapproval (Morris, 1979). A gesture taxonomy is a list of gestures. It helps to define what the gestures represent. This is important because a gesture can have several meanings across different cultures and geographical boundaries. In particular, the same thumbs up gesture, which denotes approval in most parts of the world, is seen as derogatory in the Middle East (Axtell and Fornwald, 1991). Gestures can be primarily divided into two categories: static and dynamic gestures. Static gestures are gestures in which the joints of the hand are stationary, while dynamic gestures are gestures that comprise of motion at joints in the hand. For example, a wave of the hand is a dynamic gesture, while a "thumbs-up" is a static gesture.

As illustrated in Fig. 2A, sign languages are gesture taxonomies that contain gestures that can be translated into letters or words and their respective meanings. In particular, a gesture taxonomy for sign language may comprise of static gestures that translate to letters, while another taxonomy may comprise of dynamic gestures that represent full sentences. Other taxonomies may contain gestures that represent the activities performed by the "expressor." For example, the grasp taxonomy proposed by Schlesinger depicts several hand postures that can be easily translated to the shape of the object (Heumer et al., 2007; Schwarz and Taylor, 1955). A gesture taxonomy can also illustrate a list of dynamic gestures that convey the activities performed by the user such as writing, drinking a cup of coffee, etc.

In human-computer interaction (HCI), there are various applications of hand gesture taxonomies. They are used as input commands for the control of robotic equipment in workstations and aiding doctors in performing teleoperation ( Jhang et al., 2017; Fang et al., 2015). They have enabled natural-like

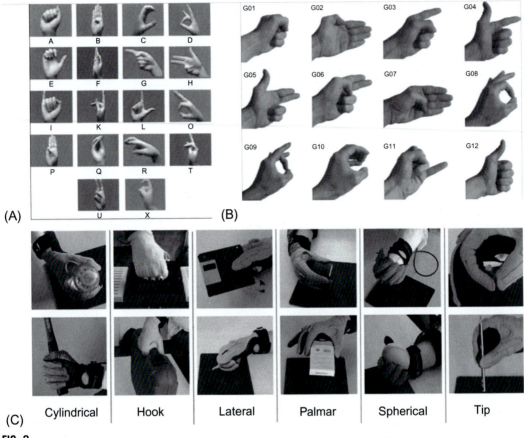

**FIG. 2**

Different gesture taxonomies. (A) Alphabets in sign language (Ibarguren et al., 2010), (B) custom gesture taxonomy (Luzanin and Plancak, 2014), and (C) Schlesinger taxonomy (Heumer et al., 2007).

interactions with virtual objects in virtual reality applications (Weissmann and Salomon, 1999). In particular, virtual rehabilitation programs contain several gestures that the patient seeks to achieve. These programs enable the healthcare professional to measure the progress of the patient's rehabilitation efficiently ( Jack et al., 2001).

## 4 Gesture classification

Gesture classification aims to accurately predict the gesture performed by the user from the acquired sensory data of the glove. For a taxonomy with a small of amount of distinct gestures, this can be manually observed from the data (Chen et al., 2016) or calculated using simple linear algorithms (Lu et al., 2012). However, machine learning is required to classify a more complex taxonomy of gestures,

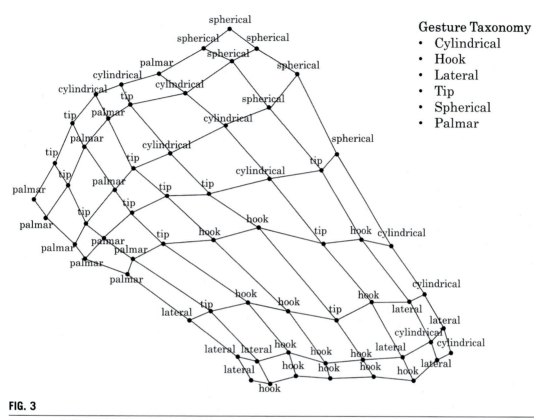

**FIG. 3**

Sammons 2-dimensional mapping of a SOM of gestures (Heumer et al., 2007).

especially gestures that are closely related. We define gestures that are closely related as gestures whose data values cannot be linearly separated. Fig. 3 illustrates a two-dimensional Sammons mapping of a self-organizing map (SOM) of a gesture data set. It illustrates the difficulty in linearly separating the different gestures. Moreover, it is impossible to linearly separate the tip, palmar, and cylindrical grasps. This data set exemplifies the relevance of machine learning in gesture classification as they can classify closely related gestures to a high accuracy.

## 4.1  Classical machine learning algorithms

Machine learning algorithm can be differentiated by their type of learning. Supervised learning occurs when correct input-output pairs are provided for the algorithm during training, while unsupervised learning requires the algorithm to determine clusters of similar input data as no target output is provided (Rautaray and Agrawal, 2015). In this section, we describe a summarized theoretical background of the popular classical machine learning algorithms used in glove-based gesture classification.

### 4.1.1 K-nearest neighbor

K-nn is a probabilistic pattern recognition technique that classifies a signal output based on the most common class of its $k$ nearest neighbors in the training data. The most common class (also referred to as the similarity function) can be computed as a distance or correlation metric (Altman, 1992). Typically, the similarity function is calculated using the Euclidean distance; however, other distance metrics such as the Manhattan distance could also be utilized. The probability density function $p(M, c_j)$ of the output data $M$ belonging to a class $c_j$ with $j$th training categories can be computed as:

$$p(M, c_j) = \sum_{n_z \in knn} d(M, n_z) V(n_z, c_j),$$ (2)

where $n_z$ is a neighbor in the training set, $V(n_z, c_j)$. The Euclidean distance $d(M, n_z)$ can be calculated as:

### 4.1.2 Support vector machine (SVM)

Traditionally, SVM was used in the linear classification of data. However, the use of a linear kernel limited its accuracy in nonlinear classification tasks. Therefore, the SVM algorithm was iterated by implementing a Gaussian kernel. This allows the algorithm to map data to an unlimited dimension space where data can become more separable in a higher dimension. The decision function for Gaussian SVM classification of an unknown pattern data $u$ can be represented as:

$$d(M, n_z) = \sqrt{\sum_{z=1}^{k} (M_z - n_z)^2}.$$ (3)

$$f(u) = \text{sign}\left(\sum_{k=1}^{h} \lambda_k c_k \exp\left(\frac{-\|u_k - u\|^2}{2\sigma^2}\right) + t\right),$$ (4)

where $c_k$ is the class label for the $k$-th support vector $u_k$, $\lambda_k$ is the Lagrange multiplier, and $t$ is the bias (Cortes and Vapnik, 1995).

### 4.1.3 Decision tree

Decision tree is a supervised learning technique that aims to split classification into a set of decisions that determine the class of the signal. The output of the algorithm is a tree whose decision nodes have multiple branches with its leaf nodes deciding the classes (Yang et al., 2016). The configuration of the algorithm is determined by specifying the maximum number of splits.

### 4.1.4 Artificial neural network (ANN)

ANN is a biologically inspired machine learning algorithm. It consists of input, hidden, and output layers that comprise of neurons. These artificial neurons simulate neurons in the brain by receiving an input, processing it using an activation function and producing an output. The output of $i$th neuron can be calculated as:

$$y_i = f_i\left(\sum_{j=1}^{n} w_{ij} x_j - \theta_i\right),$$ (5)

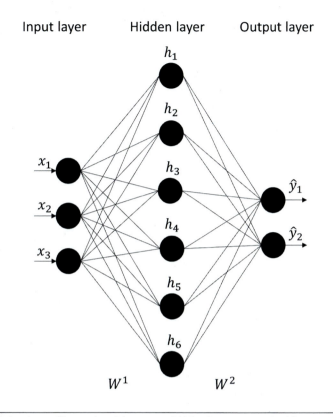

Input layer    Hidden layer    Output layer

**FIG. 4**

Example of an ANN structure with one input layer, one hidden layer, one output layer, and weight matrices **W**$^1$ and **W**$^2$ (Tang, 2019).

where $f_i$ is the transfer function, $y_i$ is the output of the neuron $i$, $x_j$ is the $j$th input to the neuron, $w_{ij}$ is the connection weight between the neurons, and $\theta_i$ is the bias of the neuron (Neto et al., 2013). Traditionally, the transfer function is either Gaussian, sigmoid, or Heaviside. Moreover, ANNs are trained by adjusting the connection weights. This can be achieved by algorithms such as backpropagation or reinforcement learning. The key factor in the operating principle of the learning algorithms is their weight-adjustment rules such as the Hebbian rule and the delta rule. Fig. 4 shows a feedforward neural network (FFNN), the simplest form of an ANN. It never feeds the output back to the output because it operates in a single forward direction.

### 4.1.5 Probabilistic neural network (PNN)

PNNs are neural networks that use the probability density function to determine the likelihood of an input data belonging to a class. They consist of four layers, which are an input layer, which contains neurons representing each data sample that are fully connected to the next layer; a hidden layer comprising of Gaussian functions centered on the data samples; a summation layer that computes the average probability of an input sample belonging to each class; and the output layer which uses Bayes rule to determine the class for the input sample (Specht, 1990). The output illustrating the classification class of the input data is computed as:

$$\hat{A}(x) = (\arg\max)_{i=1,...,d} \left\{ \frac{1}{(2\pi)^k 2\sigma^k} \frac{1}{N_i} \sum_{j=1}^{N_i} \exp\left( -\frac{\left(x - x_j^i\right)^t \left(x - x_j^i\right)}{2\sigma^2} \right) \right\}, \tag{6}$$

where $\sigma$ is the smoothing parameter, $k$ is the size of the measurement space, $N_i$ is the total number of training patterns, and $x_j^i$ is the $j$th training pattern from category $A_i$.

## 4.2 Glove-based gesture classification with classical machine learning algorithms

Several classical machine learning algorithms have been explored in the classification of gestures from data acquired by a data glove. Initially, ANN was used to classify five gestures from the American sign language (ASL) (Beale and Edwards, 1990). Thereafter, a modified version of ANN using backpropagation was implemented to recognize a taxonomy comprising of forty-two gestures from Japanese Kana (Murakami and Taguchi, 1991) acquired by a VPL data glove. Back propagation is a feedback algorithm that improves the classification results by using gradient descent to adjust the learning weights of the network. The network consisted of 16 nodes in the input layer representing 10 bend sensors and 6 positional sensors, 150 nodes in the hidden layer, and 10 nodes in the output layer representing the 10 dynamic gestures. Moreover, the input data was augmented and filtered to improve the accuracy of the network. The results show a 96% accuracy when the data was filtered and augmented; and 80% accuracy without augmentation and filtering.

Furthermore, a radial basis function (RBF) network were employed to classify twenty static gestures from five users of a Cyberglove (Weissmann and Salomon, 1999). The network was trained with four users and validated with the last user. The results showed that the average accuracy of the network was 88% during cross validation. In contrast when the validation user was included in the training set, the average accuracy was 98.3%. This study illustrates the difference in the accuracy of machine learning algorithms between "unseen" experiments and "seen" experiments. In unseen experiments, the data in the validation set is not included in the training set, while in seen experiments, some or all of the validation data is included in the training data set. We observed that machine learning algorithms are less accurate in classifying unseen data. Particularly, in glove-based gesture classification, the reduced accuracy of the machine learning algorithms in unseen experiments can be attributed to the difference in the hand dimensions of the unseen users in the validation data set and the users in the training data set. However, the difference in accuracies between unseen and seen experiments can be reduced by utilizing a large number of users in training the algorithm.

Furthermore, a feedforward ANN was utilized in classifying gestures for a VR driving application (Xu, 2006). Three hundred gestures were acquired from five participants with the Cyberglove. The gestures were split into 200 gestures for the training set and 100 gestures for the validation set. The average accuracy was 98%. This high accuracy was obtained because this was a seen experiment. In contrast, when data from three new (unseen) participants were used as a validation set, the recognition accuracy reduced to 92%.

In Luzanin's study (Luzanin and Plancak, 2014), PNN was used to classify twelve static gestures acquired with the 5DT Data Glove. Clustering algorithms were implemented to reduce the training data without affecting the performance of PNN and to maintain the representation of the actual input data. These clustering algorithms were $K$-means, $X$-means, and Expected Maximization (EM) algorithms. The classification accuracies for the seen experiment were 93.4%, 96.18%, and 95.98% for $K$-means, $X$-means, and EM algorithms, respectively. Furthermore, for an unseen validation user, the results were 63.05%, 52.48%, and 77.14% for $K$-means, $X$-means, and EM algorithms, respectively.

Two ANNs connected in series were employed in gesture classification for human-robot control (Neto et al., 2013). As depicted in Fig. 5, the first ANN was used to classify static communicative gestures, while the second ANN was used to classify noncommunicative gestures that occurred within the transition between the communicative gestures in the continuous data. The data was acquired with Cyberglove II that contains 22 sensors. Therefore, in both ANNs, the input layer and hidden layer each comprised of 44 neurons that represent two frames per sensor. Classification accuracy was up to 99.8% for 10 gestures and 96.3% for a taxonomy of 30 gestures. The aim of the study was to accurately recognize static gestures within continuous data; therefore, the authors limited the validation data set to only seen data, hence the high accuracy.

A multiclassifier approach was undertaken in (Ibarguren et al., 2010) to classify gestures acquired by a 5DT Data Glove. The gestures were eighteen ASL alphabets that do not require positional measurements of the wrist. The gestures were classified using a combination of decision tree and $k$-nn

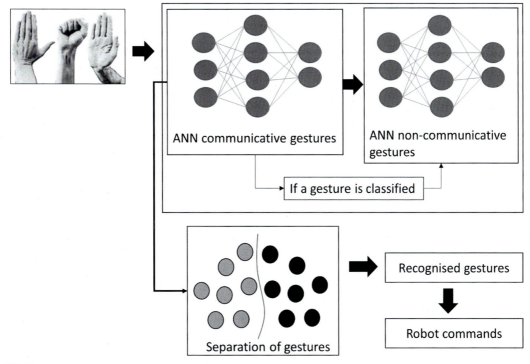

**FIG. 5**

Two serially connected ANNs for real-time gesture recognition (Neto et al., 2013).

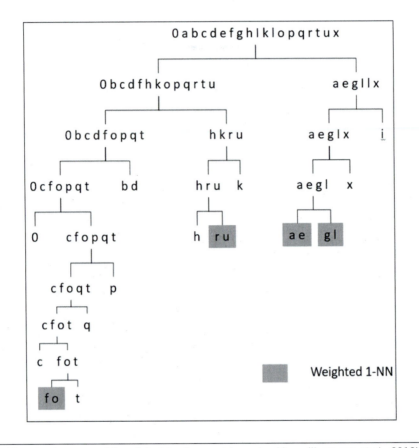

**FIG. 6**

A multiclassifier structure comprising of decision tree and *k*-nn algorithms (Ibarguren et al., 2010).

algorithms as shown in Fig. 6. A clustering method based on Euclidean distance generated a decision tree. Thereafter, *k*-nn (*k* = 1) was used to classify letters at the lowest level nodes. These letters such as a/e or f/o are very similar, and the 1-nn classifier aids in providing a more accurate classification. In addition, a segmentation layer is utilized before classification to separate the recorded gestures from the real-time continuous data. Experimental results show a 99.49% segmentation accuracy and a 94.61% classification accuracy.

A self-organizing map (SOM) was used to classify 10 static gestures acquired with a 5DT Data Glove (Jin et al., 2011). SOM is an unsupervised machine learning algorithm that aims to model the input data into a discretized lower dimension map. Training data was acquired from six participants, and the algorithm was validated with 10 participants that included two participants from the training data. The algorithm performed well with a 94.29% accuracy.

In addition, a custom IMU data was used alongside an Extreme Machine Learning (ELM) algorithm to classify 10 static gestures (Lu et al., 2016). Two sets of 44 and 45 features were extracted from the input gesture data set. The 45 feature set comprised of yaw, pitch, and roll angles of the five fingers, while the 44 feature set comprised of the 45 features of the fingers; and the yaw, pitch, and roll angles of the palm, forearm, and upper arm. ELM algorithm was utilized because of its low computational burden and reduced human reliance as its input weights and hidden layer neurons and biases are generated randomly. A modified version of ELM algorithm proposed by Huang et al. (Huang et al., 2011) that employs a kernel method was also used in the study. The original ELM algorithm, the ELM-kernel algorithm, and SVM were compared using both sets of extracted features. The classification accuracy using the 44 feature set were 68.05%, 89.59%, and 83.65% for the ELM, ELM-kernel, and SVM algorithms, respectively, while for the 45 feature set, the accuracy for ELM, ELM-kernel, and SVM algorithms were 84.40%, 85.51%, and 81.09%, respectively, thereby highlighting the superiority of the ELM-kernel algorithm for gesture classification.

A more comprehensive comparison of classical machine learning algorithms in gesture classification was illustrated in the study cited herein (Heumer et al., 2007). A Cyberglove was employed in acquiring grasp types based on Schlesinger's taxonomy. Subsequently, several classical ML algorithms were used to classify the data in six classification scenarios comprising of seen and unseen experiments. These 28 algorithms were obtained from a software package (Witten et al., 2005) and were grouped based into five categories: rule sets, trees, function approximators, lazy learners, and probabilistic methods. Rule algorithms classify the gestures by a set of logical rules, while tree algorithms (such as decision tree) classify gestures based on a pyramid of binary decisions. In addition, function approximators are supervised learning algorithms that derive an approximate function between the input data and the output class. Probabilistic algorithms produce probability models of each class and then determine (using a method such as Bayes theorem) the probability of each input data belonging to a specific class. Lazy learners delay classification of an input data until a request is received. Thereafter, the class of the data item is determined from the class of the closest data items based on the specified distance metric. The results depict that function approximating classifiers performed well with a minimum and maximum accuracy of 81.41% and 86.8%, respectively. Although the best classifier was a Lazy classifier at an accuracy of 87.61%, the average accuracy of Lazy classifiers was 78.77%. However, Bayesian, tree-based, and rule-based classifiers were poor performers. Particularly, Bayesian classifiers had a maximum and minimum accuracy of 75.31% and 61.02%, respectively. Tree-based classifiers had a maximum accuracy of 83.44% and a minimum accuracy of 31.06%, while rules-based classifiers had a maximum accuracy of 78.13% and a minimum accuracy of 30.88%. The best and worst classifier in each category is highlighted in Table 1.

## 4.3 Deep learning

Deep learning (DL) is a class of machine learning whose algorithms comprise of neural networks with several hidden layers. Examples of popular deep learning algorithms are Deep Belief Network (DBN), Deep Boltzmann Machine (DBM), Recurrent Neural Network (RNN), and Convolutional Neural Network (CNN) (LeCun et al., 2015). The advantage of deep learning algorithms over traditional machine learning algorithm is the ability of DL algorithms to automatically extract features from the input data without the bias that comes with manual feature extraction in classical machine learning algorithms as illustrated in Fig. 7. However, DL algorithms require significantly more data and computation resources than classical machine learning algorithms.

**Table 1** Summarized review of glove-based gesture classification with classical machine learning algorithms.

| Glove | Application/ taxonomy | Algorithm | Accuracy | Reference |
|---|---|---|---|---|
| VPL data glove | ASL | ANN | N/A | (Beale and Edwards, 1990) |
| VPL data glove | Japanese Kana | ANN | **96.00%** (with filtering), **80.00%** (without filtering) | (Murakami and Taguchi, 1991) |
| Cyberglove | Custom gesture set for HCI | RBF | **98.30%** (seen), **88.00%** (unseen) | (Weissmann and Salomon, 1999) |
| Cyberglove | Custom gesture for VR driving control | ANN | **98.00%** (seen), **92.00%** (unseen) | (Xu, 2006) |
| 5DT data glove | Modified NASA gesture dictionary | PNN | **95.19%** (seen), **64.22%** (unseen) | (Luzanin and Plancak, 2014) |
| Cyberglove | Human-robot interaction (HRI) | Two serially connected ANNs | **99.80%** (seen, 10 gestures), **96.30%** (seen, 30 gestures) | (Neto et al., 2013) |
| 5DT data glove | ASL | Decision tree and KNN | **94.61%** | (Ibarguren et al., 2010) |
| 5DT data glove | Custom gestures set for HCI | SOM | **94.29%** | ( Jin et al., 2011) |
| Cyberglove 2 | Schlesinger taxonomy for grasp classification | IB1 (best lazy) | **87.61%** | (Heumer et al., 2007) |
| | | MultilayerPerceptron (best FA) | **86.80%** | |
| | | LMT (best trees) | **83.44%** | |
| | | NNge (best rules) | **78.13%** | |
| | | BayesNet (best bayes) | **75.31%** | |
| | | LWL (worst lazy) | **62.95%** | |
| | | Logistic (worst FA) | **81.41%** | |
| | | DecisionStump (worst trees) | **31.06%** | |
| | | ConjuctiveRule (worst rules) | **30.88%** | |
| | | ComplementNaiveBayes (worst bayes) | **61.02%** | |
| IMU data glove | Custom gestures for HRI | ELM | **84.40%** (45 features), **68.05%** (54 features) | (Lu et al., 2016) |
| | | ELM-Kernel | **85.51%** (45 features), **89.59%** (54 features) | |
| | | SVM | **81.09%** (45 features), **83.65%** (54 features) | |

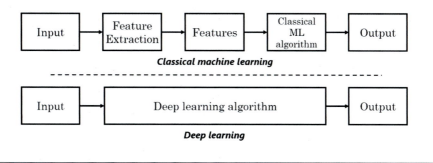

**FIG. 7**

Difference between classical machine learning and deep learning.

### 4.3.1 Convolutional neural network (CNN)

CNN is the most popular architecture used in DL applications. It became popular after *Alexnet* (a CNN algorithm) won ILSVRC 2012, a prominent computer vision classification competition. Thereafter, it has been employed in a wide variety of applications spanning from classification of images in computer vision to the classification of physiological signals (e.g., ECG, EMG) and was seen to perform excellently (Yao et al., 2020; Qin et al., 2019; Goodfellow et al., 2016; Krizhevsky et al., 2012).

A typical convolutional neural network is a feed forward deep neural network with stacks of convolutional and pooling layers and one or more fully connected layers. Features are extracted from the input data by convolving the input data with filters comprising of neurons with adjustable weights and biases in the convolutional layers. The convolution operation of the $g$th feature map on the $f$th convolutional layer located at position $(a,b)$ can be described as:

$$v_{f,g}^{a,b} = \sigma\left(b_{f,g} + \sum_{i}\sum_{x=0}^{X_{f-1}}\sum_{y=0}^{Y_{f-1}} w_{f,g,i}^{x,y} v_{f-1,i}^{a+x,b+y}\right), \tag{7}$$

where $b$ is the feature map's bias, $w$ is the weight matrix, $X$ and $Y$ are the kernel's height and width, respectively. $\sigma()$ is a nonlinear activation function such as rectified linear unit (RELU), Sigmod, or Tanh. A pooling layer is utilized to reduce the variance on the feature map due to minor changes in the input data. This is achieved by representing the spatial region as an aggregate of neighboring outputs. Although earlier studies utilized average pooling; recently, maximum pooling has become very popular. Furthermore, fully connected layers classify the input signal based on the extracted features from previous layers.

### 4.3.2 Recurrent neural network (RNN)

RNN is a deep learning algorithm that feeds back its output to its input to produce temporal memory. This internal temporal memory enables it to process dynamic input sequences. This has ensured that RNNs outperform other machine learning algorithms in sequence prediction in applications such as speech recognition and computer vision. A popular example of RNN is long short-term memory (LSTM). LSTM has outperformed general RNNs because of its error backpropagation. This eliminates the error vanishing and exploding phenomena and enables LSTM to memorize several thousands of previous time steps (Schmidhuber, 2015).

## 4.4 Glove-based gesture classification using deep learning

In this section, we review the applications that have utilized deep learning in glove-based gesture classification. Notably, a simple CNN algorithm was used to classify dynamic sign language gestures from data obtained with an IMU data glove (Fang et al., 2019). The CNN comprised of a convolutional layer, a batch normalization layer and a fully connected layer. A pooling layer was noticeably absent as the authors felt it was redundant in this architecture. The performance of the algorithm was compared to an LSTM method and a PCA-SVM method. The CNN algorithm had the highest accuracy at 99.6%, while the PCA-SVM and LSTM algorithms had accuracies of 82% and 80.8% respectively.

Furthermore, a light CNN architecture shown in Fig. 8 was implemented in a real time gesture recognition using a custom IMU data glove (Diliberti et al., 2019). The CNN was implemented using a very similar configuration to *AlexNet*. However, the authors performed a series of experiments to determine the optimal implementation of the network for their application. They achieved this by reducing the depth and width of the network till the set goal of at least 98% accuracy was met. The depth of the network was reduced by removing some layers in the network while reducing the width of the network is reducing the number of neurons in the layers. The depth percentage was measured as a percentage of the original number of layers, while the width factor, *WF*, was expressed as:

$$Neu_{new} = 2^{-WF} Neu_{old}, \qquad (8)$$

where $Neu_{old}$ and $Neu_{new}$ are the original and new number of neurons, respectively, in the layers of the network. The optimal architecture with an accuracy of 98.03% was found to have a 20% depth percentage and a width reduction factor of 4.

However, CNNs were outperformed by other deep learning algorithms. In particular, an LSTM algorithm was seen to perform better than a CNN algorithm in the classification of dynamic gestures acquired in a data glove (Simão et al., 2019). The LSTM classification accuracy was 96.5% for seen users and 89.1% for unseen users, while CNN achieved an accuracy of 81.9% and 54.7% for seen and unseen users, respectively. However, when a smaller percentage of the test users are used, CNN performs comparatively with LSTM and even outperforms it in some of these scenarios. This may have occurred because as the number of test users increases, the advantage of the memory properties of LSTM materializes.

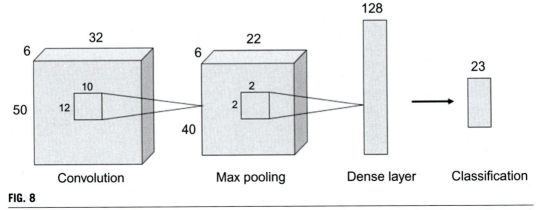

**FIG. 8**

Simple convolutional neural network architecture for gesture recognition (Diliberti et al., 2019).

Furthermore, a deep neural network (DNN) was utilized in classifying hand gestures acquired by a passive RFID data glove (Kantareddy et al., 2019). The DNN comprised of three fully connected hidden layers with 64, 128, and 32 neurons, respectively. Subsequently, its performance was compared with CNN, SVM, and random forest classifier (RFC). The CNN consisted of three 1D convolutional layers with 64, 128, and 64 filters, respectively, while the RFC had 10 trees, an average depth of 14.1 and an average number of 244.6 nodes. The DNN algorithm achieved an accuracy of 99%, while RFC, CNN, and SVM achieved an accuracy of 98%, 97%, and 86%, respectively. The CNN was outperformed by DNN because the DNN algorithm converged the global information, while the CNN algorithm only extracted the local information.

In addition, a deep learning algorithm was employed in the prediction of hand gestures. This involves predicting the next gesture to be performed by the user within a specific time frame. It helps to improve human-computer interactions by increasing the speed of gesture classification. Notably, RNN was used to predict hand gestures because of its ability to learn the temporal properties of the continuous data (Kanokoda et al., 2019). The performance of the RNN shown in Fig. 9 was compared to a time-delay neural network (TDNN) and a multiple linear regression (MLR) algorithm. Although TDNNs are proven algorithms in gesture prediction, they are limited to learning short-range dependencies and can only operate within fixed-size temporal windows (Sak et al., 2014). The results showed that the deep learning algorithm, RNN, outperformed both TDNN and MLR with a classification accuracy of 90.8% and 74.0% in predicting the next 100 ms and 300 ms of gestures, respectively.

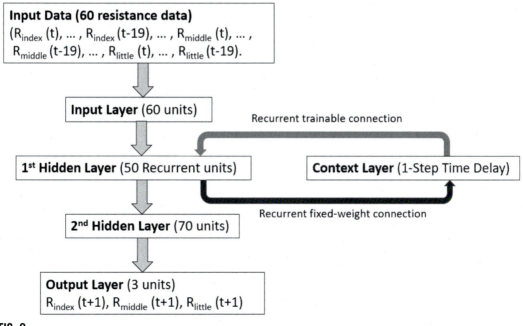

**FIG. 9**

Recurrent neural network for gesture prediction (Kanokoda et al., 2019).

## 5 Discussion and future trends

In the chapter, we have reviewed the applications of several machine learning algorithms on glove-based gesture classification. Moreover, we have shown that machine learning algorithms perform excellently in classifying hand gestures. However, the classification accuracy reduces in unseen experiments when the validation data set is made up of users that were not included in the training set. Seen experiments illustrate applications where the glove system will be used by known users, while unseen experiments illustrate commercial applications where a new user can use the glove system without re-training of the algorithm. The disparity between the accuracy in seen and unseen experiments is exemplified in Luzanin's study (Luzanin and Plancak, 2014), where the classification accuracy dropped from 95.19% in a seen experiment to 64.22% in an unseen experiment. This phenomenon can be explained mainly by the inadequate number of users in the training data set. Particularly, most studies have less than 10 participants in both the training and validation data sets. This increases the significance of the disparities in hand dimensions on the classification accuracy of the algorithm, as the training data sets do not provide a good sample size of hand dimensions.

In addition, we analyze the performance of deep learning algorithms on gesture classification. Notably, we observe that they perform better than classical machine learning algorithms. Although the number of studies illustrating the application of deep learning on glove-based gesture classification are small, we observed that deep learning algorithms were better performers than classical ML algorithms. In particular, CNN outperformed PCA-SVM by 18.8% in classifying ASL gestures (Fang et al., 2019). Moreover, a DNN algorithm outperformed an SVM algorithm by 13% (Kantareddy et al., 2019). These results show significant increases in classification accuracy by deep learning algorithms. Therefore, they increase the commercial viability of data gloves in gesture classification applications. However, the limited amount of studies makes it impossible to select the best performing deep learning algorithm, but we observe that CNN and LSTM are the most prominent among the studies reviewed as illustrated in Table 2.

A limitation to the use of deep learning algorithms in glove-based classification scenario is the lack of public data sets on which to evaluate the algorithms. This restricts researchers to creating their own experiments with a small number of participants. The use of public data sets will greatly increase contributions to the field as researchers will concentrate on developing novel deep learning algorithms to accurately classify the data. Moreover, public data sets enable the comparison of several deep learning algorithms. Thereby, ensuring that the best performing deep learning algorithms are identified.

Another potential research area is the application of deep learning in more hand gesture classification scenarios. Due to the small amount of studies utilizing deep learning, there are no applications of deep learning in scenarios such as grasp classification and other custom taxonomies. Research in this field will reveal the performance and limitations of deep learning algorithms in these scenarios.

Furthermore, the limited amount of studies illustrate that this research area is still novel and can be very fertile. Notably, hybrid models of deep learning techniques such as CNN-RNN and CNN-LSTM have shown excellent performance in the classification of surface electromyography (sEMG) signals (Hu et al., 2018; Wu et al., 2018). Furthermore, popular deep learning algorithms like Deep Boltzmann Machine and generative adversarial networks (GAN) have also shown very high classification accuracy in camera-based gesture recognition (Rastgoo et al., 2018; Zhang and Shi, 2017).

**Table 2** Summarized review of glove-based gesture classification with deep learning algorithms.

| Glove | Application | Algorithm | Accuracy | Reference |
|---|---|---|---|---|
| IMU data glove | Sign language | CNN | 99.6% | (Fang et al., 2019) |
| | | LSTM | 82.0% | |
| | | PCA-SVM | 80.8% | |
| IMU data glove | Real-time gesture recognition for HCI | CNN | 98.03 | (Diliberti et al., 2019) |
| N/A | Robot teleoperation | LSTM | 96.5% (seen) 89.1% (unseen) | (Simão et al., 2019) |
| | | CNN | 81.9% (seen) 54.7% (unseen) | |
| Passive RFID glove | Custom gestures for gesture recognition | DNN | 99% | (Kantareddy et al., 2019) |
| | | CNN | 97% | |
| | | SVM | 86% | |
| | | RFC | 98% | |
| Data glove with conductive sensors | Gesture prediction | RNN | 90.8% (100 ms) 74.0% (300 ms) | (Kanokoda et al., 2019) |
| | | TDNN | 90.4% (100 ms) 72.4% (300 ms) | |
| | | MLR | 75.4 (100 ms) 59.9 (300 ms) | |

These algorithms have not been implemented in glove-based gesture classification and present a unique research gap in significantly increasing the classification of glove-based applications.

Therefore, we propose that researchers utilize novel deep learning algorithms such as CNN-LSTM for future glove-based gesture classification studies. We recommend CNN-LSTM because our review has shown that these two algorithms provide the highest classification accuracy in glove-based gesture classification studies, and the hybrid combination of these algorithms will provide robust feature extraction and better sequence prediction especially in the classification of dynamic gestures in activity classification scenarios. Furthermore, we recommend that these studies comprise of at least 10 participants to provide a large data set for the algorithm.

# 6 Conclusion

In this study, we have provided an extensive review of classical machine learning and deep learning algorithms implemented in glove-based gesture classification. We have also shown that deep learning algorithms perform better than machine learning algorithms. Moreover, the limitations restricting the application of deep learning algorithms have been identified alongside our proposed solutions. Furthermore, we highlight potential areas of research that may increase the commercial viability of glove-based gesture classification. Finally, we recommend CNN-LSTM for future glove-based classification studies because of its accurate feature extraction and sequence prediction capabilities.

# References

5DT, 2020. 5DT Data Glove Ultra—5DT [Internet]. Available from: https://5dt.com/5dt-data-glove-ultra/.

Altman, N.S., 1992. An introduction to kernel and nearest-neighbor nonparametric regression. Am. Stat. 46 (3), 175–185.

Atalay, O., Kennon, W.R., Demirok, E., 2014. Weft-knitted strain sensor for monitoring respiratory rate and its electro-mechanical modeling. IEEE Sensors J. 15 (1), 110–122.

Axtell, R.E., Fornwald, M., 1991. Gestures: The do's and Taboos of Body Language around the World. Wiley, New York.

Beale, R., Edwards, A.D., 1990. Gestures and neural networks in human-computer interaction. In: IEEE Colloquium on neural Nets in Human-Computer Interaction. IET, pp. 1–5.

Caine, K.E., Fisk, A.D., Rogers, W.A., 2006. Benefits and privacy concerns of a home equipped with a visual sensing system: a perspective from older adults. In: Proceedings of the Human Factors and Ergonomics Society Annual Meeting. vol. 50(2). SAGE Publications, Sage CA: Los Angeles, CA, pp. 180–184.

Chen, S., Lou, Z., Chen, D., Jiang, K., Shen, G., 2016. Polymer-enhanced highly stretchable conductive Fiber strain sensor used for electronic data gloves. Adv. Mater. Technol. 1 (7), 1600136.

Conn, M.A., Sharma, S., 2016. Immersive telerobotics using the oculus rift and the 5DT ultra data glove. In: 2016 International Conference on Collaboration Technologies and Systems (CTS). IEEE, pp. 387–391.

Cortes, C., Vapnik, V., 1995. Support-vector networks. Mach. Learn. 20 (3), 273–297.

CyberGlove II, 2020. CyberGlove Systems LLC [Internet]. CyberGlove Systems LLC. Available from: http://www.cyberglovesystems.com/cyberglove-ii/.

da Silva, A.F., Gonçalves, A.F., Mendes, P.M., Correia, J.H., 2011. FBG sensing glove for monitoring hand posture. IEEE Sensors J. 11 (10), 2442–2448.

Diliberti, N., Peng, C., Kaufman, C., Dong, Y., Hansberger, J.T., 2019. Real-time gesture recognition using 3D sensory data and a light convolutional neural network. In: Proceedings of the 27th ACM International Conference on Multimedia, pp. 401–410.

Dipietro, L., Sabatini, A.M., Dario, P., 2008. A survey of glove-based systems and their applications. IEEE Trans. Syst. Man Cybern. Part C Appl. Rev. 38 (4), 461–482.

Fang, B., Guo, D., Sun, F., Liu, H., Wu, Y., 2015. A robotic hand-arm teleoperation system using human arm/hand with a novel data glove. In: 2015 IEEE International Conference on Robotics and Biomimetics (ROBIO). IEEE, pp. 2483–2488.

Fang, B., Lv, Q., Shan, J., Sun, F., Liu, H., Guo, D., Zhao, Y., 2019. Dynamic gesture recognition using inertial sensors-based data gloves. In: 2019 IEEE 4th International Conference on Advanced Robotics and Mechatronics (ICARM). IEEE, pp. 390–395.

Goodfellow, I., Bengio, Y., Courville, A., 2016. Deep Learning. MIT Press.

Heumer, G., Amor, H.B., Weber, M., Jung, B., 2007. Grasp recognition with uncalibrated data gloves—a comparison of classification methods. In: 2007 IEEE Virtual Reality Conference. IEEE, pp. 19–26.

Hsiao, P.C., Yang, S.Y., Lin, B.S., Lee, I.J., Chou, W., 2015. Data glove embedded with 9-axis IMU and force sensing sensors for evaluation of hand function. In: 2015 37th Annual International Conference of the IEEE Engineering In Medicine and Biology Society (EMBC). IEEE, pp. 4631–4634.

Hu, Y., Wong, Y., Wei, W., Du, Y., Kankanhalli, M., Geng, W., 2018. A novel attention-based hybrid CNN-RNN architecture for sEMG-based gesture recognition. PLoS One 13 (10).

Huang, G.B., Wang, D.H., Lan, Y., 2011 Jun 1. Extreme learning machines: a survey. Int. J. Mach. Learn. Cybern. 2 (2), 107–122.

Iannizzotto, G., Villari, M., Vita, L., 2001. Hand tracking for human-computer interaction with graylevel visualglove: Turning back to the simple way. In: Proceedings of the 2001 Workshop on Perceptive User Interfaces, pp. 1–7.

Ibarguren, A., Maurtua, I., Sierra, B., 2010. Layered architecture for real time sign recognition: hand gesture and movement. Eng. Appl. Artif. Intel. 23 (7), 1216–1228.

Jack, D., Boian, R., Merians, A.S., Tremaine, M., Burdea, G.C., Adamovich, S.V., Recce, M., Poizner, H., 2001. Virtual reality-enhanced stroke rehabilitation. IEEE Trans. Neural Syst. Rehabil. Eng. 9 (3), 308–318.

Jhang, L.H., Santiago, C., Chiu, C.S., 2017. Multi-sensor based glove control of an industrial mobile robot arm. In: 2017 International Automatic Control Conference (CACS). IEEE, pp. 1–6.

Jin, S., Li, Y., Lu, G.M., Luo, J.X., Chen, W.D., Zheng, X.X., 2011. SOM-based hand gesture recognition for virtual interactions. In: 2011 IEEE International Symposium on VR Innovation. IEEE, pp. 317–322.

Kanokoda, T., Kushitani, Y., Shimada, M., Shirakashi, J.I., 2019. Gesture prediction using wearable sensing systems with neural networks for temporal data analysis. Sensors 19 (3), 710.

Kantareddy, S.N., Sun, Y., Bhattacharyya, R., Sarma, S.E., 2019. Learning gestures using a passive data-glove with RFID tags. In: 2019 IEEE International Conference on RFID Technology and Applications (RFID-TA). IEEE, pp. 327–332.

Krizhevsky, A., Sutskever, I., Hinton, G.E., 2012. Imagenet classification with deep convolutional neural networks. In: Advances in Neural Information Processing Systems, pp. 1097–1105.

Kuzmanic, A., Zanchi, V., 2007. Hand shape classification using dtw and lcss as similarity measures for vision-based gesture recognition system. In: EUROCON 2007-The International Conference on "Computer as a Tool". IEEE, pp. 264–269.

Lau, D., Chen, Z., Teo, J.T., Ng, S.H., Rumpel, H., Lian, Y., Yang, H., Kei, P.L., 2013. Intensity-modulated microbend fiber optic sensor for respiratory monitoring and gating during MRI. I.E.E.E. Trans. Biomed. Eng. 60 (9), 2655–2662.

LeCun, Y., Bengio, Y., Hinton, G., 2015. Deep learning. Nature 521 (7553), 436–444.

Lin, B.S., Lee, I.J., Hsiao, P.C., Yang, S.Y., Chou, W., 2014. Data glove embedded with 6-DOF inertial sensors for hand rehabilitation. In: 2014 Tenth International Conference on Intelligent Information Hiding and Multimedia Signal Processing. IEEE, pp. 25–28.

Lu, G., Shark, L.K., Hall, G., Zeshan, U., 2012. Immersive manipulation of virtual objects through glove-based hand gesture interaction. Virtual Reality 16 (3), 243–252.

Lu, D., Yu, Y., Liu, H., 2016. Gesture recognition using data glove: an extreme learning machine method. In: 2016 IEEE International Conference on Robotics and Biomimetics (ROBIO). IEEE, pp. 1349–1354.

Luzanin, O., Plancak, M., 2014. Hand Gesture Recognition Using Low-Budget Data Glove and Cluster-Trained Probabilistic Neural Network. Assembly Automation.

Morris, D., 1979. Gestures, their Origins and Distribution. Stein & Day Pub.

Murakami, K., Taguchi, H., 1991. Gesture recognition using recurrent neural networks. In: Proceedings of the SIGCHI Conference on Human Factors in Computing Systems, pp. 237–242.

Neto, P., Pereira, D., Pires, J.N., Moreira, A.P., 2013. Real-time and continuous hand gesture spotting: an approach based on artificial neural networks. In: 2013 IEEE International Conference on Robotics and Automation. IEEE, pp. 178–183.

Qin, Z., Jiang, Z., Chen, J., Hu, C., Ma, Y., 2019. sEMG-based tremor severity evaluation for Parkinson's disease using a light-weight CNN. IEEE Signal Process Lett. 26 (4), 637–641.

Rastgoo, R., Kiani, K., Escalera, S., 2018. Multi-modal deep hand sign language recognition in still images using restricted Boltzmann machine. Entropy 20 (11), 809.

Rautaray, S.S., Agrawal, A., 2015. Vision based hand gesture recognition for human computer interaction: a survey. Artif. Intell. Rev. 43 (1), 1–54.

Sak, H., Senior, A.W., Beaufays, F., 2014. Long short-term memory recurrent neural network architectures for large scale acoustic modeling. In: INTERSPEECH-2014, pp., 338–342. https://www.isca-speech.org/archive/interspeech_2014/i14_0338.html.

Schmidhuber, J., 2015. Deep learning in neural networks: an overview. Neural Netw. 61, 85–117.

Schwarz, R.J., Taylor, C.L., 1955. The anatomy and mechanics of the human hand. Artif. Limbs 2 (2), 22–35.

Shen, Z., Yi, J., Li, X., Lo, M.H., Chen, M.Z., Hu, Y., Wang, Z., 2016. A soft stretchable bending sensor and data glove applications. Rob. Biomimetics 3 (1), 22.

Simão, M.A., Gibaru, O., Neto, P., 2019. Online recognition of incomplete gesture data to interface collaborative robots. IEEE Trans. Ind. Electron. 66 (12), 9372–9382.

Specht, D.F., 1990. Probabilistic neural networks. Neural Netw. 3 (1), 109–118.

Sturman, D.J., Zeltzer, D., 1994. A survey of glove-based input. IEEE Comput. Graph. Appl. 14 (1), 30–39.

Tang, A.T., 2019. Software Defined Networking: Network Intrusion Detection System (Doctoral dissertation). University of Leeds.

Tang, Z., Jia, S., Wang, F., Bian, C., Chen, Y., Wang, Y., Li, B., 2018. Highly stretchable core–sheath fibers via wet-spinning for wearable strain sensors. ACS Appl. Mater. Interfaces 10 (7), 6624–6635.

Watson, R., 1993. A Survey of Gesture Recognition Techniques. Trinity College Dublin, Department of Computer Science.

Weissmann, J., Salomon, R., 1999. Gesture recognition for virtual reality applications using data gloves and neural networks. In: IJCNN'99. International Joint Conference on Neural Networks. Proceedings (Cat. No. 99CH36339). vol. 3. IEEE, pp. 2043–2046.

Witten, I.H., Frank, E., Hall, M.A., 2005. Practical Machine Learning Tools and Techniques. Morgan Kaufmann, p. 578.

Wu, J., Zhou, D., Too, C.O., Wallace, G.G., 2005. Conducting polymer coated lycra. Synth. Met. 155 (3), 698–701.

Wu, Y., Zheng, B., Zhao, Y., 2018. Dynamic gesture recognition based on LSTM-CNN. In: 2018 Chinese Automation Congress (CAC). IEEE, pp. 2446–2450.

Xu, D., 2006. A neural network approach for hand gesture recognition in virtual reality driving training system of SPG. In: 18th International Conference on Pattern Recognition (ICPR'06). vol. 3. IEEE, pp. 519–522.

Yang, X., Chen, X., Cao, X., Wei, S., Zhang, X., 2016. Chinese sign language recognition based on an optimized tree-structure framework. IEEE J. Biomed. Health Inform. 21 (4), 994–1004.

Yao, Q., Wang, R., Fan, X., Liu, J., Li, Y., 2020. Multi-class arrhythmia detection from 12-lead varied-length ECG using attention-based time-incremental convolutional neural network. Inform. Fusion 53, 174–182.

Zhang, J., Shi, Z., 2017. Deformable deep convolutional generative adversarial network in microwave based hand gesture recognition system. In: 2017 9th International Conference on Wireless Communications and Signal Processing (WCSP). IEEE, pp. 1–6.

Zhang, M., Wang, C., Wang, Q., Jian, M., Zhang, Y., 2016. Sheath–core graphite/silk fiber made by dry-meyer-rod-coating for wearable strain sensors. ACS Appl. Mater. Interfaces 8 (32), 20894–20899.

# An ensemble approach for evaluating the cognitive performance of human population at high altitude

**Dipankar Sengupta[a], Vijay Kumar Sharma[b], Sunil Kumar Hota[b], Ravi B. Srivastava[b], and Pradeep Kumar Naik[c]**

*PGJCCR, Queens University Belfast, Belfast, United Kingdom[a] DIHAR, Defense Research & Development Organization, Leh, Jammu & Kashmir, India[b] School of Life Sciences, Sambalpur University, Sambalpur, Orissa, India[c]*

## Chapter outline

## 1 Introduction

Hypobaric hypoxia at high altitude can cause the loss of memory, recall, and learning resulting in cognitive impairment in addition to the acute mountain sickness (AMS), high-altitude pulmonary edema (HAPE), high-altitude cerebral edema (HACE), and neurophysiological disturbances with insomnia and dizziness (Bahrke and Shukitt-Hale, 1993; Lieberman et al., 1994; Ray et al., 2019) (Fig. 1).

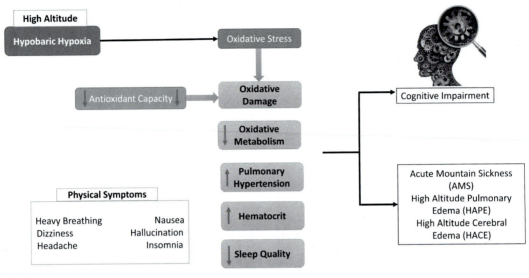

**FIG. 1**

In hypobaric hypoxia, the body is deprived of sufficient oxygen supply. At high altitude, there is fall in the atmospheric pressure and oxygen, which leads to oxidative stress. This impacts the physiology and metabolism causing oxidative damage, reduction in oxidative metabolism, and sleep quality, along with an increase in pulmonary hypertension and the hematocrit values. An individual may have an early stage cognitive impairment and develop acute mountain sickness, which if not clinically addressed may cause high-altitude pulmonary edema or high-altitude cerebral edema.

The neurological symptoms are due to lack of proper oxygen supply to brain that can alter neurotransmitter synthesis, uptake, and release and free radical generation and related excitotoxic neuronal damage (Askew, 2002; Benveniste et al., 1984; Hota et al., 2010; Rossi et al., 2000). Changes in gene expression and protein functions are also associated with hypoxia and ischemia (Chandel et al., 1998; Gorter et al., 1997; Hartman et al., 2005; Nalivaeva and Rybnikova, 2019; Pellegrini-Giampietro et al., 1992). Ascent to high altitude also increases sensory discrimination, delay in the evaluation process, and impairment of short-term memory (Hayashi et al., 2005; Nation et al., 2017; Singh et al., 2003). Chronic hypoxia exposure of volunteers residing at high altitude also revealed impairment in verbal working memory (Ray et al., 2019; Yan et al., 2011).

In the trans-Himalayan region, an early stage of cognitive impairment is commonly observed in the population who have been residing at an altitude ≥4300 m for a period of at least 12 months. This form is called the mild cognitive impairment (MCI), which is characterized by a decline in cognitive abilities [mental processes regulating perform day-to-day functions] including memory, thinking, and decision-making (Fig. 2).

Some of the cognitive domain tests commonly used for screening MCI are Multidomain Cognitive Screening Test (MDCST) (Hota et al., 2012; Sharma et al., 2014), Mini Mental State Examination (MMSE) (Folstein et al., 1975; Pan et al., 2020), Montreal cognitive Assessment (MoCA) (Nasreddine et al., 2005; Pan et al., 2020), Mini-Cog (Borson et al., 2000), Computer Administered

Control                          MCI

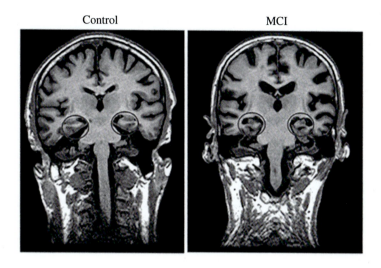

**FIG. 2**

Brain imaging studies show shrinkage of hippocampus region in MCI, which plays an important role in learning and memory (Aurtenetxe et al., 2016). Existing medical conditions like diabetes, high blood pressure, etc. increases the risk for an individual developing MCI at high altitude.

Neuropsychological Score (CANS-MCI) (Tornatore et al., 2005), and Patient Reported Outcomes in Cognitive Impairment (PROCOG) (Frank et al., 2006). Majority of these tests lack the required screening specificity and sensitivity. A few of them specifically screen for a deficit of domains, while others are bulky and time consuming. In addition, they often have a complex scoring system, which needs the expertise of a trained person. A study by Hota et al. showed MDCST to be the most effective for MCI assessment among the listed cognitive tests (Hota et al., 2012). It is most promising in particular for the demographic studies, as it exhibits excellent psychometric properties in terms of sensitivity and test-retest reliability. Considering the limitations of MMSE and MoCA, MDCST was designed to establish an easy to administer and a more reliable test for detection of MCI at early stages (Hota et al., 2012). Moreover, it is based on findings that suggest involvement of several brain regions in cognitive function. MDCST is comprehensive as it covers nine domain assessments: Orientation, Memory Registration, Visuospatial Executive, Object Recognition, Attention, Recall, Coordination & Learning, Language and Procedural Memory and, in comparison, has a better specificity with sensitivity. Thus, it provides an opportunity to increase the scope of cognitive assessment to domains like procedural memory, mindbody coordination, attention, and learning of complex tasks through improvised and customized psychometric tests. Beck Depression Inventory (BDI) with insomnia may further help in identification of hitherto concealed depression (Beck et al., 1961).

There are no demographic studies that measure the prevalence of MCI with Beck Depression Inventory (BDI), insomnia, and clinical features collected from routine assessments [like blood glucose level, blood pressure, blood cholesterol, complete blood count, kidney, and liver functionality]. A rule-based study can assist in analyzing and identifying risk factors specific to population cohorts for their cognitive decline at higher altitude ($\geq$4300 m). It has been a common practice in clinical practice to ignore the rigor and sophistication of a data mining, and rather focus on results with an interpretation

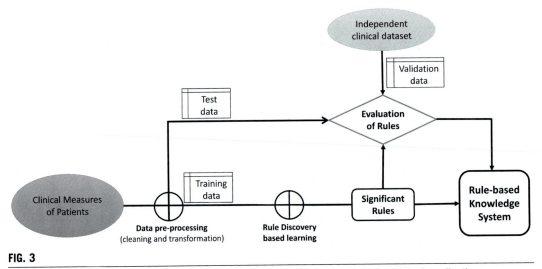

**FIG. 3**

Schematic representation for development of rule-based knowledge systems for clinical applications.

(Anhøj, 2003; Beckmann and Lew, 2016; Handelman et al., 2018). "Rule-based" analysis has been fairly promising in the domain, being a human-comprehensible knowledge system, and therefore suitable for deciphering new rules for clinical applications (Fig. 3). Association rule mining is a general-purpose rule discovery scheme of finding disease cooccurrences in electronic health record data that has been widely used to find disease-disease, disease-finding, and disease-drug cooccurrences (Agrawal et al., 1993; Brossette et al., 1998; Chen et al., 2008; Hanauer et al., 2009; Said et al., 2018; Sengupta and Naik, 2013).

In this study, we evaluate the cognitive parameters identified by MDCST along with the clinical features, which can be associated with MCI, BDI and sleep. Based on the native's residence altitude, there are two population cohorts which are been compared in this study: Highlanders (natives of altitude $\geq$1500 m but <4300 m) and Lowlanders (natives of altitude $\leq$350 m), who have been residing at an altitude $\geq$4300 m for at least 18 months. We apply an ensemble technique combining differential expression analysis with unsupervised machine learning technique to augur rules for the two cohorts. These rules help in the identification of the cognitive and clinical features which can be used for early identification of mild cognitive impairment and depression among the respective population cohorts.

## 2 Methodology

### 2.1 Data collection

Fig. 4 illustrates the overall methodology of this study in a logical flow diagram. Data used in this study was collected as a field research [August 2009–January 2011] of High-Altitude Physiology Division, Defence Institute of High-Altitude Research (DIHAR), DRDO, Leh. Data collection and subsequent studies are based on the ethical approval of the institutional ethics committee DIHAR (Hota et al., 2012).

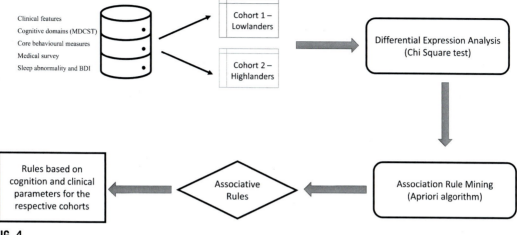

**FIG. 4**

Schematic representation of knowledge discovery process used for the identification of key cognitive parameters and clinical features for mild cognitive impairment.

The clinical features along with the parameters from MDCST were obtained from a group of volunteers in the age group of 25–40 comprising of Lowlanders and Highlanders, who have been residing at high altitude ($\geq$4300 m) (Table 1). All the participants were informed about the study purpose, protocol, and expected outcome (Hota et al., 2012). Baseline recordings were collected for both the population categories with the onset of study at an altitude of less than 350 m. Furthermore, there was a longitudinal follow-up of the cohort that ascended to high altitude ($>$4300 m) and lived there for the duration of 18 months (Hota et al., 2012).

Clinical features in this study include results from lipid profiling, kidney function test (KFT), liver function test (LFT), sugar level, blood pressure, and pulse rate. MDCST was performed independently on all the volunteers. The scores were compared to establish the subjective dependability in this scoring. Additionally, a medical survey of all the volunteers was performed via a questionnaire related to the occurrence of chronic diseases, physical and physiological ailments, heart problems, stroke, epilepsy, head injury, drug abuse, psychological disorders, and general health status (Hota et al., 2012). Data for core behavioral measures (CBM) such as the alcohol consumption, tobacco use, diet, and physical activity were also collected from all the subjects in accordance with the WHO guidelines (WHO, 2020). All the tests were administered by field investigators under the supervision of a clinical psychiatrist.

| Table 1 Inclusion criteria of human subjects for this study. | |
| --- | --- |
| **Parameter** | **Value** |
| Age (in years) (mean $\pm$ SEM) | 36.3 $\pm$ 6.84 |
| Education (in years) (mean $\pm$ SEM) | 12 $\pm$ 2 |
| Geographical location | Jammu & Kashmir, India |
| Ethnic origin of all participants | India |

## 2.2 Data processing and feature selection

Respective cohort subjects with underlying heart disease, chest pain, stroke/infarction/cerebral hemorrhage, renal failure, diabetes, viral hepatitis, chronic disease, and gastro-esophageal reflux disease (GERD) were excluded from this study. Also, subjects with previous neurologic/psychiatric symptoms, major surgery, and familial disorders were ruled out. Nevertheless, the respective elimination steps ensured inclusion of only healthy subjects in the study. Data of 200 healthy volunteers, 100 each for Lowlander, and Highlander were randomly sampled for the study.

Following clinical features were measured under the supervision of registered medical practitioner: blood glucose (BS), systolic blood pressure (SBP), diastolic blood pressure (DBP), pulse rate (PR), blood urea nitrogen (BUN), serum creatinine, serum glutamic oxaloacetic transaminase (SGOT), serum pyruvic transaminase (SGPT), total cholesterol (TC), triglycerides (TGL), high-density lipoprotein (HDL), low-density lipoprotein (LDL), very low-density lipoprotein (VLDL), TC/HDL cholesterol ratio, LDL/HDL ratio, homocysteine, vitamin B-12, and folic acid. The value for each of these parameters was normalized into an ordinal form and scaled as low, normal, and high, respectively, based upon the prescribed range (Marshall et al., 2014).

MDCST includes screening for nine cognitive domains: Orientation, Memory Registration, Visuospatial Executive, Object Recognition, Attention, Recall, Coordination & Learning, Language, and Procedural Memory (Hota et al., 2012). Each of these parameters are scored in magnitude of five with max MDCST cumulative score of 45. A cumulative MDCST score $\leq 34$ indicates onset or presence of MCI. For the subjects who qualified inclusion criterion, Sleep abnormality and Beck Depression Inventory (BDI) (Beck et al., 1961) were applied to assess activities of daily living and to investigate the presence of hitherto undetected depression. Sleep was measured in scale of 0/1, with 1 indicating abnormality, while for BDI, value $\geq 7$ indicates abnormality.

## 2.3 Differential expression analyses

The statistical significance between the anticipated and observed frequencies was assessed performing a chi-square test comparing the two cohorts. This test enables the comparison of observed and expected frequencies objectively since it is not always possible to judge from the data whether they are different enough to be considered statistically significant (Bailey et al., 1982). Multivariate statistical analysis was performed on the significant factors to identify the independent clinical and cognitive risk factors for the onset of cognitive impairment. The level of statistical significance was defined by the criteria, $P$-value $<.05$. All the statistical analysis was performed using STATISTICA DATAMINER 9.1 (StatSoft, Inc., 2010).

## 2.4 Association rule mining

Association mining, the task of finding associative rules between items in a data set, has received considerable attention, particularly since the publication of the AIS and apriori algorithms (Anand Hareendran and Vinod Chandra, 2017; Sarıyer and Öcal Taşar, 2020; Sengupta and Naik, 2013a). This study uses an apriori algorithm to obtain the information related to clinical and cognitive screening parameters to be associated with onset of cognitive impairment. It is a popular data mining technique that attempts to find interesting patterns in large databases (Agrawal et al., 1993; Borgelt, 2010; Goethals, n.d.).

The apriori algorithm exploits the downward closure property, which states that if an item-set is infrequent, all of its supersets must be infrequent (Sengupta and Naik, 2013a). Facilitates filtering item-sets but is limiting while mining infrequent item-sets. Each of the filtered item-set is backed by a statistical measure called support. For an item-set $X \subset I$, support$(X) = s$, if the fraction of transactions in the data set $D$ containing $X = s$ (Agrawal and Srikant, 1994). The classic framework for association rule mining uses support and confidence as thresholds for constraining the search space. The confidence or accuracy of an association rule $X \Rightarrow Y$ in $D$ is the conditional probability of having $Y$ contained in a transaction, given that $X$ is contained in that transaction: confidence $(X \Rightarrow Y) = P(Y \mid X) = $ support$(XY)$/support$(X)$ (Goethals, n.d.). In general, support represents the ratio of samples among the data set that simultaneously satisfies both, condition $X$ in the antecedent part and condition $Y$ in the consequent part of a rule, while confidence represents the ratio of samples that satisfy both conditions $X$ and $Y$, but only among those that satisfy condition $X$ in the antecedent part (Jung et al., 2013). A confidence value of 100 for a certain rule means that the possibility of obtaining outcome $Y$ when $X$ in a given condition $(X \rightarrow Y)$ is 100% (i.e., certain rule); if not, the possibility of $A \rightarrow B$ is defined as a value (possible rule) between 0 and 100.

## 2.5 Experimental set-up

All the experiments in this study were implemented via STATISTICA 9.1 (StatSoft, Inc., 2010) software. It is grueling to predispose appropriate criteria for any two parameters in association rule mining, since information is acquired centered on a minimum threshold for support and confidence. Therefore, the minimum confidence level was subjected to at least 30%, with a minimum support of 10%; domain specialists (human cognition and physiology) were consulted for the association rules generated, while the final confidence level was determined considering physician's opinion. Total cognitive score, BDI score, and sleep were declared as the response indicators and the remaining parameters were defined to be as categorical indicators. For maximum components for any deciphered rule, the antecedent and precedent iteration rate was set to 10.

The described experiment was set up and executed on a Dell precision workstation (M4700), with Intel(R) Core(TM) i7-3820QU CPU @ 2.70 GHz 8M cache, 4 cores and 8 threads, NVIDIA(R) Quadro(R) K1000M with 2 GB GDDR3, 32 GB RAM, and 1 TB hard disk.

# 3 Results and discussion

## 3.1 Differential analyses—Cognitive and clinical features

Table 2 represents Visuospatial Executive, Attention, and Coordination & Learning to be statistically significant screening parameters for Lowlanders in reference to the cumulative MDCST score, whereas Object recognition is significantly impaired corresponding to BDI as represented in Table 3. The Orientation parameter is found to be significantly associated with sleep abnormality (Table 4). In contrast, the results observed for Highlander population suggests Procedural Memory, Coordination and Learning, Visuospatial Executive, and Recall are statistically significant parameters against the cumulative MDCST score (Table 2), whereas no parameter is significant corresponding to BDI (Table 3) and sleep abnormality (Table 4).

Among the clinical features, the chi-square test reveals that although there is not a significant parameter for Lowlanders corresponding to either cumulative MDCST score, BDI, or sleep abnormality.

**Table 2 Cognitive screening parameters against cumulative MDCST score.**

|  | Lowlanders | | Highlanders | |
|---|---|---|---|---|
|  | Chi-square | *P*-value | Chi-square | *P*-value |
| Visuospatial executive | 22.5195 | .0002 | 15.1725 | .0044 |
| Attention | 15.2778 | .0016 | 2.0888 | .5542 |
| Coordination and learning | 14.2017 | .0067 | 16.4056 | .0058 |
| Language | 6.6546 | .1553 | 10.7607 | .0563 |
| Recall | 5.9658 | .3096 | 12.2461 | .0156 |
| Object recognition | 3.4211 | .3311 | 3.7738 | .1515 |
| Memory registration | 3.0049 | .2226 | 0.8685 | .6477 |
| Orientation | 2.2338 | .5253 | 3.9102 | .4183 |
| Procedural memory | 2.0308 | .1541 | 20.4540 | .0000 |

**Table 3 Cognitive screening parameters against BDI score.**

|  | Lowlanders | | Highlanders | |
|---|---|---|---|---|
|  | Chi-square | *P*-value | Chi-square | *P*-value |
| Object recognition | 9.5439 | .0229 | 4.7122 | .0948 |
| Coordination and learning | 6.0168 | .1979 | 6.4409 | .2657 |
| Recall | 4.7749 | .4440 | 2.2947 | .6817 |
| Visuospatial executive | 3.9827 | .4084 | 5.1914 | .2682 |
| Memory registration | 3.1067 | .2115 | 1.0602 | .5885 |
| Attention | 2.3175 | .5092 | 2.2973 | .5130 |
| Orientation | 1.9394 | .5851 | 2.6340 | .6208 |
| Language | 0.7826 | .9408 | 2.9747 | .7039 |
| Procedural memory | 0.6769 | .4106 | 0.0002 | .9880 |

**Table 4 Cognitive screening parameters against sleep abnormality score.**

|  | Lowlanders | | Highlanders | |
|---|---|---|---|---|
|  | Chi-square | *P*-value | Chi-square | *P*-value |
| Orientation | 9.1667 | .0272 | 6.1027 | .1916 |
| Attention | 4.0908 | .2518 | 3.0841 | .3788 |
| Object recognition | 3.0829 | .3790 | 1.9799 | .3716 |
| Language | 2.4253 | .6581 | 6.4835 | .2620 |
| Coordination and learning | 1.9974 | .7362 | 1.8216 | .8732 |
| Visuospatial executive | 1.7417 | .7831 | 1.3404 | .8545 |
| Recall | 1.6155 | .8994 | 1.2922 | .8627 |
| Memory registration | 1.5109 | .4698 | 1.3980 | .4971 |
| Procedural memory | 0.0677 | .7947 | 0.4686 | .4937 |

However, a significant parameter observed for Highlanders is vitamin B-12 level ($P$-value $= .0099$) that corresponded to cumulative MDCST score; total cholesterol level ($P$-value $= .0094$) that corresponded to BDI, and folic acid level ($P$-value $= .0023$) that corresponded to sleep abnormality.

## 3.2 Discovered associative rules

Table 5 enlists the associative rules observed among the Lowlander population within the defined criteria. Item-sets satisfying the support-percentage were subjected for discovery of association rules within the specified criteria. The rules suggest association of high vitamin B-12, HDL, BUN, and folic acid levels for MDCST, BDI, and sleep abnormality. Also, the alcoholic Lowlander population (alcoholic/nonalcoholic $==$ A) tend to have a low cumulative MDCST score, which indicates it may be a key factor to be analyzed in MCI screening.

While Table 6 enlists the association rules discovered within the defined criteria for the Highlander population. For Highlander population, item sets that satisfied the support-percentage were subjected to discovery of association rules within the specified mining criteria. The discovered rules showcase association of high values of vitamin B-12, HDL, VLDL, BUN, cholesterol, triglycerides, and folic acid for MDCST, BDI, and sleep abnormality. In comparison to Lowlander, the alcoholic Highlander population (alcoholic/nonalcoholic $==$ A) tend to show normal sleeping habit.

## 3.3 Discussion

Results from the study emphasizes that varied set of MDCST domains and clinical features should be used for the analyzing MCI and undetected depression (via BDI and sleep abnormality) for the respective population cohorts. MDCST considers nine different domains for analyzing cognitive performance in an individual. However, the statistical significance from our observations suggest that Visuospatial Executive, Attention, Coordination & Learning, Object recognition, and Orientation are the major cognitive screening parameters that need to be regularly monitored for Lowlanders. Whereas Procedural Memory, Coordination and Learning, Visuospatial Executive, and Recall are the key screening

**Table 5** Associative rules for the Lowlander population.

| Association rule | Support % | Confidence % | Correlation % |
|---|---|---|---|
| Alcoholic/nonalcoholic $==$ NA $==>$ BDI $==$ Normal_BDI | 40.91 | 54.55 | 68.38 |
| Alcoholic/nonalcoholic $==$ A $==>$ Abnormal_MDCST | 31.82 | 60.87 | 62.24 |
| BDI $==$ Normal_BDI $==>$ sleep $==$ Normal_Sleep | 47.73 | 87.50 | 74.62 |
| Normal_MDCST $==>$ BDI $==$ Normal_BDI | 36.36 | 48.48 | 59.38 |
| Vit-B12 $==$ High_VitB12, HDL $==$ High_HDL $==>$ Abnormal_MDCST | 50.00 | 100 | 74.16 |
| Blood Urea Nitrogen $==$ High_BUN, Vit-B12 $==$ High_VitB12, Vit-B12 $==$ High_VitB12 $==>$ Abnormal_Sleep | 52.27 | 100 | 76.79 |
| Folic Acid $==$ High_FA, Blood Urea Nitrogen $==$ High_ BUN $==>$ Abnormal_BDI | 61.36 | 64.28 | 78.73 |
| VLDL $==$ Normal_VLDL $==>$ Normal_BDI | 61.36 | 64.28 | 80.17 |

| Association rule | Support % | Confidence % | Correlation % |
|---|---|---|---|
| Normal_MDCST == > BDI == Normal_BDI | 41.30 | 76.00 | 66.15 |
| Alcoholic/Nonalcoholic == A == > sleep == Normal_Sleep | 43.48 | 58.82 | 67.27 |
| Sleep == Normal_Sleep == > BDI == Normal_BDI | 47.83 | 88.00 | 75.46 |
| Sleep == Normal_Sleep == > Normal_MDCST | 50.00 | 69.70 | 68.66 |
| HDL == High_HDL, VLDL == High_VLDL, Blood Urea Nitrogen == High_BUN, Vit-B12 == High_VitB12 == > Abnormal_MDCST | 50.00 | 58.97 | 72.22 |
| Total_Cholesterol == High_TC == > Abnormal_BDI | 52.17 | 96.00 | 73.19 |
| Creatinine == High_Creatinine, Triglycerides == High_TGL, HDL == High_HDL, Folic_Acid == High_FA, Vit-B12 == High_VitB12 == > Abnormal_Sleep | 50.00 | 58.97 | 72.22 |

**Table 6** Associative rules for the Highlander population.

parameters for the Highlanders. Furthermore, Lowlanders exhibit a higher rate of cognitive impairment and sleep abnormality compared to Highlanders at an altitude of 4300 m or more. There are no significant clinical features observed from goodness of fit for Lowlanders, whereas vitamin-B12, total cholesterol, and folic acid levels are found to be significantly associated with Highlander's cognitive performance.

Rules deduced from association mining suggests the alcoholic Lowlander population show low cognitive response with 60.87% of confidence. Also high levels of vitamin B-12 and HDL are associated with cognitive impairment (100% confidence), high vitamin B-12 and BUN are associated with sleep abnormality (100% confidence), and high levels of folic acid is associated with BDI (64.28%). Associative rules observed for Highlander population are significantly different compared to Lowlander population. The alcoholic Highlander population did not represent any significant rule corresponding to MDCST, but an important statistical observation suggests that they had normal sleep with 88% confidence. In Highlander population, high level of HDL, VLDL, BUN, and vitamin B-12 is found to be associated with cognitive impairment (58.97% confidence), while a high level of total cholesterol is associated with BDI (96%) and high level of creatinine, HDL, vitamin B-12, and folic acid to the sleep abnormality (58.97%).

## 4 Future opportunities

Data and research in this study were kindly supported by DIHAR, DRDO, India. The study identifies cognitive analyzers and clinical features for the Low ($\leq$350 m) and Highlander ($\geq$1500 m) population staying at higher altitudes ($>$4300 m) for a prolonged duration, which can be used for early screening of mild cognitive impairment and depression. Visuospatial Executive, Attention, Coordination & Learning, Object recognition, Procedural Memory, Recall, Language for Lowlander population, while Procedural Memory, Coordination and Learning, Visuospatial Executive, Recall, Language for Highlander population, respectively, are the key MDCST parameters identified for analyzing the cognitive performance with observed $P$-value $\leq.05$. These rules were evaluated by the human cognition and physiology experts from DIHAR, DRDO, India.

An interesting direction to further work upon would be longitudinal analysis of the identified features at an individual and population (Lowlander and Highlander) level, in association with early detection of mild cognitive impairment, beck depression inventory, and insomnia. Furthermore, a comparative analysis of the Lowlander and Highlander cohorts with the native population living at an altitude $\geq 4300$ m [e.g., Hikkim and Karzok in India, Dingboche in Nepal, etc.] can provide insights into the physiological and cognitive differentiation among the population.

Besides the unsupervised methodology discussed in this chapter, analyzing such biomedical longitudinal data sets using supervised learning approaches, like convolutional neural networks (CNN), random forests, gradient boosting trees (Zhao et al., 2019), regression-based linear mixed-effects model (Bandyopadhyay et al., 2011; Jensen and Ritz, 2018), or the most recent likelihood contrast model (Klén et al., 2020) can help in discovering new insights.

## 5 Conclusions

In this study, we have made first of an attempt to investigate the effects of prolonged stay at high altitudes ($\geq 4300$ m) for the respective Lowlander, as well as Highlander populations on their cognitive performance based on clinical features and cognitive screening parameters from MDCST. The parameters from MDCST are coupled with clinical features to analyze high-altitude-induced cognitive impairment and sleep abnormality. Healthy individuals with no clinical antecedents of depression were recruited to negate the influence of these factors on the cognitive performance. The subjects were recruited randomly for both the high-altitude and low-altitude location population.

Our data and the analyses identify the MDCST domains and clinical features that need to be analyzed for the identification of early onset cognitive impairment at high altitudes ($\geq 4300$ m) among Lowlander and Highlander populations. In principle, these parameters need to be further tested and validated clinically to be used for screening human subjects from their native geographical altitudes, planning their relocalization at higher altitudes.

## Acknowledgment

The work discussed in this chapter was kindly supported by DIHAR, DRDO Grant number—DIHAR/01/ASSIGN/12 (DIHAR—Leh, DRDO, Ministry of Defence, Government of India).

## References

Agrawal, R., Srikant, R., 1994. Fast algorithms for mining association rules. In: VLDB, pp. 487–499.

Agrawal, R., Imieliński, T., Swami, A., 1993. Mining association rules between sets of items in large databases. In: Proceedings of the 1993 ACM SIGMOD International Conference on Management of Data—SIGMOD '93. Association for Computing Machinery (ACM), New York, New York, USA, pp. 207–216, https://doi.org/10.1145/170035.170072.

Anand Hareendran, S., Vinod Chandra, S.S., 2017. Association rule mining in healthcare analytics. In: Lecture Notes in Computer Science (Including Subseries Lecture Notes in Artificial Intelligence and Lecture Notes in Bioinformatics). Springer Verlag, pp. 31–39, https://doi.org/10.1007/978-3-319-61845-6_4.

Anhøj, J., 2003. Generic design of web-based clinical databases. J. Med. Internet Res. 5, 158–175. https://doi.org/10.2196/jmir.5.4.e27.

Askew, E.W., 2002. Work at high altitude and oxidative stress: antioxidant nutrients. Toxicology 180, 107–119. https://doi.org/10.1016/S0300-483X(02)00385-2.

Aurtenetxe, S., García-Pacios, J., del Río, D., López, M.E., Pineda-Pardo, J.A., Marcos, A., Losada, M.L.D., López-Frutos, J.M., Maestú, F., 2016. Interference impacts working memory in mild cognitive impairment. Front. Neurosci. https://doi.org/10.3389/fnins.2016.00443.

Bahrke, M.S., Shukitt-Hale, B., 1993. Effects of altitude on mood, behaviour and cognitive functioning: a review. Sports Med. https://doi.org/10.2165/00007256-199316020-00003.

Bailey, K., Sokal, R.R., Rohlf, F.J., 1982. Biometry: the principles and practice of statistics in biological research (2nd ed.). J. Am. Stat. Assoc. https://doi.org/10.2307/2287349.

Bandyopadhyay, S., Ganguli, B., Chatterjee, A., 2011. A review of multivariate longitudinal data analysis. Stat. Methods Med. Res. https://doi.org/10.1177/0962280209340191.

Beck, A.T., Ward, C.H., Mendelson, M., Mock, J., Erbaugh, J., 1961. An inventory for measuring depression. Arch. Gen. Psychiatry 4, 561–571. https://doi.org/10.1001/archpsyc.1961.01710120031004.

Beckmann, J.S., Lew, D., 2016. Reconciling evidence-based medicine and precision medicine in the era of big data: challenges and opportunities. Genome Med. 8, 1–11. https://doi.org/10.1186/s13073-016-0388-7.

Benveniste, H., Drejer, J., Schousboe, A., Diemer, N.H., 1984. Elevation of the extracellular concentrations of glutamate and aspartate in rat hippocampus during transient cerebral ischemia monitored by intracerebral microdialysis. J. Neurochem. 43, 1369–1374. https://doi.org/10.1111/j.1471-4159.1984.tb05396.x.

Borgelt, C., 2010. Simple algorithms for frequent item set mining. Stud. Comput. Intell. 263, 351–369. https://doi.org/10.1007/978-3-642-05179-1_16.

Borson, S., Scanlan, J., Brush, M., Vitaliano, P., Dokmak, A., 2000. The Mini-Cog: a cognitive "vital signs" measure for dementia screening in multi-lingual elderly. Int. J. Geriatr. Psychiatry 15. https://doi.org/10.1002/1099-1166(200011)15:11<1021::AID-GPS234>3.0.CO;2-6.

Brossette, S.E., Sprague, A.P., Hardin, J.M., Waites, K.B., Jones, W.T., Moser, S.A., 1998. Association rules and data mining in hospital infection control and public health surveillance. J. Am. Med. Inform. Assoc. 5, 373–381. https://doi.org/10.1136/jamia.1998.0050373.

Chandel, N.S., Maltepe, E., Goldwasser, E., Mathieu, C.E., Simon, M.C., Schumacker, P.T., 1998. Mitochondrial reactive oxygen species trigger hypoxia-induced transcription. Proc. Natl. Acad. Sci. U. S. A. 95, 11715–11720. https://doi.org/10.1073/pnas.95.20.11715.

Chen, E.S., Hripcsak, G., Xu, H., Markatou, M., Friedman, C., 2008. Automated acquisition of disease-drug knowledge from biomedical and clinical documents: an initial study. J. Am. Med. Inform. Assoc. 15, 87–98. https://doi.org/10.1197/jamia.M2401.

Folstein, M.F., Folstein, S.E., McHugh, P.R., 1975. "Mini-mental state". A practical method for grading the cognitive state of patients for the clinician. J. Psychiatr. Res. 12, 189–198. https://doi.org/10.1016/0022-3956(75)90026-6.

Frank, L., Flynn, J.A., Kleinman, L., Margolis, M.K., Matza, L.S., Beck, C., Bowman, L., 2006. Validation of a new symptom impact questionnaire for mild to moderate cognitive impairment. Int. Psychogeriatr. 18, 135–149. https://doi.org/10.1017/S1041610205002887.

Goethals, B., n.d. Survey on Frequent Pattern Mining.

Gorter, J.A., Petrozzino, J.J., Aronica, E.M., Rosenbaum, D.M., Opitz, T., Bennett, M.V.L., Connor, J.A., Zukin, R.S., 1997. Global ischemia induces downregulation of GluR2 mRNA and increases AMPA receptor-mediated

CA2+ influx in hippocampal CA1 neurons of gerbil. J. Neurosci. 17, 6179–6188. https://doi.org/10.1523/JNEUROSCI.17-16-06179.1997.

Hanauer, D.A., Rhodes, D.R., Chinnaiyan, A.M., 2009. Exploring clinical associations using "-Omics" based enrichment analyses. PLoS One 4. https://doi.org/10.1371/journal.pone.0005203.

Handelman, G.S., Kok, H.K., Chandra, R.V., Razavi, A.H., Lee, M.J., Asadi, H., 2018. eDoctor: machine learning and the future of medicine. J. Intern. Med. 284, 603–619. https://doi.org/10.1111/joim.12822.

Hartman, R.E., Lee, J.M., Zipfel, G.J., Wozniak, D.F., 2005. Characterizing learning deficits and hippocampal neuron loss following transient global cerebral ischemia in rats. Brain Res. 1043, 48–56. https://doi.org/10.1016/j.brainres.2005.02.030.

Hayashi, R., Matsuzawa, Y., Kubo, K., Kobayashi, T., 2005. Effects of simulated high altitude on event-related potential (P300) and auditory brain-stem responses. Clin. Neurophysiol. 116, 1471–1476. https://doi.org/10.1016/j.clinph.2005.02.020.

Hota, S.K., Hota, K.B., Prasad, D., Ilavazhagan, G., Singh, S.B., 2010. Oxidative-stress-induced alterations in Sp factors mediate transcriptional regulation of the NR1 subunit in hippocampus during hypoxia. Free Radic. Biol. Med. 49, 178–191. https://doi.org/10.1016/j.freeradbiomed.2010.03.027.

Hota, S.K., Sharma, V.K., Hota, K., Das, S., Dhar, P., Mahapatra, B.B., Srivastava, R.B., Singh, S.B., 2012. Multidomain cognitive screening test for neuropsychological assessment for cognitive decline in acclimatized lowlanders staying at high altitude. Indian J. Med. Res. 136, 411–420.

Jensen, S.M., Ritz, C., 2018. A comparison of approaches for simultaneous inference of fixed effects for multiple outcomes using linear mixed models. Stat. Med. https://doi.org/10.1002/sim.7666.

Jung, S.J., Son, C.S., Kim, M.S., Kim, D.J., Park, H.S., Kim, Y.N., 2013. Association rules to identify complications of cerebral infarction in patients with atrial fibrillation. Healthc. Inform. Res. 19, 25–32. https://doi.org/10.4258/hir.2013.19.1.25.

Klén, R., Karhunen, M., Elo, L.L., 2020. Likelihood contrasts: a machine learning algorithm for binary classification of longitudinal data. Sci. Rep. https://doi.org/10.1038/s41598-020-57924-9.

Lieberman, P., Protopapas, A., Reed, E., Youngs, J.W., Kanki, B.G., 1994. Cognitive defects at altitude. Nature. https://doi.org/10.1038/372325a0.

Marshall, W.J., Lapsley, M., Day, A.P., Ayling, R.M., 2014. Clinical Biochemistry: Metabolic and Clinical Aspects, third ed. Elsevier Inc.

Nalivaeva, N.N., Rybnikova, E.A., 2019. Editorial: Brain hypoxia and ischemia: new insights into neurodegeneration and neuroprotection. Front. Neurosci. https://doi.org/10.3389/fnins.2019.00770.

Nasreddine, Z.S., Phillips, N.A., Bédirian, V., Charbonneau, S., Whitehead, V., Collin, I., Cummings, J.L., Chertkow, H., 2005. The Montreal Cognitive Assessment, MoCA: a brief screening tool for mild cognitive impairment. J. Am. Geriatr. Soc. 53, 695–699. https://doi.org/10.1111/j.1532-5415.2005.53221.x.

Nation, D.A., Bondi, M.W., Gayles, E., Delis, D.C., 2017. Mechanisms of memory dysfunction during high altitude hypoxia training in military aircrew. J. Int. Neuropsychol. Soc. 23, 1–10. https://doi.org/10.1017/S1355617716000965.

Pan, F.F., Huang, L., Chen, K.L., Zhao, Q.H., Guo, Q.H., 2020. A comparative study on the validations of three cognitive screening tests in identifying subtle cognitive decline. BMC Neurol. 20. https://doi.org/10.1186/s12883-020-01657-9.

Pellegrini-Giampietro, D.E., Zukin, R.S., Bennett, M.V.L., Cho, S., Pulsinelli, W.A., 1992. Switch in glutamate receptor subunit gene expression in CA1 subfield of hippocampus following global ischemia in rats. Proc. Natl. Acad. Sci. U. S. A. 89, 10499–10503. https://doi.org/10.1073/pnas.89.21.10499.

Ray, K., Kishore, K., Vats, P., Bhattacharyya, D., Akunov, A., Maripov, A., Sarybaev, A., Singh, S.B., Kumar, B., 2019. A temporal study on learning and memory at high altitude in two ethnic groups. High Alt. Med. Biol. 20, 236–244. https://doi.org/10.1089/ham.2018.0139.

Rossi, D.J., Oshima, T., Attwell, D., 2000. Glutamate release in severe brain ischaemia is mainly by reversed uptake. Nature 403, 316–321. https://doi.org/10.1038/35002090.

Said, A.A., Abd-Elmegid, L.A., Kholeif, S., Gaber, A.A., 2018. Stage – specific predictive models for main prognosis measures of breast cancer. Future Comput. Inform. J. 3, 391–397. https://doi.org/10.1016/j.fcij.2018.11.002.

Sarıyer, G., Öcal Taşar, C., 2020. Highlighting the rules between diagnosis types and laboratory diagnostic tests for patients of an emergency department: use of association rule mining. Health Informatics J. 26, 1177–1193. https://doi.org/10.1177/1460458219871135.

Sengupta, D., Naik, P.K., 2013. SN algorithm: analysis of temporal clinical data for mining periodic patterns and impending augury. J. Clin. Bioinforma. 3, 24. https://doi.org/10.1186/2043-9113-3-24.

Sharma, V.K., Das, S.K., Dhar, P., Hota, K.B., Mahapatra, B.B., Vashishtha, V., Kumar, A., Hota, S.K., Norboo, T., Srivastava, R.B., 2014. Domain specific changes in cognition at high altitude and its correlation with hyperhomocysteinemia. PLoS One 9. https://doi.org/10.1371/journal.pone.0101448, e101448.

Singh, S.B., Thakur, L., Anand, J.P., Panjwani, U., Yadav, D., Selvamurthy, W., 2003. Effect of high altitude (HA) on event related brain potentials. Indian J. Physiol. Pharmacol. 47, 52–58.

StatSoft, Inc., 2010. STATISTICA (Data Analysis Software System), Version 9.1. Available from: www.statsoft.com. (Accessed 31 July 2013). Open Access Library.

Tornatore, J.B., Hill, E., Laboff, J.A., McGann, M.E., 2005. Self-administered screening for mild cognitive impairment: initial validation of a computerized test battery. J. Neuropsychiatry Clin. Neurosci. 17, 98–105. https://doi.org/10.1176/jnp.17.1.98.

WHO, 2020. NCDs | STEPwise approach to surveillance (STEPS). WHO (WWW document). https://www.who.int/ncds/surveillance/steps/en/#:~:text=The%20WHO%20STEPwise%20approach%20to,data%20in%20WHO%20member%20countries.

Yan, X., Zhang, J., Gong, Q., Weng, X., 2011. Prolonged high-altitude residence impacts verbal working memory: an fMRI study. Exp. Brain Res. 208, 437–445. https://doi.org/10.1007/s00221-010-2494-x.

Zhao, J., Feng, Q.P., Wu, P., Lupu, R.A., Wilke, R.A., Wells, Q.S., Denny, J.C., Wei, W.Q., 2019. Learning from longitudinal data in electronic health record and genetic data to improve cardiovascular event prediction. Sci. Rep. https://doi.org/10.1038/s41598-018-36745-x.

# Machine learning in expert systems for disease diagnostics in human healthcare

**Arvind Kumar Yadav[a], Rohit Shukla[a], and Tiratha Raj Singh[b]**

*Department of Biotechnology and Bioinformatics, Jaypee University of Information Technology (JUIT), Solan, Himachal Pradesh, India[a] Centre of Excellence in Healthcare Technologies and Informatics (CHETI), Department of Biotechnology and Bioinformatics, Jaypee University of Information Technology (JUIT), Solan, Himachal Pradesh, India[b]*

## Chapter outline

## 1 Introduction

Good health is an important aspect of quality of life, as nothing is more valuable, and new technologies are continually leading to tremendous advances in healthcare. The definition of healthcare is the improvement of health through prevention, treatment, and inspection of diseases (Toli and Murtagh, 2020). Accurate diagnosis is essential for medical treatment and decision-making, but it can be difficult to identify a specific disease from the stated symptoms of a patient, due to the inexact information provided. Thus the main job in medical diagnosis is to use expert logical reasoning to make decisions. Physician control is an effective solution for diagnosis and treatment, but it is costly. Artificial intelligence (AI) seems particularly well suited for this application (Davenport and Kalakota, 2019).

A smart healthcare system for disease diagnostics can be developed using a combination of AI, Internet-of-Things (IoT), information and communication technology (ICT), along with Big Data and good decision making (Chui et al., 2017; Panigrahi and Singh, 2017). The shortage of medical personnel in the healthcare sector is a current major challenge (Liu et al., 2016), but smart healthcare systems can be developed using the available health data with increased computational power by applying AI (Shukla et al., 2021). A smart healthcare system can assist in optimizing the financial and social impact of health services having insufficient medical personnel (Du and Sun, 2015; Momete, 2016).

An expert system (ES) is a common application of AI. It is a combination of computer-based programs that employ specific information and knowledge from several human experts to resolve specific problems. An expert system basically includes a knowledge base that has stored information and a set of rules that are applied to the knowledge base to make a particular prediction (Godfrey et al., 2011; Li and Shun, 2016). This type of intelligent knowledge-based system can provide self-diagnosis to individuals. Such a self-diagnosis mechanism is still very important for early diagnosis and treatment. The most important functions of the expert system are a flexible user interface, good data representation, inference, and rapid outcomes. Results can include greater accuracy and reliability, cost savings, and minimal errors. Expert systems also have some drawbacks, such as lack of human "common sense," no effect of environment change, and no response in exceptional cases.

Expert system development has gained much attention from researchers in recent decades for medical decision-making. Expert systems can support novice medical practitioners in urban areas and, more specifically, in rural and remote areas. They are also helpful for doctors who use them to identify diseases and suggest suitable treatment options. The expert system also provides the facility to store images, sound, and videos related to disease symptoms (Ali and Saudi, 2014). The expert system appeared in medical diagnosis applications in the 1970s, when the MYCIN expert system was developed for the identification of diseases caused by bacteria. Since then, many expert systems have been used for the identification of various human diseases and are being referred to by medical practitioners globally (see Table 1).

**Table 1 Comparison of developed expert systems for human disease diagnostics.**

| Method used | Disease Diagnosed | Input | Reference |
|---|---|---|---|
| Rule-Based Expert System | Influenza | The patient data from Bangladesh collected by the influenza specialists, consultants, and disease symptoms | (Hossain et al., 2014) |
| | Memory loss | Disease symptoms | (Hole and Gulhane, 2014) |
| | Viral infection | Disease symptoms | (Patel et al., 2013) |
| | Diabetes | Lab test results, ketone, disease symptoms, obesity, age, family history | (Geberemariam, 2013) |
| | Endocrine disease | Disease symptoms | (Abu-Naser et al., 2010) |

**Table 1 Comparison of developed expert systems for human disease diagnostics—cont'd**

| Method used | Disease Diagnosed | Input | Reference |
|---|---|---|---|
| | Dehydration Viral or allergic conjunctivitis | Disease symptoms | (Patra et al., 2010) |
| | Ear problem diagnosis | Disease symptoms | (Abu-Naser and Al-Nakhal, 2016) |
| | Lower back pain | Disease symptoms | (Abu-Naser and Aldahdooh, 2016) |
| | Food disease | Disease symptoms | (Abu-Naser and Mahdi, 2016) |
| | Urination problems diagnosis | Disease symptoms | (Abu-Naser and Shaath, 2016) |
| | Breast cancer | Disease symptoms | (Abu-Naser and Bastami, 2016) |
| | Skin disease | Disease symptoms | (Abu-Naser and Akkila, 2008) |
| | Male infertility | Disease symptoms | (Abu-Naser, 2016) |
| | Mouth problem | Disease symptoms | (Abu-Naser and Hamed, 2016) |
| | Shortness of breath in infants and children | Disease symptoms | (AbuEl-Reesh and Abu Naser, 2017) |
| | Rheumatic | Disease symptoms | (El Agha et al., 2017) |
| | Genital problems in men | Disease symptoms | (Abu-Naser and Al-Hanjori, 2016) |
| | Genital problems in infants | Disease symptoms | (Naser and El Haddad, 2016) |
| Fuzzy Expert System | Hypertension disease | Body mass index, age, gender, heart rate, and blood pressure | (Abdullah et al., 2011) |
| | Liver disorders | Data collected from the trusted database, 6 entrance parameters of liver disorders | (Neshat et al., 2008) |
| | Hepatobiliary disorders | Disease symptoms | (Mitra, 1994) |
| ANN-Based Expert System | Heart disease | Disease symptoms | (Ajam, 2015) |
| | Parkinson disease | Disease symptoms | (Avci and Dogantekin, 2016) |
| Knowledge-Based Expert System | Cardiological disease | Disease symptoms | (Bursuk et al., 1999) |
| | Chest pain | Data collected from laboratory examinations, narrative texts describing the patient's condition, and chest X-ray images | (Ali et al., 1999) |
| | Bronchial asthma | Disease symptoms | (Prasad et al., 1989) |

*Continued*

**Table 1 Comparison of developed expert systems for human disease diagnostics—cont'd**

| Method used | Disease Diagnosed | Input | Reference |
|---|---|---|---|
| | Eye disease | Disease symptoms | (Ibrahim et al., 2001) |
| | Brain diseases | Disease symptoms | (Ayangbekun Oluwafemi and Jimoh Ibrahim, 2015) |
| | Spine disease | Disease symptoms | (Ghazizadeh et al., 2015) |
| | Neck pain diagnosis | Disease symptoms | (Abu-Naser and Almurshidi, 2016) |
| | Stomach pain | Disease symptoms | (Mrouf et al., 2017) |
| | Ankle disease | Disease symptoms | (Qwaider and Abu Naser, 2017) |
| | Hypertension in pregnancy | Disease symptoms | (Gudu et al., 2012) |
| | Oncology | Disease symptoms | (Shortliffe, 1986) |
| | Chest pain in infants and children | Disease symptoms | (Khella, 2017) |
| | Rickets diagnosis | Disease symptoms | (Al Rekhawi et al., 2017) |
| | Hair loss diagnosis | Disease symptoms | (Nabahin et al., 2017) |
| | Teeth and gum problems | Disease symptoms | (Abu Ghali et al., 2017) |
| | Ear disease | Disease symptoms | (Abu-Naser and Abu Hasanein, 2016) |
| | Nausea and vomiting problems | Disease symptoms | (Abu Naser and El-Najjar, 2016) |
| Adaptive Neuro-Fuzzy Inference System | Breast cancer | Disease symptoms | (Fatima and Amine, 2012) |

The amount of biomedical data is exponentially increasing and such data contain essential patient information related to diversified medical conditions (Singh et al., 2018). These datasets can provide significant hidden information if important patterns latent in the data can be extracted. This information can serve as a medical diagnostic tool to identify particular diseases (Ali and Saudi, 2014). Medical knowledge can be effectively extracted by analyzing data using various machine-learning techniques, such as genetic algorithms, (Ghaheri et al., 2015) neural networks (Lundervold and Lundervold, 2019), decision trees(Ahmed et al., 2020), and fuzzy theory (Arji et al., 2019; Sweidan et al., 2019).

These machine-learning techniques can also be helpful in automating expert systems for medical diagnosis. The aim of this chapter is to present an overview of the research and development of expert systems in the field of medical diagnosis, with the specific application of machine learning. We have provided specific case studies along with their respective algorithmic procedures, to elaborate the typical use of expert systems for diagnosis of human diseases, which include cancer and Alzheimer's disease.

## 2 Types of expert systems

There are various classes of expert systems. Several of the most prominent classes are described in the following paragraphs.

*Rule-based expert system*: The simplest form of AI is represented by the rule-based system. The rules are used as knowledge representation, for the coding of knowledge into the system, (Grosan and Abraham, 2011) as the rules can advise what to do under various conditions. The rules in the expert system can be added in the form of a simplistic model based on IF/THEN statements.

*Knowledge-based expert system*: The knowledge-based expert system uses information for the decision-making process. A knowledge-based system uses a knowledge base that consists of expert experience and applies a set of rules in particular conditions (Arbaiy et al., 2017).

*Fuzzy expert system*: Membership functions and fuzzy rules make up the fuzzy expert system. These functions and rules are applied on datasets. This system takes in numbers as an input query and the job is performed by the fuzzy inference engine (Yager and Zadeh, 2012).

*Artificial neural network (ANN)-based expert system*: The ANN is widely used for pattern recognition and regression analysis. It is an interconnected group of artificial neurons that uses a mathematical model connectionist approach for computation (Fatima and Pasha, 2017).

## 3 Components of an expert system

Expert system software consists of different components (Ghazizadeh et al., 2015). Some basic components are represented in Fig. 1 and described in the following paragraphs.

*User interface*: The user interface is the part that establishes the communication between the user and the expert system. It provides various facilities to users such as graphical interfaces, menus, etc., to establish communication. The interface must be able to represent the internal decision to the user in an understandable form. In the development of an expert system, various personnel including users, knowledge engineers, domain experts, and maintenance personnel are involved with the user interface.

*Knowledge base*: This is domain-specific information obtained from a human expert or experts and stored. Sets of rules, logic, frames, and semantic nets are used to represent the information, or knowledge. The knowledge base holds the heuristic knowledge and factual knowledge. The factual knowledge is widely shared and available knowledge from textbooks and journals. The heuristic knowledge is more experimental, more judgmental, and more difficult to collect accurately. It is the knowledge of good judgment and good practice. The achievement of a truly expert system relies on the comprehensiveness and accuracy of its knowledge base.

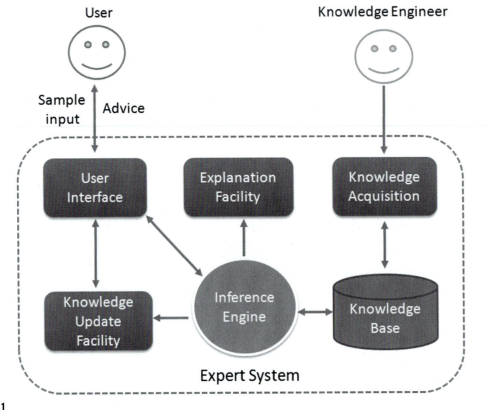

**FIG. 1**

The basic architecture of a typical expert system.

*Inference engine*: This engine performs the specific task requested, using the rules and given inputs. The main job of the inference engine is to arrive at a final decision using the forest of rules. It employs two main approaches, forward chaining and backward chaining.

*Knowledge acquisition*: This is the process of building a knowledge base. In knowledge acquisition, various techniques are used, such as protocol analysis, observation, interviews, etc. Collecting information is required to construct the knowledge pool.

*Explanation facility*: This component is helpful in explaining the reasoning process behind a recommendation made by an expert system. The explanation facility provides details about final or intermediate solutions and additional data needed. Here users can find answers to the basic question of how and why the server arrived at a conclusion or decision. Users can change the editor, if they are not satisfied with the explanation of the present reasoning. It has little flexibility in usage terms.

*Knowledge engineer*: This is a person who can design, build, and test expert systems. The knowledge engineer asks other people about their experience and knowledge and finds solutions to problems. Thus the knowledge engineer discovers the reasoning methods and implements the rules in the expert system and is also responsible for modifying, updating, and testing the expert system (Kumar, 2019).

## 4 Techniques used in expert systems of medical diagnosis

Current expert systems are composed of special software environments and are known by several names. The variations of the medical expert system depend upon their complexity. Expert systems produce situational and patient-specific suggestions. Different types of information are used by the ES to make decisions. Some techniques used in expert systems are discussed in the following paragraphs.

*AI programs*: AI programs are used by the computer to understand and implement the reasoning process. These programs attempt to mimic human reasoning, thinking, and mechanisms of learning, and, by combining all these things, to build a computational model that provides intelligent behavior and actions. AI uses both theoretical research and technology to build a model that can be implemented as a computer program. In the medical field, AI is used to build systems and tools to improve healthcare (Amisha et al., 2019; Esmaeilzadeh, 2020; Datta et al., 2019). The mechanisms and languages of AI are very costly and difficult to understand. AI can also be very hard to apply and incorporate among and within other information systems.

*Machine learning (ML)*: ML is a field of AI that solves problems by computational methods with the help of a learning process (Frank et al., 2020). The main aim of ML research is to model human learning. Based on several criteria such as learning strategy, knowledge representation, or field of application, ML methods can be categorized (Réda et al., 2020). In ML, the main methods are genetic algorithms, neural networks, instance-based learning, analytical learning, and inductive learning. ML has been used in the diagnosis of various diseases, including acute appendicitis (Godfrey et al., 2011; Li and Shun, 2016), dermatological disease (Patra et al., 2010), thyroid disease, (Ghazizadeh et al., 2015) and female urinary incontinence, (Arbaiy et al., 2017) and in the detection of bacterial pneumonia by using X-ray reports. (Abu-Naser and Al-Nakhal, 2016) The main applications of ML are in data mining and knowledge acquisition. Knowledge acquisition is a very important method in the development of expert systems, because it is needed to extract the knowledge from experts. By applying various ML methods, data mining allows nearly automatic knowledge acquisition (Fatima and Pasha, 2017).

*Data mining*: This is the process of discovering information and hidden patterns in data. Data mining is also known as knowledge discovery by ML and AI societies. In recent decades, information technologies have been frequently used for disease diagnosis to assist doctors in decision-making activity. (Joshi and Joshi, 2013) Today, a huge amount of complex data is generated by the healthcare sector on an everyday basis. To extract valid and important information from this voluminous data, data mining is used to understand the patterns in the data. In this process, suitable data is retrieved from different data sources, and then cleaned before knowledge discovery, in which the data are evaluated based on quality criteria (Fig. 2). Finally, data mining is used for the prediction and evaluation of diseases (Durairaj and Ranjani, 2013). In the healthcare sector, data mining is a promising field with major significance for better understanding the medical data. Data mining techniques are used in medical diagnostics for various diseases, including diabetes (Kazerouni et al., 2020), stroke (Panzarasa et al., 2010), cancer (Weli, 2020), Alzheimer's disease, (Panigrahi and Singh, 2012; Panigrahi and Singh, 2013) and cardiovascular diseases. (Ayatollahi et al., 2019)

*Decision tree*: Decision tree is the most commonly used classification method and is used to solve complex problems. It consists of nodes and branches and presents the knowledge structure in the form of a tree (Lopez-Vallverdu et al., 2012). The path to be followed is defined by the evaluation of

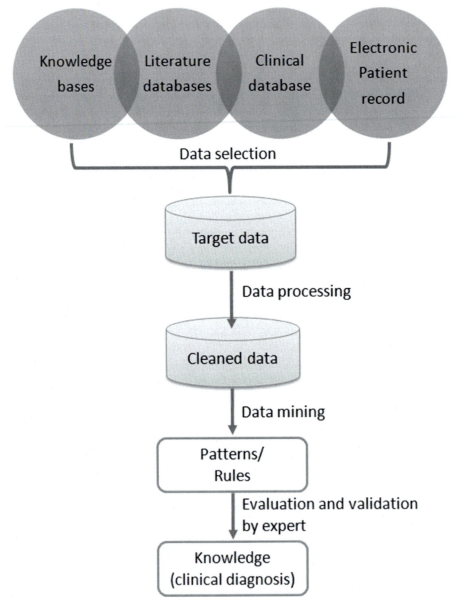

**FIG. 2**

Outline of the data mining process in medical diagnosis.

each node in the tree attributes. In this method, classification is carried out by the root node routing until the leaf node is reached. Decision tree models are best for data mining as they are simple to interpret and integrate, and have comparably better accuracy in many applications (Kumar and Singh, 2017; Lavanya and Rani, 2011).

*Neural network*: This method mimics the logic of the human brain. In neural networks, neurons and nodes are the basic components. The neural network has an input layer, one or many hidden layers, and a single output layer (Fig. 3). The neurons are connected with the network and help to decide the final output (Abiodun et al., 2018). The neural network is a widely used technique in the field of healthcare, used to diagnose various human diseases such as cancer (Shahid et al., 2019), heart disease (Reddy et al., 2017), and others.

*Genetic algorithm*: The genetic algorithm (GA) is a methodology involving an adaptive optimization search. For a heuristic search, GA supports Darwinian natural selection and genetic systems biology. The fundamentals of genetic algorithm techniques are designed to simulate the process in natural systems required for evolution (Uyar and Ilhan, 2017). The genetic algorithm has been very effective in the screening and diagnosis of several diseases (Ghaheri et al., 2015). Various medical diagnostic methods have been developed using GA for prediction of diseases such as cancer (Mansoori et al., 2014; Pereira et al., 2014), anemia (Wang, 2016), heart disease (Uyar and Ilhan, 2017), tuberculosis (Elveren and Yumuşak, 2011), and epilepsy (Kocer and Canal, 2011).

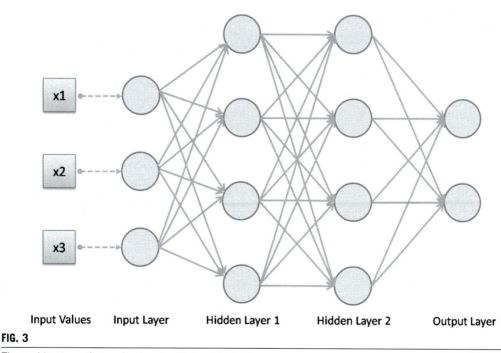

| Input Values | Input Layer | Hidden Layer 1 | Hidden Layer 2 | Output Layer |

**FIG. 3**

The architecture of neural network with two hidden layers.

## 5 Existing expert systems

A tabular compilation of the existing popular expert systems developed for a myriad of human diseases is provided in Table 1. These expert systems are based upon standard methodologies followed, such as rule based, fuzzy, ANN based, knowledge based, and adaptive hybrid.

## 6 Case studies

Specialized case studies on human diseases such as cancer and Alzheimer's disease are provided with rule-based and fuzzy-based expert systems, respectively. General descriptions, flow diagrams, internal procedures, algorithmic details, and standard measurements are provided in later sections.

### 6.1 Cancer diagnosis using rule-based expert system

Cancer is caused by uncontrolled cell proliferation in various organs. There are numerous clinical appearances and treatment methods available for cancer. Cancer is still an important health issue and a leading cause of death globally, despite advancements in modern medicine. There are many types of cancers, classified on the basis of their origin from tissue.

A web-based expert system was developed by Başçiftçi and Avuçlu that uses a reduced-rule base to diagnose cancer risk using patient symptoms (Başçiftçi and Avuçlu, 2018). This method can be used for breast cancer, lung cancer, kidney cancer, and cervical cancer. In this expert system, 13 determinant risk factors are used for the diagnosis of cancer types. Two examples are given here, showing how this expert system determines the cancer types on the basis of the 13 risk factors.

| First (Renal cancer) | Second (Breast cancer) |
|---|---|
| If<br>1. Have a certain hardness or bloody discharge in the breast end (in women) is Yes and<br>2. Coughing up blood constantly is Unimportant and<br>3. Excessive weight is Unimportant and<br>4. Taking long-term dialysis treatment >4 h is Unimportant and<br>5. Smoking is Unimportant and<br>6. Age > 50 is Yes and<br>7. Hypertension >140 mmHg is Unimportant and<br>8. Have you given birth (in women) is Yes and<br>9. Have cancer in relatives is Unimportant and<br>10. To give birth to her first child after age 30 is Yes and<br>11. The existence of vaginal bleeding is Unimportant and<br>12. Unexpected abnormal and bad-smelling vaginal discharge is Unimportant and<br>13. Pelvic pain and have spotting is Unimportant<br>  - Then the patient has renal cancer from symptoms of cancer | If<br>1. Have a certain hardness or bloody discharge in the breast end (in women) is Unimportant and<br>2. Coughing up blood constantly is Unimportant and<br>3. Excessive weight >100 is Yes and<br>4. Taking long-term dialysis treatment >4 h is Yes and<br>5. Smoking is Unimportant and<br>6. Age > 50 is Unimportant and<br>7. Hypertension >140 mmHg is Yes and<br>8. Have you given birth (in women) is Unimportant and<br>9. Have cancer in relatives is Yes and<br>10. To give birth to her first child after age 30 is Unimportant and<br>11. The existence of vaginal bleeding is Unimportant and<br>12. Unexpected abnormal and bad-smelling vaginal discharge is Unimportant and<br>13. Pelvic pain and have spotting is Unimportant<br>  - Then the patient has breast cancer from symptoms of cancer |

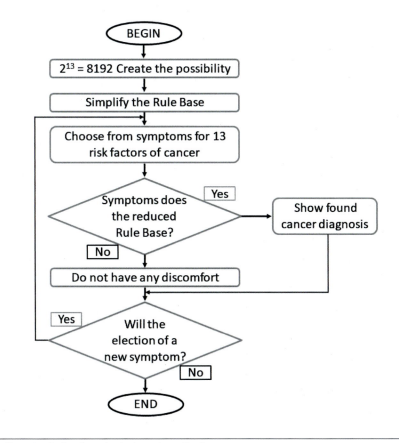

**FIG. 4**

The process flow chart of reduced rule-based application.

After performing the diagnosis using this approach, simplification of the rule-based method was carried out from all possibilities. After simplification, the expert system predicted the same results as the previous one. Diagnosis performed with the reduced-rule based system took less time. The overall process used in the reduced-rule based expert system is represented in Fig. 4.

Başçiftçi and Hatay developed a similar expert system using a reduced-rule based system by applying simplified logic functions for diabetes prediction (Başçiftçi and Hatay, 2011). In this study, they used a dataset for type 1 diabetes, type 2 diabetes, and gestational diabetes. Three datasets were downloaded from data 1 (http://www.cormactech.com/neunet/download.html), data 2 (https://www.webarchive.org.uk/wayback/archive/20180516221802/http://www.gov.scot/Publications/2003/01/16290/17629), and data 3 (http://lib.stat.cmu.edu/S/Harrell/data/descriptions/diabetes.html). The accuracy rate was observed as 97.13%, 96.5%, 98.26%, and 97.44% for diabetes patients, type 1 diabetes patients, type 2 diabetes patients, and diabetes with pregnancy, respectively.

## 6.2 Alzheimer's diagnosis using fuzzy-based expert systems

The neurological disorder called Alzheimer's disease (AD) is characterized by the two major hallmarks of β-amyloid plaques and neurofibrillary tangles (NFTs). It mainly occurs after the age of 65 and the identification of this disease in the initial stage is a critical task (Shukla et al., 2019; Shukla and Singh, 2020). AD is divided into various stages, including mild cognitive impairment (MCI), severe AD, etc. At the beginning of the disease, no critical symptoms appear, while after 5 years, when symptoms do appear, the disease has completely spread through the brain (Ewers et al., 2011). AD mainly affects the hippocampus region and destroys cognitive ability including reading, learning, etc. in patients. Hence, early identification of disease is a very important task to protect the patient's life quality from this complex disease (Weller and Budson, 2018). Expert systems come into the picture at this point, as they can participate in the early diagnosis of AD. There are several expert systems available that can diagnose CE (Hinrichs et al., 2009; Ding et al., 2018; Munir et al., 2019; Oehm et al., 2003). Two different case studies for AD are discussed here.

**Case study 1**. Here, we describe a method developed by Mallika et al., (Mallika et al., 2019) in brief, to understand how one can create an expert system that can participate effectively in AD diagnosis. In this approach, they used fuzzy logic (FL), which is a popular mathematical approach of soft computing and inferences. Set theory and crisp logic are generalized by FL, which is employed in the concept of a fuzzy set. FL is widely used with success in various fields such as image processing, medical diagnosis, knowledge engineering, and pattern recognition, etc. In this study, they developed an expert system, called a fuzzy inference system (FIS), for AD diagnosis using the hippocampus as a biomarker. This system can classify non-AD (normal control), AD, and MCI patients using image data visual features. They have taken brain MRI images from the OASIS database (https://www.oasis-brains.org/) and preprocessed them by segmenting. The segmented images were then used for the extraction of hippocampus volume and then the classification was performed by using the fuzzy inference system. The methodology is shown in Fig. 5. The accuracy, sensitivity, and precision of the three regions are shown in Table 2.

### 6.2.1 Algorithm of fuzzy inference system

Three steps are involved in the classification of the MRI images by using extracted features in the FIS. The internal structure of the FIS(Siler and Buckley, 2005) is shown in Fig. 6.

1. In the first step, the fuzzification of input variables is done.
2. A decision-making logic is built by using the fuzzy inference engine based on fuzzy rules as described in following text.
3. To crisp the value, defuzzification of the generated output was carried out.

They generated three fuzzy rules based on hippocampus volume, which is described in various research articles for AD and non-CE (Vijayakumar and Vijayakumar, 2013). These fuzzy rules are used in the previously described FIS algorithm.

The three rules that they generated are as follows:

1. If the volume $(V)$ of the hippocampus is in interval $V_{low}$ it represents AD.
2. If the volume $(V)$ of the hippocampus is in interval $V_{medium}$ it represents MCI.
3. If the volume $(V)$ of the hippocampus is in interval $V_{high}$ it represents non-AD.

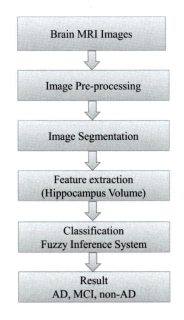

**FIG. 5**

The flow diagram of fuzzy inference system.

**Table 2 The classification evaluations of FIS.**

| Brain MRI projection | Accuracy (%) | Precision (%) | Sensitivity (%) |
|---|---|---|---|
| Sagittal | 82.21 | 91.95 | 87.43 |
| Coronal | 84.13 | 91.03 | 90.59 |
| Axial | 86.53 | 91.71 | 92.73 |

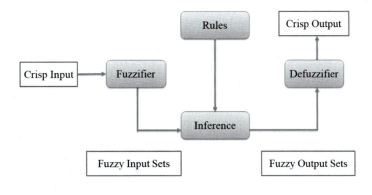

**FIG. 6**

The internal structure of fuzzy inference system (FIS).

According to these rules, the FIS classified the MRI images into AD, non-AD, and MCI classes.

**Case study 2**: Lazli et al. (2019) described a computer-aided diagnosis method on the basis of multimodal fusion (fusion of MRI and PET images). A hybrid fuzzy-genetic-possibilistic model was used to quantify the brain tissue volume and discriminate the classes using a classifier of support vector data description (SVDD). The flow diagram of the methodology is shown in Fig. 7.

This method is mainly categorized into two parts. In the first part, the fusion approach is used to quantify the brain tissue volume by using three consecutive steps: modeling, fusion, and decision.

1. The modeling is also divided into three parts. First, it is initialized by tissue cluster centroids by using a clustering algorithm of bias-corrected fuzzy C-means (BCFCM) (Ahmed et al., 2002) (Algorithm 1). Second, the optimization of the initial partition is performed by using the genetic algorithm. Finally, the possibilistic fuzzy C-means clustering algorithm (PFCM) (Pal et al., 2005) (Algorithm 2) is used for the quantification of white matter (WM), gray matter (GM), and cerebrospinal fluid (CSF) tissues.
2. In the second step, the fusion of the MRI and PET images is performed by using the possibilistic operator, which highlights the redundancies and manages the ambiguities.
3. In the third step, the decision offers the more representative anatomy-functional fusion images.

In the second part, SVDD is used to classify AD after normal aging and it automatically detects abnormal values. After that, a "divide and conquer" strategy is used to speed up the SVDD processing, which decreases the computational cost of the calculation results. The method also has proved its efficacy on synthetic datasets retrieved from Alzheimer's disease neuroimaging (ADNI) (http://adni.loni.usc.edu/), Open Access Series of Imaging Studies (OASIS) (https://www.oasis-brains.org/), and real images.

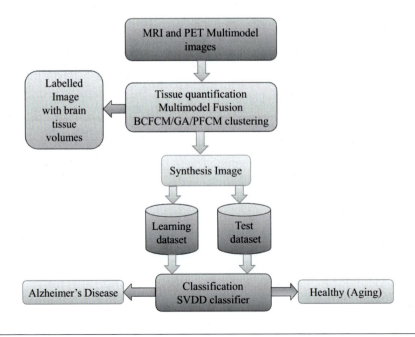

**FIG. 7**

The complete flow diagram of multimodal CAD system used for AD diagnosis proposed by Lazli et al. (2019).

The classification evaluation including accuracy, sensitivity, specificity, and area under the ROC curve for the ADNI dataset was 93.65%, 90.08%, 92.75% and 97.3%; for the OASIS dataset the values were 91.46%, 92%, 91.78% and 96.7%; and for real images they were 85.09%, 86.41%, 84.92% and 94.6%, respectively.

## ALGORITHM 1 DESCRIBES THE PSEUDOCODE FOR BCFCM

Let $X = \{x_j\}$, the voxels set; $U = \{\mu_{ij}\}$, the matrix of membership degrees; and $B = \{b_{ij}\}$, the matrix of cluster center, with $1 \leq I \leq C$, $1 \leq j \leq N$.m the degree of fuzzy, and $\mathcal{E}$ the threshold representing convergence error.

1. Initialize the center vectors $B^{(0)} = [b_j]$ and the degree of belonging matrix $U(0)$ by random values in the interval [0,1] satisfying Eq. (2).
2. At $k$-step:
   - Compute the belonging degrees matrix $U^{(k)}$ using Eq. (3).
   - Compute the center vectors $B(k) = [bj]$ using Eq. (4).
   - Estimate the bias term $\beta_j^{(k)}$ using Eq. (5).
   - Compute the objective function $J_{BCFCM}^{(k)}$ using Eq. (1).
3. Update: $B^{(k+1)}$, $U^{(k+1)}$, $\beta_j^{(k+1)}$, and $J_{BCFCM}^{(k+1)}$
4. If $\|J_{BCFCM}^{(k+1)} - J_{BCFCM}^{(k)}\| < \mathcal{E}$ then STOP otherwise return to step 2.
   Equations used in Algorithm 1:

$$J_{BCFCM}(B, U, X, \beta) = \sum_{i=1}^{C}\sum_{j=1}^{N} u_{ij}^{m}\|x_j - \beta_j - b_i\|^2 + \frac{\alpha}{N_i}\sum_{i=1}^{C}\sum_{j=1}^{N} u_{ij}^{m}\left(\sum_{x_k \in N(x_j)} \|x_k - \beta_k - b_i\|^2\right) \tag{1}$$

where:
- $B$ denotes the centroids matrix and center of cluster $i$ ($1 \leq i \leq C$) with $C$, the number of cluster.
- $X$ is the voxels vectors matrix and $xj$ ($1 \leq j \leq N$) is the observed value of log-transformed intensities at the $j$th voxel.
- $U$ denotes the matrix of degrees of membership $\mu_{ij}^{m}$ with m being a parameter controlling the degree of fuzzification.
- $\beta_j$ is the bias field value at the $j$th voxel, which helps in removing the effect of inhomogeneity.
- $N_i$ denotes the size of neighborhood that is to be considered.
- $N(x_j)$ represents the set of neighbors that exist in a window around $x_j$ and is the cardinality of $N_i$.

$$U\left\{u_{ij} \in [0, 1]\Big|\sum_{i=1}^{C} u_{ij} = 1 \forall j \text{ and } 0 < \sum_{j=1}^{N} u_{ij} < N \forall i\right\} \tag{2}$$

$$u_{ij}^{*} = \frac{1}{\sum_{k=1}^{C}\left((w_{ij} + (\alpha/N_i)\gamma_i)/(w_{kj} + (\alpha/N_i)\gamma_k)\right)^{1/(m-1)}} \tag{3}$$

where

$$w_{ij} = \|x_j - \beta_j - b_j - b_i\|^2$$

$$\gamma_i = \sum_{x_k \in N(x_j)} \|x_k - \beta_j - b_i\|^2$$

$$b_i^{*} = \frac{\sum_{j=1}^{N} u_{ij}^{m}\left((x_j - \beta_j) + (\alpha/N_i)\sum_{x_k \in N(x_j)}(x_k - \beta_j)\right)}{(1+\alpha)\sum_{j=1}^{N} u_{ij}^{m}} \tag{4}$$

$$\beta_j^{*} = x_j - \frac{\sum_{i=1}^{C} u_{ij}^{m} b_i}{\sum_{i=1}^{C} u_{ij}^{m}} \tag{5}$$

---

## ALGORITHM 2 THE PSEUDOCODE OF THE POSSIBILISTIC FUZZY C-MEANS CLUSTERING ALGORITHM (PFCM)

Let $X = \{x_j\}$ be the voxels vectors, $U = \{\mu_{ij}\}$ is the matrix of membership degrees, and $T = \{t_{ij}\}$ is the matrix of typicality degrees, and $B = \{b_{ij}\}$ is the matrix of cluster centers with $1 \leq i \leq C, 1 \leq j \leq N$. $m$ being the degree of fuzzy and $\eta$ being the weight possibilistic degree.

1. Initialization of the centers vectors $B^{(0)} = [b_j]$ and the degree of belonging matrix $U(0)$ using the hybrid BCFCM-GA method.
2. At $k$-step:
   - Compute the matrix of membership degrees $U(k)$ using Eq. (7).
   - Compute the matrix of typicality degrees $T(k)$ using Eq. (8).
   - Compute the prototype matrix $B(k)$ using Eq. (9).
   - Compute the objective function $J_{PFCM}^{(k)}$ using Eq. (6).
3. Update: $U^{(k+1)}, T^{(k+1)}, B^{(k+1)}$, and $J_{PFCM}^{(k+1)}$
4. Repeat steps [2] and [3] until the stop criterion is met: $\|J_{PFCM}^{(k+1)} - J_{PFCM}^{(k)}\| < \varepsilon$
   Equations used in Algorithm 2:

$$j_{PFCM}(u, B, m, \eta) = \sum_{i=1}^{N} \sum_{j=1}^{C} \left( au_{ij}^m + bt_{ij}^\eta \right) \|x_i - b_j\|^2 + \sum_{j=1}^{C} \gamma_i \sum_{i=1}^{N} (1 - t_{ij})^\eta \tag{6}$$

where $u_{ij}$ are constrained by the probabilistic conditions, while $t_{ij} \in [0,1]$ are subject to:

$$0 < \sum_{i=1}^{C} t_{ij} < C, \forall j$$

$$u_{ij} = \left( \sum_{k=1}^{C} \left( \frac{\|x_j - b_i\|^2}{\|x_j - b_k\|^2} \right)^{1/m-1} \right)^{-1} \quad 1 \leq j \leq N, 1 \leq i \leq C \tag{7}$$

$$t_{ij} = \frac{1}{\left( 1 + \left( \frac{b\|x_j - b_i\|^2}{y_i} \right)^{1/\eta-1} \right)} \forall i = 1.....C, \forall j = 1......N \tag{8}$$

$$bi = \sum_{j=1}^{N} \left( \left( au_{ij}^m + bt_{ij}^\eta \right) x_j \right) / \left( au_{ij}^m + bt_{ij}^\eta \right) \forall i = 1.........C \tag{9}$$

The symbols are the same as described in the previous equations.

---

# 7 Significance and novelty of expert systems

Expert systems help to enhance decision quality and reduce the cost of seeking advice from experts to solve problems. Due to the rapid enhancement of AI techniques, expert systems have been used in diverse fields of IoT and the healthcare domain such as cancer, AD, and cardiovascular disease detection. These systems are used to provide fast and efficient solutions for a particular problem and offer high reliability. Expert systems can deal with difficult problems that cannot be easily solved by human experts. It collect alters from expertise and used it proficiently to provide consistent responses for repetitive decisions. Expert systems are always available for users, even on holidays. Human experts may forget some information and make some mistakes, but expert systems use all their information consistently. As the main purpose of expert systems is to use AI technology to make better decisions to improve the health of patients, it is thus an advantage to reduce/eliminate errors and inconsistencies. The main advantage of an expert system is that of permitting nonexpert users to reach very acceptable conclusions.

Since expert systems are used as a platform for disease control, treatment, and diagnostic tools, they can be advantageous in many circumstances, as at least they will not cause harm when making decisions. It is certain that human intervention will have a better impact on the performance of expert systems. By combining technology with computing and Big Data analysis, these systems may represent an effective solution to improve healthcare services that will also enable real-time decision-making processes.

## 8  Limitations of expert systems

Although expert systems offer many advantages, there are still some limitations to consider. In the case of a large population, expert systems may not be very accurate. Expert systems will never be too accurate to replace human predictions, but they can help to alleviate some of the issues of the infrastructure of healthcare. The privacy and security of health data and personal information may be threatened, however. Expert systems can be expensive and time consuming. They are not very flexible, having no "common sense," and are unable to adapt to altering environmental conditions. Expert systems can be difficult to maintain and expensive in the area of development. There is a need for ground verification and unable to process for complex automation. They also need to be updated manually. Different expert systems need to be developed for specific domains.

## 9  Conclusion

As one of the most important applications of AI, the expert system is the best solution for diagnosing complex diseases that cannot be easily resolved using conventional methods. In fact, information-based expert systems have the advanced skills to effectively solve many problems and have proved their usefulness. The use of expert systems to monitor health is considered a major breakthrough in modern technology. Recently, AI and Big Data analysis have been applied in expert systems to provide a more effective healthcare system. In healthcare, Big Data includes medical images, MRI scans, computed tomography (CT) images, clinical data, prescriptions, doctor notes, laboratory data, pharmacy files, insurance EPR data files, and many other management operations-related data. This chapter provides an overview of different expert systems developed in the area of medical diagnostics. In the past few decades, the expert system has made great contributions to the healthcare sector. Many expert systems have been developed for the diagnosis of human diseases. The running speed of expert systems is faster than that of people, thus they provide a more rapid diagnostic facility. In healthcare research, expert systems are one of the major technological advancements. Applications of AI/machine learning with Big.

Data are considered to be significant achievements of automated diagnostic systems. However, today there is a need to develop more heart- and cancer-related expert systems, because these are the major death-causing diseases globally. We have presented the information on expert systems in a systematic way and anticipate that this chapter will be useful to academic, scientific, and medical field researchers looking for more information on expert systems.

## Acknowledgment

RS and TRS acknowledge the ICMR grant (ISRM/11 [53]/2019) for providing the Senior Research Fellowship to RS.

## References

Abdullah, A.A., Zakaria, Z., Mohamad, N.F., 2011. Design and development of fuzzy expert system for diagnosis of hypertension. In: 2011 Second International Conference on Intelligent Systems, Modelling and Simulation. IEEE, pp. 113–117.

Abiodun, O.I., et al., 2018. State-of-the-art in artificial neural network applications: a survey. Heliyon 4.

Abu Ghali, M.J., Mukhaimer, M.N., Abu Yousef, M.K., Abu-Naser, S.S., 2017. Expert system for problems of teeth and gums. Int. J. Eng. Inform. Syst. 1.

Abu Naser, S.S., El-Najjar, A.E., 2016. An expert system for nausea and vomiting problems in infants and children. Int. J. Med. Res. 1, 114–117.

AbuEl-Reesh, J.Y., Abu Naser, S.S., 2017. An expert system for diagnosing shortness of breath in infants and children. Int. J. Eng. Inform. Syst. 1, 102–115.

Abu-Naser, S.S., 2016. Male Infertility Expert System Diagnoses and Treatment. AUG Repository.

Abu-Naser, S.S., Abu Hasanein, H.A., 2016. Ear diseases diagnosis expert system using SL5 object. World Wide J. Multidiscip. Res. Devel. 2.

Abu-Naser, S.S., Akkila, A.N., 2008. A proposed expert system for skin diseases diagnosis. J. Appl. Sci. Res. 4.

Abu-Naser, S.S., Aldahdooh, R., 2016. Lower back pain expert system diagnosis and treatment. J. Multidiscip. Eng. Sci. Stud. 2.

Abu-Naser, S.S., Al-Hanjori, M.M., 2016. An expert system for men genital problems diagnosis and treatment. Int. J. Med. Res. 1.

Abu-Naser, S.S., Almurshidi, S.H., 2016. A knowledge based system for neck pain diagnosis. World Wide J. Multidiscip. Res. Devel. 2.

Abu-Naser, S.S., Al-Nakhal, M.A., 2016. A ruled based system for ear problem diagnosis and treatment. World Wide J. Multidiscip. Res. Devel. 2.

Abu-Naser, S.S., Bastami, B.G., 2016. A proposed rule based system for breasts cancer diagnosis. World Wide J. Multidiscip. Res. Devel. 2.

Abu-Naser, S.S., Hamed, M.A., 2016. An expert system for mouth problems in infants and children. J. Multidiscip. Eng. Sci. Stud. 2.

Abu-Naser, S.S., Mahdi, A.O., 2016. A proposed expert system for foot diseases diagnosis. Am. J. Innov. Res. Appl. Sci. 2.

Abu-Naser, S.S., Shaath, M.Z., 2016. Expert system urination problems diagnosis. World Wide J. Multidiscip. Res. Devel. 2.

Abu-Naser, S.S., El-Hissi, H., Abu-Rass, M., El-khozondar, N., 2010. An Expert System for Endocrine Diagnosis and Treatments Using JESS. https://scialert.net/abstract/?doi=jai.2010.239.251. https://doi.org/10.3923/jai.2010.239.251.

Ahmed, M.N., Yamany, S.M., Mohamed, N., Farag, A.A., Moriarty, T., 2002. A modified fuzzy c-means algorithm for bias field estimation and segmentation of MRI data. IEEE Trans. Med. Imaging 21, 193–199.

Ahmed, Z., Mohamed, K., Zeeshan, S., Dong, X., 2020. Artificial intelligence with multi-functional machine learning platform development for better healthcare and precision medicine. Database (Oxford) 2020.

Ajam, N., 2015. Heart diseases diagnoses using artificial neural network. IISTE Netw. Complex Syst. 5.

Al Rekhawi, H.A., Abu Ayyad, A., Abu-Naser, S.S., 2017. Rickets expert system diagnoses and treatment. Int. J. Eng. Inform. Syst. 1.

Ali, S.A., Saudi, H.I., 2014. An expert system for the diagnosis and management of oral ulcers. Tanta Dent. J. 11, 42–46.

Ali, S., Chia, P., Ong, K., 1999. Graphical knowledge-based protocols for chest pain management. In: Computers in Cardiology 1999. Vol. 26. IEEE, pp. 309–312 (Cat. No. 99CH37004).

Amisha, Malik, P., Pathania, M., Rathaur, V.K., 2019. Overview of artificial intelligence in medicine. J Family Med. Prim. Care 8, 2328–2331.

Arbaiy, N., Sulaiman, S.E., Hassan, N., Afip, Z.A., 2017. Integrated knowledge based expert system for disease diagnosis system. In: IOP Conference Series: Materials Science and Engineering vol. 226, 012097. IOP Publishing.

Arji, G., et al., 2019. Fuzzy logic approach for infectious disease diagnosis: a methodical evaluation, literature and classification. Biocybern. Biomed. Eng. 39, 937–955.

Avci, D., Dogantekin, A., 2016. An expert diagnosis system for parkinson disease based on genetic algorithm-wavelet kernel-extreme learning machine. Parkinson's Dis. 2016.

Ayangbekun Oluwafemi, J., Jimoh Ibrahim, A., 2015. Expert system for diagnosis neurodegenerative disease. Int. J. Comput. Inform. Technol. 4, 694–698.

Ayatollahi, H., Gholamhosseini, L., Salehi, M., 2019. Predicting coronary artery disease: a comparison between two data mining algorithms. BMC Public Health 19.

Başçiftçi, F., Avuçlu, E., 2018. An expert system design to diagnose cancer by using a new method reduced rule base. Comput. Methods Prog. Biomed. 157, 113–120.

Başçiftçi, F., Hatay, O.F., 2011. Reduced-rule based expert system by the simplification of logic functions for the diagnosis of diabetes. Comput. Biol. Med. 41, 350–356.

Bursuk, E., Ozkan, M., Ilerigelen, B., 1999. A medical expert system in cardiological diseases. In: Proceedings of the First Joint BMES/EMBS Conference. 1999 IEEE Engineering in Medicine and Biology 21st Annual Conference and the 1999 Annual Fall Meeting of the Biomedical Engineering Society. Vol. 2. IEEE. Cat. N vol. 2 1210.

Chui, K., et al., 2017. Disease diagnosis in smart healthcare: innovation, technologies and applications. Sustainability 9, 2309.

Datta, S., Barua, R., Das, J., 2019. Application of artificial intelligence in modern healthcare system. In: Alginates—Recent Uses of This Natural Polymer., https://doi.org/10.5772/intechopen.90454.

Davenport, T., Kalakota, R., 2019. The potential for artificial intelligence in healthcare. Future Healthc. J. 6, 94–98.

Ding, X., et al., 2018. A hybrid computational approach for efficient Alzheimer's disease classification based on heterogeneous data. Sci. Rep. 8, 9774.

Du, G., Sun, C., 2015. Location planning problem of service centers for sustainable home healthcare: evidence from the empirical analysis of Shanghai. Sustainability 7, 15812–15832.

Durairaj, M., Ranjani, V., 2013. Data mining applications in healthcare sector: a study. Int. J. Sci. Technol. Res. 2, 29–35.

El Agha, M., Jarghon, A., Abu Naser, S.S., 2017. Polymyalgia rheumatic expert system. Int. J. Eng. Inform. Syst. 1, 125–137.

Elveren, E., Yumuşak, N., 2011. Tuberculosis disease diagnosis using artificial neural network trained with genetic algorithm. J. Med. Syst. 35, 329–332.

Esmaeilzadeh, P., 2020. Use of AI-based tools for healthcare purposes: a survey study from consumers' perspectives. BMC Med. Inform. Decis. Mak. 20, 170.

Ewers, M., et al., 2011. Staging Alzheimer's disease progression with multimodality neuroimaging. Prog. Neurobiol. 95, 535–546.

Fatima, B., Amine, C.M., 2012. A neuro-fuzzy inference model for breast cancer recognition. Int. J. Comput. Sci. Inform. Technol. 4, 163.

Fatima, M., Pasha, M., 2017. Survey of machine learning algorithms for disease diagnostic. J. Intell. Learn. Syst. Appl. 9, 1.

Frank, M., Drikakis, D., Charissis, V., 2020. Machine-learning methods for computational science and engineering. Comput. Des. 8, 15.

Geberemariam, S., 2013. A Self-Learning Knowledge Based System for Diagnosis and Treatment of Diabetes. Addis Ababa University.

Ghaheri, A., Shoar, S., Naderan, M., Hoseini, S.S., 2015. The applications of genetic algorithms in medicine. Oman Med. J. 30, 406.

Ghazizadeh, A., Dehghani, M., Rokhsati, H., Fasihfar, Z., 2015. Development of a knowledge-based expert system for diagnosis and treatment of common diseases of the spine. Biomed. Pharm. J. 8, 719–723.

Godfrey, C.M., et al., 2011. Care of self–care by other–care of other: the meaning of self-care from research, practice, policy and industry perspectives. Int. J. Evid. Based Healthc. 9, 3–24.

Grosan, C., Abraham, A., 2011. Rule-based expert systems. In: Intelligent Systems. Springer, pp. 149–185.

Gudu, J., Gichoya, D., Nyongesa, P., Muumbo, A., 2012. Development of a medical expert system as an Expert-Knowledge sharing tool on diagnosis and treatment of hypertension in pregnancy. Int. J. Biosci. Biochem. Bioinform. 2, 297.

Hinrichs, C., Singh, V., Xu, G., Johnson, S., 2009. MKL for robust multi-modality AD classification. Med. Image Comput. Comput. Assist. Interv. 12, 786–794.

Hole, K.R., Gulhane, V.S., 2014. Rule-based expert system for the diagnosis of memory loss diseases. Int. J. Innov. Sci. Eng. Technol. 1, 80–83.

Hossain, M.S., Khalid, M.S., Akter, S., Dey, S., 2014. A belief rule-based expert system to diagnose influenza. In: 2014 9Th International Forum on Strategic Technology (IFOST). IEEE, pp. 113–116.

Ibrahim, F., Ali, J.B., Jaais, A.F., Taib, M.N., 2001. Expert system for early diagnosis of eye diseases infecting the Malaysian population. In: Proceedings of IEEE Region 10 International Conference on Electrical and Electronic Technology. Vol. 1. IEEE, pp. 430–432. TENCON 2001 (Cat. No. 01CH37239).

Joshi, S., Joshi, H., 2013. Applications of data mining in health and pharmaceutical industry. Int. J. Sci. Eng. Res. 4.

Kazerouni, F., et al., 2020. Type2 diabetes mellitus prediction using data mining algorithms based on the long-noncoding RNAs expression: a comparison of four data mining approaches. BMC Bioinf. 21, 372.

Khella, R., 2017. Rule based system for chest pain in infants and children. Int. J. Eng. Inform. Syst. 1.

Kocer, S., Canal, M.R., 2011. Classifying epilepsy diseases using artificial neural networks and genetic algorithm. J. Med. Syst. 35, 489–498.

Kumar, S.P.L., 2019. Knowledge-based expert system in manufacturing planning: state-of-the-art review. Int. J. Prod. Res. 57, 4766–4790.

Kumar, A., Singh, T.R., 2017. A new decision tree to solve the puzzle of Alzheimer's disease pathogenesis through standard diagnosis scoring system. Interdiscip. Sci.: Comput. Life Sci. 9, 107–115.

Lavanya, D., Rani, K.U., 2011. Performance evaluation of decision tree classifiers on medical datasets. Int. J. Comput. Appl. 26, 1–4.

Lazli, L., Boukadoum, M., Ait Mohamed, O., 2019. Computer-aided diagnosis system of Alzheimer's disease based on multimodal fusion: tissue quantification based on the hybrid fuzzy-genetic-Possibilistic model and discriminative classification based on the SVDD model. Brain Sci. 9.

Li, C.-C., Shun, S.-C., 2016. Understanding self care coping styles in patients with chronic heart failure: a systematic review. Eur. J. Cardiovasc. Nurs. 15, 12–19.

Liu, J.X., Goryakin, Y., Maeda, A., Bruckner, T., Scheffler, R., 2016. Global Health Workforce Labor Market Projections for 2030. The World Bank.

Lopez-Vallverdu, J.A., RiañO, D., Bohada, J.A., 2012. Improving medical decision trees by combining relevant health-care criteria. Expert Syst. Appl. 39, 11782–11791.

Lundervold, A.S., Lundervold, A., 2019. An overview of deep learning in medical imaging focusing on MRI. Z. Med. Phys. 29, 102–127.

Mallika, R.M., UshaRani, K., Hemalatha, K., 2019. A fuzzy-based expert system to diagnose Alzheimer's disease. In: Krishna, P.V., Gurumoorthy, S., Obaidat, M.S. (Eds.), Internet of Things and Personalized Healthcare Systems. Springer, pp. 65–74, https://doi.org/10.1007/978-981-13-0866-6_6.

Mansoori, T.K., Suman, A., Mishra, S.K., 2014. Application of genetic algorithm for cancer diagnosis by feature selection. Int. J. Eng. Res. Technol. 3, 1295–1300.

Mitra, S., 1994. Fuzzy MLP based expert system for medical diagnosis. Fuzzy Sets Syst. 65, 285–296.

Momete, D.C., 2016. Building a sustainable healthcare model: a cross-country analysis. Sustainability 8, 836.

Mrouf, A., Albatish, I., Mosa, M.J., Abu-Naser, S.S., 2017. Knowledge based system for long-term abdominal pain (stomach pain) diagnosis and treatment. Int. J. Eng. Inform. Syst. 1.

Munir, K., de Ramón-Fernández, A., Iqbal, S., Javaid, N., 2019. Neuroscience patient identification using big data and fuzzy logic–an Alzheimer's disease case study. Expert Syst. Appl. 136, 410–425.

Nabahin, A., Abou Eloun, A., Abu-Naser, S.S., 2017. Expert system for hair loss diagnosis and treatment. Int. J. Eng. Inform. Syst. 1.

Naser, S.S.A., El Haddad, I.A., 2016. An expert system for genital problems in infants. World Wide J. Multidiscip. Res. Devel. 2.

Neshat, M., Yaghobi, M., Naghibi, M.B., Esmaelzadeh, A., 2008. Fuzzy expert system design for diagnosis of liver disorders. In: 2008 International Symposium on Knowledge Acquisition and Modeling. IEEE, pp. 252–256.

Oehm, S., Siessmeier, T., Buchholz, H.-G., Bartenstein, P., Uthmann, T., 2003. A knowledge-based system for the diagnosis of Alzheimer's disease. In: Dojat, M., Keravnou, E.T., Barahona, P. (Eds.), Artificial Intelligence in Medicine. Springer, pp. 117–121, https://doi.org/10.1007/978-3-540-39907-0_17.

Pal, N.R., Pal, K., Keller, J.M., Bezdek, J.C., 2005. A possibilistic fuzzy c-means clustering algorithm. IEEE Trans. Fuzzy Syst. 13, 517–530.

Panigrahi, P.P., Singh, T.R., 2012. Computational analysis for functional and evolutionary aspects of BACE-1 and associated Alzheimer's related proteins. Int. J. Comput. Int. Stud. 1.

Panigrahi, P.P., Singh, T.R., 2013. Computational studies on Alzheimer's disease associated pathways and regulatory patterns using microarray gene expression and network data: revealed association with aging and other diseases. J. Theor. Biol. 334, 109–121.

Panigrahi, P.P., Singh, T.R., 2017. Data mining, big data, data analytics: big data analytics in bioinformatics. In: Library and Information Services for Bioinformatics Education and Research, pp. 91–111. www.igi-global.com/chapter/data-mining-big-data-data-analytics/176138. https://doi.org/10.4018/978-1-5225-1871-6.ch005.

Panzarasa, S., et al., 2010. Data mining techniques for analyzing stroke care processes. Stud. Health Technol. Inform. 160, 939–943.

Patel, M.N., Patel, A., Virparia, P.V., 2013. Rule Based Expert System for Viral Infection Diagnosis. paper/Rule-Based-Expert-System-for-Viral-Infection-Patel-Patel/426e9e630d49287901946631106a7c336c4c863c.

Patra, P.S.K., Sahu, D.P., Mandal, I., 2010. An expert system for diagnosis of human diseases. Int. J. Comput. Appl. 1, 71–73.

Pereira, D.C., Ramos, R.P., Do Nascimento, M.Z., 2014. Segmentation and detection of breast cancer in mammograms combining wavelet analysis and genetic algorithm. Comput. Methods Prog. Biomed. 114, 88–101.

Prasad, B., Wood, H., Greer, J., McCalla, G., 1989. A knowledge-based system for tutoring bronchial asthma diagnosis. In: 1989 Proceedings. Second Annual IEEE Symposium on Computer-based Medical Systems. IEEE, pp. 40–45.

Qwaider, S.R., Abu Naser, S.S., 2017. Expert system for diagnosing ankle diseases. Int. J. Eng. Inform. Syst.

Réda, C., Kaufmann, E., Delahaye-Duriez, A., 2020. Machine learning applications in drug development. Comput. Struct. Biotechnol. J. 18, 241–252.

Reddy, M.P.S.C., Palagi, M.P., Jaya, S., 2017. Heart disease prediction using ann algorithm in data mining. Int. J. Comput. Sci. Mob. Comput. 6, 168–172.

Shahid, N., Rappon, T., Berta, W., 2019. Applications of artificial neural networks in health care organizational decision-making: a scoping review. PLoS One 14.

Shortliffe, E.H., 1986. Medical expert systems—knowledge tools for physicians. West. J. Med. 145, 830.

Shukla, R., Singh, T.R., 2020. Virtual screening, pharmacokinetics, molecular dynamics and binding free energy analysis for small natural molecules against cyclin-dependent kinase 5 for Alzheimer's disease. J. Biomol. Struct. Dyn. 38, 248–262.

Shukla, R., Munjal, N.S., Singh, T.R., 2019. Identification of novel small molecules against GSK3β for Alzheimer's disease using chemoinformatics approach. J. Mol. Graph. Model. 91, 91–104.

Shukla, R., Yadav, A.K., Singh, T.R., 2021. Application of deep learning in biological big data analysis. In: Large-Scale Data Streaming, Processing, and Blockchain Security, pp. 117–148. www.igi-global.com/chapter/application-of-deep-learning-in-biological-big-data-analysis/259468. https://doi.org/10.4018/978-1-7998-3444-1.ch006.

Siler, W., Buckley, J.J., 2005. Fuzzy Expert Systems and Fuzzy Reasoning. John Wiley & Sons.

Singh, S., et al., 2018. Bioinformatics in next-generation genome sequencing. In: Wadhwa, G., Shanmughavel, P., Singh, A.K., Bellare, J.R. (Eds.), Current Trends in Bioinformatics: An Insight. Springer, pp. 27–38, https://doi.org/10.1007/978-981-10-7483-7_2.

Sweidan, S., et al., 2019. A fibrosis diagnosis clinical decision support system using fuzzy knowledge. Arab. J. Sci. Eng. 44, 3781–3800.

Toli, A.M., Murtagh, N., 2020. The concept of sustainability in Smart City definitions. Front. Built Environ. 6.

Uyar, K., Ilhan, A., 2017. Diagnosis of heart disease using genetic algorithm based trained recurrent fuzzy neural networks. Procedia Comput. Sci. 120, 588–593.

Vijayakumar, A., Vijayakumar, A., 2013. Comparison of hippocampal volume in dementia subtypes. ISRN Radiol. 2013, e174524. https://www.hindawi.com/journals/isrn/2013/174524/nn(2012.

Wang, X., 2016. The application of genetic algorithms in the biological medical diagnostic research. Int. J. Bioautom. 20, 493–504.

Weli, Z.N.S., 2020. Data mining in cancer diagnosis and prediction: review about latest ten years. Curr. J. Appl. Sci. Technol., 11–32. https://doi.org/10.9734/cjast/2020/v39i630555.

Weller, J., Budson, A., 2018. Current understanding of Alzheimer's disease diagnosis and treatment. F1000Res. 7.

Yager, R.R., Zadeh, L.A., 2012. An Introduction to Fuzzy Logic Applications in Intelligent Systems. vol. 165 Springer Science & Business Media.

CHAPTER

# An entropy-based hybrid feature selection approach for medical datasets

# 12

**Rakesh Raja and Bikash Kanti Sarkar**

*Department of Computer Science and Engineering, Birla Institute of Technology, Mesra, Ranchi, India*

## Chapter outline

## 1 Introduction

In recent years, the rapid adoption of computerized Disease Decision Support Systems (DDSS) has been shown to be a promising avenue for improving clinical research (Chen and Tan, 2012; Garg et al., 2005; Kensaku et al., 2005; Moja et al., 2014; Narasingarao et al., 2009; Syeda-Mahmood, 2015; Thirugnanam et al., 2012; Wagholikar et al., 2012; Ye et al., 2002; Srimani and Koti, 2014; Gambhir et al., 2016; Subbulakshmi and Deepa, 2016; Bhardwaj and Tiwari, 2015; Sartakhti et al., 2012; Li and Fu, 2014; Fana et al., 2011; McSherry, 2011; Marling et al., 2014; Prasad et al., 2016;

Singh and Pandey, 2014; Downs et al., 1996; Kawamoto et al., 2005; Sampat et al., 2005; Lisboa and Taktak, 2006). The reason for constructing DDSSs is that manual detection of diseases is prohibitively expensive, time consuming, and prone to error. However, there exist various *challenges* and *practical limitations* associated with clinical data. One big issue is to operate *redundant* and *noisy features*, many of which are correlated and/or of no significant diagnostic value. The redundant (and noisy) features unnecessarily increase the learning time of DDSS, and sometimes degrade the performance of the system. Feature-selection is the only solution of this issue.

## 1.1 Deficiencies of the existing models

To improve prediction accuracy of learning models by reducing feature space dimensionality, a significant number of feature-selection methods have been proposed over the years, using various schemes like probability distribution, entropy, correlation, etc. (Abdullah et al., 2014; Bhattacharyya and Kalita, 2013; Hoque et al., 2014; Swiniarski and Skowron, 2003; Breiman, 1996; Schapire, 1999). In recent years, feature selection methods are being greatly used to reduce dimensionality of data for big data analytics (Fernández et al., 2017; Kashyap et al., 2015). For comprehensive review on feature selection, one may refer the recent study (Li et al., 2017). In this chapter, it is stated that some hot topics for feature selections, e.g., stable feature selection, multiview feature selection, and multilevel feature selection have been emerged.

Although many works have been reported in the literature, there is still scope for improvement. For example, most of them are not stable and lack to select the more accurate *attributes* from dataset in linear time.

*Contribution*: Addressing the issues of the existing models, a stable linear time entropy-based feature-selection approach is introduced in the present chapter, mainly focusing on medical datasets of different sizes. In particular, stability is the *sensitivity* of the chosen feature set to variations in supplied training dataset. More specifically, how much the model is sensitive to the small changes in the dataset? Undoubtedly, such model is important, especially in medical datasets.

## 1.2 Chapter organization

The rest of the chapter is organized as follows. In Section 2, a brief discussion is given on feature selection, whereas the methodology proposed in this research is explained in Section 3. The experimental results are presented in Section 4, whereas the obtained results are analyzed in Section 5. Conclusions and future scopes are presented in Section 6.

# 2 Background of the present research

## 2.1 Feature selection (FS)

The term feature selection refers to the process of selecting the optimal features (i.e., only the most relevant features). In other words, it aims to reduce the inputs for processing and analysis. Owing to several dependent features in datasets (especially in medical datasets), feature engineering needs to be employed to select the most important ones that are likely to have a greater impact on our final model. The prime goal of any feature selection approach is to select a subset of features from the input which can efficiently describe the input data while reducing noisy or irrelevant features (accordingly reducing training time of learner and avoiding the case of overfitting model) and aims at good prediction results (Guyon and Elisseeff, 2003). In particular, when two features are perfectly correlated, only one feature is sufficient to describe the data. The dependent features provide no extra information about the classes, and thus serve as noise for the predictor. This means that the total information content can be obtained from fewer unique features which contain maximum discrimination information about the classes. Hence by eliminating the dependent variables, the amount of data can be reduced which can lead to improvement in the classification performance. More specifically, irrelevant and redundant attributes which do not have significance in classification task are reduced from the dataset.

In practice, two approaches are employed to reduce dimensionality of datasets. These are, namely feature selection and feature-extraction. Feature selection (FS) involves selection (but not transformation) of features using certain optimization function, whereas feature extraction allows transformation of features. More specifically, feature selection finds a subset of optimal features, whereas feature extraction creates a subset of new features by combinations of the existing features.

Obviously, feature selection is one of the preprocessing techniques in data mining. Several methods exist in literature for feature selection. In practice, the methods are grouped into three categories, namely filter, wrapper, and hybrid model (Witten Ian and Eibe, 2005). These are briefly explained.

- Filter method: The filter method relies on general characteristic of data to evaluate and select feature subsets without involving any mining algorithm. These are typically faster and give *an average* accuracy for all the classifiers. This method mainly focuses on elimination of feature (columns) with more missing values, elimination of features consisting of difference between maximum and minimum values of attribute with very less, and elimination of features with high correlation among themselves. Filters are usually less computationally intensive. Examples include *information gain*, *chi-square test*, *fisher score*, *correlation coefficient*, and *variance threshold*.
- The wrapper model requires one predetermined mining algorithm and uses its performance as the evaluation criteria. The wrapper methods can result high classification accuracy than filter methods for particular classifiers but they are less *cost effective*. Thus, the wrapper methods primarily focuses on the following point.
  - Selection of a set of features that result in comparatively high classification accuracy and low error rate

    In short, the wrapper methods attempt to find a subset of features and train a *learner* to get its performance. So, it is comparatively expensive. The wrapper methods usually work on recursive approach that may be of two types—forward selection and backward selection. In forward selection, features are included into a set of selected features (starting with a null set) one by one to improve the performance of the learners until no improvement is observed. This results in a set of the best features. On the other hand, the backward strategy attempts to discard the feature set (starting with the complete/original set of features) one by one to improve the performance of the learners. The process stops when no improvement of the learners is found. Here, the *worst* features are discarded from the original set. The wrapper models are comparatively computationally intensive, but it is true that selection of optimal feature subset is an NP-hard problem (Liu and Yu, 2005), which is not solvable in polynomial time. For tackling NP-hard problems, the most commonly used random search method—Genetic algorithm (GA)—is treated as the best solution (Goldberg, 1989). In a survey paper on feature selection (Chandrashekar and Sahin, 2014), Chandrashekar and Sahin have shown that GA may be treated as the best strategy for designing wrapper model to result in the best-performing feature set for that particular type of model or typical problem.

- Embedded models: These models use the algorithms that adopt built-in feature selection methods. For instance, principal component analysis (PCA) and random forest have their own feature selection methods. These approaches tend to be between filters and wrappers in terms of computational complexity.

Lastly, we may design some hybrid approaches (a specific case of ensemble approach) that are usually the combination of filter and/or wrapper models. No matter, feature-selection improves the performance of classifiers and it reduces the learning time, as there is less number of features (as compared to the original set).

Thus, any feature selection process usually consists of the following steps.

**(i)** Identification of a candidate subset of attributes from an original set of features using some searching techniques.
**(ii)** Evaluation of the subset to determine the relevancy toward the classification task using measures such as distance, dependency, information, consistency, and classifier's error rate.
**(iii)** Setting termination condition to decide the relevant subset or optimal feature subset.
**(iv)** Validation of the selected feature subset.

In the present research, feature selection technique (under filter category) is used to reduce the dimensionality of dataset.

## 3 Methodology
### 3.1 The entropy based feature selection approach

In 2000, Hall reported that the attributes having strong correlation cannot be the part of feature subset (Hall, 2000). It was also stated in his article that if the attributes are more independent among themselves, then the more information gain they have. Hence, it is expected to give improved results over unseen data. Interestingly, the present research focuses on medical datasets. As medical datasets are more sensitive, so stable feature selection approach is more effective for such datasets. With this point in mind, a stable simple entropy-based approach is introduced here and it is described below.

For better understanding the model, a conceptual model is shown in Fig. 1.

Before applying the proposed feature selection approach on any dataset (D), it is first discretized by minimum information loss (MIL) discretizer (Sarkar et al., 2011b), and each discretized dataset (D) is then split into 3 subdatasets, namely $D_1$, $D_2$, and $D_3$ based on *equi-class* distribution data-partitioning scheme as follows. The idea on equi-class distribution is first illustrated below. For understanding the effect of equi-class distribution method, one may refer to article cited herein (Sarkar, 2016).

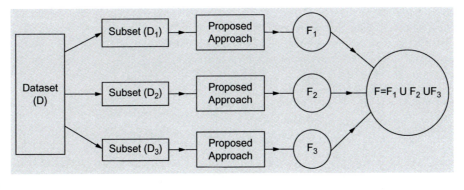

**FIG. 1**

Proposed feature selection approach.

### 3.1.1 Equi-class distribution of instances

According to the concept of equi-class distribution, same percentage of examples of each class is to be included in the training set.

*Illustration*: Suppose 30% examples of each class from a dataset (D) are to be randomly included in a set say T. Assume that there are 3 class values (say $c_1$, $c_2$, and $c_3$) and total 150 examples in D and the numbers of examples of class types: $c_1$, $c_2$, and $c_3$ are respectively 33, 42, and 75. Then 10, 13, and 23 examples of class types: $c_1$, $c_2$, and $c_3$ (based on the concept of *ceil* function, e.g., $\lceil \frac{33 \times 30}{100} \rceil = \lceil \frac{990}{100} \rceil = \lceil 9.9 \rceil = 10$) are included in T by random selection over D.

### 3.1.2 Splitting the dataset D into subsets: $D_1$, $D_2$, and $D_3$

- $D_1$ (1st subset): Here, 30% examples of each class are randomly drawn from D and included them in $D_1$ but the selected instances are not removed from D.
- $D_2$ (2nd subset): 30% examples of each class are again selected at random from D to include them in $D_2$ but attention is paid to include several distinct instances of D into $D_2$.
- $D_3$ (3rd subset): Rest of examples of D (not in $D_1$ and $D_2$) are placed in $D_3$. This is fully an independent dataset.

**Note:** Some common instances may be included in $D_1$ and $D_2$ with the intention to balance the datasets in terms of number of instances in each subset and not to ignore the informative attributes in the selected set of features. Importantly, the number of the subdatasets is here restricted to 3. However, if the number of subdatasets increases, then performance of feature selection algorithm improves but complexity increases. In many cases, the improvement of performance after certain division of data sets is negligible, and hence only three subsets are decided in the present investigation.

Suppose the dataset (D) has $n$ attributes, say $A_i$, $i = 1, \ldots n$. Let $F_s$ denote a set of features and $F_s = \{A_1, A_2, \ldots, A_n\}$.

As D is here split into 3 subsets: $D_1$, $D_2$, and $D_3$, so we will get three sets of selected features, each from a distinct subset of data. Suppose these feature sets are $F_1$, $F_2$ and $F_3$. Initially, $F_k$ ($k = 1, 2, 3$) = $F_s$. Let F be the resulting feature set obtained from $F_1$, $F_2$ and $F_3$.

Assume that P is a classification problem with $n$ attributes, say $A_i$ $_{(i=1, ...n)}$. Let F denote a set of features. Initially, $F = F_s = \{A_1, A_2, ..., A_n\}$.

1. *for* each sub-dataset ($D_k$, k = 1, 2, 3) *do*begin
2. *for* each attribute $A_i$ $_{(i=1, .. n)}$ *do*begin
3. Find information-gain for $A_i$ (i.e., Gain(S, $A_i$)) applying the formula:

$$Gain(S, A_i) = Entropy(S) - \sum_{v_j \in A_i} \frac{|S_{v_j}|}{|S|} Entropy(S_{v_j}),$$ where $v_j$ $_{(j=1,...k)}$ denotes values of attribute

$A_i$ and $Entropy(S) = \sum_{m=1}^{c} p_m \log_2 p_m$, where $S$ represents the number of examples in P, and $p_m$ is the nonzero probability of $S_m$ examples (out of $S$) belonging to class $m$, out of $c$ classes.

   *endfor*
4. Compute $r = ((max\_Gain(S, A_i) - min\_Gain(S, A_i))/n, (i = 1, ..., n)$
   // ($max\_Gain(S, A_i)$ and $min\_Gain(S, A_i)_{(i=1, ..., n)}$, are respectively *the maximum* and *the minimum information gain* among all the attributes.
5. *for* each attribute $A_i$ $_{(i=1, ..., n)}$ *do*
   begin
6. If $Gain(S, A_i)_{,(i=1,..n)} < r$, then update the feature set ($F_k$) as: $F_k = F_k - \{A_i\}$ // *discarding $A_i$ from F*
   endfor
   *endfor*
7. $F = F_1 \cup F_2 \cup F_3$
   /* F includes the common and noncommon attributes of $F_1$, $F_2$, and $F_3$. As dataset corresponding to $F_1$, $F_2$ and $F_3$ are balanced or close to balanced, so the chance of occurring common attributes in $F_1$, $F_2$ and $F_3$ increases. */.

**Note:** The computed value of $r = ((max\_Gain(S, A_i) - min\_Gain(S, A_i))/n, (i = 1, ..., n)$, is decided as the *threshold value* for filtering features. The reason is that if the difference is very high for a dataset, then the dataset may have several features possessing very less contribution in building expert system, and these may be ignored from the feature set. On the other hand, if the difference is very low, then each of them plays almost equal role in designing expert system. This strategy is a kind of *filtration technique* for feature selection based on simple search strategy. It is explained in Appendix A.

***Complexity analysis***: The algorithm is very simple and *straightforward*. Its running time is simply $O(n)$, where $n$ is the number of attributes in the dataset. The approach is implemented in Java-1.4.1.

## 4 Experiment and experimental results

This section first describes the experiments conducted in the present research over 14 real-world benchmark medical datasets drawn from UCI data repository (Blake et al., 1999). The datasets are of different sizes, e.g., comparatively large dataset with high dimension, high-dimensional but small sample-sized data, and medium-sized dataset with less number of features. The datasets are summarized in Table 1. The obtained results are arranged in tables and the results are then analyzed.

**Table 1 Summary of the selected UCI datasets (original).**

| Problem name | Number of nontarget attributes | Number of classes | Number of examples |
|---|---|---|---|
| Breast cancer Wisconsin | 10 | 2 | 699 |
| Dermatology | 34 | 6 | 366 |
| Ecoli | 8 | 8 | 336 |
| Heart (Hungarian) | 13 | 5 | 294 |
| Heart (Swiss) | 13 | 5 | 123 |
| Heart (Cleveland) | 13 | 5 | 303 |
| Hepatitis | 19 | 2 | 155 |
| Liver disorder | 6 | 2 | 345 |
| Lung cancer | 56 | 3 | 32 |
| Lymphography | 18 | 4 | 148 |
| New thyroid | 5 | 3 | 215 |
| Pima Indian diabetes | 8 | 2 | 768 |
| Primary tumor | 17 | 22 | 339 |
| Sick | 29 | 2 | 3772 |

## 4.1 Experiment using suggested feature selection approach

The implemented feature selection approach is run over 14 selected datasets. A list of selected features of the datasets is presented in Table 2. The table describes respectively the *name* of each dataset (denoted as DN), *number of instances* (NI), *number of features* (NF), *number of selected feature* (NSF), and the *selected features* (SF). The importance of the introduced approach is affirmed through the performance of the classifiers, viz., J48 (Java version of C4.5 (Quinlan, 1993)), naïve Bayes (Duda and Hurt, 1973) and JRIP (Java version of RIPPER (Cohen, 1995)) over the dataset (before and after selecting their features) shown in Tables 3 and 4, respectively.

In particular, naïve Bayes learner is chosen because it works better on datasets with independent features and the suggested feature selection approach focuses on identifying such features. On the other hand, JRIP is chosen, since it pays attention to select pure/correct rules. Further, the DT-based classifier C4.5 gives an average all datasets. For better estimation of the classifiers, 10-fold cross validation scheme is run 10 times in the WEKA toolbox.

Looking into Table 1, it is clear that the datasets, namely Breast cancer, Dermatology, Primary tumor, and Sick are comparatively large datasets with more features, whereas datasets, namely heart (Swiss), hepatitis, and lung cancer are the examples of high dimensional small-sized datasets. The remaining datasets (presented in Table 1) are the medium-sized datasets with less number of features.

## 5 Discussion
### 5.1 Performance analysis of the suggested feature selection approach

From the accuracy results yield by the selected learners over the datasets (displayed in Tables 3 and 4), the following points may be highlighted.

**Table 2** Datasets with selected features.

| Name of dataset (DN) | Number of instances (NI) | Number of features in the original datasets | Number of selected features | Selected features |
|---|---|---|---|---|
| Breast cancer Wisconsin | 699 | 10 | 6 | 1, 3, 4, 5, 6, 9 |
| Dermatology | 366 | 34 | 21 | 2, 3, 4, 5, 6, 7, 9,13,14,15,16, 19, 20, 21, 22, 26, 27, 28, 29, 30, 33 |
| Ecoli | 336 | 8 | 6 | 1, 2, 3, 5, 6, 7 |
| Heart (Hungarian) | 294 | 13 | 6 | 2, 3, 6, 9, 10, 11 |
| Heart (Swiss) | 123 | 13 | 3 | 9,10,11 |
| Heart (Cleveland) | 303 | 13 | 8 | 2, 3, 8, 9, 10, 11, 12, 13 |
| Hepatitis | 155 | 19 | 9 | 1, 2, 6, 11, 12, 14, 17, 18, 19 |
| Liver disorder | 345 | 6 | 2 | 3, 5 |
| Lung cancer | 32 | 56 | 17 | 1, 3, 5, 9, 13, 14, 15, 20, 21, 25 26, 38, 41, 45, 48, 50, 56 |
| Lymphography | 148 | 18 | 10 | 1, 2, 7, 8, 9, 11, 13, 15, 16, 18 |
| New-thyroid | 215 | 5 | 5 | 1, 2, 3, 4, 5 |
| Pima-Indians | 768 | 8 | 4 | 2, 6, 7, 8 |
| Primary tumor | 339 | 17 | 12 | 1, 2, 3, 4, 5, 7, 9, 10, 13, 15, 16, 17 |
| Sick | 3772 | 29 | 8 | 1, 8, 10, 14, 15, 20, 24, 29 |

- The accuracy (%) of the competent classifiers increases in almost all cases after removing their redundant features. In particular, the performance of naïve Bayes classifier improves significantly in almost all cases and it indicates that the introduced feature filtration method is good enough for reducing features. The reason behind the claim is that naïve Bayes classifier works better over datasets with independent features and the suggested approach aims to select such attributes. Actually, the features with very less amount of contribution (i.e., less information gain) are removed from the set when the filtration approach is applied. In other words, we may demand that the dependent features are removed from the datasets.
- The datasets with reduced features are much reliable, since standard deviation (*s.d.*) of the accuracy results yielded by the classifiers are less as compared to the standard deviation of the accuracies calculated over the original ones.

Due to feature reduction, the *learning time* of the proposed hybrid model will be reduced to a great extent, and the size of each induced rule will be small.

**Table 3** Performance of J48, JRIP, and naïve Bayes classifiers on the datasets using 10-fold cross-validation over 10 runs (*before feature selection*).

| Problem name | Number of nontarget attributes | J48 (acc. ± s.d.) | JRIP (acc. ± s.d.) | Naïve Bayes (acc. ±s.d.) |
|---|---|---|---|---|
| Breast cancer | 10 | 73.28 ± 6.05 | 71.45 ± 6.45 | 74.70 ± 7.74 |
| Dermatology | 34 | 90.11 ± 3.34 | 86.61 ± 4.89 | 91.01 ± 2.41 |
| Ecoli | 8 | 82.13 ± 5.73 | 81.41 ± 6.30 | 84.51 ± 5.46 |
| Heart (Hungarian) | 13 | 78.22 ± 7.95 | 79.57 ± 6.64 | 80.95 ± 6.27 |
| Heart (Swiss) | 13 | 36.45 ± 13.73 | 38.08 ± 9.36 | 36.38 ± 13.13 |
| Heart (Cleveland) | 13 | 76.94 ± 6.59 | 78.95 ± 6.77 | 81.34 ± 7.20 |
| Hepatitis | 19 | 77.22 ± 9.57 | 76.13 ± 9.04 | 81.81 ± 9.70 |
| Liver disorder | 6 | 62.84 ± 7.40 | 68.57 ± 7.55 | 54.89 ± 8.83 |
| Lung cancer | 56 | 68.25 ± 21.50 | 73.92 ± 19.15 | 76.42 ± 21.12 |
| Lymphography | 18 | 74.84 ± 11.05 | 75.11 ± 11.37 | 82.13 ± 8.89 |
| New-thyroid | 5 | 93.11 ± 4.32 | 94.01 ± 4.57 | 94.16 ± 3.16 |
| Pima-Indians | 8 | 73.89 ± 5.27 | 74.18 ± 4.54 | 75.75 ± 5.32 |
| Primary tumor | 17 | 41.139 ± 6.94 | 38.74 ± 5.57 | 47.71 ± 6.46 |
| Sick | 29 | 93.13 ± 0.55 | 93.29 ± 0.68 | 92.88 ± 1.36 |

*Note:* acc. *is simply* accuracy percentage, *whereas* s.d. *stands for* standard deviation.

**Table 4** Performance of J48, JRIP, and naïve Bayes classifiers on the datasets using 10-fold cross-validation over 10 run (*after feature selection*).

| Problem name | Number of nontarget attributes after reduction | J48 (acc. ± s.d.) | JRIP (acc. ± s.d.) | Naïve Bayes (acc. ± s.d.) |
|---|---|---|---|---|
| Breast cancer | 6 (10) | 78.71 ± 1.39 | 76.97 ± 2.03 | 80.13 ± 1.23 |
| Dermatology | 21 (34) | 90.88 ± 1.20 | 88.15 ± 2.18 | 92.14 ± 1.23 |
| Ecoli | 6 (8) | 82.49 ± 2.46 | 80.91 ± 1.82 | 85.61 ± 1.19 |
| Heart (Hungarian) | 6 (13) | 78.84 ± 1.19 | 80.06 ± 1.81 | 84.07 ± 1.10 |
| Heart (Swiss) | 3 (13) | 38.26 ± 3.14 | 38.02 ± 2.39 | 38.83 ± 2.82 |
| Heart (Cleveland) | 8 (13) | 78.55 ± 2.01 | 80.15 ± 2.35 | 83.81 ± 1.48 |
| Hepatitis | 9 (19) | 80.95 ± 3.38 | 78.99 ± 3.41 | 86.45 ± 2.11 |
| Liver disorder | 2 (6) | 62.15 ± 2.72 | 69.04 ± 2.07 | 56.81 ± 2.01 |
| Lung cancer | 17 (56) | 70.74 ± 7.28 | 73.24 ± 6.12 | 79.02 ± 4.37 |
| Lymphography | 10 (18) | 74.99 ± 2.03 | 74.75 ± 3.32 | 82.94 ± 1.75 |
| New-thyroid | 5 (5) | 93.08 ± 1.09 | 93.20 ± 1.42 | 94.30 ± 0.68 |
| Pima-Indians | 4 (8) | 74.43 ± 1.88 | 74.09 ± 2.31 | 77.47 ± 1.19 |
| Primary tumor | 12 (17) | 40.81 ± 1.83 | 39.22 ± 1.92 | 47.72 ± 1.12 |
| Sick | 8 (29) | 92.89 ± 0.09 | 93.19 ± 0.04 | 93.13 ± 0.08 |

*Note: Count within* parenthesis *placed in the second column gives the number of features in the original dataset.*

## 6 Conclusions and future works

At the end of this study, it may be once again pointed out that the techniques of feature selection and extraction seek to compress the dataset into a lower dimensional data vector so that classification accuracy can be increased.

The literature on feature selection techniques is very vast encompassing the applications of machine learning and pattern recognition. Comparison between feature selection algorithms is appropriate using a single dataset, since each underlying algorithm behaves differently for different data. Feature selection techniques show that more information is not always good in machine learning applications.

In this paper, an entropy-based hybrid feature selection method is introduced which combines subsets of features selected over different subsets of dataset and yields an optimal subset of features. To evaluate the performance of the model, classifiers, viz., C4.5 (decision tree-based), JRIP (sequential covering), and naïve Bayes on the datasets drawn from UCI data repository are applied. The overall performance has been found to be excellent for all these datasets.

## Conflict of interest

The study is not funded by any agency. It does not involve other human participants and/or animals. The author declares that there is *no conflict of interests* regarding the publication of this paper.

## Appendix A

*Classification problem*: A classification problem (P) is described by a set of attributes categorized as: nontarget (i.e., *feature*) attribute and class (also known as target) attribute. Each problem contains only one target attribute but many feature attributes.

For better understanding the classification problem, let us consider the "*golf-playing*" problem. The problem takes here four *feature* attributes viz., *Outlook*, *Temperature*, *Humidity* and *Windy*. The target is named *Playing-decision*. The feature attributes are denoted as respectively $A_1$, $A_2$, $A_3$ and $A_4$, whereas C is used for the class attribute. The possible nondiscretized values of the attributes are noted below.

| Name of attribute | Values |
|---|---|
| Outlook ($A_1$) | Sunny, overcast, rain |
| Humidity ($A_2$) | High, normal |
| Temperature ($A_3$) | Hot, mild, cool |
| Windy ($A_4$) | Strong, weak |
| Playing-decision (C) | No, yes |

A nondiscretized dataset of 14 days observations for this problem is shown in Table A.1. Here, $D_i$ ($i = 1, ..., 14$) represents day.

$$\text{Entropy}(S) = H(S) = -\sum_{i=1}^{c} p_i \log_2 p_i,$$ where $S$ represents the number of currently considered learn-

**Table A.1  A sample of nondiscretized "*golf-playing*" data set.**

| SI. no. | Nontarget attributes ($A_i$, $i = 1, ..., 4$) | | | | Playing-decision |
|---|---|---|---|---|---|
| | Outlook ($A_1$) | Temperature ($A_2$) | Humidity ($A_3$) | Windy ($A_4$) | |
| $D_1$ | Sunny | Hot | High | Strong | No |
| $D_2$ | Sunny | Hot | High | Strong | No |
| $D_3$ | Overcast | Hot | High | Weak | Yes |
| $D_4$ | Rain | Mild | High | Weak | Yes |
| $D_5$ | Rain | Cool | Normal | Weak | Yes |
| $D_6$ | Rain | Cool | Normal | Strong | No |
| $D_7$ | Overcast | Cool | Normal | Strong | Yes |
| $D_8$ | Sunny | Mild | High | Weak | No |
| $D_9$ | Sunny | Cool | Normal | Weak | Yes |
| $D_{10}$ | Rain | Mild | Normal | Weak | Yes |
| $D_{11}$ | Sunny | Mild | Normal | Strong | Yes |
| $D_{12}$ | Overcast | Mild | High | Strong | Yes |
| $D_{13}$ | Overcast | Hot | Normal | Weak | Yes |
| $D_{14}$ | Rain | Mild | High | Strong | No |

ing examples and $p_i$ is the nonzero probability of the examples (say $S_i$ in $S$) belonging to class $i$, out of $c$ classes. Here, number of nontarget attributes (features) is 4 and the number of classes is 2.

## A.1  Explanation on entropy-based feature extraction approach

The initial entropy (i.e., impurity) in the training set was:

$$= -(9/14)\log_2(9/14) - (5/14)\log_2(5/14) = 0.940 \text{ (since number of classes} = 2).$$

Now,

$$Gain(S, Wind) = Entropy(S) - \frac{|S_{Weak}|}{|S|} Entropy(S_{Weak}) - \frac{|S_{Strong}|}{|S|} Entropy(S_{Strong})$$

$$= 0.940 - \frac{8}{14} \cdot Entropy(S_{Weak}) - \frac{6}{14} \cdot Entropy(S_{Strong})$$

$$= 0.940 - \frac{8}{14}\left(-\frac{6}{8}\log_2\frac{6}{8} - \frac{2}{8}\log_2\frac{2}{8}\right) - \frac{6}{14}\left(-\frac{3}{6}\log_2\frac{3}{6} - \frac{3}{6}\log_2\frac{3}{6}\right) = 0.048$$

Likewise,

$$Gain(S, Outlook) = 0.246, Gain(S, Temperature) = 0.029, Gain(S, Humidity) = 0.151.$$

$Gain(S, Outlook) = 0.246$ is the *maximum information gain*, whereas $Gain(S, Temperature) = 0.029$ is the *minimum information gain*.

Thus, $r = (0.246{-}0.029)/n = (0.246{-}0.029)/4 = 0.05425$, since $n$ (number of attributes) $= 4$. Here, each of the two attributes—*Outlook* and *Humidity*—has gain-information greater than or equal to $r = 0.05425$. Now, based on the suggested *threshold criteria*, two attributes, namely, *Temperature* and *Windy*, may be removed from the dataset, since each of the attributes—*Temperature* and *Windy*—carries very less information and the *gain-information* is less than the value of $r$.

# References

Abdullah, S., Sabar, N.R., Nazri, M.Z.A., Ayob, M., 2014. An exponential Monte-Carlo algorithm for feature selection problems. Comput. Ind. Eng. 67, 160–167.

Bhardwaj, A., Tiwari, A., 2015. Breast cancer diagnosis using genetically optimized neural network model. Expert Syst. Appl. 42, 1–15.

Bhattacharyya, D.K., Kalita, J.K., 2013. Network Anomaly Detection: A Machine Learning Perspective. CRC Press, Boca Raton.

Blake, C., Koegh, E., Mertz, C.J., 1999. Repository of Machine Learning. University of California at Irvine. URL http://www.mlearn.ics.uci.edu/MLRepository.html.

Breiman, L., 1996. Bagging predictors. Mach. Learn. 24 (2), 123–140.

Chandrashekar, G., Sahin, F., 2014. A survey on feature selection methods. Comput. Electr. Eng. 40 (1), 16–28.

Chen, H., Tan, C., 2012. Prediction of type 2 diabetes based on several element levels in blood and chemo metrics. Biol. Trace Elem. Res. 147 (1–3), 67–74.

Cohen, W.W., 1995. Fast effective rule induction. In: Proceeding of Twelfth International Conference on Machine Learning, pp. 115–123.

Downs, J., Harrison, R.F., Kennedy, R.L., Cross, S.S., 1996. Application of the fuzzy ARTMAP neural network model to medical pattern classification tasks. Artif. Intell. Med. 8 (4), 403–428.

Duda, R.O., Hurt, P.E., 1973. Pattern Classification and Scene Analysis. John Wiley and Sons.

Fana, C.Y., Chang, P.C., Lin, J.J., Hsieh, J.C., 2011. A hybrid model combining case-based reasoning and fuzzy decision tree for medical data classification. Appl. Soft Comput. 11, 632–644.

Fernández, A., del Río, S., Chawla, N.V., Herrera, F., 2017. An insight into imbalanced big data classification: outcomes and challenges. Complex Intell. Syst. 3 (2), 105–120.

Gambhir, S., Malik, S.K., Kumar, Y., 2016. Role of soft-computing approaches in healthcare domain: a mini review. J. Med. Syst. https://doi.org/10.1007/S10916-016-0651. Springer.

Garg, A.X., Adhikari, N.K., McDonald, H., Arellano, M.P.R., Devereaux, P.J., Beyene, J., 2005. Effects of computerized clinical decision support systems on practitioner performance and patient outcomes: a systematic review. JAMA 293 (10), 1223–1238.

Goldberg, D.E., 1989. Genetic Algorithms in Search Optimization and Machine Learning. Addison Wesley, New York.

Guyon, I., Elisseeff, A., 2003. An introduction to variable and feature selection. J. Mach. Learn. Res. 3, 1157–1182.

Hall, M.A., 2000. Correlation-based feature selection for discrete and numeric class machine learning. In: Proceedings of Seventeenth International Conference on Machine Learning, pp. 359–366.

Hoque, N., Bhattacharyya, D., Kalita, J., 2014. Mifs-nd: a mutual information-based feature selection method. Expert Syst. Appl. 41 (14), 6371–6385.

Kashyap, H., Ahmed, H.A., Hoque, N., Roy, S., Bhattacharyya, D.K., 2015. Big data analytics in bioinformatics: a machine learning perspective. J. Latex Class Files 13 (9), 1–20. (arXiv preprintarXiv: 1506.05101).

Kawamoto, K., Houlihan, C.A., Balas, E.A., Lobach, D.F., 2005. Improving clinical practice using clinical decision support systems: a systematic review of trials to identify features critical to success. Br. Med. J. 330, 765–772.

Kensaku, K., Caitlin, A., Houlihan, E., Andrew, B., David, F.L., 2005. Improving clinical practice using clinical decision support systems: a systematic review of trials to identify features critical to success. BMJ 330 (7494), 765.

Li, X., Fu, H., 2014. PSO-based support vector machine with cuckoo search technique for clinical disease diagnoses. Sci. World J., 548483. 7 pages https://doi.org/10.1155/2014/548483.

Li, J., Tang, J., Liu, H., 2017. Recent advances in feature selection and its applications. Knowl. Inf. Syst. 53 (3), 551–577.

Lisboa, P.J., Taktak, A.F.G., 2006. The use of artificial neural networks in decision support in cancer: a systematic review. Neural Netw. 19, 408–415.

Liu, H., Yu, L., 2005. Toward integrating feature selection algorithms for classification and clustering. IEEE Trans. Knowl. Data Eng. 17 (4), 491–502.

Marling, C., Montani, S., Bichindaritz, I., Funk, P., 2014. Synergistic case-based reasoning in medical domains. Expert Syst. Appl. 41, 249–259.

McSherry, D., 2011. Conversational case-based reasoning in medical decision making. Artif. Intell. Med. 52 (2), 59–66.

Moja, L., Kwag, K.H., Lytras, T., Bertizzolo, L., Brandt, L., Pecoraro, V., Rigon, G., Vaona, A., Ruggiero, F., Mangia, M., Iorio, A., Kunnamo, I., Bonovas, S., 2014. Effectiveness of computerized decision support systems linked to electronic health records: a systematic review and meta analysis. Am. J. Public Health 104 (12), 12–22.

Narasingarao, M., Manda, R., Sridhar, G., Madhu, K., Rao, A., 2009. A clinical decision support system using multilayer perceptron neural network to assess well being in diabetes. J. Assoc. Physicians India 57, 127–133.

Prasad, V., Rao, T.S., Babu, P., 2016. Thyroid disease diagnosis via hybrid architecture composing rough data sets theory and machine learning algorithms. Soft. Comput. 20 (3), 1179–1189.

Quinlan, J.R., 1993. C4.5: Programs for Machine Learning. Morgan Kaufman, San Mateo, CA.

Sampat, M.P., Markey, M.K., Bovik, A.C., 2005. Computer-aided detection and diagnosis in mammography. In: Handbook of Image and Video Processing. Academic Press, pp. 1195–1217.

Sarkar, B.K., 2016. A case study on partitioning data for classification. Int. J. Inf. Decis. Sci. 8 (1), 73–91.

Sarkar, B.K., Sana, S.S., Chaudhuri, K.S., 2011b. MIL: a data discretization approach. Int. J. Data Min. Model. Manag. 3 (3), 303–318.

Sartakhti, J.S., Zangooei, M.H., Mozafari, K., 2012. Hepatitis disease diagnosis using a novel hybrid method based on support vector machine and simulated annealing (SVM-SA). Comput. Methods Programs Biomed. 108 (2), 570–579.

Schapire, R.E., 1999. A brief introduction to boosting. IJCAI 99, 1401–1406.

Singh, A., Pandey, B., 2014. Intelligent techniques and applications in liver disorders: a survey. Int. J. Biomed. Eng. Technol. 16 (1), 27–70.

Srimani, P.K., Koti, M.S., 2014. Rough set approach for optimal rule generation in medical data. Int. J. Conceptions Comput. Inf. Technol. 2 (2), 9–13.

Subbulakshmi, C.V., Deepa, S.N., 2016. Medical dataset classification: a machine learning paradigm integrating particle swarm optimization with extreme learning machine classifier. Sci. World J. https://doi.org/10.1155/2015/418060.

Swiniarski, R.W., Skowron, A., 2003. Rough set methods in feature selection and recognition. Pattern Recogn. Lett. 24 (6), 833–849.

Syeda-Mahmood, T., 2015. Plenary Talk: The Role of Machine Learning in Clinical Decision Support. SPIE Newsroom.

Thirugnanam, M., Kumar, P., Srivatsan, S.V., Nerlesh, C.R., 2012. Improving the prediction rate of diabetes diagnosis using fuzzy, neural network, case based approach (FNC). Procedia Eng. 38, 1709–1718.

Wagholikar, K., Sundararajan, V., Deshpande, A., 2012. Modeling paradigms for medical diagnostic decision support: a survey and future directions. J. Med. Syst. 36, 3029–3049.

Witten Ian, H., Eibe, F., 2005. Data Mining: Practical Machine Learning Tools and Techniques, second ed. Morgan Kaufmann Publishers, Elsevier Inc.

Ye, C.Z., Yang, J., Geng, D.Y., Zhou, Y., Chen, N.Y., 2002. Fuzzy rules to predict degree of malignancy in brain glioma. Med. Biol. Eng. Comput. 40 (2), 145–152.

# Machine learning for optimizing healthcare resources

# 13

**Abdalrahman Tawhid, Tanya Teotia, and Haytham Elmiligi**

*Computing Science Department, Thompson Rivers University, Kamloops, BC, Canada*

## Chapter outline

## 1 Introduction

Researchers and health administrators are always trying to explore the best options to optimize access to healthcare resources. Access to such a vital service is becoming more significant during pandemic eras. In January 2020, when the COVID-19 virus began to spread across different countries, the healthcare systems all over the world were having a stress test to ensure they have well-functioning emergency plans to deal with the COVID-19 pandemic. At early stages of the pandemic, hospitals were suffering from shortage in ventilator systems that can be used to help COVID-19 patients to breath if they have breathing difficulties. Consequently, researchers started developing machine learning models to predict the healthcare resources that will be needed in the upcoming days. Although these models were not 100% accurate, they provided a great help to decision makers to analyze the situation and to have a rough figure of resources needed during different phases of the pandemic.

Resource management during pandemics becomes more challenging when there are large population with chronic diseases. A chronic disease, in general, is a disease that lasts 3 months or more. Chronic diseases generally cannot be prevented by vaccines or cured by medication, nor do they just disappear. There are many different chronic diseases such as diabetes, kidney failure, heart, high blood pressure, etc. A study done in the New York City, United States that analyzed data of 5700 COVID-19 patients has found that nearly all of these patients had at least one major chronic health condition, and 88% of them had at least two chronic health conditions (Richardson et al., 2020).

Machine learning is a process of teaching the machine, that is, the computer, how to find common patterns in a set of data and come to a conclusion about the data correlation to conclusions without being specifically programmed to get to that result (Behera and Das, 2017). There are different types of machine learning algorithms that take different approaches in understanding the datasets and building the predictive models. Machine learning algorithms can also be used for classification or regression. In classification, the algorithm classifies the test pattern as it belongs to a specific class. In regression, the algorithm tries to predict a specific number based on the given test pattern. Machine learning problems can, sometime, be formulated as classification and/or regression problems.

Machine learning algorithms help in finding correlations between different attributes related to certain events. Hence, not only they can be used to optimize healthcare resources through predictive models, but also they can be used to provide exit strategies for pandemic situations after long lockdown. During the COVID-19 pandemic, governments started looking for an exit strategy to protect their citizens from COVID-19 virus while opening the economy after a long lockdown. In April 2020, Prof. Kostas Kostarelos at the University of Manchester suggested to deal with the COVID-19 pandemic more like a chronic disease (Kostarelos, 2020). In such a case, analyst should adopt a care model usually applied to cancer patients in order to provide a constructive way to reopen the economy while dealing with the virus. Some experts even suggested to treat COVID-19 as a chronic diseases due to the fact that many COVID-19 tested positive after recovery (Lan et al., 2020). However, there is no scientific evidence up to the time of writing this chapter that COVID-19 is a chronic disease that will keep attacking the body even after the patient has recovered over and over again.

Nevertheless, COVID-19 pandemic highlighted the significance of machine learning models in optimizing healthcare resources, predicting the number of patients that need specific care, understanding the risk factor on patients with chronic diseases, and building models that help decision makers decide when and how to return to normal life.

In this chapter, we explore how machine learning techniques could be used to help hospital administrators manage their staff and resources efficiently. Machine learning is a process used to find hidden patterns in large batches of data that can be used to teach the machine how to classify or predict certain numbers. Machine learning depends on effective data collection and warehousing as well as algorithms and computer processing. The goal of this chapter is to discuss various techniques to analyze dataset features and to develop an efficient model to predict different parameters.

## 2 The state of the art

Prior to COVID-19 pandemic, most of the previous machine learning studies that examined risk factors for hospital admissions have focused primarily on creating datasets for a specific disease or condition, a single hospital site, or even a specific patient in the population of interest. On the contrary, pandemic situations require collaborative datasets that share information from multiple sites to come up with an accurate prediction. The accuracy of traditional forecasting largely depends on the availability of admission data to base its predictions and estimates of uncertainty. In outbreaks of epidemics, and specifically at the COVID-19 pandemic, there was no data at all at the beginning and then data started to grow as time passes, making predictions widely uncertain. Although data scientists tried to come up with several models to predict the pandemic peak in each country, the accuracy of these models was not high due to the lack of data.

Based on our analysis of research papers published in this area, we managed to narrow our findings into three main categories:

1. The first category is related to resource management. This category includes research that utilizes machine learning algorithms to create models that aid in the prediction of hospital admissions in general or to the emergency department, which can cause overcrowding. We found many papers published prior to as well as during the COVID-19 pandemic.
2. The second category of interest encompasses research work that relates to the COVID-19 pandemic and its impact on people's health. This includes models that forecast mortality, and infection rates among different age groups, genders, and ethnic groups.
3. The third category is related to exploring possible exit strategies to help the economy of each country to bounce back after a long shut-down period due to the COVID-19 pandemic. This includes developing models to predict the peak time of the pandemic, the estimated time before finding a vaccine, the optimum time to lower the emergency level across the country, when to open airport to international flights, etc.

The following sections discuss the approaches taken to address these three different categories in more details.

## 2.1 Resource management

Several researchers tried to explore applying machine learning algorithms to create predictive models that address a specific problem related to a single site or a country. For example, a research work conducted by Michael LaMantia utilized a triage-based model to create a model that gives a probability of admission rates of elderly patients (LaMantia et al., 2010). This work was performed based on dataset of 4873 visits of patients to the hospital. Triage is the process of sorting and filtering out patients based on priority, it aims to determine a patient's acuity level in order to facilitate timely and effective care before their condition worsens. The work managed to predict the number of admissions in a total population of visits by elderly patients. Regression modeling is performed to identify the variables that are most significant in predicting the probability of admission. The study concluded that these variables are: age, heart rate, triage score, chief complaint, and diastolic blood pressure. However, this work only applies to elderly patients. This does not provide the broad representation which is needed to properly enable the health administrators to allocate their resources.

Another example is a study published by Weissman et al. (2020) to predict the hospital capacity needs during the COVID-19 pandemic. The study shows that using records of patients with COVID-19 alone, it would be 31–53 days before the demand for more resources exceeds existing hospital capacity. The study used the Hospital Impact Model for Epidemics (CHIME), which is a modified SIR model that is used to compute the number of people infected with COVID-19 in a closed population overtime. The CHIME model estimated that it would be 31–53 days before demand exceeds existing hospital capacity. The study identifies the needed resources in terms of the total capacity for hospital beds, the number of ICU beds and ventilators in the best-case and worst-case scenarios. Such a study is significantly important in identifying the resources that will be needed during a pandemic to help healthcare administrators plan ahead and make the most suitable decisions to optimize their resources.

A third example is the research conducted by Giacomo Grasselli in Italy, which was one of the major spots during the COVID-19 pandemic. Grasselli used historical data to predict the number of patients who will be admitted to the intensive care unit over a period of 2 weeks (Grasselli et al., 2020). This work is prevalent only to that specific hospital and its admissions. The benefit of his methodology is the ability to use real-time data specific to that hospital. The downside, however, is that his forecast does not take into account factors that account for higher infection rates and that these predictions are very region specific.

A final example is a study completed by Chen et al. In their work, authors utilized data from the Tonji Hospital in China and applied five machine learning approaches: logistic regression, partial least-squares regression, elastic net, random forest, and bagged flexible discriminant analysis to select the features and predict outcomes in severe COVID-19 patients (Chen and Liu, 2020). The authors successfully validated their results by using the area under the receiver operating characteristic curve (AUROC), which was applied to compare the model's performance. They also tested their results on 64 patients admitted to the hospital with COVID-19. The main focus was predicting the number of moralities that will result for the admitted patients. In order to have methodology that properly allows healthcare administrations to allocate resources properly, a prediction of infection rates would be a much more useful feature to work with. Also, focusing on a small hospital in a large country is not enough to give a proper representation of the virus activity. Validation of such methods needs to be established on other subjects not native to the city.

## 2.2 Impact on people's health

The second category discusses the research work that used machine learning algorithms to predict COVID-19's impact on people's health and well-being.

Before looking at the opportunity to forecast different trends of the pandemic, researchers started to think of what the global impact of the COVID-19 pandemic will be. Answering this question requires accurate prediction of the spread of confirmed cases all over the world as well as analysis of the number of deaths and recoveries in each countries.

Forecasting, however, requires ample and reliable historical data which may be a limiting factor as the virus was fairly new at the time of the study. Moreover, forecasts are influenced by the reliability of the data, vested interests, and what variables are being predicted. Also, the psychological factors play a significant role in how the population perceive and react to the danger caused by the disease and the fear that it may affect them in their own communities. Therefore, the main challenge that faced data scientists at that time is how to predict the impact on people's health using machine learning algorithms. The risks were significant because the reports generated by these algorithms were used by world leaders to make critical decisions that impact the local as well as international economy.

A study done by Fotios Petropoulos used statistical data from the John Hopkins University and analyzed preexisting graphical representations of trends to attempt and forecast future representations of the graph (Petropoulos and Makridakis, 2020). Petropoulos used exponential smoothing models, which can capture a variety of trend and seasonal forecasting patterns such as mortality, confirmed cases, and recovered cases in 10 day intervals. One of the benefits of this model is that it takes the most recent observations into account and weights them accordingly. For example, if we are looking at 4-month data in 2018, they will likely be weighted differently when considered in the same period of 2020. The exponential smoothing method takes this into account (Avercast, 2020).

In another study completed by Li, where she focused on analyzing the existing data of the Hubei epidemic situation, a corresponding model is then established, and then the simulation was carried out. Through the simulation, she studied the main factors affecting the spread of COVID-19, such as the number of basic regenerations, the incubation period, and the average number of days of cure (Li et al., 2020). This was done using a Gaussian distribution. Gaussian distribution, also known as the normal distribution, is a probability distribution that is symmetric about the mean, showing that data near the mean are more frequent in occurrence than data far from the mean. A normal distribution has two parameters: the mean and the standard deviation. An analysis of graphical representations is useful for short-term expectations of certain data, but it also limits using region-specific data.

## 2.3 Exit strategies

How did a health crisis translate to an economic crisis? Why did the spread of the COVID-19 bring the global economy to its knees? When will COVID-19 reach its peak? The answer to these questions lies in two methods by which COVID-19 stifled economic activities. First, the spread of the virus encouraged social distancing which led to the shutdown of financial markets, corporate offices, businesses, and events. Second, the exponential rate at which the virus was spreading, and the heightened uncertainty about how bad the situation could get, which led to the closure of airports, a new look at consumption and investment among consumers, investors, and even international trade partners. Preparing to open the economy once again was a very critical decision. Therefore, decision makers needed a trusted methodology to help accurately forecast the peak and termination times of the pandemic. In those circumstances, having such a methodology was an important factor to minimize the risk of further losses whether economically, or physically.

For example, a study conducted by Zahiri utilized statistical data collected from Iran and their published infection rates. The study applied the SIR model to forecast infection rate, peak times, termination times, and other parameters (Zahiri et al., 2020). An SIR model is an epidemiological model that, in this study, computed the theoretical number of people infected with a contagious illness in a closed population over time. The name of this class of models derives from the fact that they involve coupled equations relating the number of susceptible people (S), number of people infected (I), and number of people who have recovered (R) (Smith and Moore, 2004). This model may be useful in interpreting data for a specific country and under specific conditions. However, it was difficult to generalize this model and adopt it in other countries. The disease has thus far been unpredictable and this model did not also account for the wave of infection that can occur if airports and businesses reopen.

Airline business was another major industry that was impacted by the disease. In March 2020, a financial analysis study reported that Canadian airports were confronting the prospect of 2 billion dollars in losses over the next few months as borders shut and planes stay parked due to the COVID-19 pandemic (Times Colonist, 2020). This major loss encourages airport facilities to reopen, to avoid any more losses. But it is important to have methods that enable us to accurately forecast the optimum time to open airports. In our analysis of literature, this aspect seemed to be missing, with the focus primarily being on mortality and infection rates.

## 3 Machine learning for health data analysis

The healthcare sector has long been an early adopter of and benefited greatly from technological advances. These days, machine learning (a subset of artificial intelligence) plays a key role in many health-related realms, including the development of new medical procedures, the handling of patient data and records, and the treatment of chronic diseases.

As mentioned previously, a proper and reliable dataset is imperative to achieve accurate results. Data quality relies on four factors:

1. accuracy
2. completeness
3. validity
4. timeliness

Accuracy refers to how well the data describes the real-world conditions it aims to describe. Inaccurate data create clear problems, as it can cause the machine learning algorithm to come to incorrect conclusions. The actions' administrators take based on those conclusions might not have the effects they expect because they are based on inaccurate data.

Completeness encompasses how complete the dataset is and that there are no gaps in it. Everything that was supposed to be collected was successfully collected. For example, if a customer skipped several questions on a survey, the data they submitted would not be complete. If the data are incomplete, we might have trouble gathering accurate insights from it.

Validity refers to how the data are collected rather than the data itself. Data are valid if it is in the right format, of the correct type, and falls within the right range. If data do not meet these criteria, we might run into trouble organizing and analyzing it.

The final factor is timeliness, which refers to how recently the event the data represent occurred. In most cases, data should be recorded as soon as possible after the real-world event. Data typically become less useful and less accurate as time passes on. Data that reflect events that happened more recently such as the COVID-19 pandemic would be even more useful in application to the current reality. Therefore, selecting the proper dataset is a very crucial factor in any research work. The data used during this work are a secondary dataset, derived from the Public Health Agency of Canada (2015). The raw data contained data for over 10 different chronic diseases. Each disease had data for 2000–11. Within each year, there were several categories. There was the gender, 18 different age groups, prevalent cases, mortality, hospital, general, specialist visits, and much more. There were two problems that developed within this dataset. First, the dataset only provided data, for 2000–11, which left us with only one available option, to create a general formula which will be able to predict the years we do not have. The second dilemma is, the dataset cannot be used in the data mining tool as is, there would have to be preprocessing done to the data.

## 4 Feature selection techniques

In data mining applications, feature selection plays a vital role by removing irrelevant and redundant features from the dataset. This reduces the dimensionality of the dataset as well as the computational time by (1) optimizing the learning process and (2) improving the performance of machine learning algorithms (Guyon and Elisseeff, 2003; Xue et al., 2016).

Feature selection techniques can be categorized into three categories:

1. filter (Guyon and Elisseeff, 2003; Kohavi and John, 1997);
2. wrapper (Kohavi and John, 1997); and
3. embedded (Guyon and Elisseeff, 2003; Blum and Langley, 1997).

Fig. 1 shows our categorization of feature selection techniques used in the previous work. In the following sections, we discuss each approach briefly and provide examples from the literature.

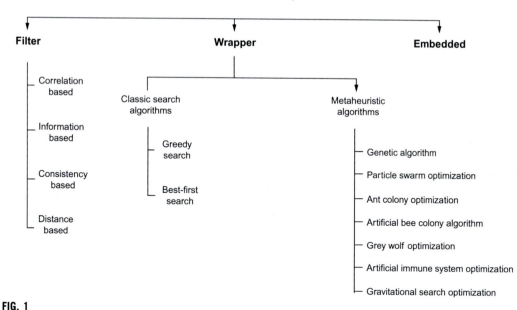

**FIG. 1**

Feature selection techniques.

## 4.1 Filter approach

In the filter approach, a ranking-based criterion is used to rank all features in the dataset. Then, a threshold value is set and all features below the threshold are removed (Chandrashekar and Sahin, 2014). The ranking methods involved in this process are known as filter methods as they filter out irrelevant features from the dataset before being evaluated by a classification algorithm. The features that are essential to construct an optimum subset are identified as highly relevant features (Yu and Liu, 2004). It is also important to ensure that there are no redundant features in the dataset to reduce the effect of *curse of dimensionality* (Chandrashekar and Sahin, 2014). The redundancy of two features can be calculated by calculating the correlation between their values. The following section discusses the major filter-based selection methods.

### 4.1.1 Correlation based

Correlation criteria are mainly based on the hypothesis *Good feature subsets contain features that are highly correlated with the class, but uncorrelated to other features* (Hall, 2000). There are two types of correlation measures: one is based on feature-feature correlation, whereas the other is based on feature-class correlation. The merit of feature subset $S$ consisting of $N$ features can be calculated as (Chen et al., 2006; Vanaja and Kumar, 2014):

$$Merit_{S_N} = \frac{N\bar{r}_{fc}}{\sqrt{N+N(N-1)\bar{r}_{ff}}} \tag{1}$$

where $\bar{r}_{ff}$ represents the average of feature-feature correlation and $\bar{r}_{fc}$ represents the average of feature-feature correlation. $N$ represents the number of features in that particular subset $S$. The feature-class and feature-feature correlations can be calculated by various correlation coefficient mathematical criteria. One of the most common criteria is based on Pearson correlation coefficient (Guyon and Elisseeff, 2003; Chandrashekar and Sahin, 2014):

$$R(i) = \frac{Cov(x_i, Y)}{\sqrt{Var(x_i)*Var(Y)}} \tag{2}$$

where $x_i$ represents the $i$th attribute of the dataset, $Y$ represents the class label, $Var()$ and $Cov()$ represent the variance and covariance. Correlation-based feature selection (CFS) is one of the most common filter approaches applied to feature selection problems (Halakou, 2013; Balagani et al., 2011; Kumar and Zhang, 2005).

### 4.1.2 Information based

Information-based feature selection is a measure that indicates the difference between prior and expected posterior uncertainty (Guyon and Elisseeff, 2003; Chandrashekar and Sahin, 2014; Liu and Setiono, 1996; Molina et al., 2002). The uncertainty of a feature $Y$ can be calculated by Shannon's definition of entropy (Chandrashekar and Sahin, 2014)

$$H(Y) = -\sum_{y} p(y) \log(p(y)) \tag{3}$$

and the conditional entropy of a random variable $Y$ given variable $X$ is computed by (Chandrashekar and Sahin, 2014)

$$H(Y|X) = -\sum_{x}\sum_{y} p(x,y) \log(p(y|x)) \tag{4}$$

The difference between Eqs. (3) and (4) describes the mutual information with respect to a random variable between $Y$ and $X$ (Chandrashekar and Sahin, 2014):

$$MI(Y,X) = H(Y) - H(Y|X) \tag{5}$$

where MI is the mutual information that measures the mutual dependence between two random variables, and

$$MI \begin{cases} = 0, & X \text{ and } Y \text{ are independent of each other,} \\ > 0, & X \text{ and } Y \text{ are dependent on each other.} \end{cases}$$

When $X$ and $Y$ are independent of each other, this results in less information gain and more uncertainty. When $X$ and $Y$ are dependent on each other, this results in more information gain and less uncertainty.

MI measures the distance between two probability distributions, whereas correlation criteria, such as Pearson correlation coefficient, measure the degree of correlation based on linear relationship between two random variables.

### 4.1.3 Consistency based

Consistency-based feature selection is used to measure the consistency of features with respect to a class value. The objective of using this measure is to find a subset of features leading to zero inconsistencies. Having two instances with the same values but belonging to two different classes indicates the occurrence of an inconsistent pattern in the dataset (Dash et al., 2000). The inconsistency count of an instance can be calculated by the number of times the same pattern is found in the dataset minus the largest number of the same pattern belonging to a single class. The inconsistency rate can be calculated by dividing the total sum of all inconsistency counts of all patterns found in a particular feature subset by the total number of patterns in the dataset with respect to that selected feature subset (Dash et al., 2000).

### 4.1.4 Distance based

Distance-based criterion is divided into two subcategories: (1) classical distance based measures and (2) probabilistic distance-based measures, also known as divergence measures.

Classical distance-based measures are used to find similarities between two feature vectors. When the distance value is small, the two vectors are considered similar, whereas when the distance value is large, they become less similar. *Relief/ReliefF*-based feature selection algorithm is an example of classical distance-based measure, which uses Euclidean and Manhattan distance measures in high-dimensional feature space (Robnik-Šikonja and Kononenko, 2003). *Relief* algorithm considers two feature vectors. One belongs to the same class, called nearest hit, whereas the other belongs to a different class, called nearest miss.

The underlying principle is that a feature is considered more relevant when the Euclidean distance between a feature and the nearest miss is large, whereas a feature is considered less relevant when the Euclidean distance between a feature and the nearest hit is small (Molina et al., 2002). Weights are given to any feature based on its relevancy. Similarly, *ReliefF* algorithm selects a feature vector of an instance randomly but searches for $k$-nearest neighbors belonging to the same class, called nearest hits, and also $k$-nearest neighbors belonging to each of the different classes, called nearest misses and computes their averages (Molina et al., 2002).

Even though filter methods, in general, are used as a preprocessing step to reduce the dimensionality of a dataset and overcome overfitting, many researchers concluded that it does not provide the best accuracy rate compared to wrapper methods as it ignores the feature subset dependency on the learning algorithm (Kohavi and John, 1997).

## 4.2 Wrapper approach

In the previous section, we discussed the filter methodology which uses an independent measure as an evaluator for subset evaluation. In this section, we discuss wrapper methodology, which uses a learning algorithm as a feature subset evaluator (Kohavi and John, 1997). This methodology uses a learning algorithm as a black box and its performance as an objective function for evaluating a selected feature subset (Chandrashekar and Sahin, 2014; Kohavi and John, 1997).

Various search techniques are used to generate different feature subsets and are evaluated using a machine learning algorithm till the optimal subset is found. These methods perform better at defining the optimal subset that is best suited to a learning algorithm. One of the key advantages of using wrapper-based feature selection approach is that it does not ignore the dependency of the selected feature subset on the overall performance of a learning algorithm (Kohavi and John, 1997). Therefore, the performance of this approach is usually superior. However, since it uses a search technique and a learning algorithm together for the subset selection and evaluation, it tends to be slower and computationally expensive.

In order to optimize the search time, different types of search algorithms have been used in the literature. Various wrapper-based experiments have been carried out by varying different search techniques and learning algorithm as a subset evaluation measure.

### 4.2.1 Classic search algorithms

In wrapper-based feature selection, sequential algorithms are used as a search technique to execute the process of feature selection sequentially. In other words, features are selected one after another in a succession fashion. They can be further divided into two basic categories, namely sequential forward selection and sequential backward selection (Chandrashekar and Sahin, 2014). In this section, we will study some search algorithms which are based on sequential search technique.

### Greedy search

In wrapper-based feature selection, the greedy selection algorithms are simple and straightforward search techniques. They iteratively make "nearsighted" decisions based on the objective function and hence, are good at finding the local optimum. But, they lack in providing global optimum solutions for large problems. Traditionally, they are divided into two categories: (1) Greedy forward selection (GFS) and (2) Greedy backward elimination (GBE).

GFS algorithm starts with an empty set and at each iteration, adds one feature to the subset until a local optimal solution is achieved. Whereas GBE algorithm starts from a complete set of features and iteratively removes one feature until a local optimal solution is achieved.

### Best first search

Best first search is a search technique which explores the nodes in a graph with a heuristic evaluation function (Kohavi and John, 1997). In feature selection, the best first search uses this evaluation function to score every candidate feature and selects the one which provides best "score" first. There are two lists which maintain the track of visited (CLOSED) and unvisited (OPEN) nodes.

This algorithm can be further divided into two subcategories: (1) best forward selection (BFS) and (2) best backward selection (BBS) (Darabseh and Namin, 2015). BFS starts with an empty set and at each iteration, adds one feature to the subset and BBS starts from a complete set of features and iteratively removes one feature from the subset.

### 4.2.2 Metaheuristic algorithms
#### Genetic algorithms
Genetic algorithm (GA) is a probabilistic search technique based on the evolutionary idea of natural selection, which mimics the process of evolution. The algorithm starts with initializing the population of chromosomes represented by a binary string, but not necessary. In feature selection, 1 and 0s of a binary string represent feature selection and rejection. At each iteration, these chromosomes are evaluated by a fitness function. A fitness function is used to score the evolving generations of these chromosomes. Pairs of chromosomes are selected at random to reproduce based on the score assigned by the fitness function.

Operations such as mutation and crossover are performed on the selected pair of chromosomes to create the next generation, new chromosome, or an offspring. Mutation involves modifying a chromosome, whereas a crossover involves merging two chromosomes of the present generation to create an offspring. After $n$ generations, this algorithm converges to the best set of chromosomes, which represent the optimal or suboptimal feature subset in a feature selection problem.

#### Particle swarm optimization
Particle swarm optimization (PSO) is a technique based on the paradigm of swarm intelligence. The intelligent behavior is inspired by the social behavior of animals like fish and bird (Liu et al., 2011). The algorithm starts with initializing a swarm of particles, where each particle represents a prospective solution to the optimization problem. At each iteration, these particles are evaluated by a fitness function.

Each particle has a position and a velocity, which describes its movement in the search space. In every iteration, position and velocity of every particle are updated based on its personal best and global best value. Each particle in the swarm has a memory of its personal best known as *pbest* value and the common global best *gbest* value that is obtained so far by any particle in the swarm. Each particle learns to accelerate toward its personal best and the global best position to reach the level of intelligence. Each particles' new velocity for acceleration is calculated based on its current velocity, the distance from its personal best, and the distance from the common global best position. After $n$ iterations, all particles converge to the best solution.

#### Ant colony optimization
Ant colony optimization (ACO) is a probabilistic search technique based on metaheuristic optimization, which mimics the process of ants foraging for food. It is used to search an optimal path in a graph between a source and a destination. The algorithm starts with all ants selecting random paths, where each path represents a prospective solution to the optimization problem. When ants start moving in search of food, they leave pheromone a chemical material on the path. An ant moving in a random direction might encounter the previously laid pheromone trail and decides to follow it based on the probability. More ants following the same path increase the pheromone deposited on it, thus reinforcing the probability of the path being followed. In a graph, the shortest path is learned via pheromone trails. But, pheromone trails gradually decrease by evaporation. At each iteration, an ant reaches a node and

selects the next path based on transition probability until its overall path converges to an effective path (Kashef and Nezamabadi-Pour, 2015). In feature selection, all features are considered as nodes of a graph and ACO is used to find the optimal path, which provides the optimal feature subset.

### Artificial bee colony

Artificial bee colony (ABC) is a stochastic search technique based on swarm intelligence, which mimics the process of honey bee swarms foraging for food. In this algorithm, each candidate solution represents the position of food source in the search space and the quality of nectar amount of the food source is used as a fitness evaluator (Schiezaro and Pedrini, 2013). It involves three group of bees: employed bees, onlookers, and scouts (Yavuz and Aydin, 2016). The number of employee bees is equivalent to food sources. Employed bees leave the hive in search of food source and collect the nectar amount of the other food sources in the vicinity of the discovered one. Once they return to their hive, they perform dance through which they provide information about the explored food source (location and quality) to the onlookers. Onlookers recruit a new food source from the information provided by the employed bees based on the selection probability of nectar amount and abandon the food source of low fitness value. Once an onlooker picks a new food source to explore, it becomes an employed bee. Once the employed bee's food source is abandoned, it converts into a scout bee which performs a random search for a food source in the search space. This process is repeated until the optimal food source is found.

### Grey wolf optimization

Grey wolf optimization (GWO) is a metaheuristic algorithm that is inspired by the behavior of grey wolves in leadership and hunting (Mirjalili et al., 2014). The algorithm classifies a population of possible solutions into four types of wolves $\alpha$, $\beta$, $\delta$, and $\omega$. The four types are ordered based on the fittest solution, which means that $\alpha$ is considered the best solution and $\omega$ is the worst. The new generation is created by updating the wolves in each one of these four groups. This update is based on the first three best solutions obtained from $\alpha$, $\beta$, and $\delta$ in the previous generation.

### Artificial immune system algorithms

Several algorithms that mimic the artificial immune system (AIS) have been published in the literature (Watkins and Boggess, 2002). There are two main approaches considered in the proposed AIS algorithms. The first approach is negative selection, in which the algorithm's main task is to define whether an instance belongs to the trained model or not. This approach has been widely used for anomaly detection (Jinquan et al., 2009). The second approach is positive selection, in which the algorithm's main task is to identify each one of the training instances as a detector and assign a radius to it. The matching phase will then examine the test instance and check if it belongs to any one of the detectors' zones.

### Gravitational search optimization

Gravitational search optimization (GSO) uses a collection of masses as a representation of candidate solutions and uses Newtonian physics theorem to create the next generation based on the gravity law and the notion of mass interactions (Rashedi et al., 2009). Based on GSO, the relative distances and masses of the candidate solutions play the major role in attracting these candidate solutions to each other in the search space. Although authors claim that mass interaction provides an effective way of communication between the possible solutions to transfer information through the gravitational force, this concept was questioned in a later study by Gauci et al. (2012). Gauci et al. (2012) spotted a fundamental inconsistency in the mathematical formulation of the GSO and showed that the distance between possible solutions was not taken into account in creating the next generation. Hence, GSO cannot be considered to be based on gravity laws.

### 4.3 Embedded approach

Embedded methodology performs feature selection as a part of the training process. In comparison to wrapper approach, these methods provide normal or extended functionality to the learning process by lowering the computational cost (Guyon and Elisseeff, 2003; Chandrashekar and Sahin, 2014). During the learning phase of the model construction, they identify the features which will be the best fit for the model based on different independent measures. Following that, these use the learning algorithm to select the final feature subset, which provides the best performance. Decision trees such as C4.5 and random forest are some of the commonly used embedded methods in classification. In regression analysis, embedded methods like Ridge Regression, Elastic Net, and LASSO are used to perform feature weighting based on different regularization models to minimize the outlines and reduce the feature coefficients to be smaller or equal to zero (Tibshirani, 1994; Zou and Hastie, 2005; Yang et al., 2015).

## 5 Machine learning classifiers

This section explores possible classification solutions. We first explain the difference between using one-class classification (OCC) versus multiclass classification. Following that, we study the feasibility of using supervised versus unsupervised learning algorithms to identify hidden patterns in health datasets.

### 5.1 One-class vs. multiclass classification

OCC or unary classification is different from binary/multiclass classification, as it trains a model with data objects belonging to only one class, called the target class, in the presence of no or limited outlier distribution. The outliers in the data objects are identified by error measurements of the feature values compared to other target class objects. OCC provides a solution for classifying new data by defining a decision boundary around the target class, such that it only accepts the target class objects while minimizing the probability of accepting outlier objects.

In literature, many machine learning applications like outlier detection, novelty detection, and anomaly detection have originated with the similar concept (Ritter and Gallegos, 1997; Bishop, 1993; Pauwels and Ambekar, 2011). Several algorithms have been developed based on SVM and ELM to address OCC problems (Tax and Duin, 2004; Schölkopf et al., 1999; Gautam and Tiwari, 2016).

In binary/multiclass classification, a model is trained to classify data objects into two or more classes, where each object is assigned to only one-class label. The trained model then classifies new data by defining a decision boundary around each class, such that it only accepts the associated class objects, while minimizing the probability of accepting other class objects. In a classification problem, the associated (optimal) class membership of a data object is predicted based on the probabilistic distribution of its association with each class.

## 5.2 Supervised vs. unsupervised learning

Supervised machine learning trains a model with an input $X$ which represents a set of data objects and a labeled output $Y$ which represents a categorical or continuous target value to construct a hypothesis function which can be later used to predict the output value for new data objects. Supervised learning algorithms address both classification and regression problems in machine learning. It is different from unsupervised learning, as the predictive model learns from the input as well as its corresponding output value.

In unsupervised learning, a model constructs a hypothesis based on input data $X$ with no labeled output. Clustering is a conventional unsupervised machine learning algorithm, which groups observations to identify hidden patterns in the input data.

## 6 Case studies
### 6.1 Experimental setup

- The raw datasets are obtained from the Public Health Agency of Canada (2020).
- Weka software is used to analyze the dataset and run machine learning algorithms (Frank et al., 2016).
- Excel software is used to visualize the data in two-dimensional (2D) format.

### 6.2 Case study 1: Diabetes data analysis

Diabetes is a disease that occurs when blood glucose reaches a very high level. The food we consume gets converted into blood glucose, which is our primary source of energy. Insulin, which is a hormone produced by the pancreas, helps glucose from food get into our cells to be utilized as energy. Sometimes our bodies do not make enough insulin or use the insulin well. The glucose stays in our blood, and cannot reach our cells (Health Information, 2016). According to the Public Health Agency of Canada, one in seven Canadians are affected by disease, and in 2050 about one in three will be afflicted (Taylor, 2016). The condition is progressing very rapidly, resulting in overflow in hospital visits. Hospitals are experiencing capacity, and resources issues that are profoundly affecting performance. Aside from hospital visits, there would be an overflow in clinic visits to the general and specialist physicians. It would be beneficial to have a reliable method for predicting how many diabetic patients are expected to be hospitalized. In a more general term, it would be very helpful to predict the future trends in the healthcare industry. Data mining is a unique method of data analysis that allows analysts to uncover hidden patterns in datasets. There are several software programs that are currently being used to conduct data analytic tasks, such as Weka, IBM Watson Analytics, and Alteryx. In this section, we used Weka to conduct our analysis. Weka is a collection of machine learning algorithms for data mining tasks. It can either be applied directly to a dataset or called from a separate Java code. Weka features include machine learning, data mining, preprocessing, classification, regression, clustering, association rules, experiments, and more. Weka is written in Java, and was developed at the University of Waikato in New Zealand.

In our case study, we downloaded raw datasets from the Public Health Agency of Canada. Although the data are huge and contain information on many prominent chronic diseases, our main focus is diabetes. Our choice to focus on diabetes in this case study was based on how prominent the disease is in today's society and the significant growth rate associated with it. Our analysis targets predicting the number of diabetic patients who are expected to visit a specific hospital 1 year ahead. The dataset contained information on visits to hospitals for 2000–11, throughout the country. The list of features includes the patients' age group, number of incident cases per year, number of GP visits per year, number of prevalent cases per year, and mortality per year. To create a generalized model that would be accepted and useful to healthcare administrators, we created six different models for 2006–11, which would effectively model the changes and fluctuations that were established throughout the years. In the data processing step, we converted all data types into strictly numerical values using the *NominaltoNumeric* filter package that is supported by the Weka software. After analyzing that dataset correlation, we decided to use seven different algorithms to predict the number of diabetic patients who are expected to visit a specific hospital 1 year ahead. These algorithms are: linear regression, decision trees, random forest, Naïve Bayes, support vector machine (SVM), and sequential minimal optimization (SMO).

- *Linear regression* is a machine learning algorithm based on supervised learning. It performs a regression task. Regression models a target prediction value based on independent variables. It is mostly used for finding out the relationship between variables and forecasting (Gupta, 2018). Different regression models differ based on the kind of relationship between dependent and independent variables under consideration and the number of independent variables being used.
- *Decision tree* algorithm belongs to the family of supervised learning algorithms (Lior and Oded, 2005). Unlike other supervised learning algorithms, the decision tree algorithm can be used for solving regression and classification problems too. The goal of using a decision tree is to create a training model that can be used to predict the class or value of the target variable by learning simple decision rules inferred from the training data.
- *Random forest* as its name implies, random forest consists of a large number of individual decision trees that operate as an ensemble. Each individual tree in the random forest spits out a class prediction and the class with the most votes becomes our models prediction.
- *Naïve Bayes* is a classification technique based on Bayes theorem with an assumption of independence among predictors (Ray, 2020). Naïve Bayes model is easy to build and particularly useful for very large datasets. Along with simplicity, Naïve Bayes is known to, sometimes, outperform other highly sophisticated classification methods.
- *SVM* is a supervised machine learning algorithm, which can be used for both classification or regression challenges. However, it is mostly used in classification problems. In the SVM algorithm, we plot each data item as a point in $n$-dimensional space (where $n$ is number of features we have) with the value of each feature being the value of a particular coordinate. Then, we perform classification by finding the hyperplane that best differentiates the two classes.
- *SMO* is a method of decomposition, by which an optimization problem of multiple variables is decomposed into a series of subproblems each optimizing an objective function of a small number of variables, typically only one, while all other variables are treated as constants that remain unchanged in the subproblem.

Table 1 shows the performance evaluation of different prediction models trained with all features using different machine learning algorithms available within the Weka software. SMO has the best performing results, in terms of accuracy as well as execution time. The great advantage of the SMO approach is that we do not need a quadratic problem solver to solve the problem and instead it can be solved

**Table 1 Overview of performance of different algorithms.**

| Classifier | Average accuracy (%) | Execution time |
|---|---|---|
| Linear regression | 85.9 | 12 min |
| SVM | 88.6 | 6 s |
| Naïve Bayes | 79 | 2 s |
| SVM | 90.3 | 3.2 s |
| SMO | 96.56 | 1.3 s |
| Random forest | 88.3 | 15 s |
| Decision trees | 70.1 | 2 s |

analytically. As a consequence, it does not need to store a huge matrix, which can cause problems with machine memory. Moreover, SMO uses several heuristics to speed up the computation, which is evident in the execution time. The SMO algorithm is, therefore, used throughout this project.

Fig. 2 shows an example model produced by the SMO algorithm to predict the number of diabetic patients who are expected to visit the hospital in the year 2006 based on records of the previous 5 years.

To evaluate the performance of a regression algorithm, we consider the following factors:

- Root mean square error (RMSE) is one of the standard ways to measure the error of a model in predicting quantitative data.

$$RMSE = \sqrt{\left(\frac{1}{n}\right)\sum_{i=1}^{n}(y_i - x_i)^2} \tag{6}$$

where $n$ represents the number of features in that particular subset. $(y_i - x_i)$ represent the differences between the experimental result and the actual value and then squared. The summation of all the values of the training set are expressed by sigma.
- Mean absolute error (MAE) measures the average magnitude of the errors in a set of predictions, without considering their direction.

$$MAE = \left(\frac{1}{n}\right)\sum_{i=1}^{n}|y_i - x_i| \tag{7}$$

where $n$ also represents the number of features in that particular subset that you are working with. $y_i - x_i$ also represents the difference between the experimental result and the actual value, but instead here it is absolute and cannot be negative.

Both MAE and RMSE express average model prediction error in units of the variable of interest. Both metrics can range from 0 to ∞ and are indifferent to the direction of errors. They are negatively oriented scores, which mean the lower the values the better the results.

Although Weka software provided the RMSE and MAE values for each model, it is still crucial to validate the models statistically, which was done in Microsoft Excel. We calculated the difference between the actual value of a given year and the predicted value for the same year. We were able to calculate the absolute error, average accuracy, and residuals. Using these values, we can manually

**SMOreg**

weights (not support vectors):
-    0.0074 * (normalized) GenderA4
-    0.0431 * (normalized) Age_Group=1 to 4
+    0.0037 * (normalized) Age_Group=5 to 9
+    0.0043 * (normalized) Age_Group=10 to 14
+    0.0066 * (normalized) Age_Group=15 to 19
+    0.0049 * (normalized) Age_Group=20 to 24
+    0.004 * (normalized) Age_Group=25 to 29
+    0.0102 * (normalized) Age_Group=30 to 34
+    0.012 * (normalized) Age_Group= 35 to 39
+    0.0137 * (normalized) Age_Group=40 to 44
+    0.0148 * (normalized) Age_Group=45 to 49
+    0.0101 * (normalized) Age_Group=50 to 54
+    0.0017 * (normalized) Age_Group=55 to 59
+    0.0035 * (normalized) Age_Group=60 to 64
+    0.0129 * (normalized) Age_Group=65 to 69
+    0.0471 * (normalized) Age_Group= 70 to 74
+    0.0712 * (normalized) Age_Group= 75 to 79
+    0.091 * (n ormalized) Age_Group= 80 to 84
+    0.0464 * (normalized) Age_Group=85+
+    0.003 * (normalized) 2001
+    0.003 * (normalized) 2002
-    0.0011 * (normalized) 2003
-    0.0029 * (normalized) 2004
-    0.0051 * (normalized) 2005
+    0.0031 * (normalized) 2006
-    0.3335 * (normalized) Incident Cases
+    0.5643 * (normalized) GP visits
+    0.3507 * (normalized) Prevalent Cases
+    0.5587 * (normalized) Mortality
-    0.6886 * (normalized) HV_2001
-    0.7397 * (normalized) HV_2002
-    0.7913 * (normalized) HV_2003
-    0.8159 * (normalized) HV_2004
-    0.8672 * (normalized) HV_2005
+    0.007

**FIG. 2**

An example model produced by the SMO algorithm to predict the number of diabetic patients who are expected to visit the hospital in 2006 based on records of the previous 5 years.

calculate RMSE and MAE. We were also able to create a graphical representation of the error and accuracy. Fig. 3 shows a graphical representation of the accuracy (top) and the error (bottom) for the 2011 model when calculated manually.

In this case study, we created an individual model to predict the number of diabetic patients who are expected to visit the hospital in a specific year based on the previous 5-year records. Since we have records from 2006 to 2011, we were able to create six different models, one to predict each year. Our goal was to create a more generalized model that can be used for any year based on the previous

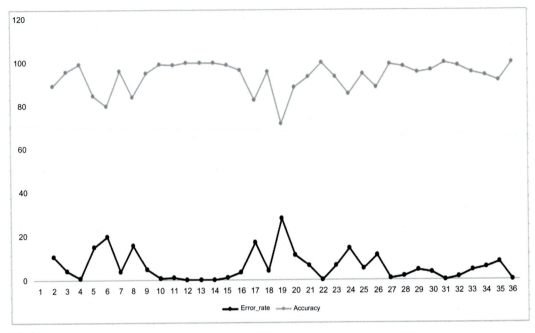

**FIG. 3**

This is an example of a graphical representation of the accuracy (*top*) and the error (*bottom*) for the 2011 model when calculated manually.

5-year records. Create such a generalized model that can maintain a low error rate was a challenging task. The normalized coefficients that were multiplied by the features were close in range, therefore, the method of choice was to average these coefficients for all the years and place the new averaged value as the new coefficient in the generalized model.

Once the generalized model is created, a cross-validation process is done to calculate the RMSE, MAE, error rates, and accuracy of this new model. We tested the new model and compared it with the individual models. Fig. 4 shows the accuracy (top) and the error (bottom) for the 2011 model when using the generalized model.

These average accuracy using the generalized model throughout the separate years is 93% compared to an average accuracy of 96% using each individualized model. When working with these types of scenarios, we expect the accuracy to drop much further when creating a general model. However, in our case, the model still shows an acceptable performance and could be used in later years.

## 7 Case study 2: COVID-19 data analysis

On December 31, 2019, a cluster of cases of pneumonia was reported in Wuhan, China, and the cause has been confirmed as a new coronavirus that has not previously been identified in humans. This virus is now known as COVID-19 (Novel Coronavirus, 2020). There are now confirmed cases of COVID-19

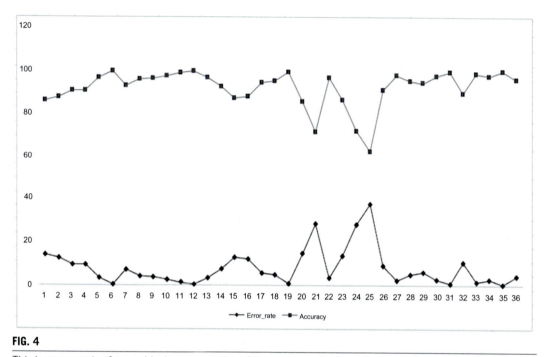

**FIG. 4**

This is an example of a graphical representation of the accuracy (*top*) and the error (*bottom*) for the generalized model when tested to predict the number of patients in 2011.

that have been identified in many countries, including Canada. The current situation is evolving every day. Therefore, new information is becoming available daily and a clearer picture is being formed as this information is analyzed by researchers in provincial, national, and international health agencies. Confirmed cases, recovered cases, and the mortality rate are varying on a daily basis. Machine learning algorithms are used to identify possible patterns of the spread of the disease and to predict the number of patients who will be hospitalized. However, it is important to understand that COVID-19 was a new disease at the time of writing this chapter, and there is very limited datasets that may help analysts to predict the numbers accurately. One of the main sources is the open source dataset by the John Hopkins University, which is used through this section of the study. The data provide a snapshot of confirmed case, recovered cases, and mortality rate for each individual country (COVID-19 Data Repository by the Center for Systems Science and Engineering (CSSE) at Johns Hopkins University, 2020). It is important to highlight that this dataset is constantly being updated. Due to the limited size of the available data records, analysts were only able to predict accurate numbers on a weekly basis. In this study, we developed a regression model to predict the number of confirmed cases for each country.

The first step, like the previous case study involved the preprocessing of the dataset, is to prepare it for use in the Weka software. We started by using the data of all previous 60-day reported cases to create our model. However, we noticed that the records were not completely accurate during the first few days of the pandemic so we focused on using the data records when countries started to conduct regular tests on citizens to spot the coronavirus. Since the original dataset included every country world-wide whether it contained cases or not, we removed all countries that did not have cases, or data were not sufficient or inconclusive, as it would interfere with the accuracy of our prediction. Our main objective was to create a model that would represent an accurate prediction of confirmed cases for each day in the week ahead. In this case study, we used linear regression, SMO, multilayer perceptron, random forest, and finally locally weighted learning (LWL).

- Multilayer perceptron (MLP) is a class of feed-forward artificial neural network (ANN). MLP utilizes a supervised learning technique called back propagation for training (Nicholson, 2019). Its multiple layers and nonlinear activation distinguish MLP from a linear perceptron. It can distinguish data that are not linearly separable.
- LWL is a class of function approximation techniques, where a prediction is done by using an approximated local model around the current point of interest. The goal of function approximation and regression is to find the underlying relationship between input and output (Rahul, 2019). In a supervised learning problem training data, where each input is associated with one output, is used to create a model that predicts values which come close to the true function.

Table 2 presents the results of applying different algorithms on the dataset to predict the number of confirmed cases 1 week ahead. Linear regression achieved the best performance because it attempts to model the relationship between two variables by fitting a linear equation to observed data. One variable is considered to be an explanatory variable, and the other is considered to be a dependent variable.

It is important to note that this prediction works well during the rising period of the pandemic but it does not predict the peak or when the confirmed cases curve will start to go down. This model was used solely as a short-term prediction model to predict only 1 week ahead data. Other models are used to predict the peak point and when the pandemic will be over.

To test our model, we compared the predicted results for the past week during the period of writing this chapter to the actual numbers that were reported by the WHO. This allowed us to compare our results to currently existing data, and confirm the accuracy of our forecast. Table 3 summarizes the results and reports the error rate.

Fig. 5 presents the accuracy and error rate when predicting the number of confirmed cases in each country for May 31, 2020. The accuracy and error rate percentages vary based on the model response to the country datasets. As shown in the figure, the model reacts efficiently to countries that have enough historical records that help the model predict future values.

**Table 2  A performance summary of different algorithms applied on the COVID-19 dataset.**

| Classifier | Average accuracy (%) | Execution time (s) |
| --- | --- | --- |
| Linear regression | 93.67 | 0.03 |
| LWL | 67.12 | 1.85 |
| Multilayer perceptron | 70.34 | 0.12 |
| SMO | 84.59 | 0.08 |
| Random forest | 46.47 | 31 |

**Table 3** **The accuracy and error rate for the dates May 25, 2020 to May 31, 2020.**

| Date | Accuracy (%) | Error rate (%) | Execution time (s) |
|------|--------------|----------------|--------------------|
| May 25, 2020 | 93.7115 | 6.2885 | 0.03 |
| May 26, 2020 | 94.536 | 5.464 | 0.04 |
| May 27, 2020 | 96.278 | 3.723 | 0.04 |
| May 28, 2020 | 92.88 | 7.124 | 0.03 |
| May 29, 2020 | 95.746 | 4.254 | 0.03 |
| May 30, 2020 | 95.7477 | 4.253 | 0.02 |
| May 31, 2020 | 93.599 | 6.401 | 0.03 |
| Average | 94.643 | 5.357 | 0.0314 |

Note: *The average accuracy of all the individualized models is 94.6%.*

At the time of writing this chapter, COVID-19 was a serious health threat, and the situation was evolving daily. The risk varies between and within communities. Having the ability to develop predictive models allows data analysts to report accurate and efficient forecasts that will assist healthcare administrators in preparing accommodations, resources, and other variables essential in the fight against this pandemic. We can also apply these methods to aid in the reopening of the economy, airlines, and other sectors affected by the disease.

## 8  Summary and future directions

The value of machine learning in health care is its ability to learn from huge datasets beyond the scope of human capability. Machine learning can then be used to uncover hidden patterns in this dataset. In healthcare applications, machine learning can be used to provide clinical insights that aid physicians in planning and providing care, ultimately leading to better outcomes, lower costs of care, and increased patient satisfaction. Health care needs to move from thinking of machine learning as a futuristic concept to seeing it as a real-world tool that can be deployed today. If machine learning is to have a role in health care, then we must take an incremental approach. Healthcare administrators should start utilizing data analytics and use predictive models as essential elements in the decision-making process. This chapter discussed and explored opportunities to apply machine learning methods in the healthcare sector. We plan to extend our analysis to analyze other datasets in the healthcare sectors and study the correlation between the quality of healthcare services and the social and economical factors within the community.

There are two possible directions that we plan to investigate. First, exploring the correlation between the rate of disease spread during pandemic and the government spending on public education. Second, analyzing the possibility of creating travel bubbles between countries without enforcing quarantine period on travelers and how that affects the public safety in each country.

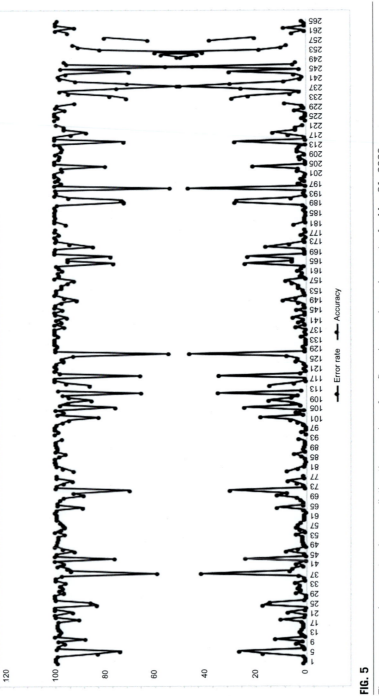

**FIG. 5**

The accuracy and error rate when predicting the number of confirmed cases in each country for May 31, 2020.

# References

Avercast, 2020. Exponential smoothing. Forecasting Methods: Exponential Smoothing. https://www.avercast.com/post/exponential-smoothing. March.

Balagani, K.S., Phoha, V.V., Ray, A., Phoha, S., 2011. On the discriminability of keystroke feature vectors used in fixed text keystroke authentication. Pattern Recogn. Lett. 32 (7), 1070–1080.

Behera, R., Das, K., 2017. A survey on machine learning: concept, algorithms and applications. Int. J. Innov. Res. Comput. Commun. Eng. 2, 1301–1309.

Bishop, C.M., 1993. Novelty detection and neural network validation. International Conference on Artificial Neural Networks (ICANN '93). Springer, London, pp. 789–794.

Blum, A.L., Langley, P., 1997. Selection of relevant features and examples in machine learning. Artif. Intell. 97 (1–2), 245–271. https://doi.org/10.1016/S0004-3702(97)00063-5.

COVID-19 Data Repository by the Center for Systems Science and Engineering (CSSE) at Johns Hopkins University, 2020. CSSEGISandData/COVID-19. GitHub. https://github.com/CSSEGISandData/COVID-19/blob/master/csse_covid_19_data/csse_covid_19_time_series/time_series_covid19_confirmed_global.csv. January.

Chandrashekar, G., Sahin, F., 2014. A survey on feature selection methods. Comput. Electr. Eng. 40 (1), 16–28. https://doi.org/10.1016/j.compeleceng.2013.11.024.

Chen, X., Liu, Z., 2020. Early prediction of mortality risk among severe COVID-19 patients using machine learning. medRxiv. https://doi.org/10.1101/2020.04.13.20064329.

Chen, Y., Li, Y., Cheng, X.-Q., Guo, L., 2006. Survey and taxonomy of feature selection algorithms in intrusion detection system. In: Information Security and Cryptology: Second SKLOIS Conference, Inscrypt 2006, Beijing, China, November 29–December 1, 2006. Proceedings. Springer, Berlin, Heidelberg, pp. 153–167.

Darabseh, A., Namin, A.S., 2015. Effective user authentications using keystroke dynamics based on feature selections. In: 2015 IEEE 14th International Conference on Machine Learning and Applications (ICMLA), December, pp. 307–312.

Dash, M., Liu, H., Motoda, H., 2000. Consistency based feature selection. In: Proceedings of the 4th Pacific-Asia Conference on Knowledge Discovery and Data Mining, Current Issues and New Applications, PADKK '00. Springer-Verlag, London, pp. 98–109. http://dl.acm.org/citation.cfm?id=646418.693349.

Frank, E., Hall, M.A., Witten, I.H., 2016. Weka software. The WEKA Workbench. Online Appendix for Data Mining: Practical Machine Learning Tools and Techniques. https://waikato.github.io/weka-wiki/downloading_weka/.

Gauci, M., Dodd, T.J., Groß, R., 2012. Why GSA, a gravitational search algorithm, is not genuinely based on the law of gravity. Nat. Comput. 11 (4), 719–720.

Gautam, C., Tiwari, A., 2016. On the construction of extreme learning machine for one class classifier. In: Proceedings of ELM-2015, Volume 1: Theory, Algorithms and Applications (I). Springer International Publishing, Cham, pp. 447–461.

Grasselli, G., Pesenti, A., Cecconi, M., 2020. Critical care utilization for the COVID-19 outbreak in Lombardy, Italy: early experience and forecast during an emergency response. JAMA 323 (16), 1545–1546. https://doi.org/10.1001/jama.2020.4031.

Gupta, M., 2018. ML: linear regression, September. https://www.geeksforgeeks.org/ml-linear-regression/.

Guyon, I., Elisseeff, A., 2003. An introduction to variable and feature selection. J. Mach. Learn. Res. 3, 1157–1182.

Halakou, F., 2013. Feature selection in keystroke dynamics authentication systems. In: International Conference on Computer, Information Technology and Digital Media (CITaDIM2013), pp. 30–33.

Hall, M.A., 2000. Correlation-based feature selection for discrete and numeric class machine learning. In: Proceedings of the Seventeenth International Conference on Machine Learning, ICML '00. Morgan Kaufmann Publishers Inc., San Francisco, CA, pp. 359–366.

Information, Health, 2016. What is diabetes? https://www.niddk.nih.gov/health-information/diabetes/. December.

Jinquan, Z., Xiaojie, L., Tao, L., Caiming, L., Lingxi, P., Feixian, S., 2009. A self-adaptive negative selection algorithm used for anomaly detection. Progress Nat. Sci. 19 (2), 261–266.

Kashef, S., Nezamabadi-Pour, H., 2015. An advanced {ACO} algorithm for feature subset selection. Neurocomputing 147, 271–279. https://doi.org/10.1016/j.neucom.2014.06.067.

Kohavi, R., John, G.H., 1997. Wrappers for feature subset selection. Artif. Intell. 97 (1–2), 273–324. https://doi.org/10.1016/S0004-3702(97)00043-X.

Kostarelos, K., 2020. COVID-19 is a chronic disease—and cancer care model is way forward. www.manchester.ac.uk. April.

Kumar, A., Zhang, D., 2005. Biometric recognition using feature selection and combination. In: Audio- and Video-Based Biometric Person Authentication: 5th International Conference, AVBPA 2005, Hilton Rye Town, NY, USA, July 20–22, 2005. Proceedings. Springer, Berlin, Heidelberg, pp. 813–822.

LaMantia, M.A., Platts-Mills, T.F., Biese, K., Khandelwal, C., Forbach, C., Cairns, C.B., Busby-Whitehead, J., Kizer, J.S., 2010. Predicting hospital admission and returns to the emergency department for elderly patients. Acad. Emerg. Med. 17 (3), 252–259. https://doi.org/10.1111/j.1553-2712.2009.00675.x.

Lan, L., Xu, D., Ye, G., Xia, C., Wang, S., Li, Y., Xu, H., 2020. Positive RT-PCR test results in patients recovered from COVID-19. JAMA 323 (15), 1502–1503. https://doi.org/10.1001/jama.2020.2783.

Li, L., Yang, Z., Dang, Z., Meng, C., Huang, J., Meng, H., Wang, D., Chen, G., Zhang, J., Peng, H., Shao, Y., 2020. Propagation analysis and prediction of the COVID-19. Infect. Dis. Model. 5, 282–292. https://doi.org/10.1016/j.idm.2020.03.002.

Lior, R., Oded, M., 2005. Decision trees. In: Data Mining and Knowledge Discovery Handbook, pp. 165–192, https://doi.org/10.1007/0-387-25465-X_9.

Liu, H., Setiono, R., 1996. A probabilistic approach to feature selection: a filter solution. In: Proc. 13th International Conference on Machine Learning. Morgan Kaufmann, pp. 319–327.

Liu, Y., Wang, G., Chen, H., Dong, H., Zhu, X., Wang, S., 2011. An improved particle swarm optimization for feature selection. J. Bionic Eng. 8 (2), 191–200. https://doi.org/10.1016/S1672-6529(11)60020-6.

Mirjalili, S., Mirjalili, S.M., Lewis, A., 2014. Grey wolf optimizer. Adv. Eng. Softw. 69, 46–61. https://doi.org/10.1016/j.advengsoft.2013.12.007.

Molina, L.C., Belanche, L., Nebot, A., 2002. Feature selection algorithms: a survey and experimental evaluation. In: Proceedings of the 2002 IEEE International Conference on Data Mining, ICDM '02. IEEE Computer Society, Washington, DC, p. 306. http://dl.acm.org/citation.cfm?id=844380.844722.

Nicholson, C., 2019. A beginner's guide to multilayer perceptrons (MLP). https://pathmind.com/wiki/multilayer-perceptron.

Coronavirus, Novel, 2020. What is COVID-19?: EOHU: Public Health. https://eohu.ca/en/covid/what-is-covid-19. May.

Pauwels, E.J., Ambekar, O., 2011. One class classification for anomaly detection: support vector data description revisited. In: Advances in Data Mining. Applications and Theoretical Aspects: 11th Industrial Conference, ICDM 2011, New York, NY, USA, August 30–September 3, 2011. Proceedings. Springer, Berlin, Heidelberg, pp. 25–39.

Petropoulos, F., Makridakis, S., 2020. Forecasting the novel coronavirus COVID-19. PLoS One 15 (3), 1–8. https://doi.org/10.1371/journal.pone.0231236.

Public Health Agency of Canada, 2015. Chronic disease datasets. https://www.canada.ca/en/public-health/services/chronic-diseases/chronic-diseases-datasets.html. March.

Public Health Agency of Canada, 2020. Open government portal. https://open.canada.ca/data/en/dataset?organization=phac-aspc.

Rahul, P., 2019. Locally weighted regression-all about analytics, June. https://medium.com/patnalarahul/locally-weighted-regression-lwl-all-about-analytics-f3107c289699.

Rashedi, E., Nezamabadi-Pour, H., Saryazdi, S., 2009. GSA: a gravitational search algorithm. Inform. Sci. 179 (13), 2232–2248.

Ray, S., 2020. Learn naive Bayes algorithm: naive Bayes classifier examples, April. https://www.analyticsvidhya.com/blog/2017/09/naive-bayes-explained/.

Richardson, S., Hirsch, J.S., Narasimhan, M., Crawford, J.M., McGinn, T., Davidson, K.W., The Northwell COVID-19 Research Consortium, 2020. Presenting characteristics, comorbidities, and outcomes among 5700 patients hospitalized with COVID-19 in the New York City Area. JAMA. https://doi.org/10.1001/jama.2020.6775.

Ritter, G., Gallegos, M.T., 1997. Outliers in statistical pattern recognition and an application to automatic chromosome classification. Pattern Recogn. Lett. 18 (6), 525–539.

Robnik-Šikonja, M., Kononenko, I., 2003. Theoretical and empirical analysis of Relieff and RReliefF. Mach. Learn. 53 (1), 23–69. https://doi.org/10.1023/A:1025667309714.

Schiezaro, M., Pedrini, H., 2013. Data feature selection based on artificial bee colony algorithm. EURASIP J. Image Video Process. 2013 (1), 47. https://doi.org/10.1186/1687-5281-2013-47.

Schölkopf, B., Williamson, R., Smola, A., Shawe-Taylor, J., Platt, J., 1999. Support vector method for novelty detection. In: Proceedings of the 12th International Conference on Neural Information Processing Systems, NIPS'99. MIT Press, Cambridge, MA, pp. 582–588.

Smith, D., Moore, L., 2004. The SIR model for spread of disease: the differential equation model. Convergence. Mathematical Association of America, Washington, DC. https://www.maa.org/press/periodicals/loci/joma/the-sir-model-for-spread-of-disease-the-differential-equation-model; 2004. (Accessed 29 April 2021).

Tax, D.M.J., Duin, R.P.W., 2004. Support vector data description. Mach. Learn. 54 (1), 45–66.

Taylor, G.W., 2016. Health Status of Canadians 2016. Public Health Agency of Canada, Canada. https://www.canada.ca/content/dam/hc-sc/healthy-canadians/migration/publications/department-ministere/state-public-health-status-2016-etat-sante-publique-statut/alt/pdf-eng.pdf.

Tibshirani, R., 1994. Regression shrinkage and selection via the lasso. J. R. Stat. Soc. B 58, 267–288.

Colonist, Times, 2020. Airports forecast 2-billion loss by June as travel halts amid COVID-19. Times Colonist. https://www.timescolonist.com/. March.

Vanaja, S., Kumar, K.R., 2014. Analysis of feature selection algorithms on classification: a survey. Int. J. Comput. Appl. 96 (17), 29–35.

Watkins, A., Boggess, L., 2002. A new classifier based on resource limited artificial immune systems. In: Proceedings of the 2002 Congress on Evolutionary Computation, 2002. CEC '02, vol. 2, pp. 1546–1551.

Weissman, G.E., Crane-Droesch, A., Chivers, C., Luong, T., Hanish, A., Levy, M.Z., Lubken, J., Becker, M., Draugelis, M.E., Anesi, G.L., Brennan, P.J., Christie, J.D., William Hanson III, C., Mikkelsen, M.E., Halpern, S.D., 2020. Locally informed simulation to predict hospital capacity needs during the COVID-19 pandemic. Ann. Intern. Med. https://doi.org/10.7326/M20-1260.

Xue, B., Zhang, M., Browne, W.N., Yao, X., 2016. A survey on evolutionary computation approaches to feature selection. IEEE Trans. Evol. Comput. 20 (4), 606–626. https://doi.org/10.1109/TEVC.2015.2504420.

Yang, W., Gao, Y., Shi, Y., Cao, L., 2015. MRM-Lasso: a sparse multiview feature selection method via low-rank analysis. IEEE Trans. Neural Netw. Learn. Syst. 26 (11), 2801–2815. https://doi.org/10.1109/TNNLS.2015.2396937.

Yavuz, G., Aydin, D., 2016. Angle modulated artificial bee colony algorithms for feature selection. Appl. Comp. Intell. Soft Comput. 2016, 7:7. https://doi.org/10.1155/2016/9569161.

Yu, L., Liu, H., 2004. Efficient feature selection via analysis of relevance and redundancy. J. Mach. Learn. Res. 5, 1205–1224.

Zahiri, A., RafieeNasab, S., Roohi, E., 2020. Prediction of peak and termination of novel coronavirus COVID-19 epidemic in Iran. medRxiv. https://doi.org/10.1101/2020.03.29.20046532.

Zou, H., Hastie, T., 2005. Regularization and variable selection via the Elastic Net. J. R. Stat. Soc. B 67, 301–320.

# Interpretable semisupervised classifier for predicting cancer stages

# 14

**Isel Grau[a], Dipankar Sengupta[a,b], and Ann Nowe[a]**

*Artificial Intelligence Lab, Free University of Brussels (VUB), Brussels, Belgium[a] PGJCCR, Queens University Belfast, Belfast, United Kingdom[b]*

### Chapter outline

## 1 Introduction

Cancer is a disease or group of diseases caused by the transformation of normal cells into tumor cells characterized by their uncontrolled growth. This is a multistage process, triggered and regulated by complex and heterogeneous biological causes (Hausman, 2019). In the process, there is a gradual invasion and destruction of healthy cells, tissues, and organs by the cancerous cells (Hausman, 2019). Therefore, a key factor in the diagnosis of cancer is identifying the extent it has spread across the body: stage and TNM grade (tumor, node, metastasis) (Gress et al., 2017). This is also important for treatment planning and patient prognosis. Clinically, the cancer stage describes the size of the tumor and how far it has spread in the body, whereas the grade of a cancer describes its growth rate, i.e., how rapidly it is spreading in the body. Usually, an initial clinical staging is made based on the laboratory (blood, histology, risk factors) and imaging (X-ray, CT scans, MRI) tests, while a more accurate pathological staging is usually performed postsurgery or via biopsy.

Clinical advancements including computational approaches based on machine learning have been developed since the 1980s, which can be used for cancer detection, classification, diagnosis, and prognosis (Cruz and Wishart, 2006; Kourou et al., 2015). With the advancement of omics-based

*Machine Learning, Big Data, and IoT for Medical Informatics.* https://doi.org/10.1016/B978-0-12-821777-1.00006-9

technologies and availability of the omics data (e.g., genome, exome, proteome, etc.) along with the clinical data, there have been impeccable improvements in these methods (Zhang et al., 2015; Zhu et al., 2020). However, mostly these developments have been for common cancer types (colon, breast, prostate, etc.), like the prostrate pathological stage predictor based on biopsy patterns, PSA (prostate-specific antigen) level, and other clinical factors (Cosma et al., 2016). In similar terms, there are staging predictors available for breast and colon cancer based on clinical factors (Said et al., 2018; Taniguchi et al., 2019). There are more than 200 types of cancer developing from different types of cells in the body; lung cancer being the most common (11.6% of total cases, 18.4% of total cancer-related deaths), followed by breast, colorectal, and prostate cancer (Bray et al., 2018; WHO, 2020). However, 27% of the cancer types, like bladder cancer, melanoma, are less common, whereas 20% of them, like thyroid cancer, acute lymphoblastic leukemia, are rare or very rare (Macmillan Cancer Support, 2020; Cancer Research UK, 2020). A major challenge with such rare cancer types is the availability of data, as they have an incidence rate of 6:100,000. The prediction performance of machine learning approaches for classification, diagnosis, prognosis, etc., involving rare cancers is thus limited by the lack of labeled data.

Semisupervised classification (SSC) constitutes an alternative approach for building prediction models in settings where labeled data are limited. The general aim of SSC is improving the generalization ability of the predictor compared to learn a supervised model using labeled data alone. The main assumption of SCC is that the underlying marginal distribution of instances over the feature space provides information on the joint distribution of instances and their class label, from where the labeled instances were sampled. When this condition is met, it is possible to use the unlabeled data for gaining information about the distribution of instances and therefore also the joint distribution of instances and labels (Zhu et al., 2020). SSC methods available in the literature are based on different views of this assumption. For example, graph-based methods (Blum and Chawla, 2001) assume label smoothness in clusters of instances, i.e., two similar instances will share their label, therefore an unlabeled instance can take the label of its neighbors and propagate this label to other neighboring instances. Semisupervised support vector machines (Joachims, 1999) assume that the boundaries should be placed on low-density areas, which is complementary to the cluster view described earlier. In this method, unlabeled instances help compute better margins for placing the boundaries. Generative mixture models (Goldberg et al., 2009) try to find a mixture of distributions (e.g., Gaussian distributions), where each distribution represents a class label. They learn the joint probability by assuming a type of distribution and adjusting its parameters using information from the labeled and the unlabeled data together. Finally, self-labeling methods use an ensemble of classifiers trained on the available labeled data for assigning labels to the unlabeled instances, assuming their classifications are correct. This assumption makes self-labeling the simplest and most versatile family of semisupervised classifiers, since they can be used with practically any base supervised classifier (Van Engelen and Hoos, 2020). Although SSC methods achieve very attractive performance in terms of accuracy in a wide variety of problems (Triguero et al., 2015), they often result in complex structures which lead to black boxes in terms of interpretability.

Nowadays, an increasing requirement in the application of machine learning is to obtain not only precise models but also interpretable ones. Interpretability is a fundamental tool for gaining insights into how an algorithm produces a particular outcome and attaining the trust of end users. Although several formalizations exist (Barredo Arrieta et al., 2020; Doshi-Velez and Kim, 2017; Lipton, 2016), interpretability is directly connected to the transparency of the machine models obtained. The transparency spectrum (see Fig. 1) starts from completely black box models which involve deep

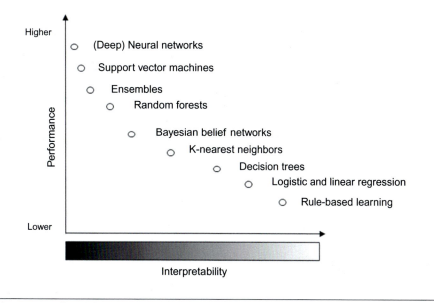

**FIG. 1**

Fictional plot representing the trade-off between accuracy and interpretability for most known machine learning families of models. The transparency spectrum is depicted along the x axis. Inspired from similar figure published by Barredo Arrieta et al. (2020).

or ensemble structures that cannot be decomposed and mapped to the problem domain. While on the opposite extreme are the white box models which are built based on laws and principles of the problem domain. This side also includes those models which are built from data, but their structure allows for interpretation, since pure white boxes rarely exist (Nelles, 2001).

White box techniques are commonly referred as intrinsically interpretable and vary in the types of interpretations they can provide as well as their limitations for prediction. Examples of intrinsic interpretable methods are linear and logistic regression (Hastie et al., 2008), k-nearest neighbors, naïve Bayes (Altman, 1992), decision trees (Quinlan, 1993), and decision lists (Cohen, 1995; Frank and Witten, 1998). On the opposite side, black boxes are normally more accurate techniques that learn exclusively from data, but they are not easily understandable at a global level. As a solution, there exist several model-agnostic post hoc methods for generating explanations which quantify the feature attribution in the prediction of certain outcomes according to the black box. Some examples of these techniques are dependency plots (Friedman, 2001), feature importance metrics (Breiman, 2001), local surrogates (LIME) (Ribeiro et al., 2016), or Shapley values (Lundberg and Lee, 2017; Shapley, 1953). While explanations provided by intrinsically interpretable models are derived from their structure and easily mappable to the problem domain, model-agnostic ones are often local or limited to feature attribution rather than a holistic view of the model.

Global surrogates or gray box models take the best of both worlds while trying to find a suitable trade-off between accuracy and interpretability. The idea behind this technique is to distill the knowledge of a previously trained black box model in an intrinsically interpretable one. In this way, the prediction capabilities are kept to some extent by the black box component, while the white box learns to mimic these predictions through a more transparent structure. In our earlier work (Grau et al., 2018,

2020a), we proposed a gray box model for SSC settings, called self-labeling gray box (SLGB). Our method uses the self-labeling strategy from SSC for assigning a label to unlabeled instances. This part of the learning process is carried out by the more accurate black box component. Once all instances have been self-labeled, then a white box model is learned from the enlarged dataset. The white box component, being an intrinsically interpretable classifier, allows for interpretable representation of the model at a global level as well as individual explanations for the prediction of instances. The SLGB outperforms several state-of-the-art SSC algorithms in a wide benchmark of structured classification problems where labeled instances are scarce (Grau et al., 2020b).

In this chapter, we illustrate the applications of self-labeling gray box models on the proteomic (reverse phase protein array) (Li et al., 2013) and the clinical dataset (Liu et al., 2018; Weinstein et al., 2013) for breast (common cancer), esophageal (less common), and thyroid (rare) cancer. In comparison to other omics datasets, we are considering the proteomics data for this study, as the activity of protein is a more relevant phenotype than its expression during pathogenesis (Lim, 2005). The target feature to predict is the cancer stage of the patient. We first study how the inclusion of features from both dimensions (clinical and proteomics) influences the prediction performance. Second, we test how accurate is the SLGB classifier when leveraging unlabeled data for predicting cancer stages. Third, we test how adding unlabeled data from more frequent types of cancers helps in the stage prediction of less common or rare cancer types. Through the experiments section, we illustrate with our interpretable semisupervised classifier, why certain cancer stages are predicted, and which information is important for predictions.

The rest of this chapter is structured as follows. Section 2 describes the SLGB approach with details on their components and learning algorithm. Section 3 describes the preprocessing steps carried out for conforming the datasets used in the analysis. Section 4 discusses the experimental results in different settings, which cover both the performance and interpretability angles. Section 5 formalizes the concluding remarks and research directions to be explored in the future.

## 2 Self-labeling gray box

In supervised classification, data points or instances $x \in X$ are described by a set of attributes or features $A$ and a decision label $y \in Y$. A function $f: X \rightarrow Y$ is learned from data by relying on pairs of previously labeled examples $(x, y)$. Later, the function $f$ can be used for predicting the label of unseen instances.

When the labeled pairs $(x, y)$ are limited, SSC uses both labeled and unlabeled instances for the learning process with the aim of improving the generalization ability. In an SSC setting, a set $L \subset X$ denotes the instances which are associated with their respective class labels in $Y$ and a set $U \subset X$ represent the unlabeled instances, where usually $|L| < |U|$. A semisupervised classifier will try to learn a function $g: L \cup U \rightarrow Y$ for predicting the class label of any instance, leveraging both labeled and unlabeled data.

Self-labeling is a family of SSC methods which uses one or more base classifiers for learning a supervised model that later predicts the unlabeled data, assuming the first predictions are correct to some extent. In the self-labeling process, instances can be added to the enlarged dataset incrementally or with an amending procedure (Triguero et al., 2015). The amending procedures select or weight the self-labeled instances which will enlarge the labeled dataset, to avoid the propagation of misclassification errors.

The SLGB method (Grau et al., 2018) combines the self-labeling strategy of SSC with the global surrogate idea from explainable artificial intelligence in one model. SLGB first trains a black box classifier to predict the decision class, based on the labeled instances available. The black box is exploited in the self-labeling step for assigning labels to the unlabeled instances. Once the enlarged dataset is entirely labeled, a surrogate white box classifier is trained for mimicking the predictions made by the black box. The aim is to obtain better performance than the base white box component, while maintaining a good balance between performance and interpretability. The blueprint of the SLGB classifier is depicted in Fig. 2.

To avoid the propagation of misclassification errors during the self-labeling, SLGB uses an amending procedure proposed by Grau et al. (2020a). The amending strategy of SLGB is based on a measure of inconsistency in the classification. This type of uncertainty emerges when very similar instances have different class labels, which can result from errors in the self-labeling process. For measuring inconsistency in the classification across the dataset we rely on *rough set theory* (Pawlak, 1982), a mathematical formalism for describing any set of objects in terms of their lower and upper approximations. In this context, an object would be an instance of the dataset, described by its attributes. The sets would be the decision classes that group these instances. The lower approximation of a given set would be all those instances that for sure are correctly classified in that class, while the upper approximation would contain instances that might belong to that class. From the lower and upper approximations of each set, positive, boundary, and negative regions of each decision class are computed. All instances in the positive region of a class are certainly classified as that class. Likewise, all instances in the negative region of a class are certainly not labeled as the given class. However, the boundary region of a decision is formed by instances that might belong to the class but are not certain. An inclusion degree measure, computed using information from these regions and similar instances (Grau et al., 2020b) is used as an indicative of how certain a prediction from the self-labeling process is. The white box component then focuses on learning from the most confident instances without ignoring the less

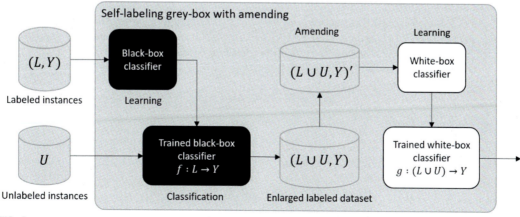

**FIG. 2**

Blueprint of the SLGB architecture using amending procedures for correcting the influence of the misclassifications from the self-labeling process.

confident ones coming from the boundary regions. This amending procedure not only improves the accuracy of SLGB, but also increases the interpretability of the surrogate white box by keeping the transparency of the white box component (Grau et al., 2020a).

The SLGB method is a general framework which is flexible for the choice of black box and white box components. In this work, random forest (Breiman, 2001) will be used as black box base classifier. Random forest is an ensemble of decision trees built from a random subset of attributes which uses bagging (Breiman, 1996) technique for aggregating the results of individual classifiers. The choice of this method as black box is supported by its well-known performance in supervised classification (Fernández-Delgado et al., 2014; Wainberg and Frey, 2016; Zhang et al., 2017) and particularly as a black box component for SLGB (Grau et al., 2020b).

Likewise, we will explore the use of several intrinsically interpretable classifiers that produces explanations in the form of *if-then* rules. In these rules, the condition is a conjunction of feature evaluations and the conclusion is the prediction of the target value. A first option for white box is decision trees learned using the C4.5 algorithm (Quinlan, 1993), which produces a tree-like structure that offers a global view of the model. The most informative attributes are chosen greedily by C4.5 for splitting the dataset on each node of the tree. In this way, the error is minimized when all instances are covered in the leaves of the tree. Decision trees are considered transparent since when traversing the tree to infer the classification of an individual instance, it produces an *if-then* rule which constitutes an explanation of the obtained classification.

A second option as white box component is decision lists of rules. In this chapter, we explore two mainstream algorithms for generating decision lists using sequential covering: partial decision trees (PART) (Frank and Witten, 1998) and repeated incremental pruning to produce error reduction (RIPPER) (Cohen, 1995). Sequential covering is a common divide-and-conquer strategy for building decision lists. These algorithms induce a rule from data and remove the covered instances before inducing the next rule, until all instances are covered by rules or a default rule is needed. Therefore, the set of rules of a decision list must be interpreted in order. PART decision lists in one of the many models implementing this strategy, where rules are iteratively induced as the most covered one from a pruned C4.5 decision tree. RIPPER is another representative algorithm that uses reduced error pruning and an optimization strategy to revise the induced rules, generally producing more compact sets. Like decision trees, decision lists are transparent and easily decomposable since the explanations that can be generated are rules using features and values of the problem domain.

## 3 Data preparation

In 12 years, the cancer genome atlas project has collected and analyzed over 20,000 samples from more than 11,000 patients with different types of cancers (Liu et al., 2018; Weinstein et al., 2013). The data in this repository are publicly available and broadly comprise genomic, epigenomic, transcriptomic, clinical (Liu et al., 2018), and proteomic (Li et al., 2013) data. In this chapter, we have focused our experiments on the prediction of the cancer stage based on two data dimensions: clinical and protein expression. We chose three types of cancers for our exploratory experiments: breast (common), esophageal (less common), and thyroid (rare) cancers.

The clinical data used in this study were downloaded from the cancer genome atlas[a] (Liu et al., 2018). In the study, we have used radiation and drug treatment information from these data. Features describing the radiation treatment include its type (i.e., external or internal), the received dose measured in grays (Gy), the site of radiation treatment (e.g., primary tumor field, regional site, distant recurrence, local recurrence, or distant site) and the response to the treatment by the patient. While features of drug treatment include the type of drug therapy (e.g., hormone therapy, chemotherapy, targeted molecular therapy, ancillary therapy, immunotherapy, vaccine, or others), the total dose, the route of administration, and the response measure to the treatment. In case a patient had more than one record for treatments, all instances are been considered. In addition, we include the age of the patient at the first event of the pathologic stage diagnosis.

The protein expression data for the three cancer types were downloaded from the cancer proteome atlas[b] (Li et al., 2013). We have used the level 4 (L4) reverse phase protein array (RPPA) data for analysis, as batch effects are been removed in L4 (Li et al., 2013). Each of these datasets have the protein expression values estimated by the RPPA high-throughput antibody-based technique, for the key proteins involved in regulation of that cancer type. It also includes the phosphoproteins, i.e., the proteins which are phosphorylated in the posttranslational processes. For example, AKT_pS473 is a phosphorylated form of AKT (serine-threonine protein kinase), having phosphorylation at an amino acid position of 473. In cancer regulation and many other diseases, the posttranslational modifications like phosphorylation, degradation, and glycosylation play a key role, for example, the role of tyrosine phosphorylation is well established in cancer biology (Lim, 2005). Therefore, all the proteins including the phosphoproteins were considered for the experiments. Data for all the phosphoproteins were normalized by subtracting their expression values from their respective parent protein. For example, AKT being the parent protein for AKT-473, to obtain the relevant phosphorylation score we compute the difference between AKT_pS473 and AKT. The phosphoproteins which did not have their parent protein expression values in the dataset have not been considered in the experiments, as they cannot be normalized.

The clinical features are stored at a patient level, whereas the protein expression data are stored at a sample level. Therefore, the patient identification was used to match each sample characterization to the corresponding patient.

The pathological stage of the patient constitutes the target feature to be predicted. After preprocessing and cleaning, a total of 3073 samples from 1789 patients are included in our experiments. The distribution of patients per type of cancer can be seen in Fig. 3, as well as the distribution of cancer stages across all types of cancers in Fig. 4. The last figure reveals imbalance in the dataset with a majority of patients labeled as stage IIA. While gathering information from the different sources of data, not all patients have information available for all the features, therefore the datasets contain missing values for some. Missing values are also present in the target feature cancer stage, leading to unlabeled instances that will be leveraged for semisupervised classification. For those patients where more than one recorded stage of the same type of cancer is available, we kept the most advanced one.

---

[a]https://portal.gdc.cancer.gov/.
[b]https://www.tcpaportal.org/.

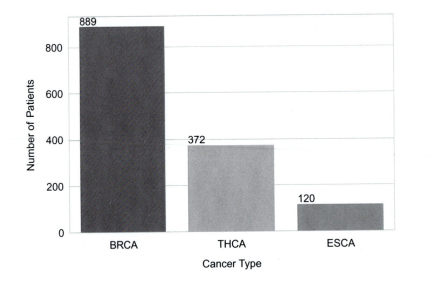

**FIG. 3**

Distribution of cancer types across patients in the dataset, showing breast cancer with the maximum number of instances. *BRCA*, breast cancer; *ESCA*, esophageal cancer; *THCA*, thyroid cancer.

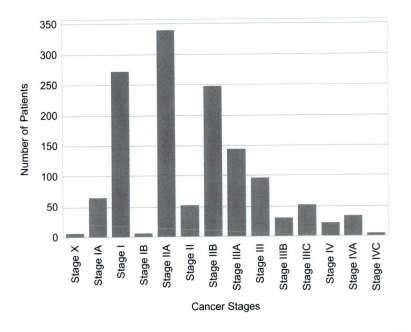

**FIG. 4**

Distribution of cancer stages across patients in the dataset shows high imbalance and stage IIA as the most common stage.

# 4 Experiments and discussion

In this section, we explore the cancer stage prediction problem for breast, esophagus, and thyroid cancer through different settings. We first explore the baseline predictions obtained by the black box and white box component classifiers when working on only the labeled data. We show the influence of adding the proteomic dimension to the clinical data for the stage prediction. Second, we explore how the unlabeled data help in the semisupervised setting where all cancer types are used to build the model. Finally, we explore how unlabeled data coming from more common cancer types can help in predicting the cancer stage of more rare ones.

For the validation of our experiments, a leave one group out cross-validation was used. In this type of cross-validation, the dataset was divided in 10 disjoint groups of patients for avoiding using samples of the same patient for training and testing. Patients with missing cancer stage are not included in the test sets, they are only added to the training sets when semisupervised classification is performed. Notice that one patient can have more than one sample record and each sample constitutes an instance in the dataset (see Tables 1–4 for the number of instances).

The Weka library (Hall et al., 2009) was used for the implementation of random forests, decision trees, and decision lists algorithms.[c] Random forests consist of 100 decision trees built using a random subset of features with cardinality equal to the base-2 logarithm of the number of features. Decision trees and PART decision lists use C4.5 algorithm for generating the trees, with a parameter $C = 0.25$ which denotes the confidence value for performing pruning in the trees (the lower the value, the more pruning is performed). The minimum number of instances on each leaf is two. In RIPPER implementation, the training data are split into a growing set and a pruning set for performing reduced error pruning. The rule set formed from the growing set is simplified with pruning operations optimizing the error

**Table 1** Classification performance change with incrementing features for random forests (RF) when using clinical and proteomic data, for each cancer type and the entire dataset.

|  | Instances | Features | RF | | | | |
|---|---|---|---|---|---|---|---|
|  |  |  | ACC | KAPPA | SEN | SPE | AUC |
| BR | 1898 | Clinical | 0.44 | 0.24 | 0.45 | 0.79 | 0.69 |
|  |  | +proteomic | 0.81 | 0.75 | 0.81 | 0.93 | 0.94 |
| ES | 124 | Clinical | 0.25 | 0.01 | 0.25 | 0.73 | 0.51 |
|  |  | +proteomic | 0.41 | 0.17 | 0.41 | 0.75 | 0.61 |
| TH | 383 | Clinical | 0.60 | 0.36 | 0.60 | 0.84 | 0.77 |
|  |  | +proteomic | 0.60 | 0.24 | 0.60 | 0.61 | 0.76 |
| All | 2405 | Clinical | 0.43 | 0.30 | 0.43 | 0.87 | 0.74 |
|  |  | +proteomic | 0.75 | 0.69 | 0.75 | 0.92 | 0.94 |

[c]For the execution of all experiments described in this section, we used a PC with Intel(R) Core(TM) i5-8350U CPU @ 1.70 GHz, 1896 MHz, 4 Cores, 8 Logical Processors, 32.0 GB RAM, and Java Virtual Machine version 8.

**Table 2** Classification performance change with incrementing features for decision tree (C4.5) when using clinical and proteomic data, for each cancer type and the entire dataset.

| | Instances | Features | C4.5 | | | | | |
|---|---|---|---|---|---|---|---|---|
| | | | ACC | KAPPA | SEN | SPE | AUC | Rules |
| BR | 1898 | Clinical | 0.46 | 0.25 | 0.46 | 0.79 | 0.70 | 94 |
| | | +proteomic | 0.75 | 0.68 | 0.75 | 0.94 | 0.86 | 222 |
| ES | 124 | Clinical | 0.30 | −0.01 | 0.30 | 0.69 | 0.47 | 4 |
| | | +proteomic | 0.23 | 0.06 | 0.23 | 0.84 | 0.46 | 28 |
| TH | 383 | Clinical | 0.65 | 0.45 | 0.65 | 0.90 | 0.77 | 4 |
| | | +proteomic | 0.59 | 0.37 | 0.59 | 0.96 | 0.64 | 40 |
| All | 2405 | Clinical | 0.51 | 0.39 | 0.51 | 0.88 | 0.78 | 299 |
| | | +proteomic | 0.67 | 0.61 | 0.67 | 0.93 | 0.82 | 325 |

**Table 3** Classification performance change with incrementing features for decision lists (PART) when using clinical and proteomic data, for each cancer type and the entire dataset.

| | Instances | Features | PART | | | | | |
|---|---|---|---|---|---|---|---|---|
| | | | ACC | KAPPA | SEN | SPE | AUC | Rules |
| BR | 1898 | Clinical | 0.39 | 0.14 | 0.39 | 0.75 | 0.61 | 78 |
| | | +proteomic | 0.77 | 0.70 | 0.77 | 0.94 | 0.86 | 149 |
| ES | 124 | Clinical | 0.29 | −0.04 | 0.29 | 0.68 | 0.48 | 10 |
| | | +proteomic | 0.28 | 0.11 | 0.28 | 0.84 | 0.45 | 17 |
| TH | 383 | Clinical | 0.65 | 0.46 | 0.65 | 0.90 | 0.78 | 12 |
| | | +proteomic | 0.62 | 0.41 | 0.62 | 0.85 | 0.67 | 28 |
| All | 2405 | Clinical | 0.46 | 0.34 | 0.46 | 0.87 | 0.73 | 277 |
| | | +proteomic | 0.68 | 0.61 | 0.68 | 0.93 | 0.80 | 229 |

on the pruning set. The minimum allowed support of a rule is two and the data are split in three folds where one is used for pruning. Additionally, the number of optimization iterations is set to two.

Given the nature of the target attribute, the prediction problem at hand is not only an imbalance multiclass classification problem, but it is also an ordinal one. The traditional approach to deal with ordinal classification is coding the decision class into numeric values and using a regression model for the prediction. However, this limits the choice of black box and white box components to regression techniques only. Instead we use the approach described by Frank and Hall (2001), which does not require any modification of the underlying prediction algorithm. With this technique, our multiclass classification problem is transformed in several binary classifications datasets where each predictor determines the probability of the class value being greater than a given label and the greatest probability is taken as the decision. This transformation is only applied in the black box component of the SLGB without affecting the interpretability of the white box component.

**Table 4** Classification performance change with incrementing features for decision lists (RIPPER) when using clinical and proteomic data, for each cancer type and the entire dataset.

| | Instances | Features | RIPPER | | | | | |
| | | | ACC | KAPPA | SEN | SPE | AUC | Rules |
|---|---|---|---|---|---|---|---|---|
| BR | 1898 | Clinical | 0.43 | 0.22 | 0.43 | 0.77 | 0.62 | 25 |
| | | +proteomic | 0.72 | 0.63 | 0.72 | 0.92 | 0.84 | 60 |
| ES | 124 | Clinical | 0.33 | 0.00 | 0.33 | 0.66 | 0.43 | 2 |
| | | +proteomic | 0.33 | 0.05 | 0.33 | 0.72 | 0.45 | 5 |
| TH | 383 | Clinical | 0.65 | 0.37 | 0.65 | 0.72 | 0.64 | 3 |
| | | +proteomic | 0.63 | 0.36 | 0.63 | 0.75 | 0.63 | 6 |
| All | 2405 | Clinical | 0.41 | 0.25 | 0.41 | 0.82 | 0.66 | 32 |
| | | +proteomic | 0.64 | 0.56 | 0.64 | 0.91 | 0.83 | 75 |

## 4.1 Influence of clinical and proteomic data on the prediction of cancer stage

In this subsection, we explore the baseline performance of the classifiers that will be later used as components of the SLGB method. This evaluation is performed in a supervised setting, i.e., only the labeled information is considered. First, we evaluate the performance of random forests (RF), decision trees (C4.5), and decision lists algorithms PART and RIPPER on the classification of cancer stages based on the clinical data only. Later, we add the protein features for comparing how much the proteomic data brings in terms of performance. We perform this analysis for each cancer type: breast (BR), esophagus (ES), and thyroid (TH), and additionally for the entire dataset. Tables 1–4 show the results using different performance metrics. Accuracy (ACC) shows the proportion of correctly classified instances, while kappa (KAPPA) (Cohen, 1960) considers the agreement occurring by chance. This makes this measure more robust in presence of class imbalance. Other measures such as sensitivity (SEN), specificity (SPE), and area under the receiver operating characteristic curve (AUC) are also included. Since the prediction problem at hand is a multiclass classification problem, the last three measures are weighted averages of these measures for each class label. For the white box classifiers, the number of rules is measured as an indication of the size of the structure and its simplicity. The number of rules is measured for the model built based on all instances instead of individual cross-validation folds.

From the Tables 1–4, we can conclude that adding proteomic information to the clinical data substantially improves the accuracy of all classifiers in the datasets, and more evidently for breast cancer. Looking at the performance across classifiers, random forests achieve the best results in terms of accuracy. Its high kappa values indicate that despite the class imbalance, the random forest can generalize further than predicting majority classes. This is supported by high true positive and true negative rates. Overall, these results make random forests a promising base black box component for self-labeling the unlabeled data in the following experiments.

Regarding the performance of the white box base classifiers, less accuracy compared to RF is observed across datasets, which is an expected result. Nevertheless, the accuracy values obtained for the entire dataset by the three white box methods are greater than 0.64 and supported by high kappa, sensitivity, specificity, and AUC values. Regarding the number of rules, C4.5 being the most accurate comes with the largest number of rules, followed by PART. RIPPER obtains slightly less accurate results with the largest reduction in the number of rules and therefore the most transparent classifier. However, the interpretation of these three white boxes differ and can be exploited according to the needs of the user.

Comparing the results across different types of cancers, there is evidence that the limitation in data of esophagus and thyroid cancer leads to poor performance. This contrasts with the performance of the predictors trained on breast cancer data which is more abundant and better balanced across classes. In the next section, we join the data for all types of cancers and explore whether the SLGB can obtain a trade-off between performance and interpretability in the semisupervised setting.

## 4.2 Influence of unlabeled data on the prediction of cancer stage

In this section, we explore the performance of SLGB in the semisupervised prediction of the cancer stage. This time we incorporate 668 unlabeled instances to the learning process, in addition to the 2405 labeled ones. As stated earlier, RF will be used as base classifier for the black box component. A weighting process based on rough sets theory measures is used for amending the errors in the self-labeling process. The three white boxes presented earlier will be explored comparing their performance and interpretability. Table 5 summarizes the experiments results.

Although the number of added unlabeled instances is not large, the SLGB still manages to improve or maintain the performance compared to their base white boxes, while reducing the number of rules needed for achieving this accuracy. The best results are observed with C4.5 as white box, where the accuracy is increased in 0.03 while the number of rules is reduced in 72%, effectively gaining in transparency.

When examining the decision tree generated by the gray box model (see pruned first levels of the tree in Fig. 5), the most informative attributes detected are the proteins FASN, EIF4G, TIGAR, ADAR1, and the clinical feature "age of the initial pathologic diagnostic." High levels of expression of FASN (fatty acid synthase) protein has been associated through several studies with the later stages of cancer, predicting poor prognosis for breast cancer among others (Buckley et al., 2017). Overexpression of EIF4G is associated with malignant transformation (Bauer et al., 2002; Fukuchi-Shimogori et al., 1997). TIGAR expression regulates the p53 tumor suppressor protein which prevents cancer

**Table 5 Classification performance and interpretability of the SLGB classifier using different white box classifiers.**

|  | ACC | KAPPA | SEN | SPE | AUC | Rules |
|---|---|---|---|---|---|---|
| SLGB (RF-C4.5) | 0.70 | 0.62 | 0.70 | 0.92 | 0.85 | 235 |
| SLGB (RF-PART) | 0.69 | 0.60 | 0.69 | 0.91 | 0.82 | 174 |
| SLGB (RF-RIPPER) | 0.63 | 0.52 | 0.63 | 0.88 | 0.83 | 26 |
| C4.5 | 0.67 | 0.61 | 0.67 | 0.93 | 0.82 | 325 |
| PART | 0.68 | 0.61 | 0.68 | 0.93 | 0.80 | 229 |
| RIPPER | 0.64 | 0.56 | 0.64 | 0.91 | 0.83 | 75 |

*The performance results of white boxes from the previous section are summarized for comparison purposes.*

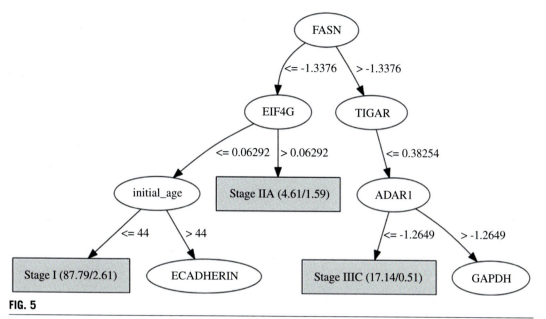

**FIG. 5**

First levels of C4.5 decision tree obtained by SLGB for classifying the stage of cancer, using data from the three types of cancer considered in this study.

development through various mechanisms (Bensaad et al., 2006; Green and Chipuk, 2006; Won et al., 2012). ADAR1 has demonstrated functional role in the RNA editing in thyroid cancer (Ramírez-Moya and Santisteban, 2020; Xu et al., 2018). PART and RIPPER rules (see Figs. 6 and 7) associate these and other features to the stages of cancer. While PART exhibits its most confident and supported rules first, RIPPER focuses in predicting the minority class. Therefore, the choice of which decision list to use must come from the need of obtaining explanations about the most common patterns or the rarest ones. These known associations support the rules learned by the machine learning models which provide potential relations that need to be further analyzed and validated clinically.

```
(X4EBP1 <= -1.05) and (CAVEOLIN1 <= -0.70)
=> pathologic_stage=Stage IVC (3.29/0.50)
(GAPDH <= -3.05) and (MEK1_pS217S221 <= -0.70)
=> pathologic_stage=Stage IB (6.23/0.0)
(PKCALPHA_pS657 >= 0.27) and (NF2 <= -0.76) and (NRAS <= 0.08)
=> pathologic_stage=Stage IV (10.53/2.51)
(...)
(BETACATENIN <= -0.43) and (X4EBP1 <= -0.44) and (CYCLIND1 <= 0.14) and (X4EBP1 >= -0.54)
=> pathologic_stage=Stage IIB (14.57/1.00)
default
=> pathologic_stage=Stage IIA (1135.03/420.95)
```

**FIG. 6**

Subset of rules obtained by SLGB using PART algorithm for classifying the stage of cancer, using data from the three types of cancer considered in this study.

```
FASN <= -1.33 AND EIF4G <= 0.062 AND initial_age <= 44:
Stage I (87.79/2.61)
FASN > -1.52 AND TIGAR > 0.38 AND TIGAR <= 0.41 AND rad_treatment_site = Primary Tumor Field:
Stage IIA (411.15/1.03)
FASN <= -1.54 AND EIF4G <= 0.027 AND SRC_pY416 <= -0.18 AND initial_age <= 67:
Stage IVC (2.79)
(...)
rad_treatment_site = Primary Tumor Field AND CASPASE7CLEAVEDD198 <= -0.52:
Stage IIB (2.58/1.07)
rad_treatment_site = Primary Tumor Field:
Stage I (2.52/1.0)
default:
Stage III (3.06/1.52)
```

**FIG. 7**

Subset of rules obtained by SLGB using RIPPER algorithm for classifying the stage of cancer, using data from the three types of cancer considered in this study.

While the SLGB approach is already able to leverage the unlabeled data for improving performance and interpretability, more impressive results are commonly obtained when the number of unlabeled instances is greater than the labeled ones. In the next subsection, we study how unlabeled instances coming from more frequent types of cancers help in the classification of more rare ones.

## 4.3 Influence of unlabeled data on the prediction of cancer stage for rare cancer types

In this subsection, we study how unlabeled instances coming from a more frequent type of cancer, such as breast, help in the classification of more rare ones. For this setting, we assume that all instances from breast cancer have the cancer stage label missing. In this manner, we are studying whether unlabeled data from breast cancer helps on improving the generalization of the classifier for thyroid and esophagus cancers. Fig. 8 shows the distribution of unlabeled instances per type of cancer in the dataset as used in the previous section (Fig. 8A) and after neglecting the labels of breast cancer for the current experiment (Fig. 8B).

Next, we test how much the performance of SLGB improves on the classification of rare cancers with regard to its interpretable supervised baseline. Table 6 shows the results of the experiment using several measures of performance and the number of rules generated as an indicative of the complexity of the model. Overall, being a very imbalanced multiclass classification problem, it is challenging to obtain a high performance in terms of accuracy even for RF classifier. Nevertheless, the accuracy obtained for all classifiers is well balanced through classes as evidenced by a fair kappa value and high specificity.

From the table we can observe that SLGB clearly outperforms its white box base classifiers for each case, with the biggest improvement using PART decision lists. At the same time, the number of rules is kept reasonably similar, without adding further complexity to the classifier and therefore keeping the transparency to some extent. The best results were obtained by SLGB using PART, and second, using RIPPER, though RIPPER needs a smaller number of rules for achieving the performance. However, the interpretation of these two classifiers differ in their focus, with PART being more appropriate for finding rules in frequent patterns and RIPPER for more rare ones as it starts from the minority class label.

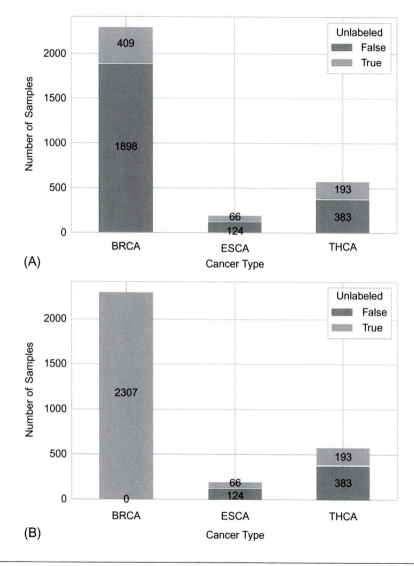

**FIG. 8**

Distribution of (A) original unlabeled samples and (B) unlabeled samples (once all labels from breast cancer are neglected) across types of cancer in the dataset. *BRCA*, breast cancer; *ESCA*, esophageal cancer; *THCA*, thyroid cancer.

# 5 **Conclusions**

In this chapter, we illustrate the application of the interpretable semisupervised classifier SLGB in the prediction of the stage of cancer patients. In a first experiment, the performance of the base classifiers conforming the self-labeling gray box indicated that joining the clinical and proteomic data from cancer patients improves the generalization ability. Later, we empirically demonstrate that the self-

**Table 6** Classification performance and interpretability of the SLGB classifier on the cancer stage classification of thyroid and esophagus cancers, using unlabeled data from breast cancer.

|  | ACC | KAPPA | SEN | SPE | AUC | Rules |
|---|---|---|---|---|---|---|
| SLGB (RF-C4.5) | 0.57 | 0.43 | 0.57 | 0.89 | 0.73 | 80 |
| SLGB (RF-PART) | **0.57** | **0.43** | **0.57** | **0.90** | **0.73** | 47 |
| SLGB (RF-RIPPER) | **0.56** | **0.41** | **0.56** | **0.89** | **0.72** | 13 |
| RF | 0.61 | 0.48 | 0.61 | 0.90 | 0.87 | – |
| C4.5 | 0.52 | 0.37 | 0.52 | 0.90 | 0.66 | 74 |
| PART | 0.48 | 0.31 | 0.48 | 0.88 | 0.67 | 51 |
| RIPPER | 0.52 | 0.32 | 0.52 | 0.83 | 0.65 | 12 |

*The performance results of base classifiers are shown as a baseline. The best results are highlighted in bold.*

labeling gray box is accurate in predicting the stage of cancer by leveraging the unlabeled data already present in the dataset. We extend this experiment in simulating that all data coming from breast cancer is unlabeled, and to study how much the SLGB is able to improve its prediction on less frequent cancers such as thyroid and esophagus. In this setting, the SLGB outperformed its white box baseline classifiers while keeping the transparency (in terms of number of rules) very similar. Using random forests as a black box component and tree different alternatives as white boxes involving decision trees and rule lists allows obtaining interpretable classifiers for different scenarios. We show the form of representation of the patterns extracted by the three different white box techniques, which detect several protein expressions features which are known to play an important role in the progression of cancer. These known associations support the rules learned by the SLGB, providing potential relations that could be further analyzed clinically. In this regard, future research will explore further the validation of the patterns detected by the interpretable models by contrasting the discovered knowledge with experts' criteria and complement it with other traditional analysis techniques. The current results pave the way for using SLGB as a tool for aiding clinicians in detecting important proteomic and clinical features that contribute to the development of advances stages in cancer.

## Acknowledgments

This work was supported by the Flemish Government (AI Research Program); the IMAGica project, financed by the Interdisciplinary Research Programs and Platforms (IRP) funds of the Vrije Universiteit Brussel; and the BRIGHT analysis project, funded by the European Regional Development Fund (ERDF) and the Brussels-Capital Region as part of the 2014–20 operational program through the F11-08 project ICITY-RDI.BRU (icity.brussels).

## References

Altman, N.S., 1992. An introduction to kernel and nearest-neighbor nonparametric regression. Am. Stat. 46, 175–185. https://doi.org/10.1080/00031305.1992.10475879.

Barredo Arrieta, A., Díaz-Rodríguez, N., Del Ser, J., Bennetot, A., Tabik, S., Barbado, A., Garcia, S., Gil-Lopez, S., Molina, D., Benjamins, R., Chatila, R., Herrera, F., 2020. Explainable artificial intelligence (XAI): concepts, taxonomies, opportunities and challenges toward responsible AI. Inf. Fusion 58, 82–115. https://doi.org/10.1016/j.inffus.2019.12.012.

Bauer, C., Brass, N., Diesinger, I., Kayser, K., Grässer, F.A., Meese, E., 2002. Overexpression of the eukaryotic translation initiation factor 4G (eIF4G-1) in squamous cell lung carcinoma. Int. J. Cancer 98, 181–185. https://doi.org/10.1002/ijc.10180.

Bensaad, K., Tsuruta, A., Selak, M.A., Vidal, M.N.C., Nakano, K., Bartrons, R., Gottlieb, E., Vousden, K.H., 2006. TIGAR, a p53-inducible regulator of glycolysis and apoptosis. Cell 126, 107–120. https://doi.org/10.1016/j.cell.2006.05.036.

Blum, A., Chawla, S., 2001. Learning From Labeled and Unlabeled Data Using Graph Mincuts., https://doi.org/10.1184/R1/6606860.V1.

Bray, F., Ferlay, J., Soerjomataram, I., Siegel, R.L., Torre, L.A., Jemal, A., 2018. Global cancer statistics 2018: GLOBOCAN estimates of incidence and mortality worldwide for 36 cancers in 185 countries. CA Cancer J. Clin. https://doi.org/10.3322/caac.21492.

Breiman, L., 1996. Bagging predictors. Mach. Learn. 24, 123–140. https://doi.org/10.1007/BF00058655.

Breiman, L., 2001. Random forests. Mach. Learn. 45, 5–32. https://doi.org/10.1023/A:1010933404324.

Buckley, D., Duke, G., Heuer, T.S., O'Farrell, M., Wagman, A.S., McCulloch, W., Kemble, G., 2017. Fatty acid synthase – modern tumor cell biology insights into a classical oncology target. Pharmacol. Ther. https://doi.org/10.1016/j.pharmthera.2017.02.021.

Cohen, J., 1960. A coefficient of agreement for nominal scales. Educ. Psychol. Meas. 20, 37–46. https://doi.org/10.1177/001316446002000104.

Cohen, W.W., 1995. Fast effective rule induction. In: Prieditis, A., Russell, S. (Eds.), Machine Learning Proceedings 1995. Elsevier, San Francisco, CA, pp. 115–123, https://doi.org/10.1016/b978-1-55860-377-6.50023-2.

Cosma, G., Acampora, G., Brown, D., Rees, R.C., Khan, M., Pockley, A.G., 2016. Prediction of pathological stage in patients with prostate cancer: a neuro-fuzzy model. PLoS One 11. https://doi.org/10.1371/journal.pone.0155856.

Cruz, J.A., Wishart, D.S., 2006. Applications of machine learning in cancer prediction and prognosis. Cancer Inform. 2. https://doi.org/10.1177/117693510600200030. 117693510600200.

Doshi-Velez, F., Kim, B., 2017. Towards a Rigorous Science of Interpretable Machine Learning. arXiv:1702.08608, pp. 1–13.

Fernández-Delgado, M., Cernadas, E., Barro, S.S., Amorim, D., Fernandez-Delgado, M., Cernadas, E., Barro, S.S., Amorim, D., 2014. Do we need hundreds of classifiers to solve real world classification problems. J. Mach. Learn. Res. 15, 3133–3181.

Frank, E., Hall, M., 2001. A simple approach to ordinal classification. In: Lecture Notes in Computer Science (Including Subseries Lecture Notes in Artificial Intelligence and Lecture Notes in Bioinformatics). Springer Verlag, pp. 145–156, https://doi.org/10.1007/3-540-44795-4_13.

Frank, E., Witten, I.H., 1998. Generating accurate rule sets without global optimization. In: Proceedings of the Fifteenth International Conference on Machine Learning, ICML '98. University of Waikato, Department of Computer Science, San Francisco, CA, USA, ISBN: 1-55860-556-8, pp. 144–151.

Friedman, J.H., 2001. Greedy function approximation: a gradient boosting machine. Ann. Stat. 1, 1189–1232. https://doi.org/10.2307/2699986.

Fukuchi-Shimogori, T., Ishii, I., Kashiwagi, K., Mashiba, H., Ekimoto, H., Igarashi, K., 1997. Malignant transformation by overproduction of translation initiation factor eIF4G. Cancer Res. 57.

Goldberg, X., Zhu, X., Goldberg, A., 2009. Introduction to semi-supervised learning. In: Synthesis Lectures on Artificial Intelligence and Machine Learning. Morgan & Claypool Publishers, https://doi.org/10.2200/S00196ED1V01Y200906AIM006.

Grau, I., Sengupta, D., Garcia Lorenzo, M.M., Nowé, A., 2018. Interpretable self-labeling semi-supervised classifier. In: IJCAI/ECAI 2018 Workshop on Explainable Artificial Intelligence (XAI).

Grau, I., Sengupta, D., Garcia Lorenzo, M.M., Nowé, A., 2020a. An interpretable semi-supervised classifier using rough sets for amended self-labeling. In: IEEE International Conference on Fuzzy Systems (FUZZ-IEEE). IEEE.

Grau, I., Sengupta, D., Garcia Lorenzo, M.M., Nowé, A., 2020b. An Interpretable Semi-Supervised Classifier Using Two Different Strategies for Amended Self-Labeling. arXiv Prepr. arXiv2001.09502.

Green, D.R., Chipuk, J.E., 2006. p53 and metabolism: inside the TIGAR. Cell. https://doi.org/10.1016/j.cell.2006.06.032.

Gress, D.M., Edge, S.B., Greene, F.L., Washington, M.K., Asare, E.A., Brierley, J.D., Byrd, D.R., Compton, C.C., Jessup, J.M., Winchester, D.P., Amin, M.B., Gershenwald, J.E., 2017. Principles of Cancer Staging., https://doi.org/10.1007/978-3-319-40618-3_1.

Hall, M., Frank, E., Holmes, G., Pfahringer, B., Reutemann, P., Witten, I.H., 2009. The WEKA data mining software: an update. ACM SIGKDD Explor. Newsl. 11, 10–18.

Hastie, T., Tibshirani, R., Friedman, J., 2008. The Elements of Statistical Learning., https://doi.org/10.1007/978-0-387-84858-7.

Hausman, D.M., 2019. What is cancer? Perspect. Biol. Med. 62, 778–784. https://doi.org/10.1353/pbm.2019.0046.

Joachims, T., 1999. Transductive inference for text classification using support vector machines. In: Proceedings of the 16th International Conference on Machine Learning (ICML).

Kourou, K., Exarchos, T.P., Exarchos, K.P., Karamouzis, M.V., Fotiadis, D.I., 2015. Machine learning applications in cancer prognosis and prediction. Comput. Struct. Biotechnol. J. https://doi.org/10.1016/j.csbj.2014.11.005.

Li, J., Lu, Y., Akbani, R., Ju, Z., Roebuck, P.L., Liu, W., Yang, J.-Y., Broom, B.M., Verhaak, R.G.W., Kane, D.W., Wakefield, C., Weinstein, J.N., Mills, G.B., Liang, H., 2013. TCPA: a resource for cancer functional proteomics data. Nat. Methods. https://doi.org/10.1038/nmeth.2650.

Lim, Y.P., 2005. Mining the tumor phosphoproteome for cancer markers. Clin. Cancer Res. https://doi.org/10.1158/1078-0432.CCR-04-2243.

Lipton, Z.C., 2016. The mythos of model interpretability. In: 2016 ICML Workshop on Human Interpretability in Machine Another Such Divergence of Real-Life and Machine Learning (WHI 2016). Association for Computing Machinery, pp. 96–100.

Liu, J., Lichtenberg, T., Hoadley, K.A., et al., 2018. An integrated TCGA pan-cancer clinical data resource to drive high-quality survival outcome analytics. Cell. https://doi.org/10.1016/j.cell.2018.02.052.

Lundberg, S.M., Lee, S.-I., 2017. A unified approach to interpreting model predictions. In: Guyon, I., Luxburg, U.V., Bengio, S., Wallach, H., Fergus, R., Vishwanathan, S., Garnett, R. (Eds.), Advances in Neural Information Processing Systems 30. Curran Associates, Inc, pp. 4765–4774.

Nelles, O., 2001. Nonlinear System Identification. Springer, Berlin, Heidelberg, https://doi.org/10.1007/978-3-662-04323-3.

Pawlak, Z., 1982. Rough sets. Int. J. Comput. Inf. Sci. 11, 341–356. https://doi.org/10.1007/BF01001956.

Quinlan, J.R., 1993. C4.5: Programs for Machine Learning. Morgan Kaufmann Publishers, San Mateo, CA.

Ramírez-Moya, J., Santisteban, P., 2020. Commentary: The oncogenic role of ADAR1-mediated RNA editing in thyroid cancer. J. Cancer Biol. 1 (1), 16–19.

Ribeiro, M.T., Singh, S., Guestrin, C., 2016. Model-Agnostic Interpretability of Machine Learning.

Said, A.A., Abd-Elmegid, L.A., Kholeif, S., Gaber, A.A., 2018. Stage-specific predictive models for main prognosis measures of breast cancer. Future Comput. Inform. J. 3, 391–397. https://doi.org/10.1016/j.fcij.2018.11.002.

Shapley, L.S., 1953. A value for n-person games. In: Kuhn, H.W. (Ed.), Contributions to the Theory Games. vol. 2. Princeton University Press, Princeton, NJ, pp. 307–317.

Taniguchi, K., Ota, M., Yamada, T., Serizawa, A., Noguchi, T., Amano, K., Kotake, S., Ito, S., Ikari, N., Omori, A., Yamamoto, M., 2019. Staging of gastric cancer with the Clinical Stage Prediction score. World J. Surg. Oncol. 17, 47. https://doi.org/10.1186/s12957-019-1589-5.

Triguero, I., García, S., Herrera, F., 2015. Self-labeled techniques for semi-supervised learning: taxonomy, software and empirical study. Knowl. Inf. Syst. 42, 245–284. https://doi.org/10.1007/s10115-013-0706-y.

Van Engelen, J.E., Hoos, H.H., 2020. A survey on semi-supervised learning. Mach. Learn. 109, 373–440. https://doi.org/10.1007/s10994-019-05855-6.

Wainberg, M., Frey, B.J., 2016. Are random forests truly the best classifiers? J. Mach. Learn. Res. 17 (110), 1–5.

Weinstein, J.N., Collisson, E.A., Mills, G.B., et al., 2013. The cancer genome atlas pan-cancer analysis project. Nat. Genet. https://doi.org/10.1038/ng.2764.

Macmillan Cancer Support, 2020. Rare cancers. Cancer information and support [WWW Document]. URL https://www.macmillan.org.uk/cancer-information-and-support/rare-cancers. (accessed 3.12.2020).

Cancer Research UK, 2020. What is a rare cancer? Rare cancers [WWW document]. URL https://www.cancerresearchuk.org/about-cancer/rare-cancers/what-rare-cancers-are. (accessed 3.12.2020).

WHO, 2020. Cancer. Fact Sheets [WWW Document]. URL https://www.who.int/news-room/fact-sheets/detail/cancer. (accessed 3.12.2020).

Won, K.Y., Lim, S.J., Kim, G.Y., Kim, Y.W., Han, S.A., Song, J.Y., Lee, D.K., 2012. Regulatory role of p53 in cancer metabolism via $SCO_2$ and TIGAR in human breast cancer. Hum. Pathol. 43, 221–228. https://doi.org/10.1016/j.humpath.2011.04.021.

Xu, X., Wang, Y., Liang, H., 2018. The role of A-to-I RNA editing in cancer development. Curr. Opin. Genet. Dev. https://doi.org/10.1016/j.gde.2017.10.009.

Zhang, P.W., Chen, L., Huang, T., Zhang, N., Kong, X.Y., Cai, Y.D., 2015. Classifying ten types of major cancers based on reverse phase protein array profiles. PLoS One 10. https://doi.org/10.1371/journal.pone.0123147.

Zhang, C., Liu, C., Zhang, X., Almpanidis, G., 2017. An up-to-date comparison of state-of-the-art classification algorithms. Expert Syst. Appl. 82, 128–150.

Zhu, W., Xie, L., Han, J., Guo, X., 2020. The application of deep learning in cancer prognosis prediction. Cancers (Basel). https://doi.org/10.3390/cancers12030603.

# Applications of blockchain technology in smart healthcare: An overview

# 15

**Muhammad Hassan Nawaz[a] and Muhammad Taimoor Khan[b]**

*Electrical Engineering Department, University of Debrecen, Debrecen, Hungary[a] Medical Department, University of Debrecen, Debrecen, Hungary[b]*

## Chapter outline

## 1 Introduction

Blockchain technology now offers excellent potential in the connected world such as information and communication technologies, and it is still expanding in various aspects. After the emergence of cryptocurrencies, blockchain technology gains massive popularity over recent years. Cryptocurrencies are the digital assets or currencies that can be used to exchange within different currencies on a digital platform (Wikipedia, 2020). Traditionally, there used to be third parties such as banks and companies which work as a mediator for exchanging currencies among participants. Due to the centralized nature of the traditional system, it had many security and financial challenges. These challenges led to the implementation of cryptocurrencies. It is found that there are more than 1500 currencies (CoinMarketCap, 2020). Bitcoin was among the first, which was controlled by a decentralized system constituting the first generation of blockchain technology known as blockchain 1.0 (Kuhn and Sommers, 1981).

Blockchain 2.0 is the second generation that was first introduced to implement the smart contract concepts and properties. Smart properties refer to the digital resources or assets. The proprietorship of these assets is controlled via a digital platform enabled by blockchain technology. However, the smart-contracts refer to software programs used to set policies regarding the management of smart properties. Some of the common examples of blockchain 2.0 in cryptocurrencies are Ethereum (Home, ethereum.org, 2020), NEO (Neo-project, 2020), and QTUM (Home—Qtum, 2020), etc.

Blockchain 3.0 is the third generation which is still under development. Presently, it is mainly focused on nonfinancial applications of various connected technologies. In the modern world, Internet of Things (IoT) has impacted our lives with many changes (Kumar and Mallick, 2018). IoT, a connected network of smart devices, allows them to generate massive data and exchange information (Al-Turjman et al., 2020). With the advent of such technologies and sharing data, there are still many challenges that are hindering its continued growth, such as security issues precisely. To tackle such challenges, blockchain technology shows excellent potential by offering a decentralized-based security system to protect data from outside forces.

Ranging from the financial applications to connected objects, blockchain technology also offers great potential in healthcare industry (Pradeep, n.d.). However, it is still a new player in the domain of healthcare. Therefore, experts need to figure out what the specific scopes are and use case scenarios in healthcare enabled by blockchain. What are the applications that have been already developed in healthcare industry based on blockchain technology (Zafar and Rajnish, 2012)? What are the challenges that are hindering its continued growth and how it can be improved?

## 1.1 Comparison to other surveys

We provided a comprehensive survey of blockchain trends to address the questions mentioned above. Also, this chapter enlightened the current and new trends in healthcare. In literature, there are some review articles regarding blockchain technology in the context of healthcare applications. A review article on blockchain-based healthcare applications was discussed in Angraal et al. (2017). Implementation of blockchain was analyzed on very few and specified healthcare applications. However, this article failed to cover other sectors of healthcare applications such as healthcare management, clinical research, and Genomics. Similarly, Engelhardt (2017) reported the existing companies which are working on healthcare applications using blockchain services. This paper also proposed other healthcare areas when blockchain technology can be implemented efficiently. Mettler (2016) also reviewed similar blockchain trends by reporting different companies which are currently working in management sectors of public health, drug counterfeiting, and pharmaceutical research in medical sector. Kuo et al. (2017) proposed the essential benefits achieved by blockchain technology in data management and discussed how these benefits could leverage healthcare industry by improving record management, clinical research, and enhancing insurance process. Again, this paper failed to discuss the other aspects of healthcare, such as genomics and neuroscience. Clauson et al. (2018) reviewed blockchain technology in the context of supply chain and pharmaceuticals in healthcare industry. However, other areas of healthcare industry were not discussed in this study and also the potential challenges of blockchain-based healthcare systems are missing. Similarly, Zhang and Ji (2018) presented reviews which are only limited to EHRs and their potential challenges.

This book chapter has overviewed a broader picture of blockchain technology in healthcare industry, as shown in Table 1. We have provided a comprehensive survey and proposed a novel

**Table 1** Summary of related surveys.

| Ref. | Blockchain-based healthcare applications | | | | | | | |
|---|---|---|---|---|---|---|---|---|
| | Healthcare data management | Clinical research | Supply chain | Neuroscience and genomics | Healthcare insurance | Pharmaceuticals | Key requirements | Potential challenges |
| Angraal et al. (2017) | ✓ | – | ✓ | – | – | – | – | ✓ |
| Engelhardt (2017) | ✓ | – | – | – | – | – | – | ✓ |
| Mettler (2016) | ✓ | ✓ | – | – | – | ✓ | – | – |
| Kuo et al. (2017) | ✓ | ✓ | – | – | ✓ | – | ✓ | ✓ |
| Clauson et al. (2018) | – | – | ✓ | – | – | ✓ | – | – |
| Zhang and Ji (2018) | ✓ | – | – | – | – | – | – | ✓ |
| [Our study] | ✓ | ✓ | ✓ | ✓ | ✓ | ✓ | ✓ | ✓ |

blockchain-enabled healthcare monitoring model as shown in Fig. 2. Various examples of blockchain technology are presented within different areas of healthcare industry. Readers can also find the current trends and future challenges of blockchain-based healthcare systems proposed in our study. Essential requirements and potential challenges were not addressed by most of the above-mentioned surveys.

Following the rest, Section 2 defines the blockchain concept by classifying the digital systems into centralized and decentralized infrastructures. This section also presents the critical factors required for the development of efficient blockchain systems. Section 3 proposes a novel patient monitoring model which is securely enabled by blockchain technology. In Section 4, applications of blockchain systems are presented within different areas of healthcare industry. Section 5 overviews the future challenges of blockchain-based healthcare systems. Finally, Section 6 concludes the chapter.

## 2 Blockchain overview

Blockchain technology is a digital ecosystem which stores series of data that are time-stamped and unchangeable. Clusters of computers manage the record of data without the ownership of single entity or any third party (decentralized). Each set of record is interlinked to each other and is fully secured using the principles of cryptography. Don and Alex Tapscott, authors of *Blockchain Revolution* (2016), defines blockchain technology as a digital ledger which has an incorruptible ability to record everything of value such as financial transactions.

Fig. 1 explains how decentralized infrastructure differs from centralized infrastructure. In centralized infrastructure, all the devices or computers are interconnected, but at the same time, they are managed by a single authority which is an internet server in Fig. 1A. It means that these devices send a request to the internet server, which in return sends back the instructions or feedback for the operation. However, blockchain technology does not work like that because it is comprised of decentralized infrastructure which connects all the devices in a chain-like series, shown in Fig. 1B. Such a structure makes blockchain a unique technology. In centralized infrastructures, hackers can easily trace single authority server and leak data; however, in decentralized infrastructure (Blockchain technology), there is no single authority, hence making impossible to hack and leak the data.

### 2.1 Key requirements

To develop a successful and efficient blockchain-based system, some required critical factors must be addressed. This section presents the essential requirements of such systems as follows:

*Nationwide interoperability*: One of the most critical requirements for blockchain-based systems is its nationwide interoperability. Nationwide interoperability can prove quite challenging to achieve, as it requires a universal standard to achieve the interoperability which current connected systems do not have (Krawiec and White, 2016; Stagnaro, 2017).

*Data security*: Another critical requirement for blockchain-based systems is sensitive data security. The data can be seen by the multiple parties that are part of the system and blockchain is expected to deliver with the appropriate level of security (Puppala et al., 2016; Al Omar et al., 2017).

*Data consistency and integrity*: Inconsistency in data or loss of the integrity of data can halt the technical process of a system and may result in higher costs to repair the inconsistencies.

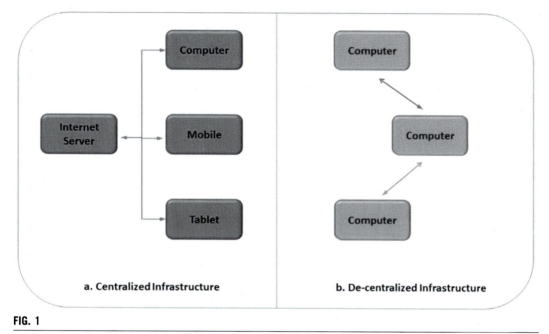

**FIG. 1**

Infrastructure of centralized and decentralized ecosystems.

A blockchain-based systems must ensure that there are no inconsistencies in the data and that it cannot be tampered with by external sources (Stagnaro, 2017; Al Omar et al., 2017).

*Cost effectiveness*: Cost effectiveness is also another critical requirement of blockchain-based systems, as current connected systems utilize resources such as intermediates that usually delay the process of particular tasks (Krawiec and White, 2016; Stagnaro, 2017). Use of blockchain may significantly reduce the costs associated that may be caused by other parties.

*Trustless and transparent*: Current connected systems are established by a mutual trust among stakeholders and concerned parties concerning safe data storage and sharing. The data stored can be seen by multiple parties, and maintaining that level of blind trust and transparency is a big obstacle (Nugent et al., 2016; Benchoufi et al., 2017; Xia et al., 2017). Block chain-based systems can build transparent and trustless data sharing and store in any scenario.

*Complexity*: A complex system can cause unnecessary delays and inconsistencies in terms of data storing, sharing and billing, which can get scattered around. This can be avoided by establishing a blockchain-based system which can prevent any further hindrances (Krawiec and White, 2016).

## 3 Proposed healthcare monitoring framework

Our model comprises scenarios in which medical staff remotely monitor the health of patients outside the hospital. In this case, wearable medical devices and sensors can be attached to the patient in which parameters such as body temperature, blood pressure, oxygen saturation, and heart rate can be measured and compared to preexisting ranges. External sensors can also be placed around the patient's residence, which can detect a change in the environment, such as movement or surrounding temperature. This live evaluation of data allows for the systems to detect abnormalities and alert the medical staff in case of emergency. All of this data are then accumulated and permanently stored in a remote database which can then be accessed in the future by healthcare professionals to evaluate the health status of the patient. Since these data are personal and sensitive to all the pertaining parties, it needs to be stored securely and should only be accessed by authorized parties. The use of blockchain technology-based systems can achieve this.

*Medical devices blockchain*: Each patient is fitted with a set of medical devices that will be monitored by our model. The data collected by the medical devices are then stored in the medical devices blockchain. The dataset for the proposed model can also be achieved from online sources as shown in Table 2. Each patient has his own Medical Devices BlockChain configured.

*Consultation BlockChain*: The Consultation BlockChain shown in the architecture contains records of the patient's history. The Consultation BlockChain is then set up across hospitals, and it includes the patient's records. This way, the medical reports become easily accessible and are exchangeable between hospitals and health workers in a confidential and secure manner. In our case, two separate BlockChains are chosen because each serves its purpose as shown in Fig. 2. Data received from sensors need to be maintained during the period of treatment. Patient records must always be accessible throughout the patient's life.

*Live monitoring device*: It is a system that manipulates data continuously and scans through various information. It is used to alert (when necessary) the healthcare professional on standby.

*Medical sensors*: Data received from the medical devices and sensors attached to the patient are stored in the BlockChain through NDN paradigm. This means that we have established a hierarchy between the medical devices to enable communication between them.

*Medical experts*: Any healthcare staff is represented by a node (e.g., computer/device) in both Medical Devices BlockChain and Consultation BlockChain. They can access the data through the Live Monitoring System based on the data stored in the Medical Devices BlockChain.

*Patient*: The patient is also represented as a node (e.g., computer/device) in the Medical Devices BlockChain. The patient collects data from the attached medical sensors and transfers them to the Medical Devices BlockChain to store it in a ledger. This allows both users (patient and healthcare staff) to interconnect with each other.

**Table 2 Datasets for proposed blockchain-enabled healthcare monitoring model.**

| Datasets | Subjects | Activity | Application | Year |
|---|---|---|---|---|
| HMD (Corbillon et al., 2017) | 59 | Head movement | Health support (monitoring paralyzed patients) | 2017 |
| USC CRCNS (Carmi and Itti, 2006) | 520 | Eye movement | Monitoring and detecting eye problems | 2004–05 |
| Harvard Dataverse (Khamis et al., 2016) | 288 | ECG recordings | Monitoring heartrate | 2016 |
| OhioT1DM (OhioT1DM Dataset, 2020) | 112 | Glucose level detection | Health monitoring of diabetes patients | 2020 |

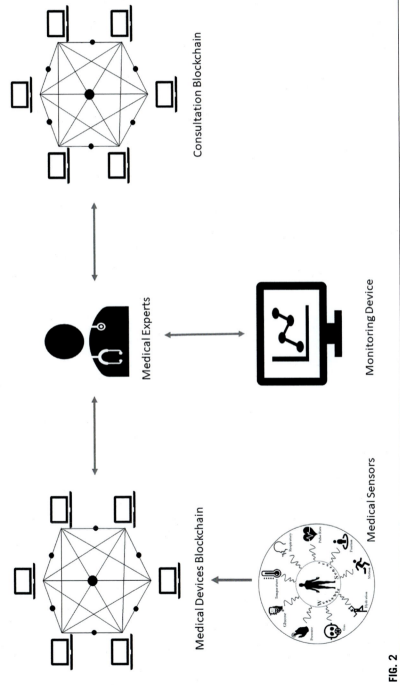

Consultation Blockchain

Medical Experts

Monitoring Device

Medical Devices Blockchain

Medical Sensors

**FIG. 2**

Blockchain-enabled healthcare monitoring framework.

## 4 Blockchain-enabled healthcare applications

Ranging from banking to supply chain logistics, it has also opened a new challenge in the healthcare industry (Fig. 3 and Table 3). Blockchain technology allows healthcare revolution to lead a digital transformation fast. There are various ways blockchain can change the healthcare industry:

*Pharmaceuticals*: One of the most rapidly expanding industries in the medical and healthcare sector is the pharmaceutical industry. It delivers new and approved drugs to the consumer markets while also maintaining supplies globally. Tracking drugs is the biggest challenge this industry is facing currently, ending up with fraudulent drugs. Screening for fraudulent drugs can be

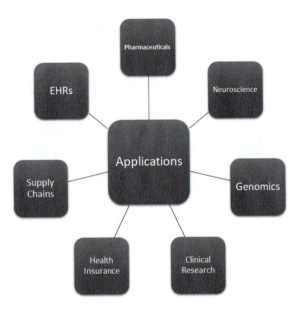

**FIG. 3**

Applications of blockchain technology in healthcare industry.

| Table 3 Examples of blockchain-enabled healthcare applications. | |
|---|---|
| **Healthcare areas** | **Examples** |
| Pharmaceuticals | Hyperledger (SecuringIndustry, 2016) |
| Electronic health records | Healthbank (HealthBank.coop, 2020), MeDShare (MedShare, 2020), MedRec (MedRec-m, 2020) |
| Neuroscience | Neurogress (Neurogress, 2020) |
| Genomics | Illumina HiSeq X Ten (Illumina, 2020) |
| Clinical research | Ethereum (Home, ethereum.org, 2020) |
| Health insurance | MIStore (Zhou et al., 2018) |

time-consuming and also potentially be hazardous toward the health of the consumer, as they are not approved; 10% of the drugs sold worldwide are counterfeits of which 30% arise from developing countries, according to the World Health Organisation (WHO, 2020). The use of blockchain technology in tracking pharmaceuticals from producer to consumer can prove the authenticity of a drug and prevent consumers from a mass-produced medication that can lead to severe consequences. Hyperledger, which is a new project, uses blockchain technology to enhance the security of pharmaceuticals from supplier to consumer (SecuringIndustry, 2016). It records timestamps such as date of production and also tracks the supplies. Another method which prevents the use of counterfeit drugs is by the use of Digital Drug Control Systems, which is also blockchain based and monitors all stages of production and supply (Plotnikov and Kuznetsova, 2018).

*Neuroscience*: The brain contains around 120 billion neurons that all interconnect and form different pathways that emit different signals. The brains neural activity can be mapped by complex sensors which can attach to regions of the head and calculate the electric impulses using complicated algorithms. All these data are stored in interfaces which can enable the user to control other pieces of technology such as drones, robotic limbs, and other neural-interactive technology through the use of blockchain systems. One example of neural blockchain technology is Neurogress (Neurogress, 2020), which uses impulses received from the brain and has a computer interface with Artificial Intelligence that assesses the information and can also learn from it and adapt to carrying out further actions. However, since it would require a massive amount of physical memory in a computer to store all the impulses from a brain, it will be almost impossible to carry out these functions. This is where the blockchain system steps in. It can form a decentralized system that can establish trust between other networks on the system which contain multiple different information over a broad user base which can also be easily accessed by the neural-interface, thus allowing full functionality. Of course, as technology improves as time goes on, different regions of the brain can be mapped, allowing for storage of a plethora of brain functions such as smell, taste, emotions, and memory. This can open up more doors to how humans can interact with artificial intelligence and be the next step in medical advancements and research.

*Genomics*: There are about 20,000–25,000 estimated human protein-coding genes which are responsible for producing multiple variations of proteins (Erdmann and Barciszewski, 2010). This is an immense amount of data which becomes very huge load upon current computer databases. These variations are then stored on a central server which poses as a problem to users who want access to the data and also becomes a privacy issue as the server becomes a single failure unit. Illumina HiSeq X Ten, a genome storing platform, has reported being able to store the sequence of the genomes of estimated 18,000 humans per year (Illumina, 2020). This corresponds to approximately 2 petabytes of data per year. To store these amounts of data, a massive infrastructure will be required to be able to handle all these data. These problems can be fixed with the implementation of blockchain technology, as they are decentralized and can be accessed by the data users and owners.

*Healthbank*: An innovation by a Swiss Digital Health startup company (HealthBank.coop, 2020) is another blockchain system that gives the patient control over their health records. With Healthbank, patients can keep a record of their history of medications, blood pressure, heart rate, sleeping patterns, etc., by integrating with other applications and wearables. This detailed information can give physicians and researchers alike a more detailed insight into patient history. Another feature of

Healthbank is that patients can provide their medical records to researchers in which they can receive payment for the information provided. This approach makes Healthbank a trading platform in which researchers can obtain detailed patient information in exchange for financial benefits. *Clinical research*: Privacy, data logging and data entry and its integrity are vital aspects to clinical research and trials. However, their opacity and misuse of the consent of trial become an issue to the patients and other stakeholders alike, as they are not informed about the full extent of the trial and the data collected. Consent between patients, researchers and stakeholders is a dynamic process and all these entities in-between need to interface with one another in a more transparent form to give more precise results in a trial. Forming a decentralized data storing and sharing is the best way to establish this, or in this case, by adopting a blockchain system. This way, all information about the trials can be seen by all the participants in a more manageable and secure fashion. An example in such a blockchain system is Ethereum (Home, ethereum.org, 2020). This system is maintained by research organizations, regulators, pharmaceutical companies that would like to test their drug, and other management systems. This forms a type of interactive datastore that can be accessed by all parties, and the trials can be monitored.

*Electronic health records (EHR)*: In this generation, digitizing data and records and storing them have been implemented in daily life as a means for more straightforward accessibility in the future. EHR is the most widely used example of blockchain technology in healthcare applications. Medical records can be in multiple institutions, and future medical references need to check on patient history, but this leaves the information dispersed in different institutions. A patients EHR contains sensitive information which is accessed by specialists, and all of this transmission of information can be scattered. This can be hazardous to the patient and impede the quality of treatment if the information is not maintained and up to date. To prevent this, blockchain technology can be acquired to maintain and manage patient records in an encrypted manner that cannot be tampered with. This can allow for a more precise diagnosis. An example of blockchain technology is MeDShare (MedShare, 2020), which shares medical records among hospitals and researchers with utmost privacy and security, maintaining the integrity of the records. Another blockchain system is a prototype called MedRec (MedRec-m, 2020), which mainly allows the patient to take control over which institutions can view their highly sensitive medial data in an easy-to-understand manner. Each medical record contains a mark in the blockchain system which guarantees authenticity. The patient can then share the respective duplicated medical data containing the mark.

*Supply chains*: Nowadays, a lot of medical companies are facing common security problems in their supply chains which are also affecting our healthcare industry negatively in terms of both business and patient care. The most affected sector in the medical industry facing such problems is pharma industries because of the kind of product they carry. Various drugs are being stolen from such companies and are being sold to consumers illegally. Blockchain technology can help pharma industries by offering close tracking of drugs in their supply chain and by eliminating falsified or fake medications. Many organizations in the world are carrying out various clinical trials and research activities to produce or check new drugs and medications. Blockchain technology can develop a single universal database gathering all the information and the data and make them available at one platform.

*Health insurance*: One of the significant problems in the healthcare industry is insurance fraud. It happens when corrupt individuals claim their payable benefits based on their fake information provided. One can imagine how serious is this problem from statistics by Boyd Insurance reporting that Medicare fraud costs about 68 billion dollars each year in the United States. This cost can be minimized significantly if Blockchain technology is utilized in the infrastructure. It helps to force individuals and providers to enter personal information to be verified first, and then the data will be stored and made accessible to the health insurance companies (Blockgeeks, 2018). In this way, the data will be recorded and managed in decentralized infrastructure, making it impossible for hackers to leak information and make fake data. One of the examples found is MIStore (Zhou et al., 2018), which is also a blockchain-based system used for medical insurance storage.

## 5 Potential challenges

This section overviews the potential challenges that are hindering the continued growth of blockchain-based healthcare systems. These challenges are discussed as follows:

*Scalability*: The most potential obstacle in blockchain healthcare is scalability. Limitations of the healthcare systems scalability are between the accessible evaluation abilities and the number of medical transactions (Xia et al., 2017).

*High costs*: Blockchain-based healthcare applications increase development and operational costs. The healthcare sector needs to assess the total cost, which includes the development, operational, and deployment costs, to present to the stakeholders involved. Optimizing these costs can substantially reduce the overall cost (Krawiec and White, 2016; Stagnaro, 2017).

*Standardization*: For a healthcare application to be successful, standardized protocols must be established (Azaria et al., 2016; Yang and Yang, 2017). This means that for data stored in a blockchain in the case of healthcare, the parameters of the information must be established such as what features, dimensions, and configuration can be sent toward the blockchain (Krawiec and White, 2016; Stagnaro, 2017; Linn and Koo, 2016)

*Cultural resistance*: The current generation is more adapted to the use of paper-based medical records or, in some rare instances, introduced to some type of online health service (Yang and Yang, 2017; Stagnaro, 2017). Establishing a cultural change toward the use of blockchain-based healthcare applications may take some time to adjust and alter the understanding of other parties interchanging patient's data.

*Regulatory uncertainty*: Creating a well-developed ecosystem between stakeholders and the current existing framework would be challenging for regulators to establish policies that would consider all the current regulations and the new regulations. Currently, the standards are already being put into place to preserve the nature of the user's medical records by the HIPAA (Health Insurance Portability and Accountability Act) (Edemekong et al., 2020).

*Security and seclusion concerns*: Security is one of the biggest concerns in blockchain technology-based healthcare applications even though they do contain security features (Azaria et al., 2016; Yli-Huumo et al., 2016). However, proper security measures need to be implemented to protect sensitive information that can only be accessed by an authorized person (Puppala et al., 2016; Al Omar et al., 2017; Linn and Koo, 2016).

*Unwillingness to share*: Stakeholders or other concerned parties, such as insurance companies, may not be inclined to share data with other parties (Beck, 2018; Mettler, 2016; Esposito et al., 2018).

This may be due to the difference in service costs provided and the actual costs of the parties concerned. A sense of trust between parties must be established to have a smooth functioning healthcare system.

## 6 Concluding remarks

We have overviewed the interdisciplinary aspects of blockchain technology while discussing its evolution that started from financing applications such as cryptocurrencies. Later, blockchain technology got a colossal intention and popularity in the digital world. Being a decentralized nature, blockchain technology offers significant benefits such as security, privacy, data provenance, robustness, and optimized data management solutions.

As our healthcare systems are lacking in terms of security and privacy, blockchain technology can do a chief role by allowing its decentralized abilities to ensure full security and integrity for healthcare systems. Due to its peer-to-peer ability, blockchain can replace third-party service providers by enabling patients and medical workers to interact with each other in a more confidential and secure manner. Besides, the integration of machine learning/artificial technology along with IoT devices can also enhance the potentials of blockchain technology in healthcare applications. The whole idea in this work is to pinpoint these benefits and propose how these potentials could improve our healthcare industry.

Different blockchain-based healthcare applications are presented in this book chapter such as EHRs, clinical research, neuroscience, genomics, and health insurance claims. However, this technology is still a new player in healthcare industry. Therefore, there are some technical challenges that are hindering its continued growth. Finally, this book chapter has presented its potential challenges that must be considered very carefully during application designing and implementation.

## Declaration of competing interest

There are no competing interests or personal relationships to be declared by authors.

## References

Al Omar, A., Rahman, M.S., Basu, A., Kiyomoto, S., 2017. Medibchain: a blockchain based privacy preserving platform for healthcare data. In: International Conference on Security, Privacy and Anonymity in Computation, Communication and Storage, pp. 534–543.

Al-Turjman, F., Nawaz, M.H., Ulusar, U.D., 2020. Intelligence in the Internet of Medical Things era: A systematic review of current and future trends. Comput. Commun. 150, 644–660. https://doi.org/10.1016/j.comcom.2019.12.030.

Angraal, S., Krumholz, H.M., Schulz, W.L., 2017. Blockchain technology. Circ. Cardiovasc. Qual. Outcomes 10 (9), e003800. https://doi.org/10.1161/CIRCOUTCOMES.117.003800.

Azaria, A., Ekblaw, A., Vieira, T., Lippman, A., 2016. Medrec: Using blockchain for medical data access and permission management. In: 2016 2nd International Conference on Open and Big Data (OBD), pp. 25–30.

Beck, R., 2018. Beyond bitcoin: the rise of blockchain world. Computer 51 (2), 54–58.

Benchoufi, M., Porcher, R., Ravaud, P., 2017. Blockchain protocols in clinical trials: transparency and traceability of consent. F1000Research 6.

Blockgeeks, December 10, 2018. Blockchain in Healthcare: The Ultimate Use Case? https://blockgeeks.com/guides/blockchain-in-healthcare/. (Accessed 08 November 2019).

Carmi, R., Itti, L., 2006. The role of memory in guiding attention during natural vision. J. Vision 6 (9), 4.

Clauson, K.A., Breeden, E.A., Davidson, C., Mackey, T.K., 2018. Leveraging blockchain technology to enhance supply chain management in healthcare: an exploration of challenges and opportunities in the health supply chain. Blockchain Healthc. Today 1 (3), 1–12.

CoinMarketCap, 2020. Cryptocurrency Market Capitalizations. https://coinmarketcap.com/. (Accessed 29 June 2020).

Corbillon, X., De Simone, F., Simon, G., 2017. 360-degree video head movement dataset. In: Proceedings of the 8th ACM on Multimedia Systems Conference, pp. 199–204.

Edemekong, P., Annamaraju, P., Haydel, M., 2020. Health Insurance Portability and Accountability Act (HIPAA). StatPearls.

Engelhardt, M., 2017. Hitching healthcare to the chain: an introduction to blockchain technology in the healthcare sector. Technol. Innov. Manag. Rev. 7 (10), 22–34. https://doi.org/10.22215/timreview/1111.

Erdmann, V.A., Barciszewski, J., 2010. RNA Technologies and Their Applications. Springer Science & Business Media.

Esposito, C., De Santis, A., Tortora, G., Chang, H., Choo, K.-K.R., 2018. Blockchain: a panacea for healthcare cloud-based data security and privacy? IEEE Cloud Comput. 5 (1), 31–37.

HealthBank.coop, 2020. https://www.healthbank.coop/. (Accessed 30 June 2020).

Home, ethereum.org, 2020. https://ethereum.org. (Accessed 29 June 2020).

Home—Qtum, 2020. https://qtum.org/en. (Accessed 29 June 2020).

Illumina, 2020. HiSeq X Series | Ultra-High-Throughput 1000 Dollar Genome Sequencing. https://www.illumina.com/systems/sequencing-platforms/hiseq-x.html. (Accessed 30 June 2020).

Khamis, H., Weiss, R., Xie, Y., Chang, C.-W., Lovell, N.H., Redmond, S.J., September 06, 2016. TELE ECG Database: 250 Telehealth ECG Records (Collected Using Dry Metal Electrodes) With Annotated QRS and Artifact Masks, and MATLAB Code for the UNSW Artifact Detection and UNSW QRS Detection Algorithms. Harvard Dataverse, https://doi.org/10.7910/DVN/QTG0EP.

Krawiec, R.J., White, M., 2016. Blockchain: Opportunities for Health Care. deLoitte.

Kuhn, M., Sommers, T., 1981. Blueprint for a new age. Geriatr. Nurs. 2 (3), 214–217. https://doi.org/10.1016/S0197-4572(81)80089-4.

Kumar, N.M., Mallick, P.K., 2018. The Internet of Things: Insights into the building blocks, component interactions, and architecture layers. Procedia Comput. Sci. 132, 109–117.

Kuo, T.-T., Kim, H.-E., Ohno-Machado, L., 2017. Blockchain distributed ledger technologies for biomedical and health care applications. J. Am. Med. Inform. Assoc. 24 (6), 1211–1220. https://doi.org/10.1093/jamia/ocx068.

Linn, L.A., Koo, M.B., 2016. Blockchain for health data and its potential use in health it and health care related research. In: ONC/NIST Use of Blockchain for Healthcare and Research Workshop. ONC/NIST, Gaithersburg, MD, United States, pp. 1–10.

MedRec-m, 2020. You Personal Electronic Health Record. https://medrec-m.com/. (Accessed 30 June 2020).

MedShare, 2020. We Improve the Quality of Life of People and Our Planet. https://www.medshare.org/. (Accessed 30 June 2020).

Mettler, M., 2016. Blockchain technology in healthcare: the revolution starts here. In: 2016 IEEE 18th International Conference on e-Health Networking, Applications and Services (Healthcom), September, pp. 1–3, https://doi.org/10.1109/HealthCom.2016.7749510.

Neo-project, 2020. Neo Smart Economy. https://neo.org/. (Accessed 29 June 2020).

Neurogress, 2020. https://neurogress.site/. (Accessed 30 June 2020).

Nugent, T., Upton, D., Cimpoesu, M., 2016. Improving data transparency in clinical trials using blockchain smart contracts. F1000Research 5. https://doi.org/10.12688/f1000research.9756.1.

OhioT1DM Dataset, 2020. http://smarthealth.cs.ohio.edu/OhioT1DM-dataset.html. (Accessed 20 October 2020).

Plotnikov, V., Kuznetsova, V., 2018. The prospects for the use of digital technology 'blockchain' in the pharmaceutical market. In: MATEC Web of Conferences, vol. 193, p. 02029, https://doi.org/10.1051/matecconf/201819302029.

A. Pradeep, n.d. Deploying popular blockchain solutions in healthcare.

Puppala, M., He, T., Yu, X., Chen, S., Ogunti, R., Wong, S.T., 2016. Data security and privacy management in healthcare applications and clinical data warehouse environment. In: 2016 IEEE-EMBS International Conference on Biomedical and Health Informatics (BHI), pp. 5–8.

SecuringIndustry, April 27, 2016. Applying Blockchain Technology to Medicine Traceability. https://www.securingindustry.com/pharmaceuticals/applying-blockchain-technology-to-medicine-traceability/s40/a2766/. (Accessed 30 June 2020).

Stagnaro, C., 2017. White Paper: Innovative Blockchain Uses in Health Care. Freed Associates.

WHO, 2020. Growing threat from counterfeit medicines. WHO. https://www.who.int/bulletin/volumes/88/4/10-020410/en/. (Accessed 30 June 2020).

Wikipedia, June 20, 2020. Cryptocurrency. (Online). Available from: https://en.wikipedia.org/w/index.php?title=Cryptocurrency&oldid=963524592. (Accessed 29 June 2020).

Xia, Q.I., Sifah, E.B., Asamoah, K.O., Gao, J., Du, X., Guizani, M., 2017. MeDShare: trust-less medical data sharing among cloud service providers via blockchain. IEEE Access 5, 14757–14767.

Yang, H., Yang, B., 2017. A blockchain-based approach to the secure sharing of healthcare data. Nisk J., 100–111.

Yli-Huumo, J., Ko, D., Choi, S., Park, S., Smolander, K., 2016. Where is current research on blockchain technology?—a systematic review. PLoS One 11 (10), e0163477.

Zafar, F., Rajnish, R., 2012. Application of blockchain technology in securing healthcare records. CSI Commun.

Zhang, M., Ji, Y., 2018. Blockchain for healthcare records: a data perspective. PeerJ. https://doi.org/10.7287/peerj.preprints.26942v1. Preprints.

Zhou, L., Wang, L., Sun, Y., 2018. MIStore: a blockchain-based medical insurance storage system. J. Med. Syst. 42 (8), 149. https://doi.org/10.1007/s10916-018-0996-4.

# Prediction of leukemia by classification and clustering techniques

# 16

**Kartik Rawal[a], Advika Parthvi[a], Dilip Kumar Choubey[b], and Vaibhav Shukla[c]**

*School of Computer Science and Engineering, Vellore Institute of Technology, Vellore, Tamil Nadu, India[a] Department of Computer Science & Engineering, Indian Institute of Information Technology, Bhagalpur, India[b] Tech Mahindra Ltd., Mumbai, Maharastra, India[c]*

## Chapter outline

## 1 Introduction

Leukemia is a cancerous growth of abnormal white cells that destroys the blood and bone marrow. Leukemia is classified by the kind of white blood cells influenced and by how rapidly the illness advances. Lymphocytic leukemia (otherwise called lymphoid or lymphoblastic leukemia) is created in the white blood cells called lymphocytes in the bone marrow. Myeloid (otherwise called myelogenous) leukemia may likewise begin in white blood cells other than lymphocytes, or in red blood cells and platelets.

Based on how rapidly it advances or deteriorates, leukemia is called either acute (quickly developing) or chronic (slow-developing). Acute leukemia advances rapidly, causing the aggregation of juvenile, functionless cells in the bone marrow. With this sort of leukemia, cells recreate and develop in the marrow, diminishing the marrow's capacity to deliver enough normal blood cells. Chronic

Machine Learning, Big Data, and IoT for Medical Informatics. https://doi.org/10.1016/B978-0-12-821777-1.00003-3

leukemia advances more gradually and results in the aggregation of generally develop, yet at the same time anomalous, white blood cells.

In diagnostic and prediction software for leukemia, different algorithms, such as support vector machine (SVM), k-nearest neighbor (k-NN), k-means, and fuzzy c-means, are implemented on datasets related to leukemia to find those having the best accuracy and the least time complexity, in order to make diagnosis faster, easier, and more accurate. This chapter uses the Konstanz Information Miner (KNIME) platform and other relevant software to implement and compare various algorithms to find the best one. Our future work will deal with analysis of leukemia patients in and around a specific area. We will specify the area having the greatest number of leukemia patients, to assist in planning, since providing a plan for the diagnosis and treatment of cancers is a key component of any overall cancer control plan. Providing doctors, equipment, and appropriate medication where it is most required, instead of distributing these resources randomly, is an important factor.

The chapter objective is to achieve better prediction of leukemia, which is a serious disease that can be cured if treated in earlier stages. The analysis of blood samples is typically done manually to determine if there are any abnormalities in the sample that are indicative of disorders. It is very beneficial for patients to be diagnosed at earlier stages, so they have a possibility of being cured. The mortality rate in India can be reduced to a certain extent if people with leukemia are treated earlier, so their disease does not prove to be fatal. If an efficient technique can be developed for the prediction of leukemia, then it will be easier for physicians to diagnose it.

The rest of the chapter is arranged as follows: motivation is stated in Section 2, a literature review is elaborated in Section 3, a description of the proposed system is provided in Section 4, simulation results and a discussion are given in Section 5, and conclusions and future directions are discussed in Section 6.

## 2 Motivation

Leukemia is a type of cancer that affects the bone marrow and is considered to be fatal. In spite of advancements in science and technology, a microscopic examination of a blood smear still remains the standard and hence most economical method for leukemia diagnosis. The technique for manual examination relies upon pathologists, that is, their experience, mental status, individual issues, etc. Thus these components can all influence the results. Due to these factors, there needs to be a viable computerized framework for screening of leukemia that yields significantly improved results. Moreover, computerized systems, when contrasted with manual analysis, can increase the precision and the speed of diagnosis. This will assist specialists in treating the disease.

## 3 Literature review

The authors have carried out a rigorous analysis and study of many research articles based on leukemia with particular focus on classification and clustering algorithms.

Since clustering and classification techniques are now being used in every medical field to obtain better outcomes, this chapter therefore emphasizes these techniques. A group of researchers (Choubey and Paul, 2015; Choubey and Paul, 2016a, b; Choubey and Paul, 2017a, b; Choubey et al., 2017; Choubey et al., 2018; Choubey et al., 2019a, 2019b; Choubey et al., 2020a; Kumar et al., 2020a) have implemented many software computing and computational intelligence methods for the prediction of diabetes. Researchers have also compared and analyzed their proposed algorithms with several existing algorithms on real-world diabetes datasets. They have evaluated the performance of each algorithm and have also discussed the future directions. In this way, Sharma et al. (2020) have discussed computational intelligence techniques for the identification of breast cancer; Parthvi et al. (2020) have done a comparative analysis using machine learning and data-mining techniques for leukemia; Pahari and Choubey (2020) have done a comparative analysis using soft computing approaches for leukemia; Kumar et al. (2018b) and Kumar et al. (2020b) have used multichannel FLANN and cat swarm optimization-based FLANN to eliminate noise from ultrasound images; Srivastava and Choubey (2020), Kumar et al. (2019), and Srivastava and Choubey (2019) have used, analyzed, and compared machine-learning and data-mining techniques for the classification of heart disease, using soft computing; Bala et al. (2017) and Bala et al. (2018) have analyzed and compared soft computing, data mining, and machine-learning techniques for the prediction of thunderstorms and lightning.

Dash et al. (2012) provided a comparison between dimensional reduction techniques like the hybrid feature selection scheme and partial least squares method. In this analysis, the relative performance of four different supervised classification procedures, including radial basis function network (RBFN), was evaluated. The results presented in the paper showed that the appropriate feature selection method was a partial least squares regression method, and a combined use of different classification and feature selection approaches made it possible to construct high-performance classification models for microarray data.

Chandrasekar et al. (2013) have presented an effective classification method. After analyzing different classification algorithms, they choose six classifiers based on simulation performance and the results showed that the random tree classifier algorithm achieved an overall classification accuracy of 98%.

Priyanga and Prakasam (2013) proposed a system called a data mining-based cancer prediction system. The main aim of this model is to give earlier warnings to patients, and it is also of both time and cost benefit to the user. This model predicts specific cancer risk. The system was validated by comparing the patient's prior medical records with the predicted result given by the model, and also this system was analyzed using the WEKA tool. This prediction system is available online.

Suji and Rajagopalan (2013) used the oral datasets of many cancer and noncancer patients; the collected data was preprocessed for duplicate and missing data. Then various classification algorithms were applied on this preprocessed dataset. The performance of all the algorithms was then analyzed. The obtained result clearly showed that for the C4.5 algorithm, the classification rate reached almost 100%, while the classification rate of the random tree algorithm and MPNN was near 98.7% and 99.5%, respectively.

Sivaraman et al. (2014) proposed a blood cancer prediction system by using a statistical approach with a fuzzy inference system and a feed-forward back-propagation neural network. Their system was implemented on a huge set of test data, and was utilized to analyze the outcomes. The proposed blood cancer prediagnosis system offered significant accuracy, sensitivity, and specificity.

Shouval et al. (2015) proposed a machine-learning algorithm that is part of the data mining (DM) approach, which may serve for transplantation-related mortality risk prediction. In the case of acute lymphocytic leukemia (ALL), the alternate decision tree model provides a robust tool for risk evaluation of patients with this disease. This method has proved useful for clinical prediction in hematopoietic stem-cell transplantation.

Daqqa et al. (2017) presented a study that predicted the existence of leukemia by determining the relationship of blood properties and leukemia to gender, health status of patient, and the age factor, using data mining identified for blood cancer classification of k-nearest neighbor (k-NN), decision tree (DT), and support vector machine (SVM). The study was performed on a dataset of about 4000 patients and the results of the study showed that the decision tree algorithm had the highest percentage in comparision with the other two algorithms. Through this study, it is also clear that the DT classifier obtains properties regarding other attributes such as cities (eastern regions) that are most vulnerable to leukemia.

Kumar et al. (2018a), using python as a key tool and k-nearest neighbor (k-NN) and naïve Bayes classifiers, depicted acceptable performance for the classification of acute leukemia by acquiring microscopic test images.

Panda and Vihar (2016) have used bioinformatics datasets for understanding the effectiveness of a proposed classification, concluding the effectiveness of the proposed approach of combining DCNN by comparing it with an FRF classifier and with the other available research in the relevant domain; they highlight the future scope of the research in their conclusions.

Vasighizaker et al. (2019) used a one-class classification support vector machine (OCSVM) method to classify an acute myeloid leukemia (AML) cancer dataset. The researchers have claimed that, compared with the traditional methods, their proposed method's experimental results indicate superiority.

Warnat-Herresthal et al. (2020) proposes a data-driven high-dimensional approach in the prediction of leukemia. The approaches used in the study are highly scalable with low marginal cost, essentially matching human expert annotation in a near-automated workflow. The results of the study show that a machine-learning approach with transcriptomics can be used as a part of an integrated omics approach where, in the risk prediction of leukemia, different diagnoses are achieved by genomics, while on the other hand the diagnosis could be assisted by transcriptomic-based machine learning.

Table 1 provides a thorough analysis of different research articles. In the table we have presented the different techniques, datasets, tools used, advantages, issues, and accuracy for cancer diseases.

**Table 1** Summary of existing works concerning leukemia.

| Authors with year | Datasets | Techniques used | Tool used | Advantages | Issues | Accuracy |
|---|---|---|---|---|---|---|
| (Kumar et al., 2018a) | Acquired digital data: Microscopic test images | K-nearest neighbor (k-NN) and naïve Bayes classifier | Python | The outcomes show that the calculation proposed accomplishes a worthy exhibition for the analysis of intense lymphocytic leukemia | Absence of forecast model improvement rules, I clung to an exacting methodologic head | 80% |

**Table 1 Summary of existing works concerning leukemia—cont'd**

| Authors with year | Datasets | Techniques used | Tool used | Advantages | Issues | Accuracy |
|---|---|---|---|---|---|---|
| (Escalante et al., 2012) | Real data such as ALL/AML dataset | Two Bayesian classification methods, which incorporate feature selection, for the classification of gene expression data derived from cDNA microarrays | – | EPSMS is an exceptionally powerful strategy for the computerized development of troupe classifiers for acute leukemia, which requires no noteworthy client mediation | There are still some open issues that call for further examination. One issue is the determination of a lot of classifiers for making a gathering | 97.68% |
| (Shouval et al., 2015) | Source not provided. | The alternating decision tree (ADT) algorithm | – | The substituting choice tree model provides a strong instrument for the chance assessment of patients with AL before HSCT | Absence of expectation model advancement guidelines, I clung to exacting methodologic principals, as opposed to the EBMT and HCT-CI scores | 70% |
| (Li et al., 2016) | The proposed method was tested on 130 ALL images taken from ALL IDB | Complete methodology is based on the dual-threshold algorithm | – | Proposed a double limit strategy for segmenting white blood cells from acute lymphoblastic leukemia images | White blood cell division, which assumes a significant job in programmed cell morphology investigation remains a difficult issue in view of the morphological variety of WBCs and the mind-boggling foundation of blood tiny pictures | 97.85% |
| (Sewak et al., 2009) | ALL and AML using the microarray gene expression data | The heuristic nature of machine-learning algorithms | – | The advisory group, through a lion's share casting a ballot, effectively ordered an aggregate of 34 of the 35 approval informational collections, | Absence of various kinds of informational indexes utilized | 97% |

*Continued*

**Table 1 Summary of existing works concerning leukemia—cont'd**

| Authors with year | Datasets | Techniques used | Tool used | Advantages | Issues | Accuracy |
|---|---|---|---|---|---|---|
| | | | | yielding an exactness of 97.14% for the three-class characterization issue | | |
| (Abdeldaim et al., 2018) | ALL-IDB1 and ALL-IDB2 | K-NN is used for classification | Python | Acceptable in terms of the segmentation performance as the accuracy of all classifiers, especially k-NN, which achieved the best accuracy | The shape features cannot be trusted because of sensitivity to segmentation errors. These features integrate together with regional features, which are less susceptible to errors | 91% |
| (Valdés and Barton, 2004) | The dataset utilized has 7129 qualities where patients are isolated into a preparation set containing 38 bone marrow tests | K-means algorithm, with a Boolean reasoning algorithm | – | Representation additionally clarified the conduct of the neural system models and recommends the potential for the presence of better arrangements | The outcomes clarify the conduct of the neural system models and propose the potential for the presence of better arrangements | 95% |
| (Do and Byrd, 2015) | The outcomes from mass cytometry were contrasted and clinical stream cytometry information, and the techniques Wrath profoundly reliable | K-means algorithm | Python | A bewildering amount of data was managed from one lot of bone marrow suctions | An astonishing amount of information was gathered and can be used for future development | 96% |
| (Panda and Vihar, 2016) | Uses bioinformatics datasets for understanding the effectiveness of our proposed classification. It uses arrhythmia, leukemia, | The goal is to develop an efficient machine learning algorithm that can help to speed up the classification process and address the | Python | We conclude with the effectiveness of our proposed approach of combining DCNN with FRF classifier compared with other available research in the | Lack of different type of datasets used | 93.7% |

**Table 1 Summary of existing works concerning leukemia—cont'd**

| Authors with year | Datasets | Techniques used | Tool used | Advantages | Issues | Accuracy |
|---|---|---|---|---|---|---|
| | lymphoma, and prostate cancer datasets for experimentation | memory constraints effectively | | relevant domain and highlight the future scope of research | | |
| (Shafique and Tehsin, 2018) | The dataset used is from Alex-Net | Zack algorithm is used for each segmentation of leukocytes, SVM classifier | – | Robotized diagnosing framework may assist in early diagnosing of leukemia so it is very well may be dealt with viably | The speed and working model can be expanded | 99.5% |
| (Fuse et al., 2019) | Niigata Group, Nagaoka Group dataset | The alternating decision tree (ADTree) algorithm is used for this, one component of the machine-learning (ML) approach based on artificial intelligence (AI) | – | The current outcomes demonstrate that ML, for example, ADTree, will add to the decision-making procedure in the expanded allo-HSCT field and be valuable for forestalling leukemia relapse | The drawback of the current examination is that the volume of patient information for ADTree to learn was generally small | 90% |
| (Wang et al., 2005) | Microarray dataset (Source not provided) | Feature selection algorithm | – | These AI calculations are actualized in IKA, a freely accessible open-source programming bundle. This product can be utilized by both experienced and inexperienced clients | Because of their high computational costs, it is difficult to consolidate wrappers with some AI calculations, for example, SMO | 85% |
| (Choudhury et al., 2013) | Source not provided | Classification, Clustering algorithms, Soft computing techniques | – | It demonstrates that all public gene expression data are potentially useful for drug discovery | Lack of different types of datasets used | 90% |

*Continued*

| **Table 1** Summary of existing works concerning leukemia—cont'd | | | | | | |
|---|---|---|---|---|---|---|
| **Authors with year** | **Datasets** | **Techniques used** | **Tool used** | **Advantages** | **Issues** | **Accuracy** |
| (Hassane et al., 2008) | The microarray gene expression data was obtained from the National Centre for Biotechnology Information (NCBI) Gene Expression Omnibus (GEO) | Isolation of CD34 AML total RNA, Microarray hybridization and analysis, Acquisition and processing of public microarray data, Query of the GEO data | – | It demonstrates that data are potentially useful for drug discovery and can be accessed by any investigator with the appropriate computational tools | Speed of prediction and visualization is too slow | 90% |

The results presented in the study show that, with existing technologies, it is potentially possible to achieve good performance in a near-automated fashion.

# 4 Description of proposed system

The proposed system is described in the following subsections.

## 4.1 Introduction and related concepts

Leukemia is a cancerous growth of abnormal white cells that damages the blood and bone marrow. Leukemia is classified by the type of white blood cells influenced and by how rapidly the illness advances. Lymphocytic leukemia (otherwise called lymphoid or lymphoblastic leukemia) appears in the white blood cells, called lymphocytes, in the bone marrow. Myeloid (otherwise called myelogenous) leukemia may likewise begin in blood cells other than lymphocytes, such as red blood cells and platelets.

Based on how rapidly it appears or advances, leukemia is called either acute (quickly developing) or chronic (slow-developing). Acute leukemia advances quickly and brings about the aggregation of juvenile, nonfunctioning blood cells in the bone marrow. With this sort of leukemia, cells recreate and develop in the marrow, diminishing the marrow's capacity to deliver enough functional blood cells.

The diagnosis of leukemia typically relies on the complete blood count (CBC), in which physicians check the complete count of white blood cells, red blood cells, and platelets. This complete blood count test can show leukemia cells, but often this is not adequate for physicians to confirm that the patient has leukemia. Other techniques are used, including bone marrow aspiration and microscopic examination of blood smears. However, all these manual methods require much effort and time. Additionally, extensively trained therapeutic experts are required to carry out this type of inspection. Despite what might be expected, computerized demonstrative frameworks can address these issues of manual

**Table 2** Descriptions of acute myeloid leukemia dataset.

| Number of features | Name of features/attributes | Number of instances/ samples | Number of class |
|---|---|---|---|
| 7 | 1. Subject identifier (id) <br> 2. Treatment arm A or B (trt) <br> 3. Time to death or last follow-up (futime) <br> 4. 1 if fulltime is a death, 0 for censoring (death) <br> 5. Time to hematopoietic stem cell transplant (txtime) <br> 6. Time to complete response (crtime) <br> 7. Time to relapse of disease (rltime) | 646 | 2 |

analysis. In addition, they can lessen the need for medical experts and can give exact and viable outcomes as compared to manual diagnosing (Table 2).

An acute myeloid leukemia dataset has been used for the analysis. The myeloid dataset is available in (Picostat, 2018) and is also found in the R package. This dataset includes seven features, including class, and 646 instances or samples. The death feature is a class (two), where 1 indicates fulltime is a death, 0 for sensoring.

## 4.2 Framework for the proposed system

The authors have used the KNIME platform in implementing this work. It is an open-source platform that has many functionalities, including data mining, statistics, etc. It also helps in analyzing the results by plotting line graphs, bar graphs, etc. There are many functionalities accessed by drag and drop to the workspace or by double clicking to select. Using KNIME, we configured the function and executed it. First, we selected the dataset by browsing files on the system. The other option is that.csv files can be directly exported to the software and then they can be executed. Next the Partitioning tool was used to partition the data in 70:30 for classification methods like SVM and k-NN, and we also applied clustering algorithms like k-means and fuzzy c-means where data partitioning was not needed.

The proposed work consists of two phases: Phase I deals with the collection and visualization of datasets and Phase II deals with machine learning and data mining techniques for the prediction of leukemia.

In Fig. 1, it can be observed that the dataset has been collected online. First, we start or run the software and then import the collected online dataset. To perform the classification algorithms, we need to partition the dataset where clustering algorithms are not needed. In this work, SVM and k-NN were used for classification algorithms, whereas k-means and fuzzy c-means have been used as clustering algorithms. Finally, this algorithm predicts leukemia and our software work is finished.

The classification algorithms are briefly explained in the following paragraphs (Fig. 2).

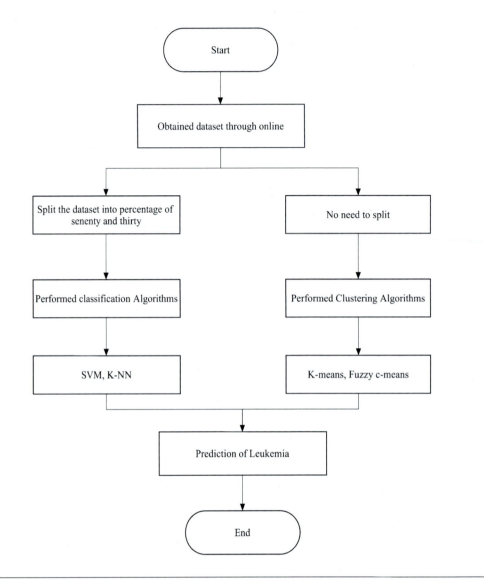

**FIG. 1**

Block diagram of proposed methodology.

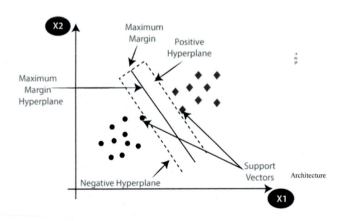

**FIG. 2**

Basic architecture of linear SVM.

### 4.2.1 Support vector machine

Vladimir N. Vapnik and Alexey Ya. Chervonenkis invented the SVM algorithm in 1963. Corinna Cortes and Vapnik's current standard incarnation (soft margin) was proposed in 1993 and published in 1995. The objective of the SVM algorithm is to find a hyperplane that best separates points in a hypercube. The nearest instances on either side of the boundary are called support vectors. The basic architecture of linear SVM is shown as:

The algorithms for SVM are noted as:

### ALGORITHM

1. SVM finds the widest street (plane) between the nearest points on either side. It may not be possible to obtain a hard decision boundary that clearly segregates the points.
2. Hard margin classifier is sensitive to outliers, one or more data points which are on the other side of the classification boundary.
3. Soft margin classifiers allow some violations of the decision boundary.
4. Smart transformation resolves many such cases, known as kernel tricks.
5. Decision boundary equation can be written as $w_1x_1 + w_2x_2 + b$, where $w_1$, $w_2$, $b$ are model parameters.
6. The training process of SVM classification will determine the values of $w_1x_1 + w_2x_2 + b$. So for any reviews, we will have the values of $x_1$ and $x_2$.
7. The decision plane will separate points based on whether $w_1x_1 + w_2x_2 + b$ is equal to or greater than 0.

### 4.2.2 K-nearest neighbor

K-NN was introduced by Fix and Hodges in 1951. K-NN is a simple, powerful, nonparametric, lazy learning method utilized for classification. In the beginning of the 1970s, k-NN was being used in statistical estimation and pattern recognition. The same algorithm was used by Choubey et al. (2020b) for the classification of diabetes (Fig. 3).

### ALGORITHM

Let $m$ be the number of training data samples. Let $p$ be an unknown point.
1. Store the training samples in an array of data points $arr[]$. This means each element of this array indicates a tuple $(x, y)$.
2. for $i = 0 to m$:
     Calculate Euclidean distance $d(arr[i], p)$.
3. Make set $S$ of $K$ smallest distances obtained. Each of these distances corresponds to an already classified data point.
4. Return the majority label among $S$.

The clustering algorithms are noted as:

### 4.2.3 K-means clustering

K-means clustering is an algorithm used to group the objects based on features into K number of groups. It works on an unlabeled dataset (unsupervised machine learning) (Fig. 4).

K-means will split a dataset into K clusters:

- Where each observation in $K_i$ is as similar to the others in that cluster as possible.
- Where the data in $K_i$ is as different as possible from the other clusters within $K_1 ............ N$.

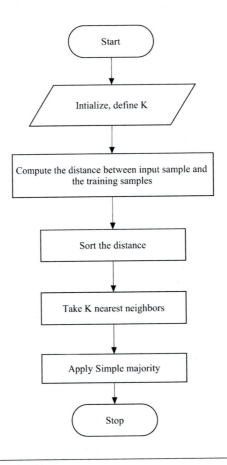

**FIG. 3**

Flowchart for K-nearest neighbor algorithm.

K-means clustering is an exploratory data analysis technique. The algorithms for k-means clustering are noted as:

### ALGORITHM

**Step 1.** Take mean value (random).
**Step 2.** Find nearest number of mean and put in cluster.
**Step 3.** Repeat steps 1 and 2 until we get the same value.

### 4.2.4 Fuzzy c-means clustering

Dunn created the fuzzy C-means clustering method in 1973 and it was improved by Bezdek in 1981. It is commonly utilized in design acknowledgments. It depends on minimization of the accompanying target work:

$$J_m = \sum_{i=1}^{N} \sum_{j=1}^{C} u_{ij}^{m} \left\| x_i - c_j \right\|^2, \quad 1 \le m < \infty$$

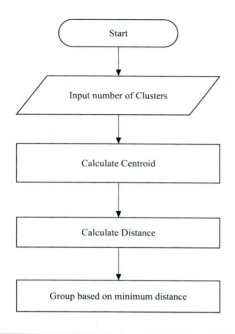

**FIG. 4**

Flowchart for K-means algorithm.

where $m$ is any real number greater than 1, $u_{ij}$ is the degree of membership of $x_i$ in the cluster $j$, $x_i$ is the $i$th of d-dimensional measured data, $c_j$ is the d-dimension center of the cluster, and $\| * \|$ is any norm expressing the similarity between any measured data and the center. Fuzzy partitioning is carried out through an iterative optimization of the objective function shown previously, with the update of membership $u_{ij}$ and the cluster centers $c_j$ by:

$$u_{ij} = \frac{1}{\sum_{k=1}^{c}\left(\frac{\|x_i - c_j\|}{\|x_i - c_k\|}\right)^{\frac{2}{m-1}}}$$

where

$$c_j = \frac{\sum_{i=1}^{N} u_{ij}^m . x_i}{\sum_{i=1}^{N} u_{ij}^m}$$

This iteration will stop when $\max_{ij}\{|u_{ij}^{(k+1)} - u_{ij}^k|\} < \varepsilon$, where $\varepsilon$ is a termination criterion between 0 and 1, whereas $k$ are the iteration steps. This procedure converges to a local minimum or a saddle point of $J_m$.

## 5 Simulation results and discussion

Every study must start with accurate data analysis. The myeloid dataset was used for the analysis, which is also available in R packages.

The performance evaluations of the classification algorithms used for leukemia are given in Table 3.

In Table 3, it may be observed that SVM performs better than k-NN classification algorithms.

The performance evaluations of the clustering algorithms used for leukemia are given in Table 4. In Table 4, it may be observed that fuzzy c-means performed better than the k-means algorithm. Now for the analysis of clustering and classification methods as shown in the following figures. Fig. 5 shows estimates of victims.

In Fig. 5, the number of patients all over the country in different states are clearly visible. Also, different graphs have been created that give an idea of the demographics of leukemia.

Fig. 6 indicates the spread of leukemia across different states in the United States.

Fig. 7 shows the overall summary of the analysis of leukemia.

Fig. 7 depicts the overall summary of the data analysis report, including doctors required average rate of get infected and many more can be understood by the picture.

Fig. 8 indicates the pivot table for the myeloid dataset.

In Fig. 9, the basic workflow of k-means and fuzzy c-means clustering methods is clearly visible.

In Figs. 10 and 11, we may clearly see k-means clustering results with different numbers of clusters.

Fig. 12 represents the clusters formed by the fuzzy c-means method.

In Fig. 12, six clusters have been formed and respectively show "futime." From this figure we can see that the clusters are forming wave-like patterns.

**Table 3 Performance evaluation of classification algorithms for leukemia.**

| Dataset | Algorithms | Sensitivity/recall | Precision | F-Measure |
|---|---|---|---|---|
| Myeloid dataset | SVM | 0.9746 | 0.9746 | 0.9746 |
| | K-NN | 0.9570 | 0.9570 | 0.9570 |

**Table 4 Performance comparison of clustering algorithms for leukemia.**

| Dataset | Algorithm | F-Measure |
|---|---|---|
| Myeloid dataset | K-means | 0.819 |
| | Fuzzy c-means | 0.829 |

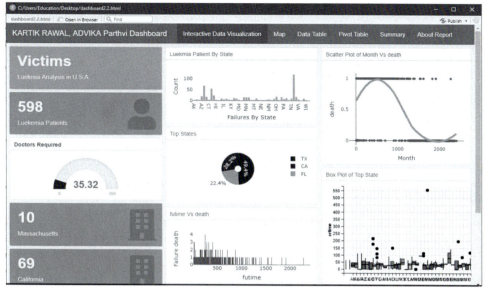

**FIG. 5**

Different graphs showing estimates of victims.

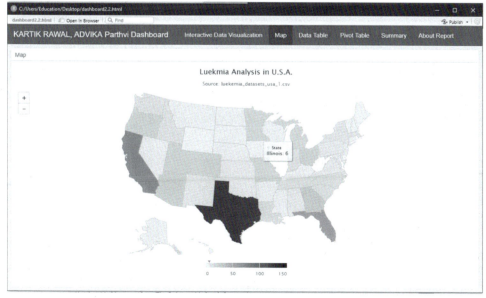

**FIG. 6**

United States map showing leukemia spread across different states.

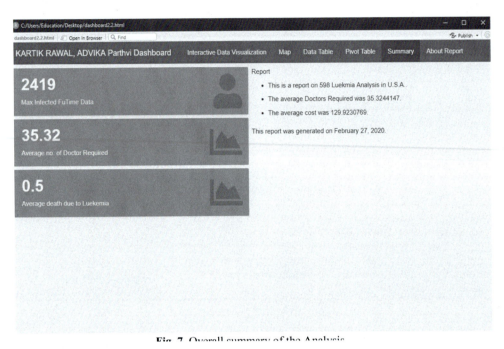

**FIG. 7**

Overall summary of leukemia analysis.

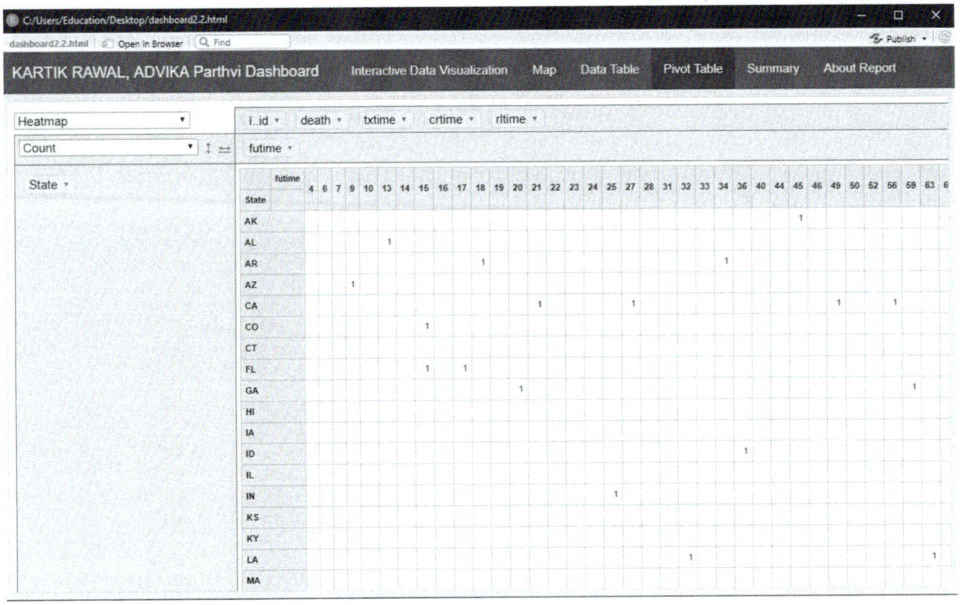

**FIG. 8**

Pivot table for myeloid dataset.

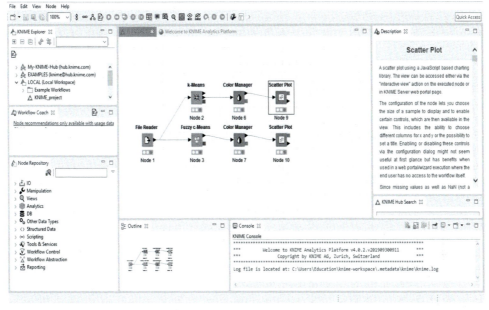

**FIG. 9**

Basic work flow diagram.

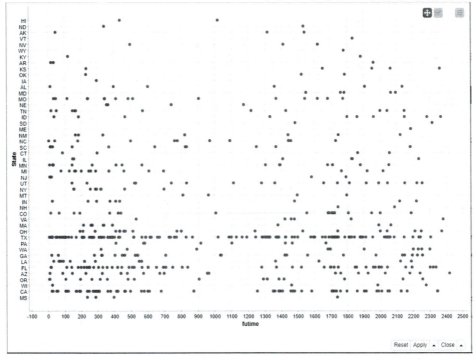

**FIG. 10**

K-means clustering plot 1.

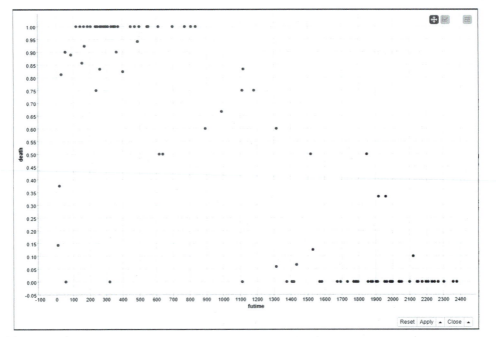

**FIG. 11**

K-means clustering plot 2.

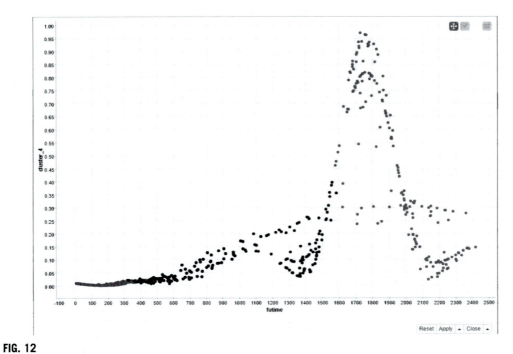

**FIG. 12**

Fuzzy c-means clustering for six clusters.

## 6 Conclusion and future directions

We have applied various algorithms to determine which one is most efficient in the diagnosis of leukemia. Results are shown in both graphical as well as tabular forms for the various algorithms that have been applied to leukemia. The KNIME was used to apply the algorithms and find an appropriate result for the classification and clustering methods of leukemia. The performance is different in each case and we have tried to find the most efficient algorithm for the diagnosis of leukemia. We have also studied the performance of various existing algorithms that have been used previously by fellow researchers. In this chapter we have utilized SVM and k-NN for classification and k-means and fuzzy c-means for clustering. Both the classification and clustering methods have been used in the prediction of leukemia.

The future directions for researchers are to deploy different deep-learning architectures for prediction of leukemia and compare these architectures to find those that perform best. We may also deploy deep-learning architectures for larger samples of datasets. Another future direction for researchers is the design of an automated detection system for leukemia blood cancer.

## References

Abdeldaim, A.M., Sahlol, A.T., Elhoseny, M., Hassanien, A.E., 2018. Computer-aided acute lymphoblastic leukemia diagnosis system based on image analysis. Stud. Comput. Intell. 730, 131–147. https://doi.org/10.1007/978-3-319-63754-9_7.

Bala, K., Choubey, D.K., Paul, S., 2017. Soft computing and data mining techniques for thunderstorms and lightning prediction: a survey. In: Proceedings of the International Conference on Electronics, Communication and Aerospace Technology, ICECA 2017, 2017-Janua., https://doi.org/10.1109/ICECA.2017.8203729.

Bala, K., Choubey, D.K., Paul, S., Lala, M.G.N., 2018. Classification techniques for thunderstorms and lightning prediction: a survey. In: Soft-Computing-Based Nonlinear Control Systems Design. IGI Global, pp. 1–17.

Chandrasekar, R.M., Palaniammal, V., Phil, M., 2013. Performance and evaluation of data mining techniques in cancer diagnosis. IOSR J. Comput. Eng. 15 (5), 39–44.

Choubey, D.K., Paul, S., 2015. GA_J48graft DT : a hybrid intelligent system for diabetes disease diagnosis. Int. J. Biosci. Biotechnol. 7 (5), 135–150.

Choubey, D.K., Paul, S., 2016a. GA_MLP NN: A Hybrid Intelligent System for Diabetes Disease Diagnosis. pp. 49–59, https://doi.org/10.5815/ijisa.2016.01.06.

Choubey, D.K., Paul, S., 2016b. Classification techniques for diagnosis of diabetes: a review. Int. J. Biomed. Eng. Technol. 21 (1). https://doi.org/10.1504/IJBET.2016.076730.

Choubey, D.K., Paul, S., 2017a. GA_SVM: a classification system for diagnosis of diabetes. In: Handbook of Research on Soft Computing and Nature-Inspired Algorithms., https://doi.org/10.4018/978-1-5225-2128-0.ch012.

Choubey, D.K., Paul, S., 2017b. GA-RBF NN: a classification system for diabetes. Int. J. Biomed. Eng. Technol. 23 (1), 71–93. https://doi.org/10.1504/IJBET.2017.082229.

Choubey, D.K., Paul, S., Dhandhenia, V.K., 2017. Rule based diagnosis system for diabetes. Biomed. Res. 28 (12).

Choubey, D.K., Paul, S., Shandilya, S., Dhandhania, V.K., 2018. Implementation and analysis of classification algorithms for diabetes. Curr. Med. Imaging Rev. 14, 340–354. https://doi.org/10.2174/1573405614666180828115813.

Choubey, D.K., Paul, S., Bala, K., Kumar, M., Singh, U.P., 2019a. Implementation of a hybrid classification method for diabetes. In: Intelligent Innovations in Multimedia Data Engineering and Management. IGI Global, pp. 201–240.

Choubey, D.K., Tripathi, S., Kumar, P., Shukla, V., Dhandhania, V.K., 2019b. Classification of diabetes by kernel based SVM with PSO. Recent Pat. Comput. Sci., 1–14.

Choubey, D.K., Kumar, M., Shukla, V., Tripathi, S., Dhandhania, V.K., 2020a. Comparative analysis of classification methods with PCA and LDA for diabetes. Curr. Diabetes Rev. 16. https://doi.org/10.2174/1573399816666200123124008.

Choubey, D.K., Kumar, P., Tripathi, S., Kumar, S., 2020b. Performance evaluation of classification methods with PCA and PSO for diabetes. Netw. Model. Anal. Health Inform. Bioinform. 9 (1), 1–17. https://doi.org/10.1007/s13721-019-0210-8.

Choudhury, T., Kumar, V., Nigam, D., 2013. Cancer research through the help of soft computing techniques: a survey. Int. J. Comput. Sci. Mob. Comput. 2 (April), 467–477.

Daqqa, K.A.S.A., Maghari, A.Y.A., Al Sarraj, W.F.M., 2017. Prediction and diagnosis of leukemia using classification algorithms. In: ICIT 2017—8th International Conference on Information Technology, Proceedings, October, pp. 638–643, https://doi.org/10.1109/ICITECH.2017.8079919.

Dash, S., Patra, B., Tripathy, B.K., 2012. A hybrid data mining technique for improving the classification accuracy of microarray data set. Int. J. Inf. Eng. Electron. Bus. 4 (2), 43–50. https://doi.org/10.5815/ijieeb.2012.02.07.

Do, P., Byrd, J.C., 2015. Mass cytometry: a high-throughput platform to visualize the heterogeneity of acute myeloid leukemia. Cancer Discov. 5 (9), 912–914. https://doi.org/10.1158/2159-8290.CD-15-0905.

Escalante, H.J., Montes-y-Gómez, M., González, J.A., Gómez-Gil, P., Altamirano, L., Reyes, C.A., Reta, C., Rosales, A., 2012. Acute leukemia classification by ensemble particle swarm model selection. Artif. Intell. Med. 55 (3), 163–175. https://doi.org/10.1016/j.artmed.2012.03.005.

Fuse, K., Uemura, S., Tamura, S., Suwabe, T., Katagiri, T., Tanaka, T., Ushiki, T., Shibasaki, Y., Sato, N., Yano, T., Kuroha, T., Hashimoto, S., Furukawa, T., Narita, M., Sone, H., Masuko, M., 2019. Patient-based prediction algorithm of relapse after Allo-HSCT for acute leukemia and its usefulness in the decision-making process using a machine learning approach. Cancer Med. 8 (11), 5058–5067. https://doi.org/10.1002/cam4.2401.

Hassane, D.C., Guzman, M.L., Corbett, C., Li, X., Abboud, R., Young, F., Liesveld, J.L., Carroll, M., Jordan, C.T., 2008. Discovery of agents that eradicate leukemia stem cells using an in silico screen of public gene expression data. Blood 111 (12), 5654–5662. https://doi.org/10.1182/blood-2007-11-126003.

Kumar, S., Mishra, S., Asthana, P., Pragya, 2018a. Automated detection of acute leukemia using K-mean clustering algorithm. Adv. Intell. Syst. Comput. 554, 655–670. https://doi.org/10.1007/978-981-10-3773-3_64.

Kumar, M., Mishra, S.K., Choubey, S.K., Tripathy, S.S., Choubey, D.K., Das, D., 2018b. Cat swarm optimization based functional link multilayer perceptron for suppression of Gaussian and impulse noise from computed tomography images. Curr. Med. Imaging 16 (4), 329–339. https://doi.org/10.2174/1573405614666180903115336.

Kumar, S., Mohapatra, U.M., Singh, D., Choubey, D.K., 2019. EAC: efficient associative classifier for classification. In: Proceedings—2019 International Conference on Applied Machine Learning, ICAML 2019, pp. 15–20, https://doi.org/10.1109/ICAML48257.2019.00011.

Kumar, S., Bhusan, B., Singh, D., Choubey, D.K., 2020a. Classification of diabetes using deep learning. In: Proceedings of the 2020 IEEE International Conference on Communication and Signal Processing, ICCSP 2020, Dl, pp. 651–655, https://doi.org/10.1109/ICCSP48568.2020.9182293.

Kumar, M., Jangir, S.K., Mishra, S.K., Choubey, S.K., Choubey, D.K., 2020b. Multi-Channel FLANN Adaptive Filter for Speckle & Impulse Noise Elimination from Color Doppler Ultrasound Images. pp. 1–4, https://doi.org/10.1109/iconc345789.2020.9117288.

Li, Y., Zhu, R., Mi, L., Cao, Y., Yao, D., 2016. Segmentation of white blood cell from acute lymphoblastic leukemia images using dual-threshold method. Comput. Math. Methods Med. 2016. https://doi.org/10.1155/2016/9514707.

Pahari, S., Choubey, D.K., 2020. Analysis of liver disorder using classification techniques: a survey. In: International Conference on Emerging Trends in Information Technology and Engineering, Ic-ETITE 2020, pp. 1–4, https://doi.org/10.1109/ic-ETITE47903.2020.300.

Panda, M., Vihar, V., 2016. Towards the Effectiveness of Deep Convolutional Neural Network Based Fast Random Forest Classifier. ArXiv, abs/1609.0.

Parthvi, A., Rawal, K., Choubey, D.K., 2020. A comparative study using machine learning and data mining approach for leukemia. In: Proceedings of the 2020 IEEE International Conference on Communication and Signal Processing, ICCSP 2020, pp. 672–677, https://doi.org/10.1109/ICCSP48568.2020.9182142.

Picostat, 2018. Leukemia, A. Myeloid. No Title. Https://Www.Picostat.Com/Dataset/r-Dataset-Package-Survival-Myeloid.

Priyanga, A., Prakasam, S., 2013. Effectiveness of data mining-based cancer prediction system (DMBCPS). Int. J. Comput. Appl. 83 (10).

Sewak, M.S., Reddy, N.P., Duan, Z.H., 2009. Gene expression based leukemia sub—classification using committee neural networks. Bioinf. Biol. Insights 3, 89–98.

Shafique, S., Tehsin, S., 2018. Acute lymphoblastic leukemia detection and classification of its subtypes using pretrained deep convolutional neural networks. Technol. Cancer Res. Treat. 17, 1–7. https://doi.org/10.1177/1533033818802789.

Sharma, D., Jain, P., Choubey, D.K., 2020. A comparative study of computational intelligence for identification of breast cancer. In: International Conference on Machine Learning, Image Processing, Network Security and Data Sciences, pp. 209–216.

Shouval, R., Labopin, M., Bondi, O., Mishan-Shamay, H., Shimoni, A., Ciceri, F., Esteve, J., Giebel, S., Gorin, N. C., Schmid, C., Polge, E., Aljurf, M., Kroger, N., Craddock, C., Bacigalupo, A., Cornelissen, J.J., Baron, F., Unger, R., Nagler, A., Mohty, M., 2015. Prediction of allogeneic hematopoietic stem-cell transplantation mortality 100 days after transplantation using a machine learning algorithm: a European group for blood and marrow transplantation acute leukemia working party retrospective data mining stud. J. Clin. Oncol. 33 (28), 3144–3151. https://doi.org/10.1200/JCO.2014.59.1339.

Sivaraman, A., Rajesh, S.A., Lakshmi, M., 2014. Optimistic diagnosis of acute leukemia based on human blood sample using feed forward back propagation neural network. Int. J. Innov. Res. Sci. Eng. Technol. 3 (3), 1046–1049.

Srivastava, K., Choubey, D.K., 2019. Soft computing, data mining, and machine learning approaches in detection of heart disease: a review. In: International Conference on Hybrid Intelligent Systems, pp. 165–175.

Srivastava, K., Choubey, D.K., 2020. Heart disease prediction using machine learning and data mining. Int. J. Recent Technol. Eng. 9 (1), 21–219. https://doi.org/10.35940/ijrte.f9199.059120.

Suji, R.J., Rajagopalan, S.P., 2013. An automatic oral cancer classification using data mining techniques. Int. J. Adv. Res. Comput. Commun. Eng. 2 (10), 3759–3765.

Valdés, J.J., Barton, A.J., 2004. Gene discovery in leukemia revisited: a computational intelligence perspective. Lect. Notes Artif. Intell. 3029, 118–127. https://doi.org/10.1007/978-3-540-24677-0_13.

Vasighizaker, A., Sharma, A., Dehzangi, A., 2019. A novel one-class classification approach to accurately predict disease-gene association in acute myeloid leukemia cancer. PLoS One 14 (12), 1–12. https://doi.org/10.1371/journal.pone.0226115.

Wang, Y., Tetko, I.V., Hall, M.A., Frank, E., Facius, A., Mayer, K.F.X., Mewes, H.W., 2005. Gene selection from microarray data for cancer classification—a machine learning approach. Comput. Biol. Chem. 29 (1), 37–46. https://doi.org/10.1016/j.compbiolchem.2004.11.001.

Warnat-Herresthal, S., Perrakis, K., Taschler, B., Becker, M., Baßler, K., Beyer, M., Günther, P., Schulte-Schrepping, J., Seep, L., Klee, K., Ulas, T., Haferlach, T., Mukherjee, S., Schultze, J.L., 2020. Scalable prediction of acute myeloid leukemia using high-dimensional machine learning and blood transcriptomics. IScience 23 (1). https://doi.org/10.1016/j.isci.2019.100780.

# Performance evaluation of fractal features toward seizure detection from electroencephalogram signals

# 17

**O.K. Fasil and R. Rajesh**

*Department of Computer Science, Central University of Kerala, Kerala, India*

## Chapter outline

## 1  Introduction

Epilepsy is an onerous disorder that causes repetitive seizures in the central nervous system. Epilepsy affected a sizeable population across the globe (Thijs et al., 2019). The analysis of the frequency, severity, and duration of the seizures are indispensable in epilepsy treatment. Among various brain scanning techniques, electroencephalogram (EEG) has been extensively used because of its high temporal resolution and low cost (Tatum et al., 2018). Long-term clinical examination is essential in most of the epilepsy cases for effective diagnosis and treatment. Manual analysis of long-term EEG recorded as part of the clinical examination is a burdensome process and error prone. Many machine learning methods have been proposed during the past decades to automate the process of EEG analysis.

The EEG signals produced by the brain are nonlinear and chaotic in nature. Most of the machine learning methods require a large amount of data and much calculation time to analyze complex EEG

*Machine Learning, Big Data, and IoT for Medical Informatics.* https://doi.org/10.1016/B978-0-12-821777-1.00005-7

signals. Dimensional complexity is mainly used to analyze the complex EEG signals. Generally, the dimensional complexity is obtained in phase space, which is only suitable to analyze long-duration events (Accardo et al., 1997). Since the seizure events are brief and in the time domain, fractal dimension (FD)-based features can be used for effective analysis of EEG. The ability of FD to analyze the irregular or complex shapes will help to characterize epileptic EEG efficiently (Lopes and Betrouni, 2009).

Many methods in literature utilized FD-based features to analyze EEG signals for various tasks. These tasks include the study of human EEG responses to odors (Şeker and Özerdem, 2018), depression detection (Mohammadi et al., 2019), analysis of states of consciousness and unconsciousness (de Miras et al., 2019), detection of Alzheimer's disease (Al-Nuaimi et al., 2017; Smits et al., 2016), sleep analysis (Asirvadam et al., 2018; Liaw et al., 2017; Al-Salman et al., 2018), emotional recognition (Xu et al., 2019; Ruiz-Padial and Ibáñez-Molina, 2018), and motor imagery analysis (Liu et al., 2017). The FD-based features are also widely used for seizure/epilepsy detection problems. Wijayanto et al. (2019b) extracted Katz FD features from subbands of EEG signals for epilepsy identification. In another work of the same authors, they have extracted Higuchi FD along with Katz FD in the same way and achieved improved results (Wijayanto et al., 2019a). Major bottleneck with this method is the subband decomposition. The algorithm will be more suitable in real-time systems if it extract features from the original signal instead of subbands. Sharma and Pachori (2017) utilized tunable-Q wavelet transform (TQWT) to decompose the signal to various subbands and extracted Higuchi FD from these subbands to detect epileptic seizures. Dautov and Özerdem (2018) also used Higuchi FD in their work. An important study by Abdulhay et al. (2017) utilized Higuchi FD with wavelet-based entropy features and higher-order spectra features for effective identification of epilepsy. Moctezuma and Molinas (2020a) extracted Higuchi and Petrosian FD from intrinsic mode function (IMFs) obtained by empirical mode decomposition (EMD). Authors extracted Teager and instantaneous energy and DFA features along with FD and used for seizure detection.

In the recent work, David et al. (2020) used multifractal detrended fluctuation analysis and Hurst exponent with FD to study the characteristics of EEG signals of epileptic patients. Wijayanto et al. (2020) extracted Higuchi FD from various EEG subbands (such as delta, theta, alpha, beta, and gamma) for classifying ictal and interictal EEG signals. Higuchi FD feature is also utilized in another work by Choubey and Pandey. Authors also extracted sample entropy with FD (Choubey and Pandey, 2020). Upadhyaya et al. (2019) used Higuchi FD to determine focal epilepsy by analyzing EEG signals. Similarly, Chakraborty et al. (2019) extracted FD features from DWT and used for classifying normal, interictal, and ictal states of epilepsy with statistical and nonlinear features. In another work, FD features are extracted from EMD and DWT used to maximize the classification result by reducing the number of channels (Moctezuma and Molinas, 2020b). In a focal identification work, Dalal et al. (2019) decomposed EEG signal into various subbands using flexible analytic wavelet transform prior to FD feature extraction.

The common factor in all studies is exposed as none of the works used FD feature alone for epilepsy detection. The works either used various features along with the FD or extracted from different transformed domains like EMD or DWT for enhanced results. The FD features extracted from the time domain will reduce the extraction time by avoiding further transformations. Moreover, the individual performance of various FD features to detect seizures is rarely studied in literature and is highly required for forthcoming research. In-depth understanding of the individual performance of FD features will ease the implementation of real-time seizure detection systems. Furthermore, it opens the door for future research.

In this work, the seizure detection efficiency of three widely used FD feature extraction methods, such as Katz, Higuchi, and Petrosian, is compared. One of the universally accepted epilepsy EEG dataset named as Bonn EEG dataset is considered for all experiments. The remaining sections of this chapter are organized as follows: Section 2 describes the details of three FD techniques. A brief description of the dataset is given in Section 3. The experimental setup of the study is explained in Section 4, and - Section 5 presents the results with discussions. Section 6 will conclude the chapter with future directions.

## 2 Fractal dimension

The fractals are self-similar patterns which appear across various scales (Lopes and Betrouni, 2009). FD is a statistical quantity of fractals complexity, which will describe how complex a self-similar pattern is. FD is widely used to characterize chaotic and nonlinear signals because of its ability to extract the complexity of signals in the time domain (Raghavendra and Dutt, 2010). In this work, three FDs, such as Katz, Higuchi, and Petrosian, are studied. Brief descriptions of each FD are given in the following sections.

### 2.1 Katz fractal dimension

The Katz FD is proposed in 1988 by Katz (1988). In this method, the FD ($D$) of the waveforms can be estimated as

$$D = \frac{\log(L/a)}{\log(d/a)} = \frac{\log(n)}{\log(n) + \log(d/L)} \tag{1}$$

where $L$ is the total length of the wave and calculated as the sum of the Euclidean distance between successive points $P_i$ and $P_{i+1}$ in the wave.

$$L = \sum_{i=1}^{N} Ed(P_i, P_{i+1}) \tag{2}$$

where $a$ is defined as the average of Euclidean distance between successive points in the wave.

$$a = \frac{1}{N} \sum_{i=1}^{N} Ed(P_i, P_{i+1}) \tag{3}$$

According to this method, $n$ is defined as the number of steps in the wave and computed as $n = L/a$. $d$ is the diameter of the wave and calculated as the maximum distance between the starting point and any other points in the wave.

### 2.2 Higuchi fractal dimension

In Higuchi method (Higuchi, 1988), the FD of the waveform $x(n)$, $n = 1, 2, 3, \ldots, N$ with length $N$ can be computed with the following steps (Sharma et al., 2017). First, from each wave $k$ subwaves can be formed as

$$x_n^k = \{x(n), x(n+k), x(n+2k), \ldots, x(n+pk)\} \tag{4}$$

where $n = 1, 2, 3, \ldots, k$, where $n$ is the starting time and $k$ is the interval time. Here, $p = \lfloor (N - n)/k \rfloor$. The average length $L_n^k$ of the obtained subwaves is calculated as

$$L_n^k = \frac{\sum_{i=1}^{\lfloor p \rfloor} |y(n+ik) - y(n+(i-1)k)|(N-1)}{\lfloor p \rfloor k} \tag{5}$$

Then, the average $L_n^k$ for $n = 1, 2, \ldots, k$ will be calculated and plot the graph of $\log(L_n^k)$ against $\log(1/k)$. After applying the least-squares linear best-fitting method, the coefficient of linear regression of the plot will be considered as the FD of the wave (Raghavendra and Dutt, 2010).

## 2.3 Petrosian fractal dimension

Petrosian method (Petrosian, 1995) computes the FD by transforming the original signal into binary sequence. The Petrosian FD of a signal $x(1), x(2), x(3), \ldots, x(N)$ with length $N$ and suppose $y_1, y_2, y_3, \ldots, y_N$ are series points in the signal, then first binary sequence $Z_i$ will be constructed as follows (Shi, 2018):

$$z_i = \begin{cases} 1, & x_i > mean(y) \\ -1, & x_i < mean(y) \end{cases}, \quad i = 1, 2, \ldots, N \tag{6}$$

Then, the total number of sign changes $N_\Delta$ in the binary sequence is calculated. Then, the Petrosian FD can be computed as

$$D = \frac{\log_{10} N}{\log_{10} N + \log_{10}\left(\frac{N}{N+0.4} N_\Delta\right)} \tag{7}$$

## 3 Dataset

A freely available benchmark dataset named as Bonn University EEG dataset is used for all experiments in this work (Andrzejak et al., 2001). Dataset consists of EEG signals from five epileptic patients and from five healthy subjects. Five sets of EEG signals (each contains 100 signals) are available in this dataset. Two sets, such as group A and group E, are considered in this study (seizure vs. nonseizure classification). Signals in group A are collected from healthy subjects in eye-open state (nonseizure signals) and signals in the group E are collected from epileptic subjects during seizure activity (seizure signals). Each signal in the dataset is 23.6 s duration and sampled at 173.61 Hz.

# 4 Experiments

The capacity of fractal features to discriminate between seizure signals (labeled as E) versus non-seizure (labeled as N) signal has experimented in this work. As a preprocessing step, signals are first filtered with sixth-order butter-worth filter to remove unnecessary frequencies. In addition to the original signals (labeled as $x$), first and the second derivative of each signal (labeled as $x'$ and $x''$, respectively) are constructed as done in Fasil and Rajesh (2019) and considered for feature extraction along with the original signal. The 23.6 s duration signals are further segmented into 10 nonoverlapping segments (2.36 s each) as suggested in Rajesh et al. (2018). FDs are computed from all segments and mean FDs across all segments are considered as features. The box plot of extracted Katz FD, Higuchi FD, and Petrosian FD features are shown in Figs. 1–3, respectively. It can be clearly seen that the feature is discriminating between seizure and nonseizure effectively. All experiments are carried out in Matlab environment on a Windows system with 4 GB RAM and Intel core i5 processor.

The features are fed to a well-known classifier support vector machine (SVM) for the classification of seizure and nonseizure. The performance in various SVM kernels (polynomial, RBF, and linear) is studied in this work. The decision boundary of SVM classifier in various kernels for Katz FD, Higuchi FD, and Petrosian FD features is shown in Figs. 4–6, respectively. A pseudo-code for the proposed epilepsy EEG signal classification method is shown in Algorithm 1.

**ALGORITHM 1 PSEUDOCODE FOR PROPOSED EPILEPSY EEG SIGNAL CLASSIFICATION METHOD.**

**Data:** EEGsignal
**Result:** Predicted label 0 for normal signal, predicted label 1 for epileptic signal

```
filteredSignal ← RemoveUnnecessaryFrequencies(EEGsignal);
firstDerivative ← ComputeFirstDerivative(filteredSignal);
secondDerivative ← ComputeSecondDerivative(firstDerivative);
for i ← (EEGsignal, firstDerivative, secondDerivative) do
    signalSegments ←
      SegmentSignalintoSubsegments(i,segmentLength);
    for j ← 1 to Count(signalSegments) do
        extractedFeature ←
          ExtractFractalDimensionFeature(signalSegments(j));
    end
end
predictedLabel ←
  ClassifySignalSVMClassifier(trainedModel,extractedFeature)
```

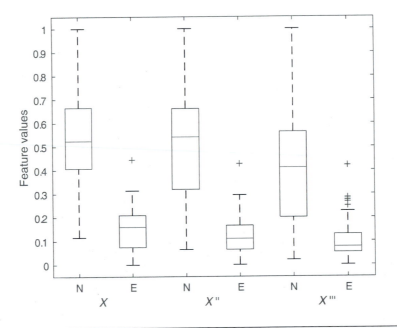

**FIG. 1**

Box plot of Katz FD feature. Box plot of Katz FD feature extracted from original signal ($x$), first derivative signals ($x'$), and second derivative signals ($x''$).

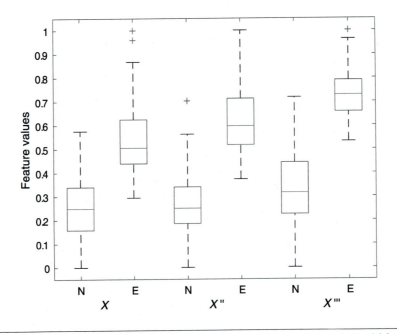

**FIG. 2**

Box plot of Higuchi FD feature. Box plot of Higuchi FD feature extracted from original signal ($x$), first derivative signals ($x'$), and second derivative signals ($x''$).

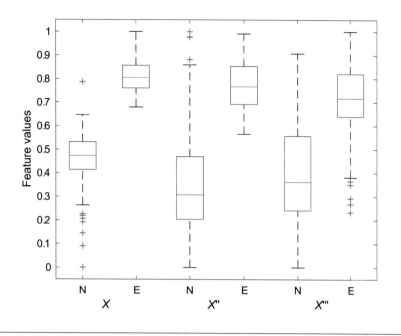

**FIG. 3**

Box plot of Petrosian FD feature. Box plot of Petrosian FD feature extracted from original signal (*x*), first derivative signals (*x'*), and second derivative signals (*x''*).

## 5 Results and discussion

The performance of FD features to discriminate seizure, and nonseizure EEG signals is evaluated with SVM classifier in various kernels. The result of the experiments in various SVM kernels is given in Table 1. It is clear that the Petrosian FD features have achieved the highest accuracy of 99.50%. Similarly, Petrosian FD features achieved 100% sensitivity in all SVM kernels. Among different kernels, polynomial kernel produces better results. The performance of Higuchi FD features is better than the Katz FD feature. In brief, all FD features have produced better results in discriminating seizure and nonseizure EEG signals. The computation of FD features is also not complicated. The results obtained in this study suggest that the FD features can be used to characterize epileptic EEG signals and can be implemented in automated detection systems.

A comparison of the results obtained from this work and previous works in the literature is presented in Table 2. The results indicate that the method experimented in this work with FD features are producing promising results.

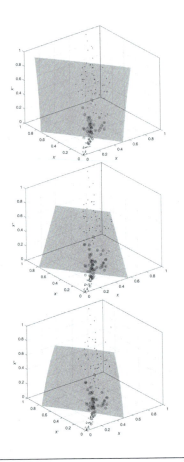

**FIG. 4**

Decision boundary of SVM classifier for Katz FD in various kernels: (A) polynomial; (B) linear; and (C) RBF.

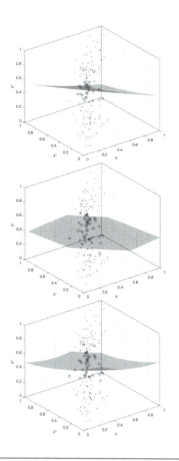

**FIG. 5**

Decision boundary of SVM classifier for Higuchi FD in various kernels: (A) polynomial; (B) linear; and (C) RBF.

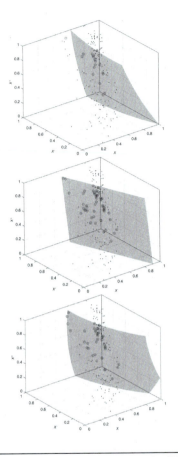

**FIG. 6**

Decision boundary of SVM classifier for Petrosian FD in various kernels: (A) polynomial; (B) linear; and (C) RBF.

**Table 1** Classification performance of FD features in SVM classifier with various kernels in terms of accuracy (Acc), sensitivity (Sen), and specificity (Spec).

| SVM kernels | Polynomial | | | RBF | | | Linear | | |
|---|---|---|---|---|---|---|---|---|---|
| Measures | Acc (%) | Sen (%) | Spec (%) | Acc (%) | Sen (%) | Spec (%) | Acc (%) | Sen (%) | Spec (%) |
| Katz FD | 94.50 | 97.00 | 92.57 | 92.50 | 94.64 | 90.93 | 92.50 | 97.05 | 89.71 |
| Higuchi FD | 96.50 | 97.99 | 95.49 | 96.50 | 99 | 94.71 | 97.00 | 100 | 94.53 |
| Petrosian FD | 99.50 | 100 | 99.05 | 98.50 | 100 | 97.23 | 97.00 | 100 | 94.46 |

**Table 2** Comparison FD-based methods in this work and previous works in literature for seizure versus nonseizure classification on Bonn University dataset.

| Reference | Features | Accuracy (%) |
|---|---|---|
| Subasi et al. (2019) | DWT coefficients | 97.87 |
| Lee et al. (2014) | WT, PSR, ED | 98.17 |
| Hassan et al. (2020) | NIG pdf | 98.33 |
| Polat and Güneş (2007) | Welch PSD | 98.72 |
| San-Segundo et al. (2019) | Raw EEG with CNN | 99.00 |
| Hassan et al. (2020) | NIG pdf | 99.00 |
| Fu et al. (2014) | TFR image | 99.125 |
| Guo et al. (2010) | ApEn | 99.38 |
| This work | Petrosian FD | 99.50 |

# 6 Conclusion

Comparison of three widely used FD-based features such as Katz, Higuchi, and Petrosian is carried out in this work. More specifically, the capacity of this feature to discriminate seizure and nonseizure EEG signals has experimented with a benchmark dataset. The results in SVM classifier show that the FD features are very effective to detect seizure EEG signals. The experiments are carried out in different kernels of SVM. Among these three FD features, Petrosian-based features in SVM classifier with polynomial kernel produced the highest accuracy. The computational simplicity of FD features will facilitate the development of a real-time system with less effort.

In future, in order to generalize, the proposed method will experiment with the various datasets. Further, the performance of fractal features to predict the chances of seizures prior to the event will be studied.

# Acknowledgments

The authors thank the Central University of Kerala for providing all research support for the work. The authors also thank the reviewers for critical review suggestions.

# References

Abdulhay, E., Elamaran, V., Chandrasekar, M., Balaji, V.S., Narasimhan, K., 2017. Automated diagnosis of epilepsy from EEG signals using ensemble learning approach. Pattern Recogn. Lett. 139, 174–181.

Accardo, A., Affinito, M., Carrozzi, M., Bouquet, F., 1997. Use of the fractal dimension for the analysis of electroencephalographic time series. Biol. Cybernet. 77 (5), 339–350.

Al-Nuaimi, A.H., Jammeh, E., Sun, L., Ifeachor, E., 2017. Higuchi fractal dimension of the electroencephalogram as a biomarker for early detection of Alzheimer's disease. In: 2017 39th Annual International Conference of the IEEE Engineering in Medicine and Biology Society (EMBC), pp. 2320–2324.

Al-Salman, W., Li, Y., Wen, P., Diykh, M., 2018. An efficient approach for EEG sleep spindles detection based on fractal dimension coupled with time frequency image. Biomed. Signal Process. Control 41, 210–221.

Andrzejak, R.G., Lehnertz, K., Mormann, F., Rieke, C., David, P., Elger, C.E., 2001. Indications of nonlinear deterministic and finite-dimensional structures in time series of brain electrical activity: dependence on recording region and brain state. Phys. Rev. E 64 (6), 061907.

Asirvadam, V.S., Hutapea, D.K.Y., Dass, S.C., et al., 2018. Comparison of EEG signals during alert and sleep inertia states using fractal dimension. In: 2018 IEEE 14th International Colloquium on Signal Processing & Its Applications (CSPA), pp. 155–160.

Chakraborty, M., Mitra, D., et al., 2019. Epilepsy seizure detection using non-linear and DWT-based features. In: 2019 International Conference on Wireless Communications Signal Processing and Networking (WiSPNET), pp. 158–163.

Choubey, H., Pandey, A., 2020. A combination of statistical parameters for the detection of epilepsy and EEG classification using ANN and KNN classifier. Signal Image Video Process., 1–9.

Dalal, M., Tanveer, M., Pachori, R.B., 2019. Automated identification system for focal EEG signals using fractal dimension of FAWT-based sub-bands signals. In: Machine Intelligence and Signal Analysis. Springer, pp. 583–596.

Dautov, Ç.P., Özerdem, M.S., 2018. Epilepsy detection using a naive signal decomposition method combined with fractal dimension. In: 2018 26th Signal Processing and Communications Applications Conference (SIU), pp. 1–4.

David, S.A., Machado, J.A.T., Inácio, C.M.C., Valentim, C.A., 2020. A combined measure to differentiate EEG signals using fractal dimension and MFDFA-Hurst. Commun. Nonlinear Sci. Numer. Simul. 84, 105170.

de Miras, J.R., Soler, F., Iglesias-Parro, S., Ibáñez-Molina, A.J., Casali, A.G., Laureys, S., Massimini, M., Esteban, F.J., Navas, J., Langa, J.A., 2019. Fractal dimension analysis of states of consciousness and unconsciousness using transcranial magnetic stimulation. Comput. Methods Programs Biomed. 175, 129–137.

Fasil, O.K., Rajesh, R., 2019. Time-domain exponential energy for epileptic EEG signal classification. Neurosci. Lett. 694, 1–8.

Fu, K., Qu, J., Chai, Y., Dong, Y., 2014. Classification of seizure based on the time-frequency image of EEG signals using HHT and SVM. Biomed. Signal Process. Control 13, 15–22.

Guo, L., Rivero, D., Pazos, A., 2010. Epileptic seizure detection using multiwavelet transform based approximate entropy and artificial neural networks. J. Neurosci. Methods 193 (1), 156–163.

Hassan, A.R., Subasi, A., Zhang, Y., 2020. Epilepsy seizure detection using complete ensemble empirical mode decomposition with adaptive noise. Knowl. Based Syst. 191, 105333.

Higuchi, T., 1988. Approach to an irregular time series on the basis of the fractal theory. Phys. D 31 (2), 277–283.

Katz, M.J., 1988. Fractals and the analysis of waveforms. Comput. Biol. Med. 18 (3), 145–156.

Lee, S.-H., Lim, J.S., Kim, J.-K., Yang, J., Lee, Y., 2014. Classification of normal and epileptic seizure EEG signals using wavelet transform, phase-space reconstruction, and Euclidean distance. Comput. Methods Programs Biomed. 116 (1), 10–25.

Liaw, S., Chen, J., et al., 2017. Characterizing sleep stages by the fractal dimensions of electroencephalograms. Biostat. Biom. 2, 555584.

Liu, Y.-H., Huang, S., Huang, Y.-D., 2017. Motor imagery EEG classification for patients with amyotrophic lateral sclerosis using fractal dimension and Fisher's criterion-based channel selection. Sensors 17 (7), 1557.

Lopes, R., Betrouni, N., 2009. Fractal and multifractal analysis: a review. Med. Image Anal. 13 (4), 634–649.

Moctezuma, L.A., Molinas, M., 2020a. Classification of low-density EEG for epileptic seizures by energy and fractal features based on EMD. J. Biomed. Res. 34 (3), 178–188.

Moctezuma, L.A., Molinas, M., 2020b. EEG channel-selection method for epileptic-seizure classification based on multi-objective optimization. Front. Neurosci. 14, 593.

Mohammadi, Y., Hajian, M., Moradi, M.H., 2019. Discrimination of depression levels using machine learning methods on EEG signals. In: 2019 27th Iranian Conference on Electrical Engineering (ICEE), pp. 1765–1769.

Petrosian, A., 1995. Kolmogorov complexity of finite sequences and recognition of different preictal EEG patterns. In: Proceedings Eighth IEEE Symposium on Computer-Based Medical Systems, pp. 212–217.

Polat, K., Güneş, S., 2007. Classification of epileptiform EEG using a hybrid system based on decision tree classifier and fast Fourier transform. Appl. Math. Comput. 187 (2), 1017–1026.

Raghavendra, B.S., Dutt, D.N., 2010. Computing fractal dimension of signals using multiresolution box-counting method. Int. J. Inf. Math. Sci. 6 (1), 50–65.

Rajesh, R., et al., 2018. Do features from short durational segments classify epileptic EEG signals effectively? In: 2018 IEEE Region 10 Humanitarian Technology Conference (R10-HTC), pp. 1–5.

Ruiz-Padial, E., Ibáñez-Molina, A.J., 2018. Fractal dimension of EEG signals and heart dynamics in discrete emotional states. Biol. Psychol. 137, 42–48.

San-Segundo, R., Gil-Martín, M., D'Haro-Enríquez, L.F., Pardo, J.M., 2019. Classification of epileptic EEG recordings using signal transforms and convolutional neural networks. Comput. Biol. Med. 109, 148–158.

Şeker, M., Özerdem, M.S., 2018. Application of Higuchi's fractal dimension for the statistical analysis of human EEG responses to odors. In: 2018 41st International Conference on Telecommunications and Signal Processing (TSP), pp. 1–4.

Sharma, M., Pachori, R.B., 2017. A novel approach to detect epileptic seizures using a combination of tunable-Q wavelet transform and fractal dimension. J. Mech. Med. Biol. 17 (7), 1740003.

Sharma, M., Pachori, R.B., Acharya, U.R., 2017. A new approach to characterize epileptic seizures using analytic time-frequency flexible wavelet transform and fractal dimension. Pattern Recogn. Lett. 94, 172–179.

Shi, C.-T., 2018. Signal pattern recognition based on fractal features and machine learning. Appl. Sci. 8 (8), 1327.

Smits, F.M., Porcaro, C., Cottone, C., Cancelli, A., Rossini, P.M., Tecchio, F., 2016. Electroencephalographic fractal dimension in healthy ageing and Alzheimer's disease. PLoS One 11 (2), e0149587.

Subasi, A., Kevric, J., Canbaz, M.A., 2019. Epileptic seizure detection using hybrid machine learning methods. Neural Comput. Appl. 31 (1), 317–325.

Tatum, W.O., Rubboli, G., Kaplan, P.W., Mirsatari, S.M., Radhakrishnan, K., Gloss, D., Caboclo, L.O., Drislane, F.W., Koutroumanidis, M., Schomer, D.L., et al., 2018. Clinical utility of EEG in diagnosing and monitoring epilepsy in adults. Clin. Neurophysiol. 129 (5), 1056–1082.

Thijs, R.D., Surges, R., O'Brien, T.J., Sander, J.W., 2019. Epilepsy in adults. Lancet 393 (10172), 689–701.

Upadhyaya, P., Bairy, G.M., Yagi, T., 2019. Computerized analysis of EEG to determine focal epilepsy. IEEJ Trans. Electron. Inform. Syst. 139 (5), 609–614.

Wijayanto, I., Hartanto, R., Nugroho, H.A., 2019a. Higuchi and Katz fractal dimension for detecting interictal and ictal state in electroencephalogram signal. In: 2019 11th International Conference on Information Technology and Electrical Engineering (ICITEE), pp. 1–6.

Wijayanto, I., Rizal, A., Humairani, A., 2019b. Seizure detection based on EEG signals using Katz fractal and SVM classifiers. In: 2019 5th International Conference on Science in Information Technology (ICSITech), pp. 78–82.

Wijayanto, I., Hadiyoso, S., Aulia, S., Atmojo, B.S., 2020. Detecting ictal and interictal condition of EEG signal using Higuchi fractal dimension and support vector machine. J. Phys. 1577 (1), 012016.

Xu, X., Cao, M., Ding, J., Gu, H., Lu, W., 2019. Emotional recognition of EEG signals based on fractal dimension. Int. J. Performabil. Eng. 15 (11), 3072–3080.

# Integer period discrete Fourier transform-based algorithm for the identification of tandem repeats in the DNA sequences

# 18

**Sunil Datt Sharma and Pardeep Garg**

*Department of Electronics and Communication Engineering, Jaypee University of Information Technology, Solan, India*

## Chapter outline

## 1 Introduction

Most of the DNA sequences possess specific repeated patterns of particular periods and hence the identification of these repeats plays a significant job to analyze the DNA sequences. There exists an association of repeated patterns with various diseases. It is well known that a string of nucleotides constitute the DNA sequences. These nucleotides are guanine (G), adenine (A), thymine (T), and cytosine (C). The respective periodicities exist in DNA sequences because of various nucleotide repeat patterns. The various biological functionalities of the living organism occur because of these repetitive patterns. Therefore, detection and analysis of repeated patterns in DNA sequences play a significant role in the field of biology, medicine, disease diagnosis, and forensic sciences (Gupta and Prasad, 2018).

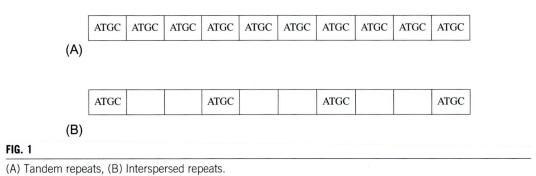

(A)

(B)

**FIG. 1**

(A) Tandem repeats, (B) Interspersed repeats.

The categorization of repeats existing in DNA sequences can be done as tandem and interspersed repeats, and it has been shown in Fig. 1A and B, respectively.

The tandem repeats (TRs) are the adjacent repeated patterns and interspersed repeats are the non-adjacent repeated patterns. Tandem repeats are also classified as satellite, minisatellite, microsatellite TRs, and these are shown in Fig. 2.

The number of copies, location, and pattern of TRs play an important role in the diagnosis of genetic diseases and cancer identification, etc. (Yin, 2017). TRs are also associated with various human diseases like Frederick's ataxia, some types of cancer, Fragile-X syndrome, Huntington's disease, and more than 40 other neuromuscular, neurodegenerative, and neurological diseases (Usdin, 2008). TRs are also applied to know about the human evolutionary history (Butler, 2003), genetic marker in microbial forensics, human identity, and for the investigation of the infectious disease irruptions

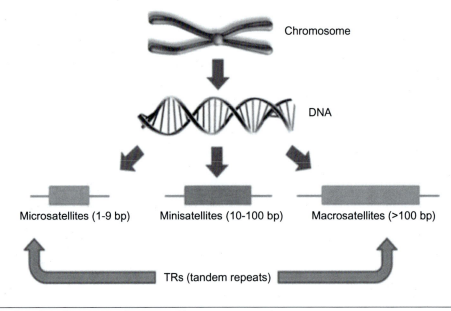

**FIG. 2**

Classification of tandem repeats (Leprae, n.d.).

(Cummings and Relman, 2002). To identify TRs in DNA sequences, periodicity present in DNA sequences has been utilized. Following are the key contributions of this chapter:

**(i)** Integer period discrete Fourier transform (IPDFT) has been applied to visualize the tandem repeats in DNA sequence.
**(ii)** Appropriate threshold selection.
**(iii)** The number of copies of tandem repeats has been enhanced.

## 2 Related work

Methods for the identification of the TRs have been classified into two categories such as string matching methods and signal processing methods. Lim et al. (2012) reviewed the string matching methods to identify the TRs. Currently, conversion of DNA characters to numerical values using numerical mapping schemes has provided the signal processing techniques a direction to analyze the genomic data (Sharma et al., 2011). Hence, the focus in this work is on the signal processing-based methods reported for the detection of TRs (Sharma et al., 2017). These methods are modified Fourier product spectrum (MFPS) (Tran et al., 2004), short time periodicity transform (STPT) (Buchner and Janjarasjitt, 2003), spectral repeat finder (SRF) (Sharma et al., 2004), Fourier product spectrum-based spectral methods for localization of tandem repeats (Pop, 2007; Pop and Lupu, 2008), exactly periodic subspace decomposition (EPSD) ( Jiang and Yan, 2011), optimized moving window spectral analysis (OMWSA) (Du et al., 2007), parametric spectral estimation (PSE) (Zhou et al., 2009), S-transform (Zribi et al., 2019), and adaptive S-transform (AST) (Sharma et al., 2014). Tran et al. proposed an MFPS for the identification of the approximate tandem repeats (Tran et al., 2004). Buchner et.al proposed a STPT to properly localize the periodicity of tandem repeat and the location of these periodicities using a periodogram. Periodicity transform is the basis of this method and multiple periodicities is the drawback of this method (Buchner and Janjarasjitt, 2003). As it is well known that Fourier analysis is a powerful tool to extract unknown periodicities in the DNA sequences in the proximity of deletion, substitution and insertion, a computer program-based method known as spectral repeat finder (SRF) has been developed by Sharma et al. the basis of which is Fourier transformation. In this method, firstly the pattern length of repeats which is obtained from the power spectrum of a DNA sequence is computed, and consequently, the identification of the location of repeats pattern has been performed using a sliding window approach (Sharma et al., 2004). Pop et al. have proposed an algorithm to detect the TRs in spectrogram using windowed discrete Fourier transform, the basis of which is the Fourier product spectrum (Pop, 2007; Pop and Lupu, 2008). As per the study from literature, it is observed that both the FT- and STPT-based methods have the drawback of multiple periodicities. Gupta et al. proposed EPSD method for the detection of TRs to find the solution to the problem of multiple periodicities ( Jiang and Yan, 2011). Liping et al. suggested an OMWSA to detect the DNA repeats, this method being perfect and more robust than Fourier transform-based spectral analysis in the proximity of deletion, substitution, and insertion; however, its drawback is that location of repeats is identified by inspecting the spectrogram (Du et al., 2007). Zhou et al. proposed the parametric spectral estimation (PSE) technique to detect the location of TRs and its pattern automatically (Zhou et al., 2009). However, PSE has limitations of order selection and selection of the appropriate window length. The S-transform-based method (Zribi et al., 2019), which employs p-nuc coding scheme, has been proposed to overcome the limitations of PSE. An adaptive S-transform-based algorithm (Sharma et al., 2014) for the TRs detection has been proposed by Sharma et al. In this chapter, an integer period discrete Fourier transform (Epps, 2009)-based algorithm for the TRs detection has been proposed. The remaining parts of this chapter have been described in the later sections.

## 3 Algorithm for detection of TRs

In this section, an algorithm based on the Integer period discrete Fourier transform (IPDFT) has been proposed to detect the tandem repeats (TRs) in DNA sequences and it has been depicted in Fig. 3. An example sequence with accession no. X64775 (NCBI, n.d) has been selected to explain the steps used in the algorithm for the TRs detection.

### 3.1 DNA sequences

DNA sequences contain the nucleotides or characters adenine (A), thymine (T), guanine (G) and cytosine (C), and these characters are considered inputs.

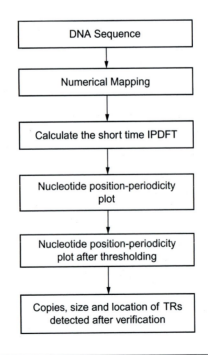

**FIG. 3**

Flow graph for the proposed algorithm.

## 3.2 Numerical mapping

Characters of the DNA sequences received from the previous step have been converted into numerical sequences using the electron-ion-interaction pseudo-potential (EIIP) mapping scheme. The EIIP mapping is preferred over other mapping schemes because it has less computational complexity (Sharma et al., 2011). The character to numerical conversion with an example has been shown in Fig. 4.

## 3.3 Short time integer period discrete Fourier transform

The IPDFT of a signal $x(n)$ is defined (Epps, 2009) using the following equation.

$$x_{IP}(p) = \sum_{n=0}^{N-1} x(n)e^{\frac{-j2\pi n}{p}}, \ p = 1,2,3,\ldots,P < N, \tag{1}$$

where $P$ is the maximum period. IPDFT is linearly related to periodicity "$p$," whereas the discrete Fourier transform (DFT) is linear with respect to the frequency.

To localize the TRs present in the DNA sequences, the short time IPDFT (STIPDFT) has been calculated using the following equation.

$$x_{IP}(p,m) = \sum_{n=0}^{N-1} x(n)*w(n-m)e^{\frac{-j2\pi n}{p}}, \tag{2}$$

where $w(n)$ is a hamming window, which is centered at nucleotides position $m=0$ initially, and further it is shifted by one nucleotide up to the end of the sequences. The 20*p window length has been selected for the experiment. Finally, nucleotides position versus periodicity plot has been plotted in Fig. 5.

## 3.4 Thresholding

Threshold has been calculated to identify the location of TRs of a particular periodicity and it is calculated using the following equation.

$$Th = mean\left(\frac{x5(p)}{\max(x5(p))}\right). \tag{3}$$

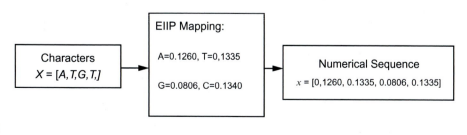

**FIG. 4**

Numerical conversion scheme.

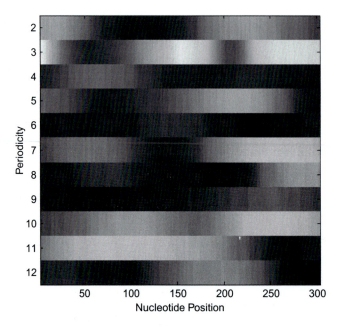

**FIG. 5**

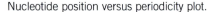

Nucleotide position versus periodicity plot.

where, $x5$ is the value of the sum of power spectrum along with position axis and it is given by –

$$x5(p) = \sum_{m=0}^{M} x_{IP}(p, m), \tag{4}$$

$$B_{IP}(p, m) = \begin{cases} 1, \text{ if } x_{IP}(p, m) \geq Th \\ 0, \text{ if } x_{IP}(p, m) \leq Th \end{cases} \tag{5}$$

Using Eq. (5), we have plotted the nucleotide position vs periodicity plot obtained postthresholding and it is shown in Fig. 6.

After thresholding, the periodicity 3, 7, 10, and 11 have been detected as candidate TRs along with their nucleotide positions 1–182 and 234–303, 234–289, 225–284, and 44–139, respectively.

## 3.5 Verification of the detected candidate TRs

The method proposed by Boeva et al. (2006) has been used to verify the candidate TRs detected after thresholding. Candidate TRs are the segments highlighted in Fig. 3, and these are located at the nucleotide positions 1–182 and 234–303, 234–289, 225–284, and 44–139. These candidate TRs after verification have been tabulated in Table 1.

In Table 1, it has been presented that the proposed algorithm has detected true TRs of periodicity 3 bps, and other falsely detected candidate TRs of periodicity 7, 10, and 11 have been removed after verification.

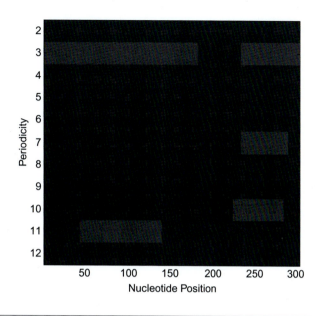

**FIG. 6**

Nucleotide position versus periodicity post-thresholding.

## 4 Performance analysis of the proposed algorithm

To assess the performance of the proposed algorithm for the TRs detections, DNA sequence having the accession number X64775 (NCBI, n.d) has been used in this study. The proposed algorithm for TRs detection has been implemented in MATLAB. The system used for simulation has 8 GB RAM, 64 bit operating system, and core i5 processor. The performance comparison of the proposed algorithm has been done with the reported methods. The comparison of results has been shown in Table 2.

From Table 2 and Fig. 7, it has been found that the proposed method has detected more number of copies as compared to other reported methods.

**Table 1** Verification of candidate TRs detected after thresholding.

| Sr. No. | Periodicity | Detected candidate TRs after thresholding | | Verification of detected candidate TRs | | |
| --- | --- | --- | --- | --- | --- | --- |
| | | Nucleotide position | Patterns | Location | Patterns | No. of copies |
| 1 | 3 | 1–182 | ATGGAGAGCGACTGCCAGTTCTTGGTGG | 19–24 | GTT CTT | 02 |
| | | | CGCCGCCCGCAGCCGCACATGTACT | 25–30 | GGT GGC | 02 |
| | | | ACGACACGGCGGCGG | 31–45 | GCC GCC GCA GCC GCA | 05 |
| | | | CGGCGGTGGACGAGGCGCAGTTCTT | | | |
| | | | GCGGCAGATGGTGGC | | | |
| | | | CGCGGCGGATCACCACGC | 50–58 | TAC TAC GAC | 03 |
| | | | GGCCGCCGCTGGGAG | 60–77 | CGG CGG CGG CGG CGG TGG | 06 |
| | | | AGGAGGCGGCGACGGCGA | | | |
| | | | CGGCGGCGGCGGCG | 78–83 | ACG AGG | 02 |
| | | | GCGGCGGCG | 89–94 | TTC TTG | 02 |
| | | | | 102–107 | TGG TGG | 02 |
| | | | | 108–116 | CCG CGG CGG | 03 |
| | | | | 117–123 | ATC ACC | 02 |

| | | | | | |
|---|---|---|---|---|---|
| 7 | 234–303 | AGACGCGTTCCACGCGCG<br>GCGGGCCAAGCTGGA<br>GCCGCGGGAGAAGGCG<br>GACGTGGCGCGGGAG<br>CTCGGG | 125–136 | GCG<br>GCC<br>GCC<br>GCT | 04 |
| | | | 142–183 | AGG<br>AGG<br>CGG<br>CGA<br>CGG<br>CGA<br>CGG<br>CGG<br>CGG<br>CGG<br>CGG<br>CGG<br>CG | 14 |
| | | | 250–255 | CGG<br>CGG | 02 |
| | | | 268–273 | CCG<br>CGG | 02 |
| | | | 274–279 | GAG<br>AAG | 02 |
| | | | Rejected | Rejected | |
| 2 | 234–289 | AGACGCGTTCCACG<br>CGCGGCGGGCCAAGCTG<br>GAGCCGCGGGGAGAA<br>GGCGGACGTGG | | | |

*Continued*

**Table 1** Verification of candidate TRs detected after thresholding—cont'd

| | | Detected candidate TRs after thresholding | | Verification of detected candidate TRs | | |
|---|---|---|---|---|---|---|
| Sr. No. | Periodicity | Nucleotide position | Patterns | Location | Patterns | No. of copies |
| 3 | 10 | 225–284 | GGTCGCTGGAGACGC<br>GTTCCACGCGCGGCGGGC<br>CAAGCTGGAGCCGCGGGA<br>GAAGGCGGA | Rejected | Rejected | Rejected |
| 4 | 11 | 11–139 | GACTGCCAGTTCTTGGTGG<br>CGCCGCCGCAGCCG<br>CACATGTACTACGACA<br>CGGCGGCGGGCGGT<br>GGACGAGGCGCAGTT<br>CTTGCGGCAGATGGTGG<br>CCGCGGCGGATCACC<br>ACGCGGCCGCGCTGGG | Rejected | Rejected | Rejected |

**Table 2** **Comparison with reported methods.**

| Periodicity | Method | Nucleotide position after thresholding | Nucleotides positions after verification | Consensus pattern | Copies | Total copies |
|---|---|---|---|---|---|---|
| 3 | Proposed method | 1–182 | 19–24 | GTT CTT | 02 | 53 |
| | | | 25–30 | GGT GGC | 02 | |
| | | | 31–45 | GCC GCC GCA GCC GCA | 05 | |
| | | | 50–58 | TAC TAC GAC | 03 | |
| | | | 60–77 | CGG CGG CGG CGG CGG TGG | 06 | |
| | | | 78–83 | ACG AGG | 02 | |
| | | | 89–94 | TTC TTG | 02 | |
| | | | 102–107 | TGG TGG | 02 | |
| | | | 108–116 | CCG CGG CGG | 03 | |
| | | | 117–123 | ATC ACC | 02 | |

*Continued*

**Table 2 Comparison with reported methods—cont'd**

| Periodicity | Method | Nucleotide position after thresholding | Nucleotides positions after verification | Consensus pattern | Copies | Total copies |
|---|---|---|---|---|---|---|
| | | | 125–136 | GCG GCC GCC GCT | 04 | |
| | | | 142–183 | AGG AGG CGG CGA CGG CGA CGG CGG CGG CGG CGG CGG CGG CGG | 14 | |
| | | | 250–255 | CGG CGG | 02 | |
| | | | 268–273 | CCG CGG | 02 | |
| | | | 274–279 | GAG AAG | 02 | |
| | AST (Sharma et al., 2014) | 19–44 | 20–25 | TTC TTG | 02 | 48 |
| | | | 25–42 | GCC | 06 | |
| | | 61–86 | 61–79 | GGC | 07 | |
| | | 89–104 | 89–94 | TTC(TTG) | 02 | |
| | | | 94–99 | GCG GCA | 02 | |
| | | 108–122 | 108–116 | CGG | 03 | |

**Table 2** Comparison with reported methods—cont'd

| Periodicity | Method | Nucleotide position after thresholding | Nucleotides positions after verification | Consensus pattern | Copies | Total copies |
|---|---|---|---|---|---|---|
| | | | 117–122 | ATC ACC | 02 | |
| | | 125–135 | 125–135 | CCG | 03 | |
| | | 141–149 | 141–149 | GAG | 03 | |
| | | 160–186 | 160–186 | CGG | 09 | |
| | | 194–207 | 194–199 | AGG AAG | 02 | |
| | | | 199–204 | GCG | 02 | |
| | | 211–223 | 211–219 | GGA | 03 | |
| | | 274–283 | 274–279 | GAG AAG | 02 | |
| | EMWD (Pop and Lupu, 2008) | 57–72 | 57–72 | CGG | 5.5 | 21 |
| | | 140–187 | 140–187 | GGC | 15.5 | |
| | Parametric spectral estimation (Du et al., 2007) | 45–90 | 49–57 | TAC | 03 | 24.7 |
| | | | 59–76 | CGG | 06 | |
| | | 140–200 | 141–188 | GGC | 15.7 | |

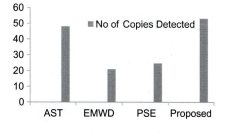

**FIG. 7**

Comparison of methods with w.r.t. total number of copies detected.

## 5 Conclusion

The proposed approach presented in this chapter has been applied successfully to identify TRs detection in the DNA sequences. It has been concluded that the performance of proposed method is better as compared to AST, EMWD, PSE, in terms of number of copies. Also, it has been concluded that fixed window length is the limitation of the proposed method and it may be overcome in future work. This chapter will also attract and motivate scientists and researchers of computer science, bioinformatics, medical sciences, and Big Data to do research in the area of genomics signal processing.

## References

Boeva, V., Regnier, M., Papatsenko, D., Makeev, V., Jan. 2006. Short fuzzy tandem repeats in genomic sequences identification and possible role in regulation of gene expression. Bioinformatics 22 (6), 676–684.

Buchner, M., Janjarasjitt, S., 2003. Detection and visualization of tandem repeats in DNA sequences. IEEE Trans. Signal Process. 51 (9).

Butler, J., 2003. Forensic DNA Typing: Biology and Technology behind STR Markers. Academic Press, London.

Cummings, C.A., Relman, D.A., 2002. Microbial forensics—cross-examining pathogens. Science 296, 1976–1979.

Du, L.P., Zhou, H.X., Yan, H., 2007. OMWSA: detection of DNA repeats using moving window spectral analysis. Bioinformatics 23 (5), 631–633. pp. 2280–2287, Sep. 2003.

Epps, J., 2009. A hybrid technique for the periodicity characterization of genomic sequence data. EURASIP J. Bioinform. Syst. Biol. 924601.

Gupta, S., Prasad, R., 2018. Searching exact tandem repeats in DNA sequences using enhanced suffix array. Curr. Bioinform. 13 (2), 216–222.

Jiang, R., Yan, H., 2011. Detection and 2-dimensional display of short tandem repeats based on signal decomposition. Int. J. Data Min. Bioinform. 5 (6), 661–690.

Lim, K.G., Kwoh, C.K., Hsu, L.Y., Wirawan, A., 2012. Review of tandem repeat search tools: a systematic approach to evaluating algorithmic performance. Brief. Bioinform. Page 1 of 15.

Leprae, n.d., Available at: https://www.jalma-icmr.org.in/LEPStr/leprae/microsatellites/leprae_micro.html (Accessesd May 2020).

NCBI, n.d., National Centre for Biotechnology Information (2020). https://www.ncbi.nlm.nih.gov (Accessed May 2020).

Pop, P.G., 2007. Tandem Repeats Localization Using Spectral Techniques [C]. IEEE Intelligent Computer Communication and Processing, Romania.

Pop, G.P., Lupu, E., 2008. DNA repeats detection using BW spectrograms. In: IEEE-TTTC International Conference on Automation, Quality and Testing, Robotics, AQTR 2008. Tome III, Romania, pp. 408–412.

Sharma, D., Issac, B., Raghava, G.P.S., Ramaswamy, R., 2004. Spectral repeat finder (SRF): identification of repetitive sequences using Fourier transforms. Bioinformatics 20 (9), 1405–1412.

Sharma, S.D., Shakya, D.K., Sharma, S.N., 2011. Advanced Numerical representation of DNA sequences. In: IEEE Proceeding of ICCET.

Sharma, S.D., Saxena, R., Sharma, S.N., 2014. Identification of microsatellites in DNA using adaptive S-transform. IEEE J. Biomed. Health Inform. 19 (3), 1097–1105.

Sharma, S.D., Saxena, R., Sharma, S.N., 2017. Tandem repeats detection in DNA sequences using Kaiser window based adaptive S-transform. Bio-Algorith. Med. Syst. 13 (3), 167–173. https://doi.org/10.1515/bams-2017-0014.

Tran, T.T., Emanuele II, V.A., Zhou, G.-T., 2004. Techniques for detecting approximate tandem repeats in DNA. In: Proceedings of IEEE International Conference on Acoustics, Speech, and Signal Processing. (ICASSP 2004). vol. 5, pp. 449–452.

Usdin, K., 2008. The biological effects of simple tandem repeats: lessons from the repeat expansion diseases. Genome Res. 18, 1011–1019.

Yin, C., 2017. Identification of repeats in DNA sequences using nucleotide distribution uniformity. J. Theor. Biol. 412, 138–145.

Zhou, H., Liping, D., Yan, H., 2009. Detection of tandem repeats in DNA sequences based on parametric spectral estimation. IEEE Trans. Inf. Technol. Biomed. 13 (5).

Zribi, S., Messaoudi, I., Oueslati, A.E., Lachiri, Z., 2019. Microsatellite's detection using the S -transform analysis based on the synthetic and experimental coding. Int. J. Adv. Comput. Sci. Appl. 10 (3).

# A blockchain solution for the privacy of patients' medical data

# 19

**Riya Sapra and Parneeta Dhaliwal**

*Department of Computer Science and Technology, Manav Rachna University, Faridabad, India*

## Chapter outline

## 1 Introduction

Healthcare has been an important industry for everyone across the globe. It always requires the best the technology to facilitate various stakeholders of the industry for the treatment of diseases. Because of the advancements and improvements in information technology, the results of medical research are proving better which helps in preventing and treating diseases. It has also resulted in conversion of the medical records into large databases of electronic health records (EHR) which can be analyzed and compared so as to reach better conclusions. EHRs can be used by patients to take advice from

Machine Learning, Big Data, and IoT for Medical Informatics. https://doi.org/10.1016/B978-0-12-821777-1.00025-2

different doctors anywhere across the globe. On the other hand, doctors can also use EHRs to consult with their peers and diagnose accordingly.

EHRs help the patients preserve their records as paper records get damaged easily. EHRs also help to keep track of medications record for the disease. But EHRs are prone to tampering and misuse as they can be easily used by hospitals or doctors without the consent of the patient. Also, while in communication, EHRs may be tampered by any intruder in the network. So the problem of security and privacy of EHRs arises. Generally, EHRs are shared using cloud services which are prone to cyber attacks where attackers can steal patient's sensitive medical data or manipulate it. Storing data on centralized data storage can also lead to data loss or single-point-of-failure.

Instead of cloud services, blockchain technology benefits in securing data from malicious users as well as data loss through single-point-of-failure. In the past few years, a significant number of blockchain-based applications for securing patient's or medical data have been designed and used successfully. These applications help bring all the healthcare stakeholders like patients, doctors, insurance agencies, hospital management, etc. under one umbrella and help in exchanging information among them in a far better way. This brings transparency among all the stakeholders. In such applications, patients are given complete access control about what is to be shared with whom. This prevents data from unauthorized access.

There are several advantages associated with using blockchain technology for maintaining EHRs. The data are stored after encryption which prevents it from any unwanted manipulation or data leakage. Blockchain (Sapra and Dhaliwal, 2021b) protects any corruption of data with the fact that data stored in network are immutable, once written, it cannot be edited. Also, in the case of permissioned blockchain, various access rights are available which makes the patients as the owner of their own medical data and they can share data with whoever they want and can also remove their access whenever required. As it is a distributed ledger technology, it does not suffer from single-point-of failure.

Many stakeholders are benefitted through EHRs and lots of data are shared among them for various purposes. This brings the need of high level of security and privacy controls in EHR applications so that no medical data are misused by anyone. Any data manipulation may lead to fatal problems as minor changes in any medical report can change the whole process of diagnosis of the patient. Few years back, healthcare industry suffered a lot due to tampering of medical data. Researchers and developers are continuously working hard to find solution for these critical problems.

Various healthcare applications are implemented using new-age technologies and upgraded continuously for better results. Combination of various technologies like Internet of Things (IoT), machine learning, big data analytics, cloud computing, blockchain, etc. are being used to provide flawless experience to various stakeholders of the industry. This chapter discusses various stakeholders in healthcare industry and challenges faced by them. Further, various laws for data protection in different countries are highlighted. This chapter also describes blockchain technology and existing applications in healthcare industry. At last, the chapter is concluded with a framework of blockchain-based application for privacy protection of patient's data.

## 2 Stakeholders of healthcare industry

In general, stakeholders are the people or organizations that are affected by any activity of the industry or affect the industry with some of their activity, i.e., they are involved in some way to that industry. Health care is a service industry meant to provide services for improving one's health by preventing, diagnosing, and treating diseases. All the stakeholders have a set of responsibilities to maintain a quality healthcare facility.

Any neglected responsibility may result in a negative impact on the goals of the industry. The major stakeholders include patients, healthcare providers (doctors, nurses, hospitals, nursing homes, clinics, etc.), government, insurance providers, pharmaceutical firms, etc. Most of the time, all of the stakeholders are dependent on one another as they need to share lots of information among themselves. Fig. 1 depicts the association of various stakeholders of healthcare industry.

Healthcare is motivated by the social and economic atmosphere. It may vary from country to country or community to community. Different countries have different laws associated with healthcare institutions. Stakeholders, in general, can be divided into three categories for any type of industry. For the healthcare industry, the stakeholders can be partitioned into three categories as follows:

1. **External stakeholders:** These stakeholders do not work for the organization but are affected by any decision made within the organization. Healthcare industry has to deal with a lot of external stakeholders. All these external stakeholders of healthcare industry fall mainly in these three categories:
   **(a)** Stakeholders who provide some input to healthcare industry: This may include patients, suppliers, and financial industry, etc. These stakeholders help the healthcare industry to survive. So it can be said that healthcare industry depends on these stakeholders to continue with their services.
   **(b)** Stakeholders who have some special interests: These may include government agencies, labor union, media, political associations, accrediting associations etc.
   **(c)** Stakeholders who compete with them: These are the competitors with the same business ideas. In healthcare industries, hospitals compete with each other to provide better services to patients.

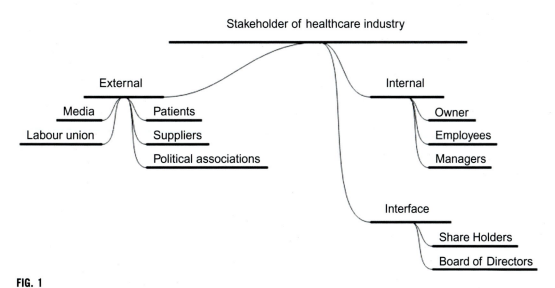

**FIG. 1**

Stakeholders of healthcare industry.

2. **Internal stakeholders:** These stakeholders work within the organization, such as owners, employees, and managers. Employees work for earning salaries. Managers too work for earning salaries. Owners work for gaining profits and improving the reputation of their organization.
3. **Interface stakeholders:** These stakeholders are an interface between the organization and the rest of the environment, such as board of directors and shareholders.

## 2.1 Patients

Healthcare industry need to be patient-centric to benefit them with quality and timely services. Various policies and programs are regularly made keeping in mind the interests and benefits of the patients. Healthcare providers may also need to understand the patient's values and culture to provide better policies for them. Few countries consider patient's suggestions also while deciding on policies for the healthcare sector.

In case of digital healthcare applications, the applications need to be patient-centric as well. All access controls must be in patients control as deciding on to share or hide any of their health records is their fundamental right. With EHRs, it has become easy for patients to share their records for insurance claims which can be directly claimed without any delay. Blockchain-based platforms facilitate patients with these services and ease their work. Patients can easily access their health records with respect to time and also share them wherever they want. They can also look at the summarized reports in the form of graphs to check for their improvement in health. This can also help them know better about the status of their health after the particular diagnosis.

## 2.2 Pharmaceutical companies

Pharmaceutical companies invest lots of money to research and produce drugs/medicines for patients. Patients and healthcare providers (doctors, nurses, hospitals, nursing homes, clinics, etc.) are all dependent on these companies for the treatment of diseases. These companies study the diseases, research, and invent new drugs/medicines for the diseases. Drug discovery and marketing are major expenses for these companies. The pharmaceutical companies require medical data and reports of patients for researching and discovering new drugs. This is made easier after medical records have gone electronic and are being stored after encryption through blockchain-based applications.

Pharmaceutical companies also face trouble during the drugs sale and purchase. As medical drugs move through various vendors in between, it becomes difficult to trace the authenticity or origin of the drug. Blockchain-based applications provide live tracing of drugs throughout its supply chain. With other technologies like Internet of Things in use, other parameters like temperature conditions of the drugs during its delivery can also be traced.

## 2.3 Healthcare providers (doctors, nurses, hospitals, nursing homes, clinics, etc.)

Healthcare providers include hospitals, doctors, nursing staff, clinics, nursing homes, medical practitioners, nutritionists and dieticians, and many more. Hospitals, clinics, and nursing homes are the places where patients come for getting diagnosis for any injury or disease. Doctors and other medical staff ensure that patients are given proper care and right diagnosis. Hospitals need to keep track of the patients, their records, diagnosis provided, medical expenses, and other details. E-platforms help manage all the details of patients and their records. These records need to be shared with insurance companies for the payments via insurance claims. Blockchain-based platforms ease the task of sharing the records and reports with the insurance companies and maintain the security of the data as well.

Many a times these records need to be shared with other health agencies or doctors to consult about a particular scenario or disease, and blockchain applications can ensure prevention of any misuse of data. The access controls of sharing data are with patients, so patients can control the use and spread of data anytime. Also with the use of applications, doctors, and nurses can track the progress of diagnosis and check for summarized reports. This helps them in better understanding of the situation in less time.

## 2.4 Government

Government has a big role to play in health care. Every country especially developing countries has government-funded hospitals for weaker sections of the society to provide good but low-priced healthcare services. Apart from hospitals, various healthcare schemes and policies are also designed by the government of every country. For every financial session, every government spares some funds to be invested in health care to ensure quality healthcare facilities to its citizens. This way, the government makes budget and other plans for the expenditure to be done in healthcare industry. Government also helps in spreading awareness about healthy practices and living styles among its citizens through various information channels.

Government also keeps a track of birth rate, death rate, and gender equality of the country or state and formulates schemes and policies for the same. It also tracks the reasons of death in the country so as to make the country aware about particular diseases. Blockchain-based application can connect all the hospitals of the country and gather all the required details very easily. Summarized reports with respect to a location or country as a whole can be analyzed and worked on.

## 2.5 Insurance companies

Insurance agencies be it government or private are a big role player in the healthcare industry nowadays. These companies provide financial plans for the expenses to be met in any illness or injury. These companies make quality healthcare facilities affordable for the people by helping them financially in the time of unpredictable events. These companies charge annual fee and provide discounted or no-cost medical services at designated hospitals or doctors. They also provide access to low-cost annual health checkups or no-cost mandatory checkups, thereby promoting quality health for the individuals.

Big organizations take collective plans for all their employees to promote the quality health within their organizations and also do annual checkups to make aware their employees of staying fit and healthy. These insurance companies also have tie-ups with hospitals for no-cost services to the people. To avail the financial help from insurance companies, people need to provide proofs of their medical records. In the past it used to be a very tedious task as copies of medical records needed to be submitted for using the insurance claims. Now with EHRs and blockchain-based applications, the process of sharing medical records with the insurance agencies is just a click task. These applications have made sharing of medical records easier for all the stakeholders of the healthcare industry.

These are some of the critical stakeholders in deciding various decisions and policies for the healthcare industry. So, any EHR platform needs to be made according to at least these above-mentioned stakeholders.

## 3  Data protection laws for healthcare industry

With all data going electronically in the healthcare industry came the need to secure it. We need to protect patient's data to prevent it from theft, misuse, and manipulation. New technologies have transformed the management of medicines and medical records throughout the world. Last decade was the decade of e-health revolution as lots of e-health applications came to the market to facilitate patients, doctors, and insurance companies. Different countries have formulated various laws to safeguard its citizen's medical data. Countries like Canada, Netherlands, United Kingdom, United States, etc. have designed and implemented privacy protection rights of medical data and many other countries are in the process for the same.

- **Australia:** In the country, an e-health system called "Personally Controlled Electronic Health Record (PCEHR)" (Andrews et al., 2014) was launched to facilitate the citizens with quality healthcare information. It is a citizen's choice to use or not to use this e-health system for maintaining or sharing its health records. With the user's permission, the data can be shared with doctors or hospitals. It abides by PCEHR Act 2012 which defines the information related to the collection of personal data by PCEHR, its purpose, and where that data are shared and used. This helps prevent personal information from manipulation, misuse, and unauthorized access.
- **Canada:** In Canada, "Personal Information Protection and Electronic Document Act (PIPEDA)" (Austin, 2006) prevents any breach or misuse of personal information. It is applicable to all the commercial sectors handling personal data. Data controllers need to specify the personal disclosure to control or maintain individual's sensitive data. The citizens can file complaint against the person or institution misusing their personal information. Disobeying PIPEDA in Canada may lead to criminal prosecution also.
- **Turkey:** Turkey came with "Data Protection Law (DPL)" (Greenleaf, 2017) in 2016 with a goal to make aware of data protection among the citizens of the nation. According to the law, the data controllers may get multiple obligations while handling any sort of sensitive data. If there is a transfer of personal data to some other country, the destination country's organization or person will also have to commit the protection of data as per DPL.
- **Qatar:** Qatar also issued "Personal Data Privacy Law" (Greenleaf, 2017) in 2016 for privacy of electronic personal data. This law is meant for organizations which use or share personal data of minors or adults. These organizations need to take permissions from the individuals or their parents (in case of minors) prior to using their personal data.
- **United Kingdom:** The citizens and organizations in United Kingdom abide by "Data Protection Act 2018" (Regulation, 2018). It controls the way of using personal information within businesses, government, or organizations. Anyone using personal information need to follow certain rules:
  - Its usage must be fair and transparent.
  - It must be used for a specified purpose only.
  - It must be accurate and need to be updated if required.
  - There should be no unlawful practice or unauthorized access.
- **United States:** "Health Insurance Portability and Accountability Act (HIPAA)" (Annas, 2003) is a medical privacy protection law, first enacted in 1996 by the United States and later revised many times. HIPAA designed the security standards to be adopted in healthcare industry while handling

electronic records. The law is meant for every entity or organization which records or shares any electronic health record. In HIPAA, they are called covered entity. These entities need to safeguard the electronic health information from any unauthorized access or modification and hence must adopt appropriate measures to protect the personal data.

- **India:** India proposes a new law called "Digital Information Security in Healthcare Act (DISHA)" (Bhavaraju, 2018) for healthcare sector. The objective of DISHA is to:
  - Organize and maintain national and state level health authority.
  - Embed privacy and security features in electronic health data.
  - Make regulations for storing and exchanging of data.

DISHA will be implemented soon in the country. This will bring data security and control of patient's sensitive information. In India, the electronic healthcare data are handled by the healthcare providers and may have control over sharing and manipulation of it as well. DISHA will help provide these data access controls to patients for their own data manipulation and sharing.

Various other countries have also formulated laws in different names with the prime motto of protecting patient's sensitive data from any unauthorized access. These laws guide the various stakeholders of healthcare industry to work in a legal manner and keep patient's data safe and secure.

## 4 Medical data management

In earlier days, patient's information or their medical records used to be restricted to patient or the hospital in paper records. No transfer or exchange of any information occurs at any end. Hence the medical records or the patient's information was safe. In the current scenario, all hospitals record the entire patient's information, their reports, and everything electronically. At any point of time, the entire historical patient's data can be seen. This helps in tracking the patient's illness for better future treatments. In this way, electronic records have so many benefits over paper records. It can help doctors in consultations with other doctors anywhere across the globe whenever required. The medical data sharing is also largely done with the insurance companies for reimbursements of loans.

Also in (Koshti et al., 2016) health monitoring systems, all the data are monitored remotely by doctors. In such scenario, the doctors are continuously monitoring the patient with the help of electronic data coming from the machines attached to the patient. The data are being shared with the doctors via internet. These remote monitoring systems help both patient and doctor to reach each other and get the diagnosis done at their respective places.

Apart from so many benefits of sharing medical data among various stakeholders of healthcare industry, it can create troubles if it gets manipulated at any point of sharing. Also there could be privacy issues if the data reach any unauthorized person. Hence information technology (IT) plays an important role in the management of medical data. Some of the popular digital technologies and techniques that are involved in management of medical data are listed below.

- **Internet of Things (IoT):** This is a technology of internet connected devices which can communicate to each other via messages. There are numerous applications using IoT (Sapra and Dhaliwal, 2020a) like self-driving cars, smart watches, smart homes, etc. In health care, the health monitoring systems are a pure application of IoT. The devices like ECG, blood pressure, blood glucose, body temperature, sweat sensor, EMG, EEG, etc. may be connected to get all the updated results which will be continuously and automatically shared to the doctors via internet. This entire task is done without any human intervention.

- **Cloud computing:** Cloud computing provides services related to hardware storage and software solutions via internet. With the help of cloud storage, one can store or backup his data over the server. Also, there are software solutions being provided via internet for the manipulation of data. In most of the healthcare applications, the medical data may be stored at various locations on some server. In health monitoring system, a lot of data processing is also done through cloud computing. Cloud computing has become the integral part of all the digital applications.

- **Cryptography:** Cryptography deals with encryption and decryption of data with the help of hashing algorithms. It helps in protecting data from any unintended user. Encrypting the data makes it difficult for anyone to know exactly what is written which protects it from any unintended access or manipulation. Cryptography is used in a lot of applications to preserve its data for cloud storage or sharing it with someone.

- **Blockchain technology:** It is a nascent technology initially meant for financial applications and now is being used by almost all areas of applications. This technology makes use of cryptography to store data in a time-stamped manner which cannot be edited. There are many healthcare applications which have started using blockchain to secure their data.

## 5 Issues and challenges of healthcare industry

With a variety of stakeholders involved in the healthcare industry, the digital scenario of the industry faces a lot of privacy and security issues. Technology experts and researchers are working on different technologies to resolve the variety of issues arising through healthcare monitoring systems and applications. Great advancements have been made in sensor technology for efficient collection of data in health monitoring systems and blockchain technology has also brought improvements in sharing of the data. Some of the major issues faced by the healthcare industry are listed in Fig. 2.

- **Data privacy:** Any healthcare application may include lots of sensitive data like patient's identity, their health records, prescriptions, bills, insurance provider details, and much more. Privacy laws and policies need to be defined for access and usage of the medical data by various stakeholders of the industry. Patients must be the owner of their own medical data and must have the right to share their data or remove someone's access to their own data.

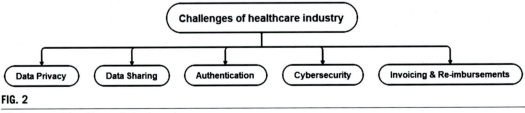

**FIG. 2**

Challenges of healthcare industry.

- **Data security:** Critical data need extra attention for their security. Cloud-based data are very prone to manipulations and thefts. In health monitoring systems, all the data are stored somewhere on any cloud servers which make them vulnerable. These data need to be well-preserved to prevent data breaches and cyber attacks.
- **Authentication:** The digital content brings the risk of availability to anyone. There is always a need for good authentication mechanism with the digital content. Medical records contain critical data so their storage and sharing require a good authentication system so that the data are not visible to any unintended user. Biometric authentication is also possible while logging in by doctors, patients, and insurance providers to provide better level of security.
- **Cyber security:** Applications related to health care involves patient's sensitive data whether it is their identity or their medical records. Any manipulation to such data can cause havoc. So handling such type of data makes the application very critical. As the cases of data theft and data manipulation is very normal these days, utmost care needs to be taken while handling such important data. The application need to be secured enough to protect from cyber crime.
- **Invoicing and reimbursement:** Invoicing and reimbursements is a very big challenge of healthcare applications. Majority of patients have a health insurance plan with them, so whenever there are any doctor's visits or checkups or hospital admissions, all bills need to be provided to insurance providers with the proofs. In earlier days, the patients need to give all the bills-related proofs to the insurance providers themselves by scanning the documents and sharing it with them. This was a big trouble for patients as it involves delay in payment and there were also chances of fraud documents being shared. Now with the healthcare applications, the bills are directly shared with insurance providers by the hospitals, and all settlements are done directly, which has eased patient's work.

## 6 Blockchain technology

Blockchain (Sapra and Dhaliwal, 2021a) is a distributed ledger technology which stores transactions in chronological order and does not allow any modification to it. Its features make the technology robust which is the reason for its popularity. The technology is being used in majority of application areas like banking (Guo and Liang, 2016), insurance (Crawford, 2017), entertainment (Liao and Wang, 2018), retail (Chakrabarti and Chaudhuri, 2017.), etc. Initially, blockchain technology was being used only in financial applications. This resulted in a huge number of cryptocurrencies. In today's market, there are more than 4000 cryptocurrencies (List of all cryptocurrency|CoinLore, 2020) available. After few years, the technology was adopted by a large number of nonfinancial applications (Sapra and Dhaliwal, 2018) to record the transfer and storage of data. Few of the important terms related to blockchain technology are listed below:

**Peers/Nodes:** In a blockchain network, the participants in the network are called as peers or nodes and hence it is also called a peer-to-peer (P2P) technology. P2P provides a transparent communication system among the peers and does not involve any third party to verify the transactions. There can be three types of nodes in any blockchain network:

- **Simple node:** These nodes participate in the network by doing transactions within the network. They neither validate any transactions nor maintain any copy of the blockchain ledger.

- **Full node:** These nodes store the copy of blockchain and validate the transactions happening in the blockchain network. There are many full nodes in the network. So if few nodes are down, it does not impact the efficiency of the network.
- **Miner node:** Miner nodes are the creator of blocks in the network. They store the whole copy of blockchain, validate transactions, and mine (create) the blocks. The mining process for blockchain networks differ from one blockchain network to another depending on the type and requirement of blockchain network.

**Transactions:** Transactions are generally referred to any financial transfer. In blockchain applications, transactions can be a financial transfer, data transfer, data storage, automatic code execution, etc. depending on the blockchain platform.

**Hash:** Hash is a fixed value output for any sized input after getting processed by a hash function. A hash function is meant for the encryption of data using an algorithm so that it cannot be understood by anyone. There are a variety of hash functions like SHA-1, SHA-256, RSA, MD5, etc. Every hash function takes a string and a key as input to convert the string to a fixed size hash. Table 1 shows some hash function conversions for SHA-256 hash function. A small change in the input string totally changes the output hash value. This makes it nearly impossible for anyone to know the input string. This process of hashing is used while creating a block. All the transactions are first converted to hashes and then stored on block which makes it hard to tamper.

**Block:** Blockchain contains a long chain of blocks. A block consists of a predefined number of transactions happening in real time as per the blockchain application. Apart from transactions, every block has a block header which contains the following elements:

- **Root hash:** Root hash is evaluated as a hash value obtained by combining the hashes of all the transactions present in a block. It follows a bottom up process of evaluation as shown in Fig. 3. In step 1, all the transactions in a block are converted to their corresponding hashes. In step 2, two consecutive hashes combine to form a single hash. Step two is repeated again and again till a single hash is created. This hash is called as Merkle root hash or root hash of the block.
- **Nonce:** Nonce is an arbitrary number which acts as a significance of the difficulty level for the miners of the block. The miners need to evaluate nonce as a part of mining.
- **Timestamp:** Timestamp signifies the time of creation of block.
- **Previous block hash:** Every block in the network stores the root hash of previous block so as to connect to it. The first block of every blockchain is called genesis block. It does not have any previous root hash and stores the basic details of the network.

| Table 1 SHA-256 hash conversions. | |
|---|---|
| **Input** | **Output** |
| A sends 100 dollars to B | 7fe48bd557e0a4b65f2fc590e5b69031069aeaac868efba4511c1c60a06f93dd |
| C sends 100 dollars to B | 52c5eedf4c1210887cbe258d9b10cf66f469c20d45a97901944fdd93817fc344 |
| C sends 10 dollars to A | 5fd875e9fff1d86b5b96041260989147fd46b27562a9c6267ba85b5d4ff3a104 |

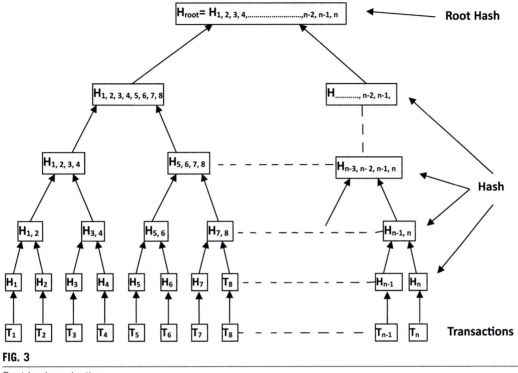

**FIG. 3**

Root hash evaluation.

**Mining:** The miner nodes in a blockchain network gather all validated transactions, convert to hashes, evaluate root hash and nonce to create a block, this is called mining of blocks in a blockchain network. In a blockchain network, there are a number of miners who mine the same block at the same time and compete with each other to mine first and gets rewarded with the mining fee.

**Consensus Protocol:** Blockchain network includes a variety of nodes. A lot of protocols need to be finalized to bring trust within the network. Consensus protocol or algorithms include the procedure for choosing miner, participants, their access rights, block creation, etc. Proof of work (POW) (Gramoli, 2020) was the first consensus protocol defined for Bitcoin. Other algorithms include Proof of Stake (PoS) (Kiayias et al., 2017), Proof of Burn (PoB) (Karantias et al., 2019), Proof of Elapsed Time (PoET) (Chen et al., 2017).

**Smart Contract:** Smart contract (Sapra and Dhaliwal, 2020b) is the programming attached to the blockchain system for automatic working. They have brought a new revolution to the digital scenario of the transactions and payments. They automate processes in blockchain system. Applications like supply chain management (Saberi et al., 2019), voting systems (Hjálmarsson et al., 2018), mortgage payments (Gout, 2017), etc. are employing smart contracts for their automatic transaction processes.

## 6.1 Features of blockchain

Blockchain technology has been popular from the very beginning because of its features like decentralized, append only, anonymity, etc. The technology is designed to bring trust in the network without adding any third party client and hidden user's identity. Some of the important features listed in Fig. 4 are as follows:

- **Decentralized:** The data in blockchain are stored at multiple locations which make them better for any centralized storage system. Whenever a particular number of transactions happen, a block is created and shared with all the peers of the network. All the full nodes and miner nodes store the same copy of the blockchain, so if a node gets down, the blockchain network keeps on running with the remaining nodes.
- **Anonymity:** In blockchain network, the nodes of the network are assigned a unique user ID which helps in keeping the identity of the user hidden. Also, every transaction is digitally signed to verify the identity of the node.
- **Transparent:** In public blockchain, anyone can join the blockchain network, read, write, or monitor the transactions. This makes the transactions of the blockchain network transparent to all the users with the user's identity hidden with unique user ID.
- **Immutability:** Blockchain works on the principle of append only transactions. Any transaction cannot be edited or rolled back in time. Even any intruder cannot make any changes to any transaction as it will require the root hash to change which is stored in the next block too, making it immutable.
- **Time-stamped:** The time of happening of any transaction or creation of a block is stored in block. This brings another level of transparency and clarity of happening of any event in blockchain network.
- **Autonomous:** With the advancements in blockchain technology, smart contracts have been designed for many applications. Smart contract are the programmable part of blockchain which executes after it meets certain criteria or condition. These contracts are of big use in automatic payments, insurance reimbursements, loan payments etc.

## 6.2 Types of blockchain

In the initial years of blockchain technology, public blockchain was majorly used for cryptocurrencies and some financial applications. With time, lots of changes were adopted to use blockchain in various application areas and various types of blockchain network were created and used. As per access rights, there can be majorly three types of blockchain network as shown in Table 2.

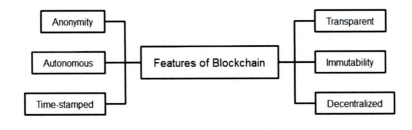

**FIG. 4**

Features of blockchain.

**Table 2  Private vs. public vs. federated blockchain.**

| Property/type | Private | Federated | Public |
|---|---|---|---|
| Read access | Public/restricted | Public/restricted | Public |
| Write access | Restricted | Restricted | Public |
| Architecture | Partially decentralized | Partially decentralized | Decentralized |
| Identity | Known | Known | Anonymous |
| Transaction frequency | Low | Low | High |
| Transaction cost | Less | Less | High |
| Transaction commit speed | Fast | Fast | Slow |
| Network scope | Everyone belongs to an organization | Only few organizations participate in network | Anyone can join the network |
| Miner | Miners are within the organization | Miners are selected among the designated set of organizations | Anyone can be miner |
| Data tempering | Possible | Possible | Not possible |
| Energy consumption | Less | Less | High |
| Consensus algorithms | Proof of authority, proof of elapsed time, Raft etc. | Proof of authority, delegated proof of stake etc. | Proof of work, proof of stake, proof of activity etc. |
| Examples | Monax, BankChain | EWF, R3 | Litecoin, Bitcoin |

- **Public blockchain:** Public blockchain is transparent to everyone. Anyone from outside can join the network and become part of the blockchain network. After joining the network, anyone can read, transact or mine in the network. The number of transactions in the network is high with a high transaction cost. Most of the cryptocurrencies are public blockchain.
- **Federated blockchain:** Federated blockchain is a partially decentralized blockchain with access to restricted people say few organizations. The identity of the participants is generally known as the number of participants is less as compared to public blockchain. Also the frequency of transaction and transaction cost is low as compared to federated blockchain.
- **Private blockchain:** Private blockchain is generally restricted to a small group like employees of an organization. The identity of the participants is known. Transaction frequency is less and few selected participants are only allowed to mine the block. The system is partially decentralized.

The above categorization of blockchain is according to the access control for the participants of a blockchain network. There can be another categorization of blockchain network on the basis of selection of miners. If anyone is allowed to mine the blocks, it is permissionless blockchain network, else it is permissioned network. Both of the blockchain networks are distributed networks and use consensus algorithms. The difference between both categories is shown in Table 3.

| Table 3 Permissioned vs. permissionless blockchain. | |
|---|---|
| **Permissioned blockchain** | **Permissionless blockchain** |
| Partially decentralized | Decentralized |
| Fast transaction execution | Slow transaction execution |
| Low transaction cost | High transaction cost |
| Restricted participants | Anyone can be part of network |
| Network can be administered | Network is transparent |

- **Permissionless blockchain:** In this blockchain system, anyone can elect himself or herself to be the miner for the blockchain network. It is similar to public blockchain network. This network is difficult to monitor but provides high level of transparency. E.g., Bitcoin.
- **Permissioned blockchain:** In permissioned blockchain, participants are selected within the network to be the miner on the basis of some criteria as per the consensus algorithm of the blockchain network. This network can be monitored easily via an administrator or a group of administrators. E.g., Ripple.

## 6.3 Working of blockchain

Blockchain works in a decentralized manner. The network is always running even if few nodes are down at a particular point of time. All the nodes in the network are given a unique ID to keep them anonymous in the network. So if anyone wants to transact in the network, he needs the unique ID of the receiver. Also, the transactions in the network are signed digitally by the sender. The working of blockchain network is shown in Fig. 5.

Creation of a block and appending to the existing blockchain network is a step-by-step process. It starts with a request of a transaction by any of the peers in the network. Whenever any peer wants to do any financial or non-financial transaction to any other peer, the transaction is first broadcasted in the network. It will be validated by the full nodes and the miner nodes. More than 50% of the nodes must validate the transaction, so that the transaction can be considered for addition to the blockchain. After the validation of the transaction, it will be added to the new block in the process.

Once a certain number of transactions are added to the block, root hash will be evaluated. Nonce will be calculated by the miners and one of the miners with required nonce will be selected for proposing the new block to the blockchain network. This selected block will be added to the existing blockchain and all the transactions of the new block will be confirmed/committed. The time for a transaction to confirm depends on the type of the blockchain network and the consensus protocol used by the blockchain network.

## 7 Blockchain applications in healthcare

Blockchain technology is being adopted in a wide range of application areas because of its features like distributed computing, encryption, no appending, etc. It is also being used in healthcare applications to store and share medical data of patients like Medrec (Ekblaw and Azaria, 2016), MedShare

Blockchain works in a decentralized manner. The network is always running even if few nodes are down at a

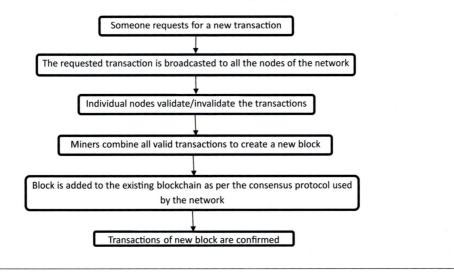

**FIG. 5**

Working of blockchain.

(Fan et al., 2018), etc. These blockchain-based healthcare applications have proved to be better in authentication, identity management, data sharing, and automatic transactions. Some of the blockchain-based healthcare applications are listed in Table 4.

Medrec (Ekblaw and Azaria, 2016) is an Ethereum blockchain-based medical platform for patient's medical record management. It provides complete access controls to patients for the sharing of their medical records. It facilitates the patients with the complete historical log of data exchange done with any of the users of the application. Patients can receive their records from any of medical service

**Table 4** Blockchain applications in health care.

| Application | Blockchain type | Smart contract | Data encryption |
|---|---|---|---|
| Medrec | Public | Yes | No |
| MeDShare | Federated | Yes | No |
| MedBlock | Public | No | Yes |
| Gem health network | Federated | Yes | Yes |
| OmniPHR | Federated | No | No |
| PSN | Federated | No | Yes |
| Healthcare data gateway | Public | No | Yes |
| BBDS | Federated | No | Yes |
| Smart Care | Federated | Yes | No |
| MedSBA | Private | Yes | Yes |
| ModelChain | Private | Yes | Yes |

provider through the application which can be viewed or shared further, if required. Hence, Medrec is a patient-centric decentralized electronic medical record management platform for accessing and sharing of patient's medical records.

Gem Health Network (Mettler, 2016) is another Ethereum-based blockchain platform meant for synchronizing electronic health information with various stakeholders of the healthcare industry. It focuses on a patient-centric approach to electronic record retrieving and sharing, keeping data security at its best. It combines individuals, healthcare experts, and businesses to provide transparent access to everyone. OmniPHR (Roehrs et al., 2017) is also a distributed platform for synchronizing all electronic health information of patients at one place from various healthcare organizations. It allows patients to maintain their historical personal health records (PHR) and keep a track on data sharing at the same time.

Another approach (Zhang et al., 2016) uses blockchain technology for pervasive social network (PSN) of medical sensors. In a PSN, medical sensors act as nodes and collect data continuously. These data need to be shared among other nodes as well as to the data clouds. These scenarios are used especially in disease monitoring or remote health care. This approach creates a health blockchain with medical sensors as nodes of the blockchain network. The sensor nodes share data among themselves which is written to the blocks after encryption. This ensures secure sharing of medical data within the network.

A smartphone application Healthcare Data Gateway (Yue et al., 2016) has been proposed for patients to access, share, and manage their medical data on the ease of a smartphone. All the medical data are stored on the blockchain platform and any request to access the data is evaluated using a purpose-centric access control mechanism. This makes the whole process simple and secure. Another Blockchain-based data sharing (BBDS) approach (Xia et al., 2017b) for EHRs has been proposed for cloud environments. It allows only verified users to enter the blockchain network and everyone's log of actions is also stored in the blockchain system to ensure high-end security of the medical data. BBDS also uses encryption mechanism to encrypt the data in the blockchain network. This keeps all access to the sensitive data under control.

Similarly, MedShare (Xia et al., 2017a) focuses on secure data sharing among the various stakeholders of the industry. It uses a blockchain-based platform with the cloud services for keeping the medical data safe and secure. MedShare monitors data accesses and ensures that the data do not reach any malicious user by tracking data's behavior and detecting any violation of permissions. MedBlock (Fan et al., 2018) is also a blockchain-based electronic health records information management system with focus on the protection of sensitive medical data. Asymmetric cryptography and access control mechanisms are used while sharing data. The platform also eases the patient by integrating its medical records from various hospitals at one location.

ModelChain (Kuo and Ohno-Machado, 2018) uses machine learning and blockchain technology for privacy preservation of the patient's medical data. The framework used the metadata of the transactions to find out the existing scenario of privacy in the blockchain and then used it to design the privacy model for the blockchain. It used private blockchain and proof of information consensus algorithm to provide security of medical data. SmartCare (Duong-Trung et al., 2020) is a patient-centric blockchain-based healthcare system for security and privacy of patient's medical data. A patient can give access to his/her own medical data and can also remove the data at any point of time. It uses smart contracts to provide access control mechanisms which introduces trust among the patients and the receivers (doctors, insurance providers, hospitals etc.) of his/her data.

MedSBA (Pournaghi et al., 2020) uses private blockchain and attribute-based encryption techniques to store the medical data of patients. The proposed system provides user privacy and secured access control mechanism for patients to exchange their medical data. The main motto of all the applications is the security and privacy of the medical data of the patients. Different types of blockchain network and encryption techniques are used to improve the efficiency of the existing application scenarios.

## 8 Blockchain-based framework for privacy protection of patient's data

In healthcare industry, patients mostly deal with doctors and hospitals for their treatments. They also have to deal with insurance providers for their medical reimbursements or payments. When patients visit doctors and hospitals, they are generally given paper visiting slips or paper medical records for their checkups or follow-ups. Few hospitals provide e-visiting slips or e-medical records also. The patient can also scan the documents and keep it safe with them. In some cases, patient may need to change the doctor or want to take some medical advice; these documents are to be shared with other doctors or hospitals also. Also these e-records are shared with the insurance providers for bill payments or medical reimbursements. All the sharing of documents is done at patient's level. In case, the patient is not able to share the records with other doctors or insurance companies, there can be big problems too.

An ecosystem for maintaining patient's records is required in current scenario of medical treatments where the insurance companies directly pay the hospitals for all the medical expenses. The insurance companies may also consider the e-records shared by hospitals to be genuine. This also reduces the patient's burden. For creating and maintaining e-database of medical records, patient's privacy must be taken care. Also data need to be secured so that no intruder is able to view or change any of the e-records. Medical data are very critical as minor changes to data may result in different medications for the patient. So it must be handled carefully.

In this scenario, a blockchain-based framework can be used for maintaining and sharing e-records among patients, hospitals, and insurance providers. In the proposed framework, a federated blockchain network will be used to include various stakeholders in the blockchain network. So, whenever anyone wants to join the blockchain network, it will have to ask for the permission to join the network. It will only be able to join network after permissions are granted. In this way, the blockchain network will have trusted nodes only. An example scenario of the blockchain network is as shown in Fig. 6.

In the blockchain network, all the hospitals will be the full nodes and will maintain the copy of the blockchain with them. Patients and insurance providers will act as simple nodes in the network. Hospital authorities will assign a miner for mining of the blocks. So hospitals will be full nodes as well as miner nodes. Mining process will be assigned to hospitals on a rotation basis. The medical records will be stored after encryption. While adding records to the block, the data will be encrypted. The patients can provide access to his/her records and doctor/insurance provider will be able to view the records only if they have the permissions for it.

Whenever a patient visits a hospital, he is assigned a unique id which will be recorded on blockchain platform and will be used for updating his/her records. Patient's records will be updated in data structure as shown in Fig. 7. So whenever there is any medical checkup or doctor's follow-up visit, the whole

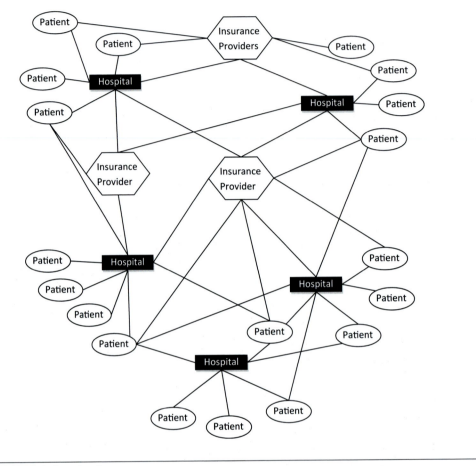

**FIG. 6**

Proposed blockchain network.

data structure will be updated. The parameters in the data structure are the various medical checkups associated with patients like vitamin D3, hemoglobin, etc. It will act like a physical checkup booklet for the patient. So whichever parameter is not required, -NA- will be written.

The patients will be given all the access controls for their data with permissions to share or remove access from anyone. So if the patient wants to consult his medical history with any other doctor, he can easily show his historic medical conditions. Also his records will be updated every time there is a visit to the doctor; it can be shared with the insurance providers as a proof for the same. This will solve the big problem of medical reimbursements between the insurance providers and hospitals/patients. Whenever a patient wants to apply for a medical reimbursement, he will just need to raise a request for the same with the access to his stored copy of medical records on blockchain. This will enable the smart contract for automatic payment by the insurance providers. This smart contract is stored on the blockchain network and is invoked whenever there is a request from the patient's end

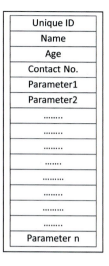

**FIG. 7**

Patient's record structure.

for medical claims. Fig. 8 shows the process of smart contract between the insurance providers and hospitals/patients.

The smart contract ensures automatic payment to the hospitals so that the patient need not suffer. The proposed framework will ensure the privacy of the patient via unique IDs, restricted access controls, and data encryption. This framework will be patient-centric where patients have complete control over their data. Their task of claiming insurance will be reduced through smart contract and they can remove or provide any accesses to their data anytime to anyone. This framework will also provide an insight to the health trends of the patient by checking their historical records.

## 9  Conclusion

Health industry requires the best of technology for serving the patients with the best of services. Any glitch due to technology can cause havoc for the patient, doctor or hospital. In today's world, sharing of data is not a problem but protecting it from the intruders is a big issue. As the industry is dependent on various information technologies like cloud computing, machine learning, internet of things, blockchain technology, cryptography, etc., researchers are looking for security solutions to protect critical medical data. The major problem with data sharing is its authenticity, data privacy, and security. Many applications have been proposed for maintaining the privacy and security of the healthcare data.

The proposed framework will provide a secure solution for sharing of electronic medical records. It will also help patients in processing of their medical claims and can also provide historical insights of the medical records which is extremely helpful in case of chronic diseases like heart problems, diabetics etc. The framework uses blockchain technology to ensuring privacy of medical data. It also employs smart contract for medical reimbursements by the insurance providers. By encrypting the data,

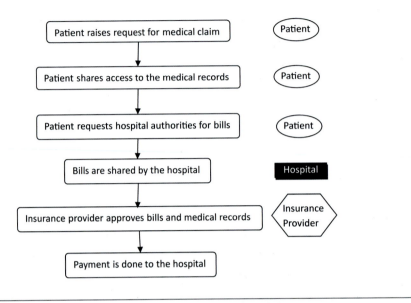

**FIG. 8**

Process of smart contract between insurance providers and patients/hospitals.

the framework ensures that no intruder can read or update the patient's medical data. The framework can also be used to analyze the historical medical data and keep track of any updates happening. Blockchain technology will ensure the authentication and security of data.

# References

Andrews, L., Gajanayake, R., Sahama, T., 2014. The Australian general public's perceptions of having a personally controlled electronic health record (PCEHR). Int. J. Med. Inform. 83 (12), 889–900.

Annas, G.J., 2003. HIPAA regulations-a new era of medical-record privacy? N. Engl. J. Med. 348 (15), 1486–1490.

Austin, L.M., 2006. Reviewing PIPEDA: control, privacy and the limits of fair information practices. Canadian Business Law J. 44, 21.

Bhavaraju, S.R., 2018. From subconscious to conscious to artificial intelligence: a focus on electronic health records. Neurol. India 66 (5), 1270.

Chakrabarti, A., Chaudhuri, A.K., 2017. Blockchain and its Scope in retail. Int. Res. J. Eng. Technol. 4 (7), 3053–3056.

Chen, L., Xu, L., Shah, N., Gao, Z., Lu, Y., Shi, W., 2017, November. On security analysis of proof-of-elapsed-time (poet). In: International Symposium on Stabilization, Safety, and Security of Distributed Systems. Springer, Cham, pp. 282–297.

Crawford, M., 2017. The insurance implications of blockchain. Risk Manage. 64 (2), 24.

Duong-Trung, N., Son, H.X., Le, H.T., Phan, T.T., 2020, January. Smart care: integrating blockchain technology into the design of patient-centered healthcare systems. In: Proceedings of the 2020 4th International Conference on Cryptography, Security and Privacy, pp. 105–109.

Ekblaw, A., Azaria, A., 2016. Medrec: Medical Data Management on the Blockchain. Viral Communications.

Fan, K., Wang, S., Ren, Y., Li, H., Yang, Y., 2018. Medblock: efficient and secure medical data sharing via blockchain. J. Med. Syst. 42 (8), 136.

Gout, B., 2017. Block and Mortar: A Blockchain-Inspired Business Model for Mortgage Funding Market Place.

Gramoli, V., 2020. From blockchain consensus back to byzantine consensus. Futur. Gener. Comput. Syst. 107, 760–769.

Greenleaf, G., 2017. Global data privacy laws 2017: 120 national data privacy laws, including Indonesia and Turkey. In: Including Indonesia and Turkey (January 30, 2017). vol. 145, pp. 10–13.

Guo, Y., Liang, C., 2016. Blockchain application and outlook in the banking industry. Financ. Innovation 2 (1), 24.

Hjálmarsson, F.Þ., Hreiðarsson, G.K., Hamdaqa, M., Hjálmtýsson, G., 2018, July. Blockchain-based e-voting system. In: 2018 IEEE 11th International Conference on Cloud Computing (CLOUD). IEEE, pp. 983–986.

Karantias, K., Kiayias, A., Zindros, D., 2019. Proof-of-burn. In: International Conference on Financial Cryptography and Data Security.

Kiayias, A., Russell, A., David, B., Oliynykov, R., 2017, August. Ouroboros: a provably secure proof-of-stake blockchain protocol. In: Annual International Cryptology Conference. Springer, Cham, pp. 357–388.

Koshti, M., Ganorkar, S., Chiari, L., 2016. IoT based health monitoring system by using raspberry pi and ecg signal. Int, J. Innov. Res. Sci. Eng. Technol. 5 (5), 8977–8985.

Kuo, T.T., Ohno-Machado, L., 2018. ModelChain: decentralized privacy-preserving healthcare predictive modeling framework on private blockchain networks. arXiv preprint arXiv: 1802.01746.

Liao, D.Y., Wang, X., 2018, December. Applications of blockchain technology to logistics management in integrated casinos and entertainment. In: Informatics. vol. 5(4). Multidisciplinary Digital Publishing Institute, p. 44.

List of all cryptocurrency | CoinLore 2020, Cryptocurrency List, viewed 22 May 2020, https://coinmarketcap.com/.

Mettler, M., 2016, September. Blockchain technology in healthcare: the revolution starts here. In: 2016 IEEE 18th international conference on e-health networking, applications and services (Healthcom). IEEE, pp. 1–3.

Pournaghi, S.M., Bayat, M., Farjami, Y., 2020. Med SBA: a novel and secure scheme to share medical data based on blockchain technology and attribute-based encryption. J. Ambient. Intell. Humaniz. Comput., 1–29.

Regulation, P., 2018. General data protection regulation. In: Intouch.

Roehrs, A., da Costa, C.A., da Rosa Righi, R., 2017. OmniPHR: a distributed architecture model to integrate personal health records. J. Biomed. Inform. 71, 70–81.

Saberi, S., Kouhizadeh, M., Sarkis, J., Shen, L., 2019. Blockchain technology and its relationships to sustainable supply chain management. Int. J. Prod. Res. 57 (7), 2117–2135.

Sapra, R., Dhaliwal, P., 2018, December. Blockchain: the new era of technology. In: 2018 Fifth International Conference on Parallel, Distributed and Grid Computing (PDGC). IEEE, pp. 495–499.

Sapra, R., Dhaliwal, P., 2020a. Blockchain for security issues of internet of things (IoT). In: Principles of Internet of Things (IoT) Ecosystem: Insight Paradigm. Springer, Cham, pp. 599–626.

Sapra, R., Dhaliwal, P., 2020b. MissingChain: a novel blockchain system for missing or found cases. Test Eng. Manag. 83, 12670–12677.

Sapra, R., Dhaliwal, P., 2021a. Blockchain: the perspective future of technology. Int. J. Healthc. Inf. Syst. Inform. 16 (2), 1–20. https://doi.org/10.4018/IJHISI.20210401.oa1.

Sapra, R., Dhaliwal, P., 2021b. PlasmaBlock: a plasma donation Blockchain system in COVID-19 (In press).

Xia, Q.I., Sifah, E.B., Asamoah, K.O., Gao, J., Du, X., Guizani, M., 2017a. MeDShare: trust-less medical data sharing among cloud service providers via blockchain. IEEE Access 5, 14757–14767.

Xia, Q., Sifah, E.B., Smahi, A., Amofa, S., Zhang, X., 2017b. BBDS: blockchain-based data sharing for electronic medical records in cloud environments. Information 8 (2), 44.

Yue, X., Wang, H., Jin, D., Li, M., Jiang, W., 2016. Healthcare data gateways: found healthcare intelligence on blockchain with novel privacy risk control. J. Med. Syst. 40 (10), 218.

Zhang, J., Xue, N., Huang, X., 2016. A secure system for pervasive social network-based healthcare. IEEE Access 4, 9239–9250.

# A novel approach for securing e-health application in a cloud environment

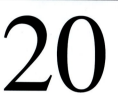

**Dipesh Kumar[a], Nirupama Mandal[a], and Yugal Kumar[b]**

*Department of ECE, IIT(ISM), Dhanbad, India[a] Department of CSE & IT, JUIT, Solan, Himachal Pradesh, India[b]*

## Chapter outline

## 1 Introduction

With the rapid increase in convergence technologies, the world is able to get lot of information through the portable mobile devices (Mumrez et al., 2019). Due to development of internet and its users across the world, there is a demand of centralized healthcare information system. Rapid increase in chronic diseases and various disease aspects, disease prevention, and various government policies of providing a better healthcare facility to its citizens steadily increased the demand for intelligent and portable mobile-based services (Sravani et al., 2017). In the past one decade, the use of smart phones has increased and the same can be utilized for e-Health services and can be used for providing personal health record (PHR), disease-related information and other self-heathcare facilities ( Jung and Chung, 2016).

In the current scenario, the use of Information Communication Technologies (ICT)-based intelligent system such as smart mobile devices gives ample opportunity for the growth and development of e-Health services. Irrespective of geographical barriers, the use of ICT helps to deliver mobile-based e-Health services to its users. Nowadays, the mobile health (m-health) applications directly address the problems of sudden rise in chronic diseases and help patients and their families for self-care (Xiong, 2019; Chung et al., 2015).

ICT-based intelligent system can be seen as a combination of person device assistant (PDA) (such as mobile phones, electronic/smart watches, and i-pad) with the application of IoT and Cloud computing services (Mumrez et al., 2019; Vishwakarma et al., 2019). Intelligent personal devices (IPD) are software agents that help the users in doing their day-to-day work (such as shopping, online bill payments, making appointments, and attending meetings) with ease of simplicity. Now, with the advancement and inclusion of IoT and cloud computing with IPD, the capabilities and demands of such devices are increasing at an alarming rate. Researchers have created many dynamic and static gateways to enable portable/personal devices to work with IoT or Cloud-based intelligent systems (Nanayakkara et al., 2019).

The emergence of Internet of Things (IoT) has made all the addressable devices/objects to communicate and cooperate with each other in order to further increase the capabilities of IPD. By providing an easy gateway path, we can easily extend the accessibility of intelligent devices on different dynamic scenarios. Further, building of smart cities, homes, transportation, and healthcare services are some applications where IoT can be used along with the IPD (Atzori et al., 2010).

The convergence of cloud computing with mobile devices and other computing technologies has allowed us to build an intelligent system for providing a better e-Healthcare services (Selvaraj and Sundaravaradhan, 2020). The innovative idea of cloud technology, which came up with a new and extended infrastructure facilities, has made intelligent system like portable computing/mobile devices to provide more reliable services to its end users. As mentioned earlier, like other technologies, cloud computing can help in empowering the healthcare services in the most efficient way. It offers a fast, reliable, and cost-effective infrastructure and application. The concept of cloud can help in management of data-centric health facilities and can help in removing the complexity involved in storing and retrieval of health-related data. Only challenges that cloud technologies currently facing are security, confidentiality, and trust issue. Weak security factor in cloud hinders its complete application in health industry. Further, measures were taken to remove security challenges for cloud to enable its application in healthcare industry (Malhotra et al., 2019).

As stated earlier, with the rapid increase in chronic diseases and intelligent devices to monitor those diseases, there is a need to develop systems for monitoring personal healthcare record (PHR) using cloud computing techniques (Kadhim et al., 2020). To provide continuous healthcare facility to an individual, a tool known as PHR needs to be created which can monitor and manage health-related information. It may also help us to maintain and view medical information that can be needed while a patient visits hospitals for treatment. This development of PHR is only possible when we have an intelligent system for recording and monitoring healthcare information of an individual in a convenient way. Apart from intelligent system, many hospitals also maintain a centralized cloud-based system to record day-to-day information of their patient situated at distant places (Silva et al., 2015; Santos et al., 2016; Kaur and Chana, 2014; Kanrar and Mandal, 2017).

A PHR or e-Health application utilizes patient's clinical data. Security of clinical data is an important concern while sending it to cloud environment. Data can be secured using https protocol using ciphers. Cipher is used to encrypt and decrypt data using encryption and decryption algorithm. While sending patient's clinical data to the cloud server, data should be encrypted. Encryption of data hides the actual message and converts it to hypothetical text so that the data are not easily read by hackers. At destination, i.e., cloud server, the encrypted data are decrypted by using decryption algorithm to fetch the actual data.

With increasing technology usage, various steps have been taken to secure the data in transport layer, and also various technologies have been developed by hackers to decode the secured data to get the original message. The PHR's or e-Health application stores very sensitive data. The data include patient's clinical information, patient's medical history, bank account details used for transactions with hospitals, etc. These data are very private and can cause major impact if it is hacked by any hacker and can be used for any unusual activities. So, there is a need to implement new ciphers as the already existing ciphers can be decoded by hackers. So, existing ciphers must be updated, and new ciphers must be developed with course of time. The proposed work includes introduction of new improved cipher for encrypting the message at the senders' end and decrypting the message at the receivers' end to allow end-to-end secured connectivity and transmission of message securely for an e-Health application. In the proposed work, an improved reverse transposition cipher is proposed which provides new improved encryption and decryption algorithm.

## 1.1 Contribution

The major contribution of the proposed work is to develop new algorithm to be used in cipher to encrypt the message at the senders' end and decrypt the message at the receivers' end to retrieve the original message. The proposed algorithm allows to develop new cipher to be used in digital certificates in e-Health application and cloud servers. The proposed cipher will be effective to secure the messages and prevent any unauthorized access by hackers. In the proposed work, the improved reverse transposition cipher will provide encryption of messages at the senders' end and decryption of messages at the receivers' end to retrieve the original message.

## 2 Motivation

The increase in the growth of e-services between users and enterprises is one of the most interesting and considerable topics for researchers. In the current scenario, the diseases are being transformed from acute stage to chronic stage in a quick span of time due to rapid increase in population, lack of knowledge, etc. It has been studied in the literature (Mumrez et al., 2019; Sravani et al., 2017; Jung and Chung, 2016; Xiong, 2019; Chung et al., 2015; Vishwakarma et al., 2019; Nanayakkara et al., 2019; Atzori et al., 2010; Selvaraj and Sundaravaradhan, 2020; Malhotra et al., 2019; Kadhim et al., 2020; Silva et al., 2015) that many healthcare intelligent system use cloud and IoT-based applications for providing e-Health services. However, both cloud and IoT is inefficient to handle, store, and process health-related data due to its complex structure, hardware capacity limitations, and -security-related issues (Shin et al., 2016). A reliable healthcare system is the need of the hour which can be used to manage and monitor public health and can provide suitable treatment as and when required. The motivation behind this work is to develop an intelligent system-based platform that provides an uninterrupted and scalable cloud service interface, which can easily provide healthcare facilities to its users. The interface between portable devices and cloud technologies often faces the problem related to security and privacy. In the proposed work, we have developed a uniform platform to centralize user data that can be shared and accessed across various platforms by preserving the security and privacy of user personal data (Lee and Kim, 2014).

## 2.1 **Related works**

With increase in the uses of mobile phones, e-Health care becomes one of the most important factors in today's growing life. In the past few years, the world has witnessed a rapid increase in population and because of this, it is hard to provide a smooth and better healthcare facilities to all the individuals situated at different remote locations. Therefore, there is a need to provide medical facilities and healthcare services via mobile technologies. In the current era of mobile revolution, it is easier to develop a mobile-based online application which can easily be accessed through personal smart mobile phones or portable devices where a user can maintain and update their health-related information and the same can also be accessed and managed by maintaining a centralized database through cloud or IoT-based application (Santos et al., 2015).

It has been observed that ICT-based e-Health services are gaining popularity among its user and medical practitioners across the world (Ogasawara, 2006). ICT-based intelligent devices have the potential to provide high-quality, low-cost and error-free healthcare facility to all its user in a convenient and efficient way. But, still, these intelligent devices lack in providing some basic services due to data complexity, storage limitation, less infrastructure and proper coordination of distributed databases. In the studies cited herein (Shojania et al., 2009; Deutsch et al., 2004; Wang et al., 2009) different solutions have been suggested to overcome this limitation. Due to increase in the use of smart mobile phones or other portable devices, many healthcare applications (Patients Like Me (Wicks et al., 2010), Sugar Stats (Sugarstats, 2019), Cure Together (Curetogether, 2020), TU Diabetes (Tudiabetes, 2019)) are available where users can maintain their own health data and can seek medical advices as and when required.

It has been seen in the literature (Mumrez et al., 2019; Sravani et al., 2017; Jung and Chung, 2016; Xiong, 2019; Chung et al., 2015; Vishwakarma et al., 2019; Nanayakkara et al., 2019; Atzori et al., 2010; Selvaraj and Sundaravaradhan, 2020; Malhotra et al., 2019; Kadhim et al., 2020; Silva et al., 2015; Santos et al., 2016; Kaur and Chana, 2014; Kanrar and Mandal, 2017; Shin et al., 2016; Lee and Kim, 2014; Santos et al., 2015; Ogasawara, 2006; Shojania et al., 2009; Deutsch et al., 2004; Wang et al., 2009; Wicks et al., 2010; Sugarstats, 2019; Curetogether, 2020; Tudiabetes, 2019; Apple Siri Webpage, 2015; Google Now Webpage, 2015; Samsung, 2015; Microsoft, 2015; Rodrigues et al., 2013; Komninos and Stamou, 2006) that ICT-based intelligent devices can easily be interfaced with other applications to assist patients, doctors, and hospitals. Further, many applications such as Apple's Siri (Apple Siri Webpage, 2015), Google Now (Google Now Webpage, 2015), Samsung's S Voice (Samsung, 2015), and Microsoft's Cortana (Microsoft, 2015) are currently being used to monitor personal healthcare information which includes medicine reminder, day-to-day change in health condition, monitoring heart beat and blood pressure, etc. Authors in the referred study here (Rodrigues et al., 2013) presented a similar kind of mobile-based health application where patient's weight is getting monitored to prevent obesity. Apart from maintaining weight information, the application also keeps record of body mass index, health meal planning, and basal metabolic rate. As we are considering the use of intelligent devices, authors in the referred study here (Komninos and Stamou, 2006) made an application where peripheral device such as thermometer interact with PDA of the patient and a notification of the temperature will be sent to the doctor or the care taken if there is any variation in patient body temperature beyond the prescribed limit (Santos et al., 2016).

As we have seen in literature and in the above paragraph, cloud technology will help in developing an intelligent portable platform to perform the exchange of healthcare services to its service providers.

Further, authors in the referred study here (Pandey et al., 2012) used data mining technique to build an intelligent system with a strong focus on the quality of services with respect to cost, infrastructure, and security. The same strategy is followed by the authors in the study cited herein (Kuo, 2011) which use cloud computing techniques to provide the services suggested in the other study (Pandey et al., 2012).

As stated earlier in this chapter, there is a need to look upon the security requirements of cloud applications. In this view, Xie et al. (Xie et al., 2019) presented an approach for the security aspect of cloud technology, which consists of prospective threats and the preventative measure need to be followed in the deployment of cloud application. Before using cloud application for healthcare industry, we should have a complete knowledge of the work being done in the same field. Avancha et al. (Avancha et al., 2012) provided a complete review of the application of cloud in healthcare industry and also presented a privacy framework for e-Health sector. Ibrahim et al. (Ibrahim and Singhal, 2016) provided a secure sharing on e-Health data with different service providers using cloud computing. Along the line, Abbas and Khan (2014) presented related studies which aim to contrast the privacy-preserving approaches employed in e-Health clouds.

Authors in the studies referred herein (Ferna'ndez et al., 2013; Dong et al., 2012; Metri and Sarote, 2011; Seol et al., 2018) also presented various security-related issues and mechanism to overcome the same for e-Health cloud environment. We introduce the summary of the most existing technique that is commonly being adopted by various health sectors for cloud environment. With reference to the various literature studies (Chenthara et al., 2019; Abbas and Khan, 2014; Wang et al., 2019; Zhang et al., 2018; Ayofe et al., 2019), there is no inclusive survey available independently at a point of concentration on confidentiality issues of e-Health cloud. As per the survey, it is clearly indicated that privacy and security of the personal health and medical related data are very much important. Various authors (Dong et al., 2012; Metri and Sarote, 2011; Seol et al., 2018; Chenthara et al., 2019; Abbas and Khan, 2014) introduced the architectural view of cloud for handling applications related to biomedical with respect to security and privacy issues.

## 2.2 Challenges

The major challenge in e-Health application is to maintain confidentiality and integrity of the data retrieved from IoT device which is continuously monitoring a patient. There are multiple ways to breach data by hackers. Transport layer is very prone to attack by hackers the reason why data encryption is a very challenging task. Various ciphers are available in today's world, but hackers' attacks are also increasing day by day. To avoid such kind of attacks, proper steps need to be taken for securing the data. With the advancement of technology, attackers use new techniques to steal or hack data. So, there is a need to introduce new improved encryption and decryption technique which provides an efficient solution to save data from various types of security threats and attacks. In the upcoming section, a new approach to secure e-Health application using improved reverse transposition cipher is discussed.

## 3 Proposed system

In this section, a new approach to secure e-Health application using improved reverse transposition cipher is proposed. In the architecture shown in Fig. 1, the IoT device with MP5700AP pressure sensor to record patients' blood pressure is used, which records and sends data to e-Health mobile application.

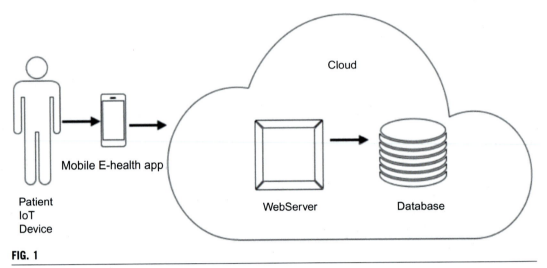

**FIG. 1**

IoT-based mobile e-Health architecture.

The e-Health mobile application is developed to interact and receive data from IoT sensor and send it to web server in cloud environment securely with https protocol using cipher. The e-Health mobile application is developed using android studio version 3.6.3 in 64 bit windows platform which supports Android version jelly beans and above android versions. After receiving the data from e-Health mobile application, the web server sends the data to the app server and the app server sends that data to cloud database. The web server is apache Tomcat and the database is Microsoft SQL Server. In Fig. 1, patient's clinical data are sent to web server by e-Health mobile application using https protocol. The https protocol requires ciphers to encrypt data while sending and to decrypt data after receiving it.

The improved reverse transposition cipher provides encryption algorithm to encrypt the data while sending it from e-Health mobile application to web server. Also, it provides decryption algorithm to decrypt the received data at the web server end. The encryption and decryption technique is explained in detail in the next section.

### *Improved reverse transposition Cipher:*

Improved reverse transposition cipher is explained in the following sections:

### *Encryption of message:*

The data recorded by the IoT device is encrypted by using the below encryption algorithm while sending to the cloud web server:

- Select a key value of any length say N.
- Create a two dimensional table with column length N and row length depends on the length of message to be encrypted.
- Assign each alphabet (including blank spaces) of the message to each cell of the table.
- Create a new empty table of size same as the original table.
- Move the elements of last column of the table and first column of new table vertically.

- Repeat this until all the elements of the original table are moved to new table in the reverse order.
- Note down the elements of first two columns of new table. Then jump by two columns and note down elements of 5th and 6th columns of the table and again jump by two columns and repeat the process.
- If there is no column further left in the table. Then end the loop and note the elements of 3rd and 4th columns and again jump 2 places and note the elements of next two columns and continue the same process till all the columns are covered.
- Place all the elements together to obtain the encrypted message.

The above encryption algorithm is explained in detail below:

Let us assume that below message is recorded by IoT device and sent to e-Health application for saving it securely in cloud database.

Recorded message:

*"Systolic blood pressure:120, Diastolic blood pressure:80"*.

**Step 1:** Let us assume we have selected a key value as 10.

**Step 2:** Create two-dimensional table with column length as 10 and assign each alphabets to each cell (Fig. 2)

**Step 3:** Create a new empty table. Move all the elements of last column of the table shown in Fig. 1 to the first column of new table. Then, move all the elements of the second last column of the old table to the second column to the new table. Repeat this step until all the elements of old table are assigned to the new table in reverse order. This step is explained in Fig. 3. After assigning all the elements of the old table to the new table in reverse order, name the columns of the new table as C1, C2, ... C10 as shown in Fig. 3.

**Step 4:** In this step, note down all the alphabets (including space for empty cells) from C1 and C2. Jump two columns and note down all the alphabets (including space for empty cell) from C5 and from C6. Again, jump two columns and note down all the alphabets (including space for empty cell) from C9 and C10. This step is explained in Fig. 4.

Below message is obtained from this step:

*bsilu sobs lp2ir o 1lp0yorsoesluaor.*

When the execution reaches the last column, then, stop the iteration and go back and note the alphabets (space for empty cell) from C3 and from C4. Again jump two columns and note down all the

| S | y | s | t | o | 1 | i | c |  | b |
|---|---|---|---|---|---|---|---|---|---|
| 1 | o | o | d |  | p | r | e | s | s |
| u | r | e | : | 1 | 2 | 0 | , | D | i |
| a | s | t | o | 1 | i | c |  | b | 1 |
| o | o | d |  | p | r | e | s | s | u |
| r | e | : | 8 | 0 |  |  |  |  |  |

**FIG. 2**

Received messages assigned row-wise to create a table.

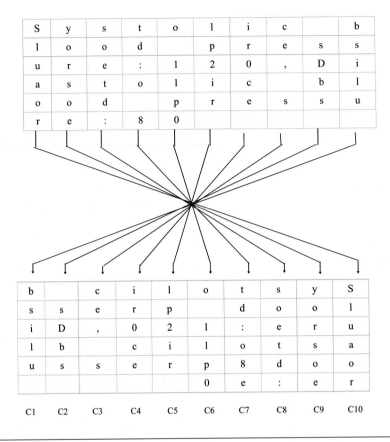

**FIG. 3**

Mapping process to create new table with elements in reverse order.

alphabets (space for empty cell) from C7 and from C8. Since there is no column after this to jump the iteration, the execution will be stopped.

The below message is obtained from this step:

*ce, s ir0ce td:o 8soetd:*

Now, combine these two messages to obtain the final encrypted message as below:

*bsilu sDbs lp2ir o 1lp0yorsoesluaorce, s ir0ce td:o 8soetd:*

The encryption process is explained in flowchart (Fig. 5) below:

### Decryption of received message:

The encrypted message received at the server's end in cloud environment is decrypted by using the decryption algorithm shown here:

- Count the total number of alphabets in the received encrypted message (including blank spaces).
- Divide the total count by key value N to get K.
- Create a table with row size as K and column size as N.

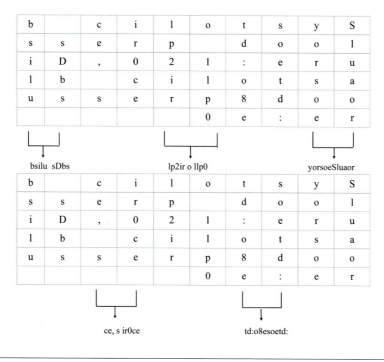

**FIG. 4**

Reverse transposition method to encrypt message.

- Fill first two column of the table with alphabet from encrypted message received. Once all the cells of first two columns got filled, then leave the two columns empty and jump to 5th columns and fill cells of the next two columns with alphabets. After filling the 5th and 6th columns, again leave two columns blank and jump to the 9th column and fill the alphabets from encrypted message to the 9th and 10th columns. After this, return back to the 3rd column which was left empty and fill the cells of the 3rd and 4th columns with alphabets and jump to the 7th column and fill the cells of 7th and 8th columns.
- Create a new table. Starting from last column, move all the elements of the last column of old table to the first column of the new table. Continue this process to make sure that all the elements of old table are moved to the new table in reverse order.
- Place the alphabets of this table row wise to get the decrypted message.

The decryption algorithm is explained below:

    Below is the message received at the server's end:

      *bsilu sDbs lp2ir o 1lp0yorsoesluaorce, s ir0ce td:o 8soetd:*

**Step 1:** Count the length of received encrypted message.

      Length of encrypted message is 60 (including blank spaces).

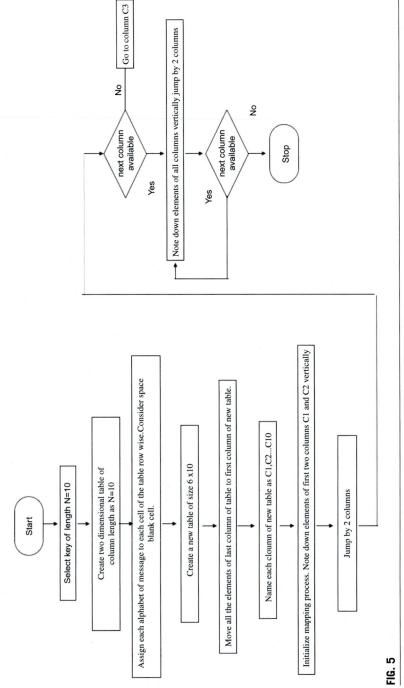

**FIG. 5**

Flowchart of encryption process using improved reverse transposition method.

**Step 2:** Calculate N.

$$N = \text{Message length}/K$$
$$N = 60/10$$
$$N = 6$$

**Step 3:** Create a table of row length as N, i.e., 6 and assign the first 12 letters in the first two columns C1 and C2 vertically. Then skip two columns and assign another 12 letters in the next two columns C5 and C6. Again skip two columns and assign another 12 letters in the next two columns, i.e., C9 and C10, respectively.

When all the columns get filled, then return back to the 3rd column C3 and fill letters in two consecutive columns, i.e., C3 and C4. Jump two times to columns C7 and C8 and fill the cells of C7 and C8 with remaining letters as shown in the table below to create a table.

**Step 4:** Create a new table. In Fig. 6, starting from the last column, i.e., C10, move all the elements of column C10 to the first column of the new table. Repeat this process so that all the elements of the above table get assigned to the new table in reverse order vertically as shown in Fig. 7.

**Step 5:** Note all elements from each cell row wise as shown in Fig. 8.

Combine all the elements got from the table and retrieve original message as below: ***"Systolic blood pressure: 120, Diastolic blood pressure: 80".***

The Decryption process is explained in the flowchart (Fig. 9).

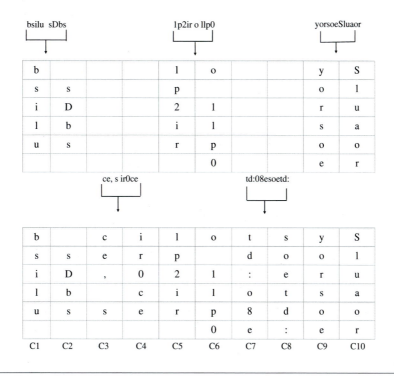

| bsilu sDbs | | | | 1p2ir o llp0 | | | | yorsoeSluaor | |
|---|---|---|---|---|---|---|---|---|---|
| b | | | | 1 | o | | | y | S |
| s | s | | | p | | | | o | l |
| i | D | | | 2 | 1 | | | r | u |
| l | b | | | i | 1 | | | s | a |
| u | s | | | r | p | | | o | o |
| | | | | | 0 | | | e | r |

| | | ce, s ir0ce | | | | td:08esoetd: | | | |
|---|---|---|---|---|---|---|---|---|---|
| b | | c | i | 1 | o | t | s | y | S |
| s | s | e | r | p | | d | o | o | l |
| i | D | , | 0 | 2 | 1 | : | e | r | u |
| l | b | | c | i | 1 | o | t | s | a |
| u | s | s | e | r | p | 8 | d | o | o |
| | | | | | 0 | e | : | e | r |
| C1 | C2 | C3 | C4 | C5 | C6 | C7 | C8 | C9 | C10 |

**FIG. 6**

Inverse transposition method to decrypt message.

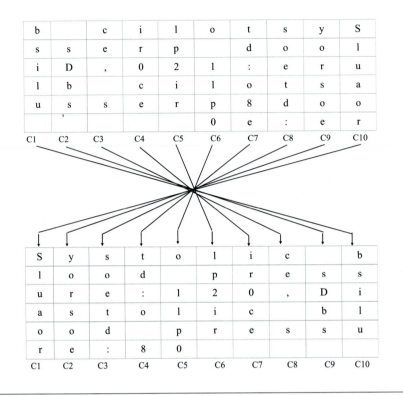

**FIG. 7**

Mapping process.

| C1 | C2 | C3 | C4 | C5 | C6 | C7 | C8 | C9 | C10 |
|---|---|---|---|---|---|---|---|---|---|
| S | y | s | t | o | l | i | c |  | b |
| l | o | o | d |  | p | r | e | s | s |
| u | r | e | : | 1 | 2 | 0 | , | D | i |
| a | s | t | o | l | i | c |  | b | l |
| o | o | d |  | p | r | e | s | s | u |
| r | e | : | 8 | 0 |  |  |  |  |  → re:80 |

The arrows to the right read:
- Systolic b
- lood press
- ure:120,Di
- astolic bl
- ood pressur
- re:80

**FIG. 8**

Fetching original message from the table.

## 4 Conclusion

The development of e-Health mobile application using cloud environment has proved to be very useful in monitoring and managing patient's clinical data. The security of patient's data using e- Health mobile application is an important area of concern. The e-Health mobile application interacts with cloud environment to save patients' critical health data in cloud database securely. The study in this paper

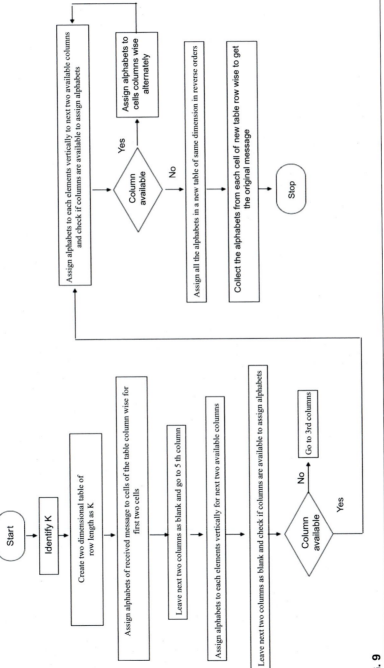

**FIG. 9**

Flowchart of decryption process using improved reverse transposition method.

shows that the connectivity between e-Health mobile application and cloud web server can be secured using ciphers. The reverse transposition cipher can be used to secure data in cloud environment. The effectiveness of encryption and decryption technique depends on the difficulty level it presents to hackers to decode the original message. The improved reverse transposition cipher has suggested an effective technique to encrypt and decrypt data. In further studies, this cipher can be compared with other ciphers available in today's world in terms of efficiency. The proposed improved transposition cipher can be used for performing encryption, decryption, hashing, or digital signatures. The proposed cipher can be used in digital certificates used in e-Health application and cloud server for authentication and handshaking to initiate https connectivity between the client and the server.

## References

Abbas, A., Khan, S.U., 2014. A review on the state-of-the-art privacy-preserving approaches in the e-health clouds. IEEE J. Biomed. Health Inform. 18 (4), 1431–1441.

Apple Siri Webpage, 2015. "Apple Siri Webpage." [Online]. Available: https://www.apple.com/ios/siri/.

Atzori, L., Iera, A., Morabito, G., October 2010. The internet of things: a survey. Comput. Netw. 54 (15), 2787–2805.

Avancha, S., Baxi, A., Kotz, D., 2012. Privacy in mobile technology for personal healthcare. ACM Comput. Surv. 45 (1), 1–54.

Ayofe, N., Charles, A., Vyver, V., 2019. Security and privacy issues in e-health cloud-based system: A comprehensive content analysis. Egypt. Inform. J. 20 (2), 97–108.

Chenthara, S., Ahmed, K., Wang, H., Whittaker, F., 2019. Security and privacy-preserving challenges of e-health solutions in cloud computing. IEEE Access 7.

Chung, K., Kim, J.C., Park, R.C., 2015. Knowledge based health service considering user convenience using hybrid Wi-Fi P2P. Inf. Technol. Manag. https://doi.org/10.1007/s10799-015-0241-5.

Curetogether, 2020. http://curetogether.com/.

Deutsch, T., Gergely, T., Trunov, V., 2004. A computer system for interpreting blood glucose data. Comput. Methods Programs Biomed. 76, 41–51.

Dong, N., Hugo, J., Pang, J., 2012. Challenges in e-Health: From enabling to enforcing privacy. In: Foundations of Health Informatics Engineering and System. Springer, Berlin, Germany, pp. 195–206.

Ferna'ndez, A.J.L., Senõr, I.C., Lozoya, P.Á.O., Toval, A., 2013. Security and privacy in electronic health records: a systematic literature review. J. Biomed. Inform. 46, 541–562.

Google Now Webpage, 2015. "Google Now Webpage." [Online]. Available: http://www.google.com/landing/now/.

Ibrahim, B.M., Singhal, M., 2016. A secure framework for sharing electronic health records over clouds. In: IEEE International Conference on Serious Games and Applications for Health (SeGAH), Kyoto, Japan, pp. 1–8.

Jung, H., Chung, K., 2016. PHR based life health index mobile service using decision support model. Wirel. Pers. Commun. 86, 315–332. https://doi.org/10.1007/s11277-015-3069-8.

Kadhim, K.T., Alsahlany, A.M., Wadi, S.M., Kadhum, H.T., 2020. An overview of patient's health status monitoring system based on internet of things (IoT). Wirel. Pers. Commun. 114, 2235–2262.

Kanrar, S., Mandal, P.K., 2017. E-health monitoring system enhancement with Gaussian mixture model. Multimed. Tools Appl. 76, 10801–10823.

Kaur, P.D., Chana, I., 2014. Cloud based intelligent system for delivering health care as a service. Comput. Methods Programs Biomed. 113, 346–359.

Komninos, A., Stamou, S., 2006. HealthPal: an intelligent personal medical assistant for supporting the self-monitoring of healthcare in the ageing society. In: 4th International Workshop on Ubiquitous Computing for Pervasive Healthcare Applications (UbiComp 2006), California, USA, September 17-21.

Kuo, A.M., 2011. Opportunities, challenges of cloud computing to improve health care services. J. Med. Internet Res. 13 (3), e67.

Lee, E., Kim, C., 2014. An intelligent green Service in Internet of things. J. Converg. 5 (3), 4–8.

Malhotra, A., Som, S., Khatri, S.K., 2019, February. IoT based predictive model for cloud seeding. In: 2019 Amity International Conference on Artificial Intelligence (AICAI). IEEE, pp. 669–773.

Metri, P., Sarote, G., 2011. Privacy issues and challenges in cloud computing. Int. J. Adv. Eng. Sci. Technol. 5 (1), 001–006.

Microsoft, 2015. "Microsoft Cortana Webpage." [Online]. Available: http://www.windowsphone.com/en-us/how-to/wp8/cortana/meetcortana.

Mumrez, A., Tariq, H., Ajmal, U., Abrar, M., 2019. IOT-based framework for E-health monitoring system. In: International Conference on Green and Human Information Technology (ICGHIT).

Nanayakkara, N., Halgamuge, M., Syed, A., 2019. Security and Privacy of Internet of Medical Things (IoMT) Based Healthcare Applications: A Review. International Conference on Advances in Business Management and Information Technology, Istanbul, Turkey.

Ogasawara, A., 2006. Energy issues confronting the ICT sector. Sci. Technol. Trends 21. Quarterly Review No. 20.

Pandey, S., Voorsluys, W., Niu, S., Khandoker, A., Buyya, R., 2012. An autonomic cloud environment for hosting ECG data analysis services. Futur. Gener. Comput. Syst. 28, 147–154.

Rodrigues, J.J.P.C., Lopes, I.M.C., Silva, B.M.C., La Torre, I.D., 2013. A new mobile ubiquitous computing application to control obesity. SapoFit. Inform. Health Soc. Care 38 (1), 37–53.

Samsung, 2015. "Samsung S Voice Webpage." [Online]. Available: http://www.samsung.com/global/galaxys3/svoice.html.

Santos, P., Varandas, L., Alves, T., Romeiro, C., Casal, J., Lourenço, S., Santos, J., 2015. A pervasive system architecture for smart environments in internet of things context. In: ICMI 2015: XVII International Conference on Multimodal Interaction, London, United Kingdom, January 19–20.

Santos, J., Rodrigues, J.J.P.C., Silva, B.M.C., Casal, J., Saleem, K., Denisov, V., 2016. An IoT-based mobile gateway for intelligent personal assistants on mobile health environments. J. Netw. Comput. Appl. 71, 194–204. https://doi.org/10.1016/j.jnca.2016.03.014.

Selvaraj, S., Sundaravaradhan, S., 2020. Challenges and opportunities in IoT healthcare systems: a systematic review. SN Appl. Sci. 2 (1), 139.

Seol, Y.-G., Kim, E.L., Seo, Y.-D., Baik, D.-K., 2018. Privacy-preserving attribute-based access control model for XML-based electronic health record system. IEEE Access 6, 9114–9128.

Shin, D., Shin, D., Shin, D., 2016. Health: Ubiquitous healthcare platform for chronic patients. In: International Conference on Platform Technology and Service (PlatCon).

Shojania, K.G., Jennings, A., Mayhew, A., Ramsay, C.R., Eccles, M.P., Grimshaw, J., 2009. The effects of on-screen, point of care computer computer reminders on processes and outcomes of care. Cochrane Database Syst. Rev. https://doi.org/10.1002/14651858.CD001096.pub2, CD001096.

Silva, B.M.C., Rodrigues, J.J.P.C., de la Torre Díez, I., López-Coronado, M., Saleem, K., 2015. Mobile-health: a review of current state in 2015. J. Biomed. Inform. 56, 265–272.

Sravani, D., Vinod Nayak, B., Ravindra Babu, J., 2017. IoT based patient health monitoring system. Int. J. Sci. Eng. Technol. Res. 5 (35), 7327–7330.

Sugarstats, 2019. https://sugarstats.com/.

Tudiabetes, 2019. http://www.tudiabetes.org/.

Vishwakarma, S.K., Upadhyaya, P., Kumari, B., Mishra, A.K., 2019, April. Smart energy efficient home automation system using IoT. In: 2019 4th International Conference on Internet of Things: Smart Innovation and Usages (IoT-SIU). IEEE, pp. 1–4.

Wang, T., Shao, K., Chu, Q., et al., 2009. Automics: an integrated platform for NMR-based metabonomics spectral processing and data analysis. BMC Bioinform. 10, 83.

Wang, F., Shi, T., Li, S., 2019. Authorization of searchable CP-ABE scheme with attribute revocation in cloud computing. In: IEEE 8th Joint International Information Technology and Artificial Intelligence Conference (ITAIC).

Wicks, P., et al., 2010. Sharing health data for better outcomes on patients like me. J. Med. Internet Res. 12 (2), e19.

Xie, Y., Wen, H., Wu, B., Jiang, Y., Meng, J., 2019. A modified hierarchical attribute-based encryption access control method for mobile cloud computing. IEEE Trans. Cloud Comput. 7 (2).

Xiong, N., 2019. Application of artificial intelligence technology in decision support software. In: International Conference on Virtual Reality and Intelligent Systems (ICVRIS) IEEE.

Zhang, C., Zhu, L., Xu, C., Lu, R., 2018. PPDP: an efficient and privacy-preserving disease prediction scheme in cloud-based e-healthcare system. Futur. Gener. Comput. Syst. 79, 16–25.

CHAPTER

# An ensemble classifier approach for thyroid disease diagnosis using the AdaBoostM algorithm

# 21

**Giuseppe Ciaburro**

*Department of Architecture and Industrial Design, Università degli Studi della Campania Luigi Vanvitelli, Aversa, Italy*

## Chapter outline

Machine Learning, Big Data, and IoT for Medical Informatics. https://doi.org/10.1016/B978-0-12-821777-1.00002-1

# 1 Introduction

Thanks to digital technologies we can extract knowledge from data by attributing intelligence to objects, through a connection between them. This new way of thinking about data has revolutionized processes and services, providing a new reading key to information from various sectors, so much so that the world of health has also been affected by this revolution (Ward, 2013; Mosavi et al., 2019). The healthcare sector is characterized by a series of problems and critical issues that have often affected its efficiency, offering patients a poor-quality service with significant costs (Hassan et al., 2019). To tackle this problem, a clear transformation of the system was required that would make it possible to respond to requests for improvement in the service provided (Wan, 2006; Beam et al., 2020).

The use of Information Technology (IT) in healthcare products, services, and processes accompanied by organizational changes and the development of new skills has introduced significant improvements in efficiency and productivity in the healthcare sector, as well as greater economic and social value of the health (Wan et al., 2020). IT is applied to medicine for personal care, which is at the center of the therapeutic, diagnostic, or preventive project, and as such receives or requires medical, health, or socio-sanitary acts (Dua et al., 2014; Liyanage et al., 2019).

Personal care, understood as the relationship between the person and the health system, has not changed. What has undergone is a clear transformation by the way in which health care is provided, both in terms of performing a medical service and in terms of organizing related services. The introduction of Information Technology has made health care more convenient from an economic point of view, as it reduces waste and inefficiencies with greater citizen involvement (Van Calster et al., 2019). IT allows a substantial reduction in the consumption of resources, both for the healthcare professional and for the citizen-user. The increase in productivity derives from the reduction of medical errors, from the attenuation or elimination of unnecessary treatment, from the reduction of waiting lines, from the limitation of the movements of citizens in the territory, from the reduction of waiting lists, and from the simplification of access to patient data and facilitating disease treatment (Siau and Shen, 2006; Kwak and Hui, 2019; Jewell et al., 2020).

A digital report without leaving home, paying for a specialist reservation without going to the office, or changing your doctor from the comfort of your PC are just some examples of improvements introduced using new technologies. The use of IT allows a tracking of operations to guarantee respect for privacy and the tracking of any access to clinical documents (Steil et al., 2019; Lanzing, 2019). The economic convenience introduced by the use of IT is closely connected with the increase in productivity and derives from the reduction of medical errors, from the mitigation or elimination of unnecessary treatment, through greater communication between the different healthcare institutions and the same professionals (Gu et al., 2019; Iftikhar et al., 2019). Another saving is obtained by reducing and/or eliminating paper material (Usak et al., 2020).

In this work, we used ensemble methodologies to preventively diagnose endocrinologic disorders such as those related to the thyroid. The data used as input derive from tests carried out on a population sample with the collection of numerous indicators. The term ensemble refers to a set of basic learning machines whose predictions are combined to improve the overall performance. The ensemble methods can be divided into two categories: generative and nongenerative. The nongenerative ones try to combine in the best possible way the predictions made by the machines, while the generative ones generate new sets of learners, to generate differences between them that can improve the overall performance. An ensemble method is a technique that combines predictions from multiple machine-learning algorithms to make predictions more accurate than any single model. By using multiple methods in modeling, prediction skills are improved as each contribution seeks to reinforce the weaknesses of the others.

The first part of the paper introduces the basics of the techniques based on Machine Learning with particular attention to the methods used in the field of Medical Informatics. Subsequently, the main algorithms based on Ensemble Learning are treated in detail and then move on to a rich review of the main works that have used a Machine Learning-based model for disease diagnosis. Finally, a specific case is treated: Predicting thyroid disease using ensemble learning.

## 2  Data analytics

Health care supported by digital technologies has generated in recent years a large volume of useful data on the clinical history of patients, on the treatment plans to which they have undergone, on the costs that the therapies applied have produced, and finally on the insurance coverage which the patients enjoyed. This amount of data has attracted the attention of data analysis experts who have been concerned with developing methodologies to analyze them (Zikopoulos and Eaton, 2011).

Data Analytics are tools that are based on statistical inference to examine in depth the raw data and knowledge available to identify correlations, trends or verify existing theories and models. They answer questions precisely and start from hypotheses formulated from the beginning, focusing on sectors, with the aim of obtaining the best practices that lead to an improvement of the system. These tools allow you to make future forecasts and what-if simulations to verify the effects of certain changes on the system, as well as to obtain more detailed and in-depth analyses. Using more sophisticated techniques and tools, they can analyze much larger datasets. Analysis tools help analysts turn data into knowledge. The ability to analyze a large amount of information, often unstructured, represents a clear source of competitive advantage and differentiation. Big Data, combined with sophisticated data analysis, have the potential to provide researchers with unprecedented insights into patient behavior and health system conditions, enabling decisions to be made faster and more effectively (Raghupathi and Raghupathi, 2014).

The data analysis examines the data with the aim of extracting knowledge from the information. In emergency assistance, data analysis helps emergency teams to efficiently select raw data, message traffic and news feeds from the Internet to instantly define where and when a health emergency is occurring. In preventive care, data analysis identifies outbreaks, trends, and prepares health specialists for the challenges they will face in the future (Kambatla et al., 2014).

Medical research also benefits greatly from data analysis. The ability to collect research, filter results, and stay abreast of the latest research-based best practices helps teams collaborate, improve test methods, and successfully apply for grants based on updated needs and information. Data analysis is more than just a hypothesis, but a determination of future events based on current facts and trends. Data analysis can be divided into two different spectra: exploratory data analysis and confirmation data analysis (Palanisamy and Thirunavukarasu, 2019). Exploratory data analysis, also known as EDA, is used to determine new trends in a market or sector. The analysis of confirmation data, or CDA, is used to demonstrate or refute existing hypotheses. In the medical field, the CDA is used in various sectors, from identifying the origin of a specific disease to which common drugs are most useful in the treatment of current symptoms. This is generally the way new drugs are developed, where research over time uses a combination of products and drugs to test and improve treatments. After years of research and combined data, the researcher can perform a complete analysis of the data, to determine whether the medical combination can cure the disease (Martinez et al., 2010).

Effective health analysis requires much more than extracting information from a database, applying a statistical model, and passing results to various end users. The process of transforming the data acquired in the source systems into information used by the health organization to improve quality and performance requires specific knowledge, adequate tools, quality improvement methodologies, and management commitment. Healthcare transformation efforts require decision makers to use information to understand all aspects of an organization's performance. In addition to knowing what happened, decision makers now need information on what is likely to happen, what the organization's improvement priorities should be, and what the expected impacts of the process and other improvements will be. Simply producing reports and visualizations of data from the health data repository is not enough to provide the information decision makers need (Reddy and Aggarwal, 2015).

Data Analytics can help decision makers achieve understanding of quality and operational performance by transforming the way information is used and decisions are made across the organization. Data Analytics is the system of tools and techniques necessary to generate understanding of data. The effective use of analysis within an organization requires that the necessary tools, methods, and systems have been applied appropriately and consistently and that the information generated by the analysis is accurate, validated, and reliable (Strome and Liefer, 2013).

## 3  Machine learning

Recently, a new tool for knowledge extraction has appeared in the panorama of Data Analytics: It is Machine Learning, a class of algorithms that using optimization techniques manage to retrieve useful information from data automatically. Machine Learning is a branch of Artificial Intelligence that includes all the studies on algorithms capable of performing a task with better performance as the experience grows. What makes this field extremely innovative is that it makes the machine an entity capable of carrying out inductive reasoning based on experience, in a completely analogous way to how man himself does it (Alpaydin, 2020).

Therefore, based on a training set of data from a certain probability distribution, the machine must be able to deal with new problems, therefore not known a priori, by building a probabilistic model of the occurrence space (Ciaburro, 2020). The computational analysis of machine learning algorithms is one of the works performed in learning theory, a field of study that aims to solve with various approaches, although never being able to offer certainties about the results, both for the finished quantity of data for training and for any underfitting and overfitting problems, essentially due to a disproportion between the required parameters and the number of observations (Marsland, 2015).

With the progress of studies and with the recognition of the various facets of the problems faced, there is a subdivision of the Machine Learning field into various branches that differ in the approach to solving the problems faced, for the type of data processed and for the task to be performed by the algorithm (Ciaburro and Venkateswaran, 2017).

Several paradigms have been developed, based on which to classify this type of algorithm:

- Supervised learning: The model is trained by collecting input data, to then obtain outputs that allow one to formulate a general rule to correctly associate inputs and outputs.
- Unsupervised learning: The model takes unlabeled inputs as an input and tries to generate a structure common to these input data.
- Reinforcement learning: The model interacts with a dynamic environment and is notified or rewarded only if the goal to be accomplished is accomplished.

In this field there are numerous approaches, which are based both on the type of strategies adopted and on the models generated. Moving from decision trees, graphs that allow decision-making through paths that lead to the prediction of a given variable by classification, to genetic algorithms, algorithms that emulate the phenomenon of natural selection and genetic evolution through techniques such as mutation and crossover, from inductive logic programming, an approach that links propositional logic to symbolic learning and that makes extensive use of entailment starting from knowledge bases, to Bayesian networks, graphical representations of the dependency relationships between the variables of a system that provide a specific of any complete joint probability distribution. Among the algorithms based on Machine Learning, ensemble learning has proved particularly effective in supervised classification (Ciaburro, 2017).

## 4  Approaching ensemble learning

Artificial intelligence studies the reproducibility of complex mental processes through the use of computers and pays particular attention to how they perceive the external environment, how they interact with it, and how they are able to learn and solve problems, elaborate information, and reach decisions. Of great importance is the learning activity, which allows to increase the knowledge of the machine and to make adaptive changes, so that the decision-making process in a later period is more efficient (Polikar, 2012).

Therefore, the realization of an inductive as well as deductive learning is important, that is, a process that starting from a collection of examples concerning a specific sphere of interest, he arrives at the formulation of a hypothesis capable of predicting future examples. The conceptual difficulty in formulating a hypothesis consists in the impossibility of establishing whether it is a good approximation of the function that it must emulate or not, but it is possible to draw qualitative considerations, so a hypothesis that will be able to make a good generalization, so he will be able to correctly predict examples he has not seen so far. Furthermore, it is possible to arrive at the formulation of several hypotheses, with similar predictive capacity, all consistent. In this case, the optimal choice will be the simplest solution (Zhang and Ma, 2012).

A substantial difference between deductive and inductive inference is that the former guarantees logical correctness, as it does not alter the reality of interest, while the latter can tend toward excessive generalization and therefore carry out incorrect selective processes. Artificial intelligence systems are reflected in a vast domain of applications concerning a high quantity and heterogeneity of sectors, from the interpretation of natural language, to games, to the demonstration of mathematical theorems, to robotics. Furthermore, machine learning has great relevance in Data Mining, that is, the extraction of data and knowledge from an enormous wealth of information through automated methods. To reproduce typical activities of the human brain, such as the recognition of shapes and figures, the interpretation of language, and the perception of the environment in a sensorial way, neural networks have been created, with the aim of simulating the functioning of the animal brain on the computer (Krawczyk et al., 2017).

Ensemble learning methods are very powerful techniques for obtaining more correct decision-making processes, at the expense of greater complexity and a loss of interpretability, compared to learning systems based on single hypotheses. The ensemble learning combines the predictions of hypothesis collections to obtain greater performance efficiency. For explanatory purposes, it is useful to compare this type of learning to an executive committee of a company, in which several people with certain skills present their ideas to reach a final decision. It is evident that the knowledge of a group of people can lead to a more thoughtful solution than the decision of a single director. Also, this type of analogy allows us to make qualitative considerations that will be applicable in the domain of artificial intelligence (Gomes et al., 2017).

In fact, it is easy to imagine that if the directors all have very similar knowledge and therefore limited to the same area, the analyses and decisions of the individuals will not be very heterogeneous and we will obtain benefits to a lesser extent in the use of the ensemble. If, on the other hand, the knowledge of each director is highly sectored, so that each participant on the committee adds knowledge that is not replicated, the final decision will be more appropriate. If we assume that there is a director at the board's management, who once had taken into consideration the individual opinions (votes), comes to a solution, it is reasonable to think that he trusts most of those who made more correct choices in the past, in the case I therefore practice advisors who he deems most reliable (Wang et al., 2016).

Similarly, in committee learning, the votes of the individual hypotheses are weighted to emphasize the predictions of those deemed most correct. In conclusion, ensemble learning combines different models derived from the same training set to produce a combination of them that widens the space of hypotheses. The term ensemble means a set of basic learning machines whose predictions are combined to improve overall performance (Akyuz et al., 2017).

Ensemble methods can be divided into two categories: generative and nongenerative. The nongenerative ones try to combine the predictions made by the machines in the best possible way, while the generative ones generate new sets of learners, to generate differences among them that can improve overall performance.

As for nongenerative techniques, in the classification, for example, the technique of major voting is used, possibly refined by weighing the votes proposed by the machines. Predictions can be combined by means of possibly weighted, median, product, sum, or by choosing the minimum or the maximum. Generative methods attempt to improve system performance by attempting to use diversity between learners. To do this, different sets are generated with which to train the machines using the resampling technique, or the aggregation of classes is manipulated differently through the feature selection technique, or even learners can be trained who specialize on specific parts of the set of learning with the mixture of expert techniques. Resampling techniques, such as bootstrapping, allow you to generate new sets from the original one (Wang et al., 2018).

The most common and efficient ensemble learning methods are:

- bagging
- boosting
- stacking

However much they can improve the actual performance of the system, it is necessary to take into account a greater difficulty of analysis, since they can be composed of a substantial number of single models, which is why it will be difficult to intuitively understand which factors contributed to the improvement and which ones instead can be considered redundant or degrading.

For example, several decision trees generated on the same dataset could be considered and a vote by each of them on the classification of new data. The final predictive capacity will easily be more correct than that of the individual models and this could be significantly affected even by a subset of the trees involved in the choice, but intuitively it will be difficult to recognize this subset (Ciaburro and Iannace, 2020).

The simplest technique for combining the responses of individual classifiers into a single prediction is that of weighted votes and is used by both boosting and bagging, the substantial difference of which is in the way in which these models are generated (Alam et al., 2019).

# 5 Understanding bagging

Bagging is an ensemble method that takes its name from the union of the words Bootstrap AGGregat-ING and provides for the assignment of identical weights for each individual model applied to a specific set of training. It may be thought that if several training sets of equal cardinality are extracted starting from the same domain of a problem and a decision tree is built for each one, then these trees will be similar and will arrive at identical predictions for a new test example. Bootstrapping consists of the extraction with replacement of its elements to create new training sets that are different from each other. The probability of extraction of each example, in bagging, is equal to that of the others. The basic algorithm involves the creation of models for each training set and subsequently the combination of the various predictions on the test set through an average operation (Baskin et al., 2017).

This assumption is usually incorrect due to the instability of the decision trees, which owing to small changes in the input attributes can correspond to large changes in terms of ramifications and therefore lead to different classifications. It is implicit that if starting from the same basic set, one achieves remarkably different results, then the outputs can be both correct and wrong. In a system where there is a hypothesis for each training set and whose response to a new example is determined by the votes of the individual hypotheses (majority vote), a correct prediction will be more necessary than that which we would obtain starting from a single model. Nonetheless, it will always be possible to find an incorrect answer, as no learning scheme is affected by error. An estimate of the expected error in the architecture assumed can be calculated as the average of the errors of the individual classifiers. To better understand the characteristics of bagging, it is good to analyze bias errors, variance errors, and bootstrap first (Yaman and Subasi, 2019).

Given the following initial dataset:

$$C = \{(x1; y1), \ldots, (xn; yn)\} \tag{1}$$

A few new datasets $C_k$ (with $k = 1, \ldots, m$) are extracted from the set $C$ using the replacement technique. For each $C_k$ dataset obtained, a predictive model is elaborated, according to the following function:

$$f(x, C) = \frac{1}{m} \sum_{i=1}^{m} f_k(x, C_k) \tag{2}$$

The algorithm brings improvements, thanks to the diversity of the various $f_k$ models (Fig. 1). For this reason, less stable basic models are recommended, that is, capable of producing consistent differences also starting from similar training sets. This does not mean that the basic machines must necessarily be different. Bagging improves overall prediction performance because it reduces variance if the machines that are part of it have low bias (Subasi and Qaisar, 2020).

Recall that in an algorithm based on machine learning, we can identify two error components: the first due to the particular learning algorithm used, called bias, and the second relating to the peculiar training set used, indicated with the name of variance. The bias represents a deviation from the current value and cannot be calculated accurately, but can only be approximate, it is also independent of the number of training sets used and is an indicator of the persistence of the error of a specific algorithm.

The variance, on the other hand, is closely related to the training set used and is a measure of the variability of the learning model. In practical terms, if we use different training sets to repeat the training several times, the variance will be the difference between the values predicted by each model.

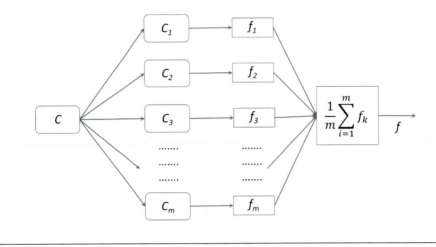

**FIG. 1**

Bagging operating scheme.

The choice of the type of architecture to be used in bagging is based on the evaluation of the best performance obtained on the test set: An evaluation of the error of the basic machines in terms of bias and variance can be carried out. Mediating low bias models allows you to obtain a low bias model by reducing the variance. Although the bias-variance analysis of the machines has not been addressed, the choice to consider the model with better performance on the test set proves to be consistent (Ditzler et al., 2017).

You can further criticize the choice by thinking that the best machines are optimal for the original training set and it is not known if they can be used for the various sets generated by the random extraction. The hope is that the best ones have characteristics of complexity suitable for the characteristics of the data to be approximated.

As for the dimensions of the $C_k$ sets, there is no theory that indicates what the optimal value should be. This depends on the quantity and type of data available. Bagging is a parallelizable algorithm since the training of a single machine does not influence in any way that of the others.

This bootstrap aggregation technique tends to neutralize the instability of the learning algorithms and is more useful precisely in learning schemes where there is a high instability, as this implies a greater diversity obtainable with small input variations. Consequently, when bagging is used, attempts are made to make the learning algorithm as unstable as possible. The operation of this method can be summarized in two steps:

1. the generation of individual models, in which m instances are selected from the training set and the learning algorithm is applied
2. the combination of the models obtained to produce a classification

The error due to the bias turns out to be the mean square deviation obtained by averaging the numerical classifications of the individual models, while the variance is the distance between the predictions of the individual models and depends on the training set used. Bias and variance are closely related to the complexity of the learning model, so as the parameters added to it increase, the bias component will decay while the variance component will increase exponentially (Singhal et al., 2018).

## 6 Exploring boosting

The basic idea of the Boosting techniques is to build a list of classifiers by assigning, in an iterative way, a weight to each new classifier. Considering, in this way, its ability to recognize samples not correctly identified by the other classifiers already involved in the training. At each phase of the algorithm, a new classifier is trained using the dataset, in which the weighted coefficients are adjusted based on the performance of the previously trained classifier, so as to assign a greater weight to the incorrectly classified data points (Liu et al., 2018).

The algorithm focuses on the most difficult samples to classify, which are therefore weighted more. The final classifier is obtained with a weighted vote of the built models. As with other ensemble techniques, combining multiple models is particularly effective when they achieve a high percentage of correct predictions and are quite different from each other, i.e., presenting a high rate of variability. The ideal situation to which boosting aims is the maximum sectorization of the models, so that each of them is a specialist in a part of the domain in which the other classifiers fail to arrive at accurate predictions. Therefore, boosting attributes greater weight to instances that have not been correctly predicted, to build high models, in subsequent iterations, capable of filling this gap. In analogy with bagging, only learning algorithms of the same type are combined and their outputs are combined by vote or by averaging the individual responses, in the case of classification or numerical prediction, respectively (Ghojogh and Crowley, 2019).

The algorithm consists of the following steps:

1. A tree is produced with a process that considers instances with greater weight to be more relevant
2. The product tree is used to classify the training set
3. The weight of instances correctly classified is reduced, while that of instances incorrectly classified is increased
4. Steps 1 to 3 are repeated until a specified number of trees have been produced
5. A weight proportional to its performance on the training set is assigned to each tree.

For the classification of new instances, a weighted voting system is used, usually majority voting, by all trees. The purpose of this algorithm is to produce different trees, to cover a wider set of types of instances. The defect with which the boosting method is often accused is the susceptibility to noise. If there are incorrect data in the training set, the boosting algorithm will tend to give greater weight to the instances that contain them, inevitably leading to a deterioration in performance. To overcome this problem, boosting algorithms have also been proposed, in which instances that are repeatedly classified incorrectly are interpreted as containing incorrect data and consequently their weight is reduced (Ng et al., 2018).

## 7 Discovering stacking

Stacked generalization, from whose abbreviation the term stacking derives, is the most recent ensemble technique, conceived to generate a scheme that minimizes the error rate of classifiers. Stacking, by virtue of its functioning, can be considered as a process that evolves the behavior of cross-validation to combine different individual models more efficiently. Stacking is a technique used to obtain high precision in generalization. This method tries to evaluate the reliability of the trees produced and is usually used to combine trees produced by different algorithms. The idea is to extract a new dataset containing an instance for each instance of the original dataset, in which however the original attributes are replaced with the classifications produced by each tree, while the output remains the original class. These new instances are then used to produce a new classifier that combines the different predictions into one. It is suggested to divide the original training set into two subsets. The first used to create the dataset and the second used to produce the base classifiers (Divina et al., 2018).

The new classifier's predictions will therefore reflect the actual performance of the basic induction algorithms. While classifying a new instance, each base tree produces its prediction. These predictions will constitute a new instance which will be classified by the new classifier. If trees produce a probability classification, it is possible to increase the stacking performance by inserting in the new instances the probabilities expressed by each tree for each class. Stacking performance has been shown to be at least comparable to that of the best classifier chosen by cross-validation (Sun and Trevor, 2018).

## 7.1 Machine learning applications for healthcare analytics

In recent years, algorithms based on Machine Learning have been applied to extract knowledge in many fields. In HealthCare, these algorithms have been used to improve the quality of life by supporting researchers in activities aimed at diagnosing diseases, analyzing clinical data, in the process of drug discovery, to name a few (Panesar, 2019).

## 7.2 Machine learning-based model for disease diagnosis

In the last 10 years, there has been a significant and growing use of Machine Learning in HealthCare, which is gaining great interest thanks also to publications that have revealed a precision in specific clinical contexts. Some algorithms have managed to show a diagnostic accuracy comparable to that of doctors experienced in different disciplines. Some examples of applications of machine learning in HealthCare that lead to a benefit of diagnostic accuracy were detection of cancers through the analysis of radiological images, detection of diabetic retinopathy, and algorithms capable of predicting future cardiovascular events (Rojas et al., 2019).

## 7.3 Machine learning-based algorithms to identify breast cancer

Cancer is a very complex genetic disease, the appearance of which is attributable to certain unwanted genetic mutations. Knowing how to recognize these genetic mutations could be useful for the identification and prevention of tumor development in individuals. Even more useful would be to be able to identify tumor development from a limited number of mutations. Fine-needle aspiration (FNA) of a breast lump allows us to take a sample of cells to be studied under the microscope to discriminate whether a breast lump is of a benign nature or if it is a malignant tumor. A thin needle is inserted into the breast, until it reaches the lump, from where a part of the content to be examined in the laboratory is sucked. The sampling is done simultaneously with an ultrasound scan to locate the nodule. The aspirated biological liquid is subsequently substituted for cytological examination, which consists in the observation under an optical microscope of cells taken to characterize their content through the extraction of features. Agarap (2018) applied six machine learning-based algorithms to identify breast cancer based on features extracted from FNA tests. The dataset used by Agarap for training the algorithm contains the features obtained through the cytological examination. Six algorithms have been used in this study: Linear Regression, Multilayer Perceptron (MLP), Nearest Neighbor (NN), Softmax Regression, Support Vector Machine (SVM), and finally a combination of recurrent neural network (RNN) and the SVM. All the algorithms used have returned satisfactory results with high performance on the binary classification of breast cancer, with an accuracy that has exceeded 90%.

## 7.4 Convolutional neural networks to detect cancer cells in brain images

Sawant et al. (2018) used an algorithm based on convolutional neural networks (CNNs) to detect cancer cells in brain images obtained by the Magnetic resonance imaging (MRI) test. MRI is a test carried out with an implant that nowadays plays an important role in the health sector and allows you to perform a whole range of diagnostic tests, from traditional to functional neuroradiology, from internal diagnostics to obstetrics and gynecology and pediatrics. The machine is equipped with a magnet that creates a strong and stable magnetic field to align all the protons in the same field and determine their rotation, all in the same direction. A frequency signal is subsequently sent within the magnetic field which determines the misalignment of the protons; at the end of the same, the protons return to their equilibrium position, release energy, which is detected by a receiving coil. From the detection, the time it takes for the protons to return to their aligned position is measured, providing information regarding the type of tissue and reconstructing the image of the site in question. In this study, the authors used the Tensorflow platform to develop the CNN-based algorithm, obtaining 98.6% accuracy on validation data.

## 7.5 Machine learning techniques to detect prostate cancer in Magnetic resonance imaging

Prostate cancer originates from the cells of the prostate gland. Many forms of prostate cancer grow slowly and are unlikely to spread, but some can proliferate faster. The precise causes of prostate cancer are unknown and early stage prostate cancer is often asymptomatic. Prostate cancer is the second most common malignant neoplasm in the world in men and mainly affects men of advanced age. In fact, over half of prostate cancer cases are diagnosed in men over the age of 70. Early stage prostate cancer is typically asymptomatic. Symptoms that can manifest themselves as the disease progresses are often caused by the compression exerted by the cancerous mass on the urethra and include an increase in the frequency with which you urinate, have difficulty urinating, or feel an urgent need to urinate. Normally, the diagnosis of prostate cancer is based on the results of the clinical examination of the prostate, a blood test that measures the levels of a protein called prostate-specific antigen (PSA) and biopsy. Further investigations may help determine how advanced the cancer is. For example, imaging tests are called the magnetic resonance imaging (MRI). Prostate cancer is diagnosed based on the size of the tumor, the presence or absence of involvement of the lymph nodes, and the presence or absence of spread to other parts of the body. This information is used to facilitate the choice of the optimal therapeutic strategy. The images obtained with the MRI test have a high resolution and require adequate diagnostic tools for a correct interpretation. Hussain et al. (2018) applied an algorithm based on several Machine Learning techniques to detect prostate cancer in images obtained from the Magnetic resonance imaging (MRI) test. To support the radiologist in detecting anomalies, the authors developed algorithms based on the Bayesian approach, on the Support vector machine (SVM), on the radial base function (RBF), and on the Gaussian and Decision Tree. The algorithms were trained using the invariant feature transform (SIFT), and elliptic Fourier descriptors' (EFDs') features, among others. The results obtained in the automatic diagnosis of prostate cancer have been satisfactory, returning an accuracy that has reached 98.3% in the SVM Gaussian Kernel case.

## 7.6 Classification of respiratory diseases using machine learning

Respiratory diseases are diseases that affect the lungs and/or respiratory tract. These include asthma, chronic obstructive pulmonary disease (COPD), allergic rhinitis, work-related lung disease, and pulmonary hypertension. To diagnose these diseases, the doctor carries out a thorough physical examination and an interview. The characteristics of the disease and respiratory problems will also be examined and evaluated. Typical examination performed by the doctor is auscultation. It is a diagnostic system that consists of listening to the internal sounds of the body. The part of interest refers to the term with the meaning of listening, through a stethoscope, to the sounds produced by the respiratory system. The stethoscope can be placed in various parts of the chest, back, and neck. The normal sounds that can be heard on a subject's chest during the inhalation phase are mainly generated in the lobar part of the respiratory tract. The respiratory sounds are generated by air turbulence in the airway. The characteristics of the sounds are very variable, you can notice differences from person to person that depend on weight, age, health, and other factors. There is also a variability with respect to the density of the gas breathed. Abnormal or pathological respiratory sounds are accidental sounds that are not part of the normal breathing cycle. In recent years, the classic stethoscope has been replaced by an electronic version that records the sounds from the lungs. Poreva et al. (2017) studied lung sounds to classify them automatically using some algorithms based on Machine Learning. The authors used the sounds recorded by the patients by extracting the coefficient of bicoherence that was used to train the algorithms. Five algorithms were tested: Support Vector Machine, Logistic regression, Bayes Classifier, k-Nearest Neighbors, and Decision tree. The results showed that the SVM classifier and the decision tree classifier returned the best performances of 88% and 77% accuracy, respectively.

## 7.7 Parkinson's disease diagnosis with machine learning-based models

Parkinson's disease is a degenerative disease of the central nervous system that affects 7 to 10 million people worldwide, with an average age of onset around 60 years. The prevalence of this disease is expected to double over the next 20 years mainly due to the growing aging of the population. This pathology manifests itself with various symptoms that can be motor or nonmotor and that can lead to various problems that are reflected in daily life. Quantitatively, the number of symptoms is very high, and it is difficult to consider all the subjective signs and symptoms. As a result, research often focuses on a certain aspect, leaving out or in any case not considering everything else, thus losing the overall vision of the subject. A motor symptom of this disease is the difficulty of language: The voice may be feebler, or it may present a loss of tonality and modulation, which leads the patient to speak in a rather monotonous way. Sometimes, a palilalia appears which manifests itself in a repetition of syllables, and there is a tendency to accelerate the emission of sounds and not to pronounce all the syllables. Mostafa et al. (2019) developed a methodology for the identification of Parkinson's disease by classifying voice disorders using algorithms based on. The authors first extracted features from the dataset of recorded vocal sounds and then filtered these features through a Multiple Feature Evaluation Approach (MFEA) with a multi-agent system. They later used several Machine Learning-based algorithms to classify voice disorders: Decision Tree, Naïve Bayes, Neural Network, Random Forest, and Support Vector Machine. The models returned an accuracy ranging from 74% to 86%.

## 8  Processing drug discovery with machine learning

Drug research and development is an expensive, long, and inefficient process, which takes more than 10 years to transfer a new drug to the market, with a cost of several billion dollars and a high risk of failure. The need to overcome the limits in the development of new therapies is made even more evident in the light of the global health needs' data. Half of the failures are due to lack of efficacy, while a quarter of the failures are due to problems of tolerability, both causes expressing the difficulty of selecting the right target for the disease under study (Stephenson et al., 2019). To optimize the process of discovery and development of new therapeutic molecules, it is therefore necessary to use the knowledge hidden in the complexity of the data made available by biomedical research in the most efficient way. However, thanks to the computational skills and methodologies of computer science and machine learning techniques, it is possible to manage and analyze the volume of biomedical data in an automated way, to extrapolate significant relationships, generate new hypotheses to be subjected to experimental verification, and predict with statistical method the occurrence of future phenomena, including efficacy and toxicity associated with drugs (Vamathevan et al., 2019).

The search for new drugs is long and complex. First, some molecule candidates for therapy are identified and tested on cell cultures. Those that are most effective go to the next stages, in vivo tests. Finally, clinical trials are conducted on human patients. This process often requires years of research and significant economic investments. In recent times, the development of technology is revolutionizing the process of finding new drugs (Ekins et al., 2019).

In most cases, the targets of drug action are functional proteins such as receptors, enzymes, transport proteins, and a cascade of intracellular events derived from the drug-substrate interaction that culminates in the final biological effect. In a smaller number of cases, the methods of interaction between drug and living matter are carried out differently without affecting macromolecular complexes. Finally, some categories of drugs interact directly with DNA (Klambauer et al., 2019).

Generally, the birth of a drug starts precisely from the identification of a pharmacological target in the context of a clinical condition of interest. Once a project has been planned for the creation of a new drug starting from a real therapeutic need, researchers must focus attention on a pharmacological target to treat a pathological condition. Thus, begins the process of developing a drug, a long journey in stages that requires the use of huge human and economic resources (Xiao and Sun, 2019).

In this long process, the use of artificial intelligence can play a crucial role in speeding up the process by identifying the essential characteristics and leaving out the superfluous ones. Machine learning can be of assistance in many activities used in the modeling of new drugs. Identification of protein sequences, virtual screening, prediction of bio activators, chemical synthesis, and prediction of toxicity are just some examples of activities that can be dealt with taking the help of algorithms based on Machine Learning (Zoffmann et al., 2019).

## 8.1 Analyzing clinical data using machine learning algorithms

Electronic devices connected to an intensive care unit (ICU) patient produce a large amount of data on the patient's status. These data are often only used to activate alerts in the event of an emergency that alert medical personnel who in this way go to the patient to check their health. Currently, thanks to the algorithms based on Machine Learning, these data could be used to extract knowledge on the patient's clinical path and help medical staff in predicting the evolution of the disease. The historical data of patients who have undergone a similar course of the disease could be used to train a model capable of predicting the future situation of a patient in hospital. A Machine Learning-based model can be developed to predict mortality of ICU patients using Medical Information Mart's diagnostic codes (Jaworska et al., 2019).

This example is only an application that is well suited to the use of patient clinical data to generate predictive scenarios that support medical personnel in the decision-making process related to the therapy to be given to a patient. Other possible applications are the use of wearable sensors to manage a patient's rehabilitation path. The collected data can be used to develop a model to recognize a patient's behavior based on a recurrent neural network using collected sequential data (Khan et al., 2020).

A further source of data is represented by the Electronic Health Records (EHRs). EHR is a tool used to collect patient's medical history data, data that are collected during meetings with healthcare professionals, for prevention or on episodes of illness. The data present in it, suitably reworked, will subsequently constitute a source of historical data useful for the management of the health system, alongside the more strictly administrative and organizational data. These data can be used to develop a model to predict future patient health based on the past EHR data (Wang et al., 2020).

## 8.2 Predicting thyroid disease using ensemble learning

The thyroid is an endocrine gland capable of secreting and synthesizing two hormones such as thyroxine (T4) and triiodothyronine (T3) which control numerous metabolic functions, act on the development of the central nervous system, and allow the organism to grow. The thyroid consists of two lobes connected by an isthmus and is located in the neck between the second and third tracheal rings, and inferior to the thyroid cartilage. The synthesis of thyroid hormones is divided into three phases (Cooper and Biondi, 2012).

- Iodine uptake. Follicular thyroid cell-mediated iodine uptake is the first step in the synthesis of thyroid hormones.
- Synthesis of thyroglobulin. The thyroglobulin synthesized in the endoplasmic reticulum is transferred to the Golgi apparatus where it is glycosylated, then stored in exocytotic vesicles and released into the cavity of the follicle.
- Iodide organization and iodotyrosine condensation. This process involves numerous reactions catalyzed by thyroid oxidase (TPO). TPO is an enzyme containing a heme group thanks to which it oxidizes the iodine collected by follicular cells.

Synthesis and secretion of thyroid hormones are regulated by extrathyroid factors that act on the processes according to a feedback-negative mechanism and intrathyroid factors of self-regulation dependent on iodine intake.

Thyroid diseases include both benign and functional pathologies that can be traced back to normal- and hyperfunctioning forms (depending on the quantity of thyroid hormones produced), as well as inflammatory and neoplastic pathologies.

The term hyperthyroidism refers to a clinical situation characterized by an increase in circulating thyroid hormones T3 and T4. Since thyroid hormones are the main regulators of metabolism, this condition leads to an increase in many metabolic reactions (Vanderpump, 2011).

Hypothyroidism is a clinical syndrome due to an insufficient action of the thyroid hormones at the tissue level and causes a slowdown of all metabolic processes. Hypothyroidism that develops during fetal and/or neonatal life determines an important and often permanent reduction of growth and neurological development processes, while hypothyroidism in adults, which has a high frequency (20.6%–20.8%), with greater frequency in the female sex, in old age and, in most cases, a consequence of the autoimmune pathology, causes a generalized slowdown of the metabolic processes (Fatourechi, 2001).

## 8.3 Machine learning-based applications for thyroid disease classification

The diagnosis of thyroid disorder requires experience and knowledge from the doctor. The diagnosis is made through a physical examination of the patient and a simultaneous interview to collect the symptoms he feels and subsequently examining blood tests from laboratory tests. Despite all these tests, it is not easy to diagnose and predict thyroid disorder with accuracy.

Shankar et al. (2018) have developed an algorithm for classifying thyroid disorders based on the kernel classifier process. To start with, they carried out a process of selecting features to reduce the number of variables to be used in the model to reduce the processing time of the algorithm and focus attention only on the most significant predictors. The authors used a multikernel SVM for the classification of the thyroid disorder. Support vector machines (SVMs) are a set of supervised learning methods that can be used for both classification and regression. Given two classes of multidimensional linearly separable patterns, among all possible separation hyperplanes, SVM determines the one capable of separating the classes with the greatest possible margin. In practice, the linear case is not easily identifiable, whereas nonlinear models or a combination of linear and nonlinear models are used to solve this problem. The authors used a combination of linear kernel and radial basis function kernel. The results obtained were satisfactory with an accuracy of 97%.

Tyagi et al. (2018) studied the classification of thyroid disorders using different machine learning-based algorithms. First, they used the Artificial Neural Networks, then a model based on Support Vector Machine, then they used Decision Tree, and finally they applied the k-Nearest Neighbor. In Decision Tree-based algorithms, classification functions are learned in the form of a tree where: each internal node represents a variable, an arc toward a child node represents a possible value for that property, and a leaf represents the predicted value for a class starting from the values of the other properties, which in the tree is represented by the path from the root node to the leaf node. The k-Nearest Neighbor algorithm is based on the concept of classifying an unknown sample considering the class of the k closest samples of the training set. The new champion will be assigned to the class to which most of the nearest k champions belong.

Ma et al. (2019) used single-photon emission computed tomography (SPECT) images to train a model based on convolutional neural networks to diagnose thyroid disorders. SPECT is a recent diagnostic test that allows you to reconstruct scintigraphy images relating to the distribution of a radioactive tracer substance in small doses into the patient's organism to measure some biological and biochemical processes on the computer. Three types of disorders are classified: Graves' disease, Hashimoto's disease, and subacute thyroiditis. The authors developed a model based on a DenseNet architecture. A DenseNet network is made up of a series of dense blocks interspersed with pooling layers. A dense block consists of a sequence of convolutional feature maps, without polling, where the input of a map is the concatenation of the outputs of all the previous maps.

Poudel et al. (2019) used ultrasounds of the thyroid for the classification of the disorders adopting a methodology based on the combination of machine learning algorithms and autoregressive features. Thyroid diseases change their size and shape, and these changes are appreciably noticeable with the course of the disease. With the ultrasound of the thyroid it is possible to study the position, shape, structure, and size of this gland. Therefore, it is used in the study of chronic thyroid diseases. The analysis of ultrasound of the thyroid gland is not simple as it deals with low contrast images, with a consistent presence of noise and an uneven distribution. To automate the classification process of thyroid ultrasounds, the authors used three machine learning algorithms: Support Vector Machine, Artificial Neural Network, and Random Forest. For the extraction of the features to be used in the training of the model, a methodology based on autoregressive modeling was adopted, identifying 30 spectral functions. The proposed technology returned an accuracy of approximately 90% with all three methods.

Ouyang et al. (2019) classified thyroid nodules through linear and nonlinear machine learning algorithms. Early treatment of thyroid cancer through analysis of malignant thyroid nodules is crucial in the treatment of thyroid disorders. In this task, algorithms based on machine learning can support the work of clinicians in the classification of nodules based on the information contained in pathological reports or from data obtained with fine-needle aspiration (FNA). The authors compared the results obtained in the classification of nodules using linear and nonlinear algorithms. Ridge regression, Lasso-penalty, and Elastic Net (EN) were applied among the linear methods. As nonlinear methods the authors used random forest (RF), kernel-Support Vector Machines (k-SVMs), Neural Network (Nnet), kernel nearest neighborhood (k-NN), and Naïve Bayes (NB). The linear and nonlinear methods returned comparable results, among which the methods that returned the best performances were Random Forest and Kernel-Support Vector Machines.

## 8.4 Preprocessing the dataset

The goal of this work is to identify a thyroid disorder among three a priori defined classes. To do this, we will use the data contained in the dataset called Thyroid Disease Data Set from the Garavan Institute. These data were taken from the UCI Repository of Machine Learning databases (Dua and Graff, 2019). The database contains 7200 instances with 21 predictors, including 15 categorical and 6 real attributes. The response variable contains three classes: 1-normal (nonhypothyroid), 2-hyperthyroid, and 3-hypothyroid. The variables contained in the dataset are the following:

1. Age: real
2. Sex: categorical
3. On_thyroxine: categorical
4. Query_on_thyroxine: categorical
5. On_antithyroid_medication: categorical
6. Sick: categorical
7. Pregnant: categorical
8. Thyroid_surgery: categorical
9. I131_treatment: categorical
10. Query_hypothyroid: categorical

11. Query_hyperthyroid: categorical
12. Lithium: categorical
13. Goiter: categorical
14. Tumor: categorical
15. Hypopituitary: categorical
16. Psych: categorical
17. TSH: real
18. T3: real
19. TT4: real
20. T4U: real
21. FTI: real
22. Class: categorical

The ability of an algorithm to perform well on inputs never observed previously is called generalization. During the training phase, the efficiency of the network is evaluated by sending test data as input, to calculate the error associated with the test. The algorithm's performance is improved by trying to minimize this error. This is a simple optimization problem. What separates machine learning from optimization is the minimization not of the training error, but of the error on generalization. The generalization error is defined as the expected value of the error on a new input. The expectation value is assessed on a series of different inputs, extracted from the distribution of inputs that we expect the system to meet in practice (Kawaguchi et al., 2019).

To guarantee the generalization of the algorithm, it is necessary to appropriately divide the available data into two subsets: training set and test set. The training set will be used for training the algorithm, while the test set will be authorized in the test phase. In this way, in the test phase the properly trained algorithm will be tested on data it has never seen before (Tabassum, 2020).

There are several techniques for splitting the dataset into the two-subset training and test sets. The most used are: Simple random sampling (SRS), Systematic sampling, Trial-and-error methods, Convenience sampling, and Stratified sampling. In this work, we have used the Simple random sampling (SRS) method (Reitermanova, 2010).

This is the most used method, given its efficiency and simplicity of implementation. Through this method, the samples are randomly selected with a uniform distribution: Each sample has the same probability of selection. Random selection ensures that there are no datasets with similar characteristics that are selected in one subset. In this study, 70% of the data (5040 samples) was used for the training set and the remaining 30% of the data (2160 samples) for the test set.

The hardware and software described in Tables 1 and 2 were used to tackle the problem of predicting thyroid disorders with the use of ensemble methods.

| Table 1 Hardware requirements for the simulation. | |
|---|---|
| Central Processing Unit (CPU): | Intel Core i5 6th Generation processor or higher, and AMD equivalent processor |
| RAM: | 8 GB minimum, 16 GB or higher is recommended |
| Graphics Processing Unit (GPU): | NVIDIA GeForce GTX 960 or higher |
| Operating System: | Ubuntu or Microsoft Windows 10 |

| Table 2 Software requirements for the simulation. | |
|---|---|
| Programming Platform: | Python |
| | R |
| Library: | TensorFlow |
| | Scikit-Learn |
| | Keras |

## 8.5 AdaBoostM algorithm

The AdaBoostM algorithm is one of the most used variants of boosting. This method is indicated if our set of inputs is discreet and therefore you want to solve a classification problem. This algorithm sequentially trains individual models, encouraging them at each iteration to provide correct predictions regarding the most important instances, that is, those to which the greatest weight is attributed.

AdaBoostM initially assigns to each of the instances of the training set the same weight, after which the specific learning algorithm chosen to generate a classifier is applied and new weights are attributed, which will be decremented as regards the aforementioned training set instances correctly and incremented for those that are not (Freund and Schapire, 1996).

The AdaBoostM algorithm elaborates a complex classifier starting from simple classifiers:

$$f(x) = \sum_{t=1}^{T} w_t * h_t(x)$$

Here,

- $w_t$ is the weight of the $t$th observation
- $h_t(x)$ is the function that indicates the diversity between the hypothesis, that is, the prediction made by the classifier and the actual value of the predicted class

Since at each iteration of the learning algorithm a redistribution of the weights is carried out, from time to time we will obtain sets of instances that can be defined easier and others more difficult, that is, not yet correctly classified, on the basis of which the following classifiers will be built.

At each iteration ($t$), the new weights are updated only for correctly classified instances, while the weight of the unclassified instances initially remains unchanged. Subsequently, the distributed weights are normalized, so that their total sum remains unaltered. This is accomplished by multiplying and dividing the weight of each instance respectively by the sum of the old and new weights. This operation increases the importance of the features not yet classified.

Once the iterative construction of the individual models has been established, it is necessary to understand how to combine them together to obtain a prediction, so even the individual responses of the classifiers will be weighed, giving greater emphasis to those believed to make better predictions (Burduk et al., 2020).

The estimate that allows us to evaluate the performance of each element belonging to the ensemble is the prediction error, which, if it is close to zero, is an indicator of high accuracy.

The algorithm consists of the following steps:

- **Input**: training set $x_i \in X$, $y_i \in Y$
- Initialization $D_1(i) = \frac{1}{N}$
- **For $t = 1, ..., T$:**
  1. Train the weak $h_t$ classifier using $t$th distribution $D_t$ minimizing the following error:
     $$\epsilon_t = \sum_i D_t(i) * h_t(x_i, y_i)$$
  2. Set $w_t = \dfrac{\epsilon_t}{1 - \epsilon_t}$
  3. Update $D$ using the following equation:

  $$D_{t+1}(i) = D_t(i) \frac{e^{-w_t(h_t(x_i, y_i) - h_t(x_i, y))}}{Z_t}$$

Here, $Z_t$ is a constant used for the $D_{t+1}$ normalization

- **Output**: Set the final classifier $H(x)$ as follows:

$$H(x) = \arg \max_{y \in Y} f(x, y) = \arg \max_{y \in Y} \left( \sum_{t=1}^{T} w_t * h_t(x) \right)$$

To reach a conclusive prediction, the weighted votes in favor of each output class are added and the most quoted is chosen.

After training the algorithm using the training dataset, the model obtained is used to make the forecast on the test dataset. Finally, a comparison is made between the predicted and expected values. The results are proposed using a confusion matrix. A confusion matrix is a square matrix $n \times n$, with $n$ number of classes to predict. This matrix tells us how a classifier works with respect to the different classes, in fact the correctly predicted class number is positioned on the main diagonal. In this way, all values outside the main diagonal represent classification errors. Table 3 shows the results of the classification:

From the analysis of the confusion matrix we can see that the classifier returned an excellent result on the test dataset. Recall that these data had not previously been provided to the classifier during the training phase. Out of 2160 observations, only 6 h were committed with a correct recognition of 2154 requests, obtaining an accuracy of 99.7%.

**Table 3 Confusion matrix.**

| | | Predicted class | | |
|---|---|---|---|---|
| | | Class 1 | Class 2 | Class 3 |
| True class | Class 1 | 53 | 0 | 0 |
| | Class 2 | 0 | 95 | 2 |
| | Class 3 | 4 | 0 | 2006 |

# 9 Conclusion

In this chapter, we have studied ensemble learning algorithms and how these algorithms can be used for the classification of health disorders. Ensemble learning methods provide decision-making processes with superior performance, compared to basic methods. This improvement in performance is due to greater complexity and a loss of interpretability compared to learning systems based on individual hypotheses. Learning the ensemble combines the predictions of hypothesis collections to achieve greater performance efficiency. We initially introduced the topic by analyzing various bibliographic contributions that used Machine Learning-based models in the context of HealthCare. Subsequently, we deepened the methodologies underlying Ensemble learning by showing different algorithms. Finally, we applied these methods to classify thyroid problems.

The techniques based on Ensemble Learning record ranking results superior to those of other algorithms, which recommends their use. On the other hand, the models obtained with the use of these techniques are difficult to interpret, as the output of the model is difficult to explain. This makes such methodologies less popular in the business world. Furthermore, ensemble methods are difficult to learn for technicians and any wrong selection can lead to lower predictive accuracy than an individual model. Finally, the training process with such methodologies is expensive both in terms of computation time and memory space. These weaknesses represent starting points for improving technologies based on Ensemble Learning. They also pose challenges to the scientific community to spread the use of these technologies more widely in the world of work.

# References

Agarap, A.F.M., 2018. On breast cancer detection: an application of machine learning algorithms on the Wisconsin diagnostic dataset. In: Proceedings of the 2nd International Conference on Machine Learning and Soft Computing, pp. 5–9.

Akyuz, A.O., Uysal, M., Bulbul, B.A., Uysal, M.O., 2017. Ensemble approach for time series analysis in demand forecasting: ensemble learning. In: 2017 IEEE International Conference on INnovations in Intelligent SysTems and Applications (INISTA). IEEE, pp. 7–12.

Alam, K.M.R., Siddique, N., Adeli, H., 2019. A dynamic ensemble learning algorithm for neural networks. Neural Comput. Applic., 1–16.

Alpaydin, E., 2020. Introduction to Machine Learning. MIT Press.

Baskin, I.I., Marcou, G., Horvath, D., Varnek, A., 2017. Bagging and boosting of classification models. In: Tutorials in Chemoinformatics, pp. 241–247.

Beam, A.L., Manrai, A.K., Ghassemi, M., 2020. Challenges to the reproducibility of machine learning models in health care. JAMA 323 (4), 305–306.

Burduk, R., Bożejko, W., Zacher, S., 2020. Novel approach to gentle AdaBoost algorithm with linear weak classifiers. In: Asian Conference on Intelligent Information and Database Systems. Springer, Cham, pp. 600–611.

Ciaburro, G., 2017. MATLAB for Machine Learning: Practical Examples of Regression, Clustering and Neural Networks. Packt Publishing.

Ciaburro, G., 2020. Sound event detection in underground parking garage using convolutional neural network. Big Data Cogn. Comput. 4 (3), 20. https://doi.org/10.3390/bdcc4030020.

Ciaburro, G., Iannace, G., 2020. Improving smart cities safety using sound events detection based on deep neural network algorithms. Informatics 7 (3), 23.

Ciaburro, G., Venkateswaran, B., 2017. Neural Networks with R: Smart Models Using CNN, RNN, Deep Learning, and Artificial Intelligence Principles. Packt Publishing Ltd.

Cooper, D.S., Biondi, B., 2012. Subclinical thyroid disease. Lancet 379 (9821), 1142–1154.

Ditzler, G., LaBarck, J., Ritchie, J., Rosen, G., Polikar, R., 2017. Extensions to online feature selection using bagging and boosting. IEEE Trans. Neural Netw. Learn. Syst. 29 (9), 4504–4509.

Divina, F., Gilson, A., Goméz-Vela, F., García Torres, M., Torres, J.F., 2018. Stacking ensemble learning for short-term electricity consumption forecasting. Energies 11 (4), 949.

Dua, S., Acharya, U.R., Dua, P. (Eds.), 2014. Machine Learning in Healthcare Informatics. Vol. 56. Springer, Berlin.

Dua, D., Graff, C., 2019. UCI Machine Learning Repository. University of California, School of Information and Computer Science, Irvine, CA. http://archive.ics.uci.edu/ml.

Ekins, S., Puhl, A.C., Zorn, K.M., Lane, T.R., Russo, D.P., Klein, J.J., Hickey, A.J., Clark, A.M., 2019. Exploiting machine learning for end-to-end drug discovery and development. Nat. Mater. 18 (5), 435.

Fatourechi, V., 2001. Subclinical thyroid disease. Mayo Clin. Proc. 76 (4), 413–417. Elsevier.

Freund, Y., Schapire, R.E., 1996. Experiments with a new boosting algorithm. In: ICML. Vol. 96, pp. 148–156.

Ghojogh, B., Crowley, M., 2019. The Theory Behind Overfitting, Cross Validation, Regularization, Bagging, and Boosting: Tutorial. arXiv preprint arXiv:1905.12787.

Gomes, H.M., Barddal, J.P., Enembreck, F., Bifet, A., 2017. A survey on ensemble learning for data stream classification. ACM Comput. Surv. (CSUR) 50 (2), 1–36.

Gu, D., Li, T., Wang, X., Yang, X., Yu, Z., 2019. Visualizing the intellectual structure and evolution of electronic health and telemedicine research. Int. J. Med. Inform. 130, 103947.

Hassan, M.K., El Desouky, A.I., Elghamrawy, S.M., Sarhan, A.M., 2019. Big data challenges and opportunities in healthcare informatics and smart hospitals. In: Security in Smart Cities: Models, Applications, and Challenges. Springer, Cham, pp. 3–26.

Hussain, L., Ahmed, A., Saeed, S., Rathore, S., Awan, I.A., Shah, S.A., Majid, A., Idris, A., Awan, A.A., 2018. Prostate cancer detection using machine learning techniques by employing combination of features extracting strategies. Cancer Biomark. 21 (2), 393–413.

Iftikhar, S., Saqib, A., Sarwar, M.R., Sarfraz, M., Arafat, M., Shoaib, Q.U.A., 2019. Capacity and willingness to use information technology for managing chronic diseases among patients: a cross-sectional study in Lahore, Pakistan. PLoS One 14 (1), e0209654.

Jaworska, N., de la Salle, S., Ibrahim, M.H., Blier, P., Knott, V., 2019. Leveraging machine learning approaches for predicting antidepressant treatment response using electroencephalography (EEG) and clinical data. Front. Psychol. 9, 768.

Jewell, N.P., Lewnard, J.A., Jewell, B.L., 2020. Predictive mathematical models of the COVID-19 pandemic: underlying principles and value of projections. JAMA 323 (19), 1893–1894.

Kambatla, K., Kollias, G., Kumar, V., Grama, A., 2014. Trends in big data analytics. J. Parallel Distrib. Comput. 74 (7), 2561–2573.

Kawaguchi, K., Bengio, Y., Verma, V., Kaelbling, L.P., 2019. Generalization in machine learning via analytical learning theory. Statistics 1050, 6.

Khan, S.A., Zia, K., Ashraf, S., Uddin, R., Ul-Haq, Z., 2020. Identification of chymotrypsin-like protease inhibitors of SARS-CoV-2 via integrated computational approach. J. Biomol. Struct. Dyn., 1–10.

Klambauer, G., Hochreiter, S., Rarey, M., 2019. Machine learning in drug discovery. Nat. Rev. Drug Discov. 18.

Krawczyk, B., Minku, L.L., Gama, J., Stefanowski, J., Woźniak, M., 2017. Ensemble learning for data stream analysis: a survey. Inform. Fusion 37, 132–156.

Kwak, G.H., Hui, P., 2019. DeepHealth: Review and Challenges of Artificial Intelligence in Health Informatics. arXiv preprint arXiv:1909.00384.

Lanzing, M., 2019. "Strongly recommended" revisiting decisional privacy to judge hypernudging in self-tracking technologies. Philos. Technol. 32 (3), 549–568.

Liu, Y., Browne, W.N., Xue, B., 2018. Adapting bagging and boosting to learning classifier systems. In: International Conference on the Applications of Evolutionary Computation. Springer, Cham, pp. 405–420.

Liyanage, H., Liaw, S.T., Jonnagaddala, J., Schreiber, R., Kuziemsky, C., Terry, A.L., de Lusignan, S., 2019. Artificial intelligence in primary health care: perceptions, issues, and challenges: primary health care informatics working group contribution to the yearbook of medical informatics 2019. Yearb. Med. Inform. 28 (1), 41.

Ma, L., Ma, C., Liu, Y., Wang, X., 2019. Thyroid diagnosis from SPECT images using convolutional neural network with optimization. Comput. Intell. Neurosci. 2019.

Marsland, S., 2015. Machine Learning: An Algorithmic Perspective. CRC Press.

Martinez, W.L., Martinez, A.R., Solka, J., Martinez, A., 2010. Exploratory Data Analysis with MATLAB. CRC Press.

Mosavi, A., Ardabili, S., Varkonyi-Koczy, A.R., 2019. List of deep learning models. In: International Conference on Global Research and Education. Springer, Cham, pp. 202–214.

Mostafa, S.A., Mustapha, A., Mohammed, M.A., Hamed, R.I., Arunkumar, N., Ghani, M.K.A., Jaber, M.M., Khaleefah, S.H., 2019. Examining multiple feature evaluation and classification methods for improving the diagnosis of Parkinson's disease. Cogn. Syst. Res. 54, 90–99.

Ng, W.W., Zhou, X., Tian, X., Wang, X., Yeung, D.S., 2018. Bagging–boosting-based semi-supervised multi-hashing with query-adaptive re-ranking. Neurocomputing 275, 916–923.

Ouyang, F.S., Guo, B.L., Ouyang, L.Z., Liu, Z.W., Lin, S.J., Meng, W., Huang, X.Y., Chen, H.X., Qiu-Gen, H., Yang, S.M., 2019. Comparison between linear and nonlinear machine-learning algorithms for the classification of thyroid nodules. Eur. J. Radiol. 113, 251–257.

Palanisamy, V., Thirunavukarasu, R., 2019. Implications of big data analytics in developing healthcare frameworks–a review. J. King Saud Univers. Comput. Inform. Sci. 31 (4), 415–425.

Panesar, A., 2019. Machine Learning and AI for Healthcare. Apress.

Polikar, R., 2012. Ensemble learning. In: Ensemble Machine Learning. Springer, Boston, MA, pp. 1–34.

Poreva, A., Karplyuk, Y., Vaityshyn, V., 2017. Machine learning techniques application for lung diseases diagnosis. In: 2017 5th IEEE Workshop on Advances in Information, Electronic and Electrical Engineering (AIEEE). IEEE, pp. 1–5.

Poudel, P., Illanes, A., Ataide, E.J., Esmaeili, N., Balakrishnan, S., Friebe, M., 2019. Thyroid ultrasound texture classification using autoregressive features in conjunction with machine learning approaches. IEEE Access 7, 79354–79365.

Raghupathi, W., Raghupathi, V., 2014. Big data analytics in healthcare: promise and potential. Health Inform. Sci. syst. 2 (1), 3.

Reddy, C.K., Aggarwal, C.C., 2015. Healthcare Data Analytics. Chapman and Hall/CRC.

Reitermanova, Z., 2010. Data Splitting. WDS'10 Proceedings of Contributed Papers,745 Part I., ISBN: 978-80-7378-139-2, pp. 31–36.

Rojas, E.M., Moreno, H.B.R., Ramirez, M.R., Palencia, J.S.M., 2019. Contributions of machine learning in the health area as support in the diagnosis and care of chronic diseases. In: Innovation in Medicine and Healthcare Systems, and Multimedia. Springer, Singapore, pp. 261–269.

Sawant, A., Bhandari, M., Yadav, R., Yele, R., Bendale, M.S., 2018. Brain cancer detection from MRI: a machine learning approach (tensorflow). Brain 5 (04).

Shankar, K., Lakshmanaprabu, S.K., Gupta, D., Maseleno, A., De Albuquerque, V.H.C., 2018. Optimal feature-based multi-kernel SVM approach for thyroid disease classification. J. Supercomput., 1–16.

Siau, K., Shen, Z., 2006. Mobile healthcare informatics. Med. Inform. Internet Med. 31 (2), 89–99.

Singhal, Y., Jain, A., Batra, S., Varshney, Y., Rathi, M., 2018. Review of bagging and boosting classification performance on unbalanced binary classification. In: 2018 IEEE 8th International Advance Computing Conference (IACC). IEEE, pp. 338–343.

Steil, J., Hagestedt, I., Huang, M.X., Bulling, A., 2019. Privacy-aware eye tracking using differential privacy. In: Proceedings of the 11th ACM Symposium on Eye Tracking Research & Applications, pp. 1–9.

Stephenson, N., Shane, E., Chase, J., Rowland, J., Ries, D., Justice, N., Zhang, J., Chan, L., Cao, R., 2019. Survey of machine learning techniques in drug discovery. Curr. Drug Metab. 20 (3), 185–193.

Strome, T.L., Liefer, A., 2013. Healthcare Analytics for Quality and Performance Improvement. Wiley, Hoboken, NJ, USA.

Subasi, A., Qaisar, S.M., 2020. Surface EMG signal classification using TQWT, bagging and boosting for hand movement recognition. J. Ambient. Intell. Humaniz. Comput. https://doi.org/10.1007/s12652-020-01980-6.

Sun, W., Trevor, B., 2018. A stacking ensemble learning framework for annual river ice breakup dates. J. Hydrol. 561, 636–650.

Tabassum, H., 2020. Enactment ranking of supervised algorithms dependence of data splitting algorithms: a case study of real datasets. Int. J. Comput. Sci. Inform. Technol. (IJCSIT) 12.

Tyagi, A., Mehra, R., Saxena, A., 2018. Interactive thyroid disease prediction system using machine learning technique. In: 2018 Fifth International Conference on Parallel, Distributed and Grid Computing (PDGC). IEEE, pp. 689–693.

Usak, M., Kubiatko, M., Shabbir, M.S., Viktorovna Dudnik, O., Jermsittiparsert, K., Rajabion, L., 2020. Health care service delivery based on the internet of things: a systematic and comprehensive study. Int. J. Commun. Syst. 33 (2), e4179.

Vamathevan, J., Clark, D., Czodrowski, P., Dunham, I., Ferran, E., Lee, G., Li, B., Madabhushi, A., Shah, P., Spitzer, M., Zhao, S., 2019. Applications of machine learning in drug discovery and development. Nat. Rev. Drug Discov. 18 (6), 463–477.

Van Calster, B., Wynants, L., Timmerman, D., Steyerberg, E.W., Collins, G.S., 2019. Predictive analytics in health care: how can we know it works? J. Am. Med. Inform. Assoc. 26 (12), 1651–1654.

Vanderpump, M.P., 2011. The epidemiology of thyroid disease. Br. Med. Bull. 99 (1).

Wan, T.T., 2006. Healthcare informatics research: from data to evidence-based management. J. Med. Syst. 30 (1), 3–7.

Wan, S., Qi, L., Xu, X., Tong, C., Gu, Z., 2020. Deep learning models for real-time human activity recognition with smartphones. Mob. Netw. Appl. 25 (2), 743–755.

Wang, T., Zhang, Z., Jing, X., Zhang, L., 2016. Multiple kernel ensemble learning for software defect prediction. Autom. Softw. Eng. 23 (4), 569–590.

Wang, Z., Wang, Y., Srinivasan, R.S., 2018. A novel ensemble learning approach to support building energy use prediction. Energy Build. 159, 109–122.

Wang, Y., Zhao, Y., Therneau, T.M., Atkinson, E.J., Tafti, A.P., Zhang, N., Amin, S., Limper, A.H., Khosla, S., Liu, H., 2020. Unsupervised machine learning for the discovery of latent disease clusters and patient subgroups using electronic health records. J. Biomed. Inform. 102, 103364.

Ward, R., 2013. The application of technology acceptance and diffusion of innovation models in healthcare informatics. Health Policy Technol. 2 (4), 222–228.

Xiao, C., Sun, J., 2019. Tutorial: data mining methods for drug discovery and development. In: Proceedings of the 25th ACM SIGKDD International Conference on Knowledge Discovery & Data Mining. ACM, pp. 3195–3196.

Yaman, E., Subasi, A., 2019. Comparison of bagging and boosting ensemble machine learning methods for automated EMG signal classification. Biomed. Res. Int. 2019.

Zhang, C., Ma, Y. (Eds.), 2012. Ensemble Machine Learning: Methods and Applications. Springer Science & Business Media.

Zikopoulos, P., Eaton, C., 2011. Understanding Big Data: Analytics for Enterprise Class Hadoop and Streaming Data. McGraw-Hill Osborne Media.

Zoffmann, S., Vercruysse, M., Benmansour, F., Maunz, A., Wolf, L., Marti, R.B., Heckel, T., Ding, H., Truong, H.H., Prummer, M., Schmucki, R., 2019. Machine learning-powered antibiotics phenotypic drug discovery. Sci. Rep. 9 (1), 1–14.

# A review of deep learning models for medical diagnosis

# 22

Seshadri Sastry Kunapuli[a] and Praveen Chakravarthy Bhallamudi[b]

*Xinthe Technologies PVT LTD, Visakhapatnam, India*[a] *Lumirack Solutions, Chennai, India*[b]

## Chapter outline

## 1 Motivation

Brain tumor detection/segmentation is the most challenging, as well as essential, task in many medical-image applications, because it generally involves a significant amount of data/information. There are many types of tumors (sizes and shapes). Artificial intelligence-assisted automatic/semiautomatic detection/segmentation is now playing an important role in medical diagnosis. Prior to therapies such as chemotherapy, radiotherapy, or brain surgery, the medical practitioners must validate the limits and the regions of the brain tumor as well as determine where specifically it lies and the exact affected locations. This chapter reviews various algorithms for brain tumor segmentation/detection and compares their Dice similarity coefficients (DSCs). Finally, an algorithm for brain tumor segmentation is proposed.

Machine Learning, Big Data, and IoT for Medical Informatics. https://doi.org/10.1016/B978-0-12-821777-1.00007-0

## 2 Introduction

This chapter reviews various deep learning models for tumor segmentation and proposes a technique for more efficient tumor segmentation. Magnetic resonance imaging (MRI) is a popular noninvasive technique of choice for structural brain analysis and visualization of different abnormalities in the brain. MRI provides images with high contrast and spatial resolutions for soft tissues and accessibility of multispectral images and presents no known health risks. However, identifying the pixels of organs or injuries in MRI images is among the most challenging of medical image analysis tasks, but is needed in order to deliver crucial data about the shapes and volumes of these organs or injuries.

Many researchers have examined various automated segmentation systems by applying different technologies. Researchers are employing deep learning techniques increasingly to automate these applications. Nowadays, numerous computer vision applications based on deep learning have shown improved performance, sometimes better than humans, and the applications range from recognizing objects or recognizing indicators for blood cancer and tumors in MRI scans.

Deep neural networks (DNNs) are capable of learning from unstructured data by using fine-tuning done by the backpropagation technique. The architecture of DNN has several levels to represent the features. In addition, more general information is provided at a higher level. Deep learning has progressed during the digital era, due to the availability of more massive amounts of data.

Earlier systems were built on traditional methods, such as edge detection filters and mathematical methods. Later, machine learning (ML) approaches extracting hand-crafted features became a dominant technique for an extended period. Designing and extracting appropriate features is a big concern in developing ML-assisted systems, and due to the complexities of these procedures, ML-based systems are not widely deployed. Recently, deep learning approaches came into the picture and started to demonstrate their considerable capabilities in image-processing tasks. The promising ability of deep learning approaches has placed them as the first option for image segmentation, and particularly for medical image segmentation.

Deep learning is being widely used because of its recent superior performance in many applications, such as object detection, speech recognition, facial recognition, and medical imaging.(Bar et al., 2015). Many researchers have pursued works on applications of deep learning in ultrasound (Shen et al., 2017), medical imaging (Baumgartner et al., 2017; Bergamo et al., 2011; Cai et al., 2017; Chen et al., 2017, 2015, 2016a), magnetic resonance imaging (Chen et al., 2016b, c), medical image segmentation, such as (Litjens et al., 2017) and (Shen et al., 2017), and electroencephalograms (Cheng et al., 2016). Recurrent neural network (RNN) is an alternative DL technique that is perfect for evaluating sequential data (for example, text and speech) because it has an inner state of memory that can be used for storage of data about prior data points. LSTM (Hochreiter and Schmidhuber, 1997) is a variation of RNN with better memory retention, as compared to conventional RNN. It is used for recognition of speech, captioning of images, and machine translations. Generative adversarial networks (GANs) and their various forms are another rising DL architecture containing generator and discriminator networks that are trained by backpropagation. The generator network artificially generates more realistic data cases that attempt to imitate the training data, whereas the discriminator network attempts to determine whether the artificially generated samples belong to training samples. GANs have shown great possibilities in medical image applications, like the reconstruction of medical imaging, e.g., compressed sensing MRI reconstruction (Mardani et al., 2017). Shen et al. (Shen et al., 2017) reviewed applications of deep learning on different kinds of medical image analysis problems. In the process,

Zhou (2019) has reviewed deep learning architectures for different multimodality datasets as they can provide multiinformation of a specific tissue or a cell or an organ.

Before automated analysis can be carried out, preprocessing steps are needed to make the images appear more similar. Typical preprocessing steps for structural brain MRI include: (1) registration, (2) registration, (3) bias field correction, (4) intensity normalization, (5) noise reduction.

Registration is the alignment of the images to a common coordinate system/space (Shen et al., 2017). Interpatient registration is a process to align the images of different sequences, to obtain a multichannel representation for each location within the brain. Interpatient image registration aids in standardizing the MR images onto a standard stereotaxic space, commonly the Montreal Neurological Institute (MNI) space. Klein et al. (2009) ranked 14 algorithms applied to brain image registration according to three completely independent analyses (permutation tests, one-way ANOVA tests, and indifference-zone ranking). They derived three almost identical top rankings of the methods. The algorithms ART, SyN, IRTK, and SPM's DARTEL Toolbox gave the best results based on overlap and distance measures.

Skull stripping is an important step in MRI brain imaging applications, referring to the removal of the noncerebral tissues. The main problem in skull-stripping is the segmentation of the noncerebral and intracranial tissues due to their homogeneous intensities. Many researchers have proposed algorithms for skull-stripping. Smith (2002) proposed and developed an automated method for segmenting magnetic resonance head images into the brain and nonbrain, called Brain Extraction Tool (BET). Iglesias et al. (2011) developed a robust, learning-based brain extraction system (ROBEX). Statistical Parametric Mapping (SPM), with a number of improved versions, is open source software commonly used in MRI analysis (Iglesias et al., 2011; Ashburner and Friston, 2005). The process of mapping intensities of all images into a standard reference scale is known as intensity normalization, with intensities generally scaled between 0 and 4095. Nyúl and Udupa (1999) proposed a two-step postprocessing method for standardizing the intensity scale in such a way that for the same MR protocol and body region,

Noise reduction is the reduction of the locally variant Rician noise observed in MR images (Coupe et al., 2008). With the advent of deep learning techniques, some of the preprocessing steps became less critical for the final segmentation performance. Gondara (2016) proposed convolutional denoising autoencoders to denoise images.

Akkus et al. (2017) surveyed various segmentation algorithms used for MRI scans and presented them. Razzak et al. (2018) presented an overview of various deep learning methods proposed under medical image processing in the literature. Vovk et al. (2007) has reviewed a paper on different image enhancement techniques based on correction of intensity inhomogeneity for MRI images with different qualitative and quantitative approaches. Menze et al. (2014) proposed the multimodal brain tumor image segmentation benchmark (BRATS) for brain tumor segmentation, which in turn used by many researchers for Image Segmentation from basic Convolution Methods to advanced U-Nets. One such a paper is proposed by Pereira et al. (2016). Işın et al. (2016) presented a review of MRI-based brain tumor image segmentation using deep learning methods. Hall et al. (1992) compared neural network and fuzzy clustering techniques in segmenting magnetic resonance images of the brain. Krizhevsky et al. (2012) proposed deep learning architecture for image classification. Litjens et al. (2017) presented a survey on deep learning in medical image analysis. Xian et al. (2018) proposed algorithms on automatic breast ultrasound image segmentation. Kitahara et al. (2019) proposed a deep learning approach for dynamic chest radiography. Chang et al. (2019) proposed a deep learning method for the detection of complete anterior cruciate ligament tear. Ronneberger et al. (2015) proposed U-Net, convolutional networks for biomedical image segmentation. Long et al. (2015) proposed fully convolutional networks for semantic segmentation. Dong et al. (2017) proposed automatic brain tumor detection and segmentation using U-Net based fully convolutional networks. Çiçek et al. (2016) proposed the 3D U-Net: learning dense volumetric segmentation from the sparse annotation. Ioffe and Szegedy (2015) proposed accelerating deep network training by reducing the internal covariate shift. Wang et al. (2018) proposed automatic brain tumor segmentation using cascaded anisotropic convolutional neural networks.

A review of all these deep learning algorithms for medical image segmentation has been done previously (Ronneberger et al., 2015) with explanations as to how they can be useful in segmenting even the minor regions of the incoherent or fuzzy structures of the tumors in the medical image, along with their challenges in implementation for limited annotated datasets. But the main challenge in designing a deep neural network architecture is the vanishing gradient problem during the training of deep networks. So, to overcome this problem, a feed-forward connection from one layer to all the subsequent layers has been done using Densenets, which not only adds regularization effects but also reduces the problem of overfitting on small datasets. Inspired by the Densenets, Dolz (2019) proposed a multi-modal technique called HyperDense-Net to improve the accuracy of brain lesion segmentation with the help of multimodal settings in the network. In dealing with the overfitting or vanishing gradients problem, An (2019) proposed an adaptive dropout technique in his spliced convolution neural network for image depth calculation and segmentation and he measured his model accuracy using the Dice score and Jaccard index for the spine web dataset. As no rigid segmentation is required for PET images, Cheng and Liu (2017) has proposed a combination of Convolution Neural Networks (to extract internal features) and Recurrent Neural Networks (to classify these features) is used for Alzheimer's disease diagnosis.

However, the traditional strided convolution techniques (such as in deep convolution networks (DCNs) or fully connected neural networks (FCNNs) (An, 2020)) are being replaced for image segmentation by atrous (i.e., dilated) kernels or convolution, with holes (which introduces a dilation rate to the convolution layers that defines the spacing between the kernel values). This technique can be used in DCNs (Zhou, 2020) in order to achieve a maximum accuracy in segmenting medical images, with a trade-off of greater memory and segmentation time. However, the usage of this atrous convolution layer in a simple encoder network has been proposed by Gu (2019), in which the network consists of a simple decoder with pretrained Resnet32 and a dense atrous convolution (DAC) block with use of a residual multikernel pooling (RMP) layer instead of a dense U-Net architecture to improve the segmentation accuracy. In recent research, different models with U-Net architecture, such as single U-Net architecture with atrous spatial pyramidal pooling (ASPP) (Pengcheng, 2020) and double U-Net architecture ( Jha, 2020) with a connection of VGG-19 squeeze and excite block with ASPP network architectures, have been proposed and that outperformed medical image segmentation, with better accuracy and low false positive rate. Dice ratio or Jaccard index can be used to find the accuracy of the segmented image, or it can be done with the help of modern machine learning parameters such as precision and recall.

The results of the preceding papers mostly confirmed that the use of atrous, a.k.a. dilated, convolution techniques, or convolution with holes, in medical image segmentation along with the U-Net architecture brings up the most probabilistic detection on medical image segmentation or tumor segmentation, even though they are in a coherent or incoherent structure, when compared to the other techniques. So, in this review, we strongly suggest that the structure of multiscale atrous convolution in the U-Net architecture gives better and more accurate results in detecting minute tumors in real time, with the trade-off of time and memory.

# 3  MRI Segmentation

Image segmentation is an essential step for brain tumor analysis of MRI images. In the present scenario, the human expert performs tumor segmentation manually. This manual segmentation is a very time-consuming, tedious task, usually involving lengthier procedures, and the results are very dependent on human expertise. Moreover, these results vary from expert to expert and generally are not reproducible by the same expert. Thus automatic segmentation and reproducible segmentation methods are very much in demand. MRI segmentation is used to provide a more accurate classification for the subtypes of brain tumors and inform the subsequent diagnosis. It allows precise delineation that is crucial in radiotherapy or surgical planning. In this chapter, we review various architectures used to segment brain tissues and compare their Dice sensitivity coefficient (DSC). Table 1 shows the list of datasets available: T1 (spin-lattice relaxation), T1_1mm (3D T1-weighted scan), T1_IR (multislice T1-weighted inversion recovery scan registered to the T2 FLAIR), T1C (T1-contrasted), T2 (spin-spin relaxation), proton density (PD) contrast imaging, diffusion MRI (dMRI), and fluid attenuation inversion recovery (FLAIR) pulse sequences. The BraTS dataset provides four modalities for each patient: T1, T2, T1c, and FLAIR diffusion-weighted imaging (DWI) are designed to detect the random movements of water protons. DWI is a suitable method for detecting acute stroke. Computed tomography (CT), T1-DUAL (in-phase) (40 datasets), and T2-SPIR (opposed phase) The contrast between these modalities gives an almost unique signature to each tissue type. MRBrainS13 and ISLES2015 provide four and five modalities, respectively.

**Table 1  MRI datasets.**

| S. no. | Dataset | Task | Modality |
|--------|---------|------|----------|
| 1 | Brats2012 | Brain tumor | T1, T1C, T2, FLAIR |
| 2 | Brats2013 | Brain tumor | T1, T1C, T2, FLAIR |
| 3 | Brats2014 | Brain tumor | T1, T1C, T2, FLAIR |
| 4 | Brats2015 | Brain tumor | T1, T1C, T2, FLAIR |
| 5 | Brats2016 | Brain tumor | T1, T1C, T2, FLAIR |
| 6 | Brats2017 | Brain tumor | T1, T1C, T2, FLAIR |
| 7 | Brats2018 | Brain tumor | T1, T1C, T2, FLAIR |
| 8 | ISLES2015 | Ischemic stroke lesion | T1, T2, TSE, FLAIR, DWI |
| 10 | MRBrainS13 | Brain tissue | T1, T1_1 mm, T1_IR, FLAIR |
| 11 | NeoBrainS12 | Brain tissue | T1, T2 |
| 12 | iSeg-2017 | Brain tissue | T1, T2 |
| 13 | CHAOS | Abdominal organs | CT, T1-DUAL, T2-SPIR |
| 14 | IVD | Intervertebral disc | In-phase, Opposed-phase, Fat, Water |

# 4 Deep learning architectures used in diagnostic brain tumor analysis

## 4.1 Convolutional neural networks or convnets

Convolutional neural networks are also deep feedforward networks that are widely used in classification, recognition, and detection tasks, such as object detection, object recognition ( Jiang et al., 2013; Wang et al., 2019), handwriting recognition (Havaei, 2017), and image classification (Dong, 2017; Pinto et al., 2015; Havaei et al., 2016; Kamnitsas et al., 2017). The difference between the fully connected feedforward neural networks (FCNs) and the deep convolution neural networks (DCNNs) is that the adjacent layers are connected in different ways. The DCNN only has some nodes connected between the adjacent two layers, while the FCN has all nodes connected between the adjacent two layers. The biggest problem with using an FCN is that there are too many parameters/features for the network. Increasing the features will only lead to increased complexity, reduced speed, and overfitting problems. To reduce overfitting, it is required to reduce the parameters given to the network. Therefore convolutional neural networks were proposed to achieve this goal. Convolutional neural networks consist of convolutional and pooling layers. In the convolutional layer, only a small patch of the previous layer is used as the input of each node in the convolutional layer, and the size of the small patch is often 3*3 or 5*5. The convolutional layer attempts to analyze each small patch of the neural network in depth, which results in the higher abstraction of feature representation—the pooling layer followed by the convolutional layer. The pooling layer reduces the size of the output of the convolutional layer; thus this combination of convolutional layers and the pooling layer can reduce the number of parameters in the network. So, pooling layers not only speed up the calculation but also prevent overfitting. In general, there are two types of convolution neural network architectures, according to the different connection modes of the different convolutional layers. One is to connect 2D convolutional layers in series, such as VGG-16, VGG-19 (Zhou, 2020), ResNET (Gu, 2019), and INCEPTION-NETt (Pengcheng, 2020). Fig. 1 shows an example architecture of the convolutional neural network and the other is 3D Multi-Scale CNN for MRI brain lesion segmentation which is proposed by Kamnitsas et al. (2016) and Kleesiek et al. (2016).

## 4.2 Stacked autoencoders

An autoencoder is a type of artificial neural network used to learn efficient data coding in an unsupervised manner. There are two parts in an autoencoder: the encoder and the decoder. The encoder is used to generate a reduced feature representation from an initial input x by a hidden layer h. The decoder is used to reconstruct the initial input from the encoder's output by minimizing the loss function. The autoencoder converts high-dimensional data to low-dimensional data. Therefore the autoencoder is

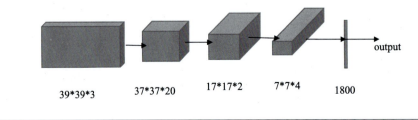

39*39*3          37*37*20          17*17*2     7*7*4          1800          output

**FIG. 1**

An example of a deep convolutional network.

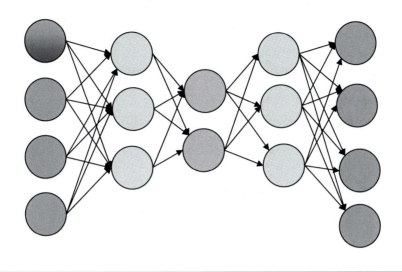

**FIG. 2**

Example of an autoencoder.

especially useful in noise removal, feature extraction, compression, and similar tasks. There are three types of autoencoder: the sparse autoencoder (Zhou, 2020), the denoising autoencoder (Gu, 2019; Majumdar, 2019; Vaidhya, 2015) and the contractive autoencoder (Pengcheng, 2020). Sparse autoencoders are typically used to learn features for another task such as classification. Denoising autoencoders create a noisy copy of the input data by adding some noise to the input. This prevents the autoencoders from copying the input to the output without learning features of the data. The objective of a contractive autoencoder is to have a robust learned representation that is less sensitive to small variations in the data. Robustness of the data description is created by applying a penalty term to the loss function. A contractive autoencoder is another regularization technique, just like sparse and denoising autoencoders. However, this regularizing corresponds to the Frobenius norm of the Jacobian matrix of the encoder activations concerning the input. The Frobenius norm of the Jacobian matrix for the hidden layer is calculated concerning input, and it is the sum of the squares of all elements. Fig. 2 shows an autoencoder example.

## 4.3 Deep belief networks

The Boltzmann machine (Ioffe and Szegedy, 2015; Wang et al., 2018; Ronneberger et al., 2015) is derived from statistical physics and is a modeling method based on energy functions that describe the high-order interaction between variables. Although the Boltzmann machine is relatively complex, it has a relatively complete physical interpretation and a strict mathematical statistics theory. The Boltzmann machine is an asymmetric coupled random feedback binary unit neural network, which includes a visible layer and multiple hidden layers. The nodes of the Boltzmann computer can be divided into visible units and hidden units. In a Boltzmann machine, the visible and invisible units represent the random neural network learning model. The weights between two units in the model are used to describe the correlation between the corresponding two units. A restricted Boltzmann machine (Dolz, 2019; An, 2019) is a unique form, which only includes a visible layer and a hidden layer. Unlike feedforward neural networks, the connections between the nodes of the hidden layer and the visible layer's nodes in the restricted Boltzmann machines can be bidirectionally connected. Compared to Boltzmann machines, since the restricted Boltzmann machines only have one hidden layer, they have faster calculation speed and better flexibility. In general, restricted Boltzmann machines have two main functions: (1) Similar to autoencoders, restricted Boltzmann machines are used to reduce the dimension of data; (2) Restricted Boltzmann machines are used to obtain a weight matrix, which is used as the initial input of other neural networks. Similar to stacked autoencoders, deep belief networks (An, 2020; Zhou, 2020; Gu, 2019; Pengcheng, 2020) are also neural networks with multiple restricted Boltzmann machine layers.

Furthermore, in deep belief networks, the next layer's input comes from the previous layer's output. Deep belief networks adopt the hierarchical unsupervised greedy pretraining method (An, 2020) to pretrain each restricted Boltzmann machine hierarchically. The obtained results in this study were used as the initial input of the supervised learning probability model, whose learning performance improved significantly. In addition to the segmentation tasks, a classification model of various brain tumors on MRI images have been done with the help of Deep Belief Networks have been done by Ahmed (2019).

## 4.4 2D U-Net

The U-Net was proposed by Olaf Ranneberger et al. for biomedical image segmentation (Ronneberger et al., 2015). It is an improvement on the fully convolutional neural networks for semantic segmentation (Hesamian et al., 2019; Dong, 2017). U-Net follows the idea of an autoencoder to find a latent representation of a lower dimension than the input used for the segmentation task architecture, containing two parts. The first part is the encoder part or contraction path, used to capture the image's context. An encoder consists of convolutional and pooling layers. The second path, known as a decoder, is an expanding path, which is used to enable localization using transposed convolutions. U-Net contains only fully convolutional layers and does not contain any dense layer, because it can accept images of any size (Hesamian et al., 2019). Fig. 3 shows an example of the U-Net architecture.

## 4.5 3D U-Net

The 3D U-Net architecture is similar to the U-Net (He, 2016). It comprises an analysis path to the left and a synthesis path to the right. The whole image is analyzed in a contracting way, and subsequent expansions produce the final segmentation. In the analysis path of U-Net, each layer contains two $3 \times 3 \times 3$ convolution layers, each followed by a ReLU layer, and then a $2 \times 2 \times 2$ max pooling layer with strides of two in each dimension. In the synthesis path of U-Net, each layer consists of a $2 \times 2 \times 2$ up-convolution by strides of value two in each dimension, followed by two $3 \times 3 \times 3$ convolution layers, each followed by a ReLU activation function. Shortcut connections from the analysis path to the synthesis path provide the high-resolution features. In the last segment, a convolution of size $1 \times 1 \times 1$ reduces the number of output channels to three labels. 3D U-Net has all the operations in 3D and uses batch normalization, which was shown to improve the training convergence. An example of this separable 3D U-Net Architecture on MRI images for brain tumor segmentation has been proposed by Chen et al. (2018) which has shown a good result in tumor segmentation when comparing to the 2D architectures.

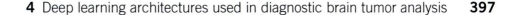

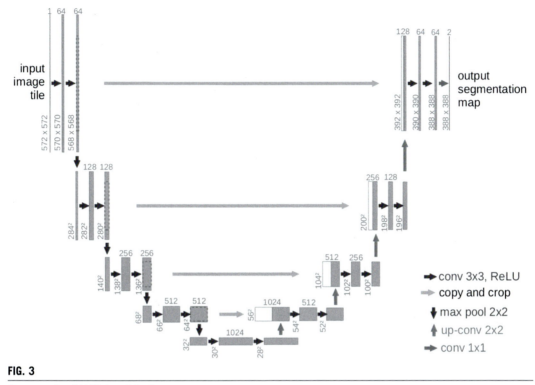

**FIG. 3**

An example of U-Net architecture.

## 4.6 Cascaded anisotropic network

The cascaded anisotropic network (Wang et al., 2017) consists of three convolutional neural networks (CNNs) that segment each of three subregions sequentially: 1. tumor, 2. tumor core, and 3. enhancing tumor. Hence, anisotropic convolutions perform well on 3D MRI, but result in higher complexity and memory consumption. The fusion of the CNN outputs in three orthogonal views is used to enhance the brain tumor segmentation. The cascaded anisotropic network uses three CNNs to hierarchically and sequentially segment whole tumor, tumor core, and enhancing tumor core. These CNNs are referred to as WNet, TNet, and ENet, respectively, and they follow the hierarchical structure of the tumor sub-regions. WNet and TNet have the same architecture, while ENet only uses one down-sampling layer due to the smaller input size. The WNet takes the full MRI. As input and segments, the first region: whole tumor. A corresponding bounding box is computed and used as the input of the TNet that segments the tumor core similarly used for the ENet. The bounding boxes allow a restriction of the segmentation region and minimize false positives and false negatives. One of the cascade's drawbacks is that it is not an end-to-end method and thus training and testing time are more extended than with the other methods. Fig. 4 shows the architecture of the cascaded anisotropic network.

Table 2 shows a comparison of the Dice sensitivity coefficient (DSC) of the complete tumor, the core of the tumor, and the enhanced core of tumors. TP- True Positives, FP- False Positives, FN- False Negatives. The formula for DSC is given by $DSC = \frac{2TP}{2TP + FP + FN}$.

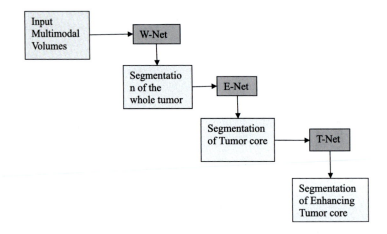

**FIG. 4**

Cascaded anisotropic network.

| **Table 2 DSC comparison of different architectures on BraTS dataset.** | | | | |
|---|---|---|---|---|
| **S. no.** | **Architecture** | **Complete** | **Core** | **Enhancing** |
| 1 | CNN | 0.78 | 0.63 | 0.68 |
| 2 | Input Cascade CNN | 0.88 | 0.79 | 0.73 |
| 3 | U-Net | 0.88 | 0.87 | 0.81 |
| 4 | Extremely Randomized Forest | 0.88 | 0.76 | 0.73 |
| 5 | Deep Neural Networks | 0.88 | 0.79 | 0.73 |
| 6 | 3D CNN | 0.85 | 0.67 | 0.63 |
| 7 | 3D U-Net | 0.899 | 0.684 | 0.867 |
| 8 | Deep Belief Network | 0.8038 | 0.953 | 0.976 |
| 9 | Cascaded Anisotropic CNN | 0.9050 | 0.8378 | 0.7859 |
| 10 | Stacked Autoencoders | 0.815 | 0.643 | 0.68 |

## 5 Deep learning tools applied to MRI images

In recent years, based on the previously described general deep learning methods, some deep learning tools applied to MRI have also been developed. They are briefly introduced as follows.

*BrainNet*: This tool was developed based on TensorFlow and aims to train deep neural networks to segment grey matter and white matter from brain MRIs.

*LiviaNET*: LiviaNET (Dolz et al., 2018) was developed using Theano, aiming to train 3D fully convolutional neural networks to segment subcortical brain on MRI.

*DIGITS*: This tool was also developed to rapidly train accurate deep neural networks for image segmentation, classification, and tissue detection tasks. For example, DIGITS is used to perform Alzheimer's disease prediction by using MRI and obtains good results (Sarraf and Tofigh, 2016).

*resnet CNN MRI adni*: This tool was developed to train residual and convolutional neural networks (CNNs) to perform automatic detection and classification of MRIs.

*mrbrain*: This tool was developed to train convolutional neural networks by using MRIs to predict the age of humans.

*DeepMedic*: DeepMedic was developed using Theano and aims to train multiscale 3D CNNs for brain lesion segmentation from MRI.

## 6 Proposed framework

Based on a comparison of DSCs of various architectures in Table 2, cascaded anisotropic CNN performed well on the BraTs dataset compared to other architectures. Further, U-Net also performed reasonably well on all three types of data: complete, core, and enhanced. We are confident that enhancing the architecture of U-Net would improve its performance. We propose a U-Net architecture with atrous, a.k.a. dilated, convolution layers (convolution with holes) for medical image segmentation. The proposed technique exhibits the most accurate probabilistic detection on medical image segmentation/tumor segmentation even though they are incoherent structures, when compared to the other techniques. Hence, we propose a multiscale atrous convolution U-Net architecture with batch normalization and he-norm as a kernel initializer (as the dataset contains fewer images and different tumor sizes in each image). The architecture of our proposed model is shown in Fig. 5.

In this architecture, we used an exponential increase of receptive fields with an increased kernel parameter linearly, without losing the characteristics of the image, i.e., resolution or coverage. Let $f_1, f_2, f_3, \ldots, f_n$ be the discrete functions such that they belong to any real dimension (R) of data and $k_1, k_2, \ldots, k_n$ are the kernels such that in a multiscale atrous convolution the size of each element in the receptive field increases exponentially with a linear increase of n elements by the factor of $(2n+2-1) \times (2n+2-1)$, such that if $n=0$ the size of the kernel becomes 3*3 and if $n=1$ the size becomes 7*7, and so on. This exponential increase of the kernel does not affect the resolution or coverage of the image and it works well if we have a less image segmentation dataset.

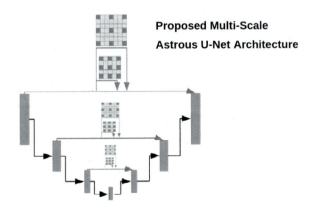

**Proposed Multi-Scale Astrous U-Net Architecture**

**FIG. 5**

Proposed multiscale atrous U-Net architecture (without batch normalization layer).

In general, the activation functions, such as either relu or tanh, may sometimes lead to either vanishing gradients or saturation problems. We generally preferred he-normalization as a kernel initializer, as it introduces zero mean and common variance between the predecessors when compared to other initializers, such as "Xavier normal/uniform" and "uniform/random" initializers. To optimize our network, we used a batch normalization between every multiscaling dilated convolution layer to converge faster, even though with high learning rates this causes the gradients to move towards the direction of the prediction faster. In the proposed U-Net architecture, instead of up-sampling, we used atrous convolution transpose. Up-sampling has no trainable parameters and it only repeats the rows and columns in the data. In the convolution transpose layer, both convolution and up-sampling are used. In our proposed technique, we used multiscale atrous convolution transpose, which would utilize different filter sizes in transpose convolution and finds the depth of the image with greater detail. The proposed algorithm, as expected, performed well on the BraTS dataset compared to U-Net and cascaded anisotropic CNN. The Dice sensitivity coefficient (DSC) of the proposed architecture complete tumor was 0.91, the core of the tumor was 0.89, and the enhanced core of tumors was 0.82.

## 7 Conclusion and outlook

In summary, this chapter has aimed to provide valuable insights for researchers about applying deep learning architectures in the field of MRI research. Deep learning architectures are widely applied to MRI processing and analysis in registration, bias field correction, intensity normalization, noise reduction, image detection, image segmentation, and image classification. Although deep learning approaches perform well on MRI, there are still many limitations and challenges that need to be met and overcome. In designing deep learning approaches, significant limitations are dataset size and class imbalance. Generally, deep learning approaches require larger datasets for better results—namely, the size of the MRI. The dataset is limited due to its cost in image acquisition processes and privacy considerations; further, many disease-related MRIs are rarely found. Therefore the size of the datasets with MRIs are often small. So, it is overly complicated to train deep neural networks and get the desired performance with the class imbalance in the images.

However, there are many strategies for dealing with imbalanced datasets, such as resampling techniques, which include random undersampling and random oversampling. Random undersampling removes examples randomly in the majority class, aiming to balance class distribution by indiscriminantly eliminating majority class examples. This elimination of examples is done until the majority and minority class examples are balanced out.

Oversampling increases the number of examples in the minority class by randomly copying and replicating them to increase samples of the minority class in the dataset. In cluster-based oversampling, the K-means unsupervised algorithm is applied to the minority and majority classes separately. This process is done to identify groups/clusters in the dataset. Subsequently, each group is oversampled, such that all groups of the same class have the same number of examples, and all classes have the same size. Due to replicating sample model overfits, to avoid overfitting in informed oversampling, new synthetic similar instances of the minority class are created and added to the dataset.

Transfer learning is an approach used in deep learning to learn new tasks based on knowledge earned on older tasks. Transfer learning is widely applied to deal with limited dataset size and class imbalance. Transfer learning consists of selecting a pretrained network, followed by a fine-tuning process, i.e., choosing a suitable pretrained deep learning architecture and tuning its corresponding hyperparameters for a particular application. It is difficult to select an architecture straightaway and tune its hyperparameters for a particular application. This remains an unsolved problem. Presently, most researchers are pursuing experimental experience to address the previously mentioned problems—the size of the MRI. The dataset may no longer be a problem due to the continuous advancements of medical data. Moreover, new progress and understanding of deep learning concepts may result in choosing a suitable deep learning architecture and its corresponding hyperparameters for a particular application more appropriately. Shortly, we may expect more remarkable achievements through deep learning on MRI analysis.

## 8  Future directions

Despite the many improvements in artificial intelligence/machine learning, there are still many inadequacies. Mostly these issues are identified with the current methods, which are not adjusted to the larger, more varied, and increasingly complex datasets, which may affect the accuracy of tumor segmentation. Further research should investigate and propose new architectures, layers, or even activations to develop a next-generation segmentation for tumor detection.

## References

Ahmed, K., 2019. Classification of brain tumors using personalized deep belief networks on MRImages: PDBN-MRI. In: Eleventh International Conference on Machine Vision (ICMV 2018).

Akkus, Z., Galimzianova, A., Hoogi, A., Rubin, D.L., Erickson, B.J., 2017. Deep learning for brain M.R.I. segmentation: state of the art and future directions. J. Digit. Imaging 30 (4), 449–459.

An, F.-P., 2019. Medical image segmentation algorithm based on optimized convolutional neural network-adaptive dropout depth calculation. Complexity. https://doi.org/10.1155/2020/1645479.

An, F.-P., 2020. Medical Image Segmentation Algorithm Based on Feedback Mechanism CNN. https://doi.org/10.1155/2019/6134942.

Ashburner, J., Friston, K.J., 2005. Unified segmentation. NeuroImage 26 (3), 839–851.

Bar, Y., Diamant, I., Wolf, L., Greenspan, H., 2015. Deep learning with non-medical training used for chest pathology identification. In: Medical Imaging 2015: Computer-Aided Diagnosis. vol. 9414.

Baumgartner, C.F., Koch, L.M., Pollefeys, M., Konukoglu, E., 2017. An exploration of 2D and 3D deep learning techniques for cardiac MR image segmentation. In: International Workshop on Statistical Atlases and Computational Models of the Heart. Springer, pp. 111–119.

Bergamo, A., Torresani, L., Fitzgibbon, A.W., 2011. Picodes, learning a compact code for novel-category recognition. In: Advances in Neural Information Processing Systems, pp. 2088–2096.

Cai, J., Lu, L., Xie, Y., Xing, F., Yang, L., 2017. Improving Deep Pancreas Segmentation in C.T. and M.R.I. Images via Recurrent Neural Contextual Learning and Direct Loss Function. arXiv. 1707.04912.

Chang, P.D., Wong, T.T., Rasiej, M.J., 2019. Deep learning for detection of complete anterior cruciate ligament tear. J. Digit. Imaging 32, 1–7.

Chen, H., Ni, D., Qin, J., Li, S., Yang, X., Wang, T., Heng, P.A., 2015. Standard plane localization in fetal ultrasound via domain transferred deep neural networks. IEEE J. Biomed. Health Inform. 19 (5), 1627–1636.

Chen, H., Qi, X., Cheng, J.Z., Heng, P.A., et al., 2016a. Deep contextual networks for neuronal structure segmentation. In: Proceedings of the AAAI Conference on Artificial Intelligence, pp. 1167–1173.

Chen, H., Qi, X., Yu, L., Heng, P.A., 2016b. DCAN: deep contour-aware networks for accurate gland segmentation. In: Proceedings of the IEEE Conference on Computer Vision and Pattern Recognition, pp. 2487–2496.

Chen, J., Yang, L., Zhang, Y., Alber, M., Chen, D.Z., 2016c. Combining fully convolutional and recurrent neural networks for 3D biomedical image segmentation. In: Advances in Neural Information Processing Systems, pp. 3036–3044.

Chen, H., Dou, Q., Yu, L., Qin, J., Heng, P.A., 2017. Voxresnet, Deep voxelwise residual networks for brain segmentation from 3D M.R. images. NeuroImage 170, 446–455.

Chen, W., et al., 2018. S3D-UNet: Separable 3D U-Net for Brain Tumor Segmentation.

Cheng, D., Liu, M., 2017. Combining convolutional and recurrent neural networks for Alzheimer's disease diagnosis using pet images. In: 2017 IEEE International Conference on Imaging Systems And Techniques (I.S.T.). IEEE, pp. 1–5.

Cheng, J.Z., Ni, D., Chou, Y.H., Qin, J., Tiu, C.M., Chang, Y.C., Huang, C.S., Shen, D., Chen, C.M., 2016. Computer-aided diagnosis with deep learning architecture: applications to breast lesions in U.S. images and pulmonary nodules in C.T. scans. Sci. Rep. 6, 24454.

Çiçek, Ö., Abdulkadir, A., Lienkamp, S.S., Brox, T., Ronneberger, O., 2016. 3D U-Net: learning dense volumetric segmentation from sparse annotation. In: International Conference on Medical Image Computing and Computer-Assisted Intervention, pp. 424–432.

Coupe, P., Yger, P., Prima, S., Hellier, P., Kervrann, C., Barillot, C., 2008. An optimized blockwise nonlocal means denoising filter for 3-D magnetic resonance images. IEEE Trans. Med. Imaging 27 (4), 425–441.

Dolz, J., 2019. HyperDense-Net: A Hyper-Densely Connected CNN for Multi-Modal Image Segmentation. arXiv. 1804.02967v2.

Dolz, J., Desrosiers, C., Ayed, I.B., 2018. 3D fully convolutional networks for subcortical segmentation in MRI: a large-scale study. Neuroimage 170, 456–470. https://doi.org/10.1016/j.neuroimage.2017.04.039.

Dong, H., 2017. Automatic brain tumor detection and segmentation using u-net based fully convolutional networks. In: Annual Conference On Medical Image Understanding and Analysis.

Dong, H., Yang, G., Liu, F., Mo, Y., Guo, Y., 2017. Automatic brain tumor detection and segmentation using U-Net based fully convolutional networks. In: Annual Conference on Medical Image Understanding and Analysis, pp. 506–517.

Gondara, L., 2016. Medical image denoising using convolutional denoising autoencoders. In: 2016 IEEE 16th International Conference on Data Mining Workshops (ICDMW).

Gu, Z., 2019. CE-Net: Context Encoder Network for 2D Medical Image Segmentation. arXiv. 1903.02740v1.

Hall, L.O., Bensaid, A.M., Clarke, L.P., Velthuizen, R.P., Silbiger, M.S., Bezdek, J.C., 1992. A comparison of neural network and fuzzy clustering techniques in segmenting magnetic resonance images of the brain. IEEE Trans. Neural Netw. 3 (5), 672–682.

Havaei, M., 2017. Brain tumor segmentation with deep neural networks. Med. Image Anal. 35, 18–31.

Havaei, M., et al., 2016. Brain tumor segmentation with deep neural networks. Med. Image Anal. 35, 18–31.

He, K., 2016. Deep residual learning for image recognition. In: Proceedings of the IEEE Conference on Computer Vision and Pattern Recognition.

Hesamian, M.H., et al., 2019. Deep learning techniques for medical image segmentation: achievements and challenges. J. Digit. Imaging. https://doi.org/10.1007/s10278-019-00227-x.

Hochreiter, S., Schmidhuber, J., 1997. Long short-term memory. Neural Comput. 9 (8), 1735–1780.

Işın, A., Direkoğlu, C., Şah, M., 2016. Review of MRI-based brain tumor image segmentation using deep learning methods. Procedia Comput. Sci. 102, 317–324.

Iglesias, J.E., Liu, C.-Y., Thompson, P.M., Tu, Z., 2011. Robust brain extraction across datasets and comparison with publicly available methods. IEEE Trans. Med. Imaging 30 (9), 1617–1634.

Ioffe, S., Szegedy, C., 2015. Batch Normalization: Accelerating Deep Network Training by Reducing Internal Covariate Shift. arXiv. preprint arXiv:1502.03167.

Jha, D., 2020. DoubleU-Net: A Deep Convolutional Neural Network for Medical Image Segmentation. arXiv. 2006.04868v2.

Jiang, X., et al., 2013. A novel sparse auto-encoder for deep unsupervised learning. In: 2013 Sixth International Conference on Advanced Computational Intelligence (I.C.A.C.I.).

Kamnitsas, K., et al., 2016. Efficient multi-scale 3D CNN with fully connected C.R.F. for accurate brain lesion segmentation. Med. Image Anal. 36, 61–78.

Kamnitsas, K., Ledig, C., Newcombe, V.F.J., Simpson, J.P., Kane, A.D., Menon, D.K., Rueckert, D., Glocker, B., 2017. Efficient multi-scale 3D CNN with fully connected C.R.F. for accurate brain lesion segmentation. Med. Image Anal. 36, 61–78.

Kitahara, Y., Tanaka, R., Roth, H.R., Oda, H., Mori, K., Kasahara, K., Matsumoto, I., 2019. Lung segmentation based on a deep learning approach for dynamic chest radiography. Proc. SPIE 10950, Medical Imaging: Computer-Aided Diagnosis.

Kleesiek, J., et al., 2016. Deep M.R.I. brain extraction: a 3D convolutional neural network for skull stripping. NeuroImage 129, 460–469.

Klein, A., et al., 2009. Evaluation of 14 nonlinear deformation algorithms applied to human brain M.R.I. registration. NeuroImage 46 (3), 786–802.

Krizhevsky, A., Sutskever, I., Hinton, G.E., 2012. ImageNet classification with deep convolutional neural networks. In: Advances in Neural Information Processing Systems, pp. 1097–1105.

Litjens, G., Kooi, T., Bejnordi, B.E., Setio, A., Ciompi, F., Ghafoorian, M., Van Der Laak, J.A., Van Ginneken, B., S'anchez, C.I., 2017. A survey on deep learning in medical image analysis. Med. Image Anal. 42, 60–88.

Long, J., Shelhamer, E., Darrell, T., 2015. Fully convolutional networks for semantic segmentation. In: Proceedings of the IEEE Conference on Computer Vision and Pattern Recognition, pp. 3431–3440.

Majumdar, A., 2019. Blind denoising autoencoder. IEEE Trans. Neural Netw. Learn. Syst. 30 (1), 312–317.

Mardani, M., Gong, E., Cheng, J.Y., et al., 2017. Deep Generative Adversarial Networks for Compressed Sensing Automates M.R.I. arXiv. 1706.00051.

Menze, B.H., Jakab, A., Bauer, S., Kalpathy-Cramer, J., Farahani, K., Kirby, J., Burren, Y., Porz, N., Slotboom, J., Wiest, R., et al., 2014. The multimodal brain tumor image segmentation benchmark (BRATS). IEEE Trans. Med. Imaging 34 (10), 1993–2024.

Nyúl, L.G., Udupa, J.K., 1999. On standardizing the M.R. image intensity scale. Magn. Reson. Med. 42 (6), 1072–1081.

Pengcheng, G., 2020. A Multi-Scaled Receptive Field Learning Approach for Medical Image Segmentation.

Pereira, S., Pinto, A., Alves, V., Silva, C.A., 2016. Brain tumor segmentation using convolutional neural networks in M.R.I. images. IEEE Trans. Med. Imaging 35, 1240–1251.

Pinto, A., Pereira, S., Correia, H., Oliveira, J., Rasteiro, D.M.L.D., Silva, C.A., 2015. Brain tumor segmentation based on extremely randomized forest with high-level features. In: 2015 37th Annual International Conference of the IEEE Engineering in Medicine and Biology Society (E.M.B.C.), pp. 3037–3040.

Razzak, M.I., Naz, S., Zaib, A., 2018. Deep learning for medical image processing: overview, challenges and the future. In: Classification in BioApps, pp. 323–350.

Ronneberger, O., Fischer, P., Brox, T., 2015. U-net: convolutional networks for biomedical image segmentation. In: International Conference on Medical Image Computing and Computer-Assisted Intervention, pp. 234–241.

Sarraf, S., Tofigh, G., 2016. Deep learning-based pipeline to recognize Alzheimer's disease using fMRI data. FTC 2016—Future Technologies Conference 20166-7, December 2016.

Shen, D., Wu, G., Suk, H.I., 2017. Deep learning in medical image analysis. Annu. Rev. Biomed. Eng. 19, 221–248.

Smith, S.M., 2002. Fast robust automated brain extraction. Hum. Brain Mapp. 17 (3), 143–155.

Vaidhya, K., et al., 2015. Multi-modal brain tumor segmentation using stacked denoising autoencoders. In: BrainLes 2015.

Vovk, U., Pernus, F., Likar, B., 2007. A. review of methods for correction of intensity inhomogeneity in M.R.I. IEEE Trans. Med. Imaging 26 (3), 405–421.

Wang, G., et al., 2017. Automatic brain tumor segmentation using cascaded anisotropic convolutional neural networks. In: International MICCAI Brainlesion Workshop.

Wang, G., Li, W., Ourselin, S.'e., Vercauteren, T., 2018. Automatic Brain Tumor Segmentation Using Cascaded Anisotropic Convolutional Neural Networks, volume 10670 LNCS of Lecture Notes in Computer Science. pp. 178–190.

Wang, C., et al., 2019. Pulmonary Image Classification Based on Inception-v3 Transfer Learning Model. IEEE Access 7, 146533–146541.

Xian, M., Zhang, Y., Cheng, H.-D., Xu, F., Zhang, B., Ding, J., 2018. Automatic breast ultrasound image segmentation: a survey. Pattern Recogn. 79, 340–355.

Zhou, T., 2019. A review: deep learning for medical image segmentation using multi-modality fusion. Array 3, 100004.

Zhou, X.-Y., 2020. ACNN: a Full Resolution DCNN for Medical Image Segmentation. arXiv. 1901.09203v4.

# Machine learning in precision medicine

# 23

**Dipankar Sengupta**

*PGJCCR, Queens University Belfast, Belfast, United Kingdom*

## Chapter outline

## 1 Precision medicine

Sir William Osler described, "Variability is the law of life, and as no two faces are the same, so no two bodies are alike, and no two individuals react alike and behave alike under the abnormal conditions which we know as a disease" (Osler, 1903). This impeccably summarizes the challenge of understanding the overlaying mechanism for disease, its regulation, and treatment in medicine or associated sciences. Diseases like cancer involve complex underlying causes among the biological processes ranging from the molecular to the cellular level. These genetic variations may not always be one-to-one with the patient phenotype. Different genetic aberrations may result in similar or different phenotype, making it difficult to recognize the specific cause of the disease (Kim et al., 2016; Mardinoglu and Nielsen, 2012). Therefore, often a treatment used against a particular disease may not work on all the patients (Fig. 1).

In 1999, Francis Collins, one of the pioneers of the Human Genome Project, gave the foundation document for precision medicine (Collins, 1999). The following year, he briefed in a news conference, how the completion of the Human Genome Project is going to accelerate precision medicine leading to the complete transformation of therapeutic medicine (Wade, 2010). This gave the base concept for

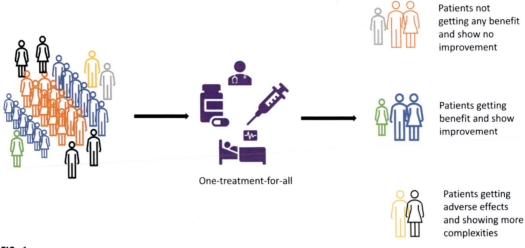

**FIG. 1**

Majority of the current treatment protocols follow one-treatment-for-all, i.e., the treatment is available for a standard patient based on the knowledge base of the particular disease. In this scenario, a few get the benefit, whereas there are sub-groups in the population who are not relieved or may have adverse side-effects.

improvising patient care, by planning the treatment based on the maximum information gained for a patient along with the existing knowledge base of the disease. In the last 20 years or so, the study of genomes and other omics disciplines (proteomics, metabolomics, transcriptomics, etc.) has rapidly advanced the scenario and is being routinely adapted along with the clinical examinations for decision-making.

Precision Medicine can be best described as "an emerging approach for disease treatment and prevention that takes into account individual variability in genes, environment, and lifestyle for each person" (Ashley, 2015; Collins and Varmus, 2015; Hodson, 2016). Besides the patient-doctor relationship being the core, the new biomedical information might add substantial information beyond the observable signs and symptoms (König et al., 2017). Thus, Precision Medicine implies the novelty of harnessing this wide array of patient's data, including clinical, poly-omics (genomic, transcriptomic, proteomic, metabolomic, epigenomic, etc.), and lifestyle information (Pinho, 2017) (Fig. 2). This gives the opportunity of identifying sub-populations who vary in their prognosis and treatment response, by understanding their difference in biology for that particular disease (Uddin et al., 2019).

The major contribution for this has been the rapid advancement of genomic and computational technologies, and with the costs of genetic tests plunging, the new targeted therapies are making it increasingly possible to prevent or treat illnesses based on an individual patient's characteristics (Love-Koh et al., 2018; Weil, 2018). It provides the opportunity to the clinicians, bioinformaticians, biomedicine, and associated researchers to develop new approaches for detection and diagnosis, prognosis, and other applications by analyzing a wide range of biomedical data—including molecular, genomic, cellular, clinical, behavioral, physiological, and environmental features. For example, in "precision oncology," i.e., precision medicine for cancer, a few of the obstacles currently been addressed are: the unexplained drug resistance observed in certain patient cohorts, genomic heterogeneity of tumor, risk assessment

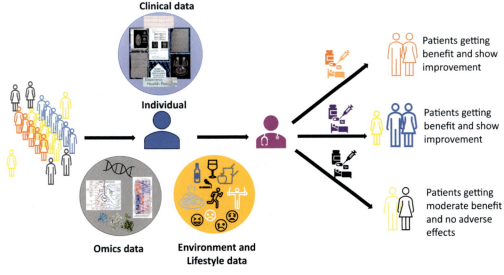

**FIG. 2**

Precision medicine aims to harness patient's clinical data along with the poly-omics, environment, and lifestyle data, to develop treatment strategies for the sub-cohorts, which benefits or has no adverse side-effects. The aim is to deliver the right treatment to a patient by identifying the differences in underlying biology.

and means for monitoring responses, tumor recurrence, and drug combinations to be used for treatment (Collins and Varmus, 2015).

Machine learning combines the strengths of computer science, mathematics, and statistics, providing the computational capabilities to learn from the data, and thus has the competency to provide a platform aiding precision medicine for learning from massive sets of clinical, poly-omics, and other datasets. Thus, in this chapter, we review and discuss the basic applications of machine learning on the heterogeneous datasets comprising poly-omics and clinical data, focusing on methods in use and its opportunities in precision medicine. In the following sections, firstly we discuss machine learning in brief; thereafter, the use of machine learning in precision medicine and along with discussing example applications showing its potential use in the detection and diagnosis, prognosis, therapy response, and in the discovery of new biomarkers and drug candidates; we conclude looking into the opportunities for addressing a few other challenges that can be addressed using precision medicine.

# 2 Machine learning

As modern computing evolved in the early part of the 20th century, the inception of "thinking machines" was aroused by the advent and evolution of the "electronic or digital computer" (Turing, 1950). The aim was to apply this computational capacity toward elucidating patterns and inferences from the dataset which is difficult to achieve by conventional statistical methods. In 1959, Arthur Samuel coined the term "Machine Learning," explaining how from a given set of minimum parameters a computer can be programmed, so that it will learn to play a better game of checkers in comparison to the humans (Samuel, 1959). Thereafter, since the 1960s, machine learning has been at the forefront, enabling learning from data. Furthermore, in the 1990s, Tom Mitchell explained, the focus for machine learning to be, "*developing a computer program, which is said to learn from experience* E *with respect to some class of tasks* T *and performance measure* P, *if its performance at tasks in* T, *as measured by* P, *improves with experience* E" (Mitchell, 1997). A simple example of this would be a computer program that could predict what kind of television program a person likes, based on the parameters like age, gender, occupation, and geographical location. Or based on customer's bank transaction history, a program could identify and/or predict fraudulent transactions. In both these scenarios, the computer program is considered to learn from the available data and its prediction performance improves as more data are made available to it.

Machine learning aims to provide learning algorithms (computer programs), which can be applied for analysis on the input data, for predicting the corresponding output values, identify patterns and trends within an acceptable performance range, and improvise based on experience (Fig. 3).

Depending on how the algorithm makes this learning, machine learning can be broadly categorized into supervised, unsupervised, and semisupervised learning (Ayodele, 2010; Brownlee, 2016; Maetschke et al., 2014). Supervised learning can be defined as learning a function, which given a sample of labeled data (i.e., data with known outputs), approximates a function that maps inputs to outputs (example—classification or regression-based learning) (Caruana et al., 2008; Caruana and Niculescu-Mizil, 2006). Unsupervised learning can be defined as learning a function in data that does not have any labeled outputs; therefore, it goals to infer the natural structure present within a set of data points [example—clustering learning] (Celebi and Aydin, 2016; Ghahramani, 2004). Whereas, in semisupervised learning, the learning can be defined as labeling the unlabeled data points using knowledge learned from a few labeled data points [example—reinforcement learning] (Sinha, 2014; Xu et al., 2012).

## 3 Machine learning in precision medicine

Technological advancements aiding the development of new omics-based diagnostics and therapeutics have the potential of creating the unprecedented ability for detection, prevention, treatment planning, and monitoring of diseases. Cancer is one such heterogeneous disease having complex biological relationships, involving key molecules across the omics space, some of which are uncharacterized while some have unknown context-specific functions. In almost all cancer types, the available treatments are beneficial only for a patient sub-population, whereas for others, it may have adverse effects, or no improvements are observed. Considering the genetic variations at the granularity of an individual can thereof help in a better understanding of the disease and lead in the facilitation of better patient management. Thus, the need for this hour is the technological interventions that can guide for individualized prevention diagnostics and therapeutics leading to improved outcomes for all.

In the last 15–20 years, with the completion of the Human Genome Project and advancement in omics-based technologies, the data have been ever-increasing. Like, the cancer genome atlas program, a joint initiative by National Cancer Institute, USA and the National Human Genome Research Institute, USA, which commenced in 2006, and over a period has generated ~2.5 PB (PetaBytes) of genomic, epigenomic, transcriptomic, proteomic, and clinical data for different cancer types. For clinical

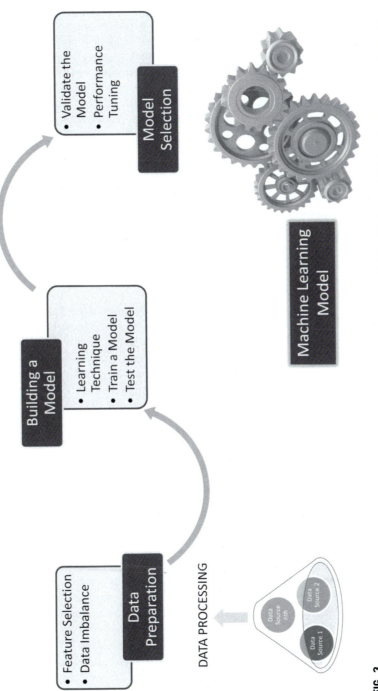

**FIG. 3**

Developing a machine learning model involves varied steps: data preparation (data cleaning, selection of features), build models using different learning techniques, validate and select a model by analyzing its performance on test dataset.

advancements and research objectives, the data in this program have been made publicly available via the genomics data portal [https://portal.gdc.cancer.gov/] that handles genomic, epigenomic, transcriptomic, and clinical data (Akbani et al., 2014; Liu et al., 2018; Weinstein et al., 2013); and the cancer proteome atlas portal [https://www.tcpaportal.org/], which manages the protein expression datasets (Li et al., 2013). This poly-omics data is complex in nature, and along with clinical data provides an opportunity for exploring new insights via data-driven approaches (Filipp, 2019). Learning from this data can have multifold applications in diagnostics, prognostics, and as well as the discovery of new biomarkers or drug candidates. Spurred by the advancement in computer technologies, machine learning for precision medicine has therefore been a growing area of interest (Handelman et al., 2018; Holzinger, 2014). Supporting these objectives are initiatives like Project Data Sphere [https://data.projectdatasphere.org/projectdatasphere/html/home], which is promoting the development of new cancer therapies by providing an open access data sharing platform for sharing and analysis of patient-level data, giving access to more than 150 datasets (Green et al., 2015; Hede, 2013). It also offers an opportunity to collaborate in research programs using machine learning and big data analytics for oncology (Fig. 4).

Machine learning can be used for analyzing the omics (genome, epigenome, transcriptome, proteome, metabolome, and microbiome) data together with the clinical data and prior knowledge, inferring relationships or finding patterns or deciphering causal associations, giving insight into pleiotropy, complex interactions, and context-specific behavior. The multidimensional poly-omics datasets along with the clinical and other relevant data can be trained using machine learning algorithms to find the relevant genotypic structures which could be subsequently mapped to the observed phenotype. This model may then be used for diagnostic (predict risk, stage of disease), prognostic (chances of the patient treated successfully), and other outcomes for individual patients based on their characteristics (Fig. 5).

In comparison to the current process of treatment based on the symptoms-based classification (Fig. 1), this would provide clinicians the opportunity to tailor-made interventions for patients (Fig. 2).

Globally, various research groups and companies like Google and IBM are already exploring the opportunities of machine learning-centered advances for precision medicine. And, of late, there have been ground-breaking studies describing these approaches illustrating exemplary outcomes, for example, the prognosis of lung cancer patients based on 9879 histopathological and image-based features, distinguishing short-term from long-term survivors (Yu et al., 2016). In further sub-sections, we embellish applications discussing machine learning in precision medicine for the detection and diagnosis, prognosis, and the discovery of new biomarkers and drug candidates.

## 3.1 Detection and diagnosis of a disease

In precision medicine, data heterogeneity forms a major challenge in the development of early diagnostic applications. This can be addressed with the aid of machine learning, as it assists in extracting relevant knowledge from clinical and omics-based datasets, like disease-specific clinical-molecular signatures or population-specific group patterns. One such explicatory example is the recent development of a classifier for predicting skin lesions (skin cancer) using a single CNN (convolutional neural network), with its competency comparable to a dermatologist (Esteva et al., 2017). Detection and diagnosis of any disease shapes the ground for clinicians to plan and provide a targeted treatment ensuring minimal/no side-effects, along with consideration of the patient's past clinical history and medications. In the past five years, numerous machine learning-based efforts have been made for a better understanding of diseases facilitating predictive diagnosis in cancer, cardiac arrhythmia,

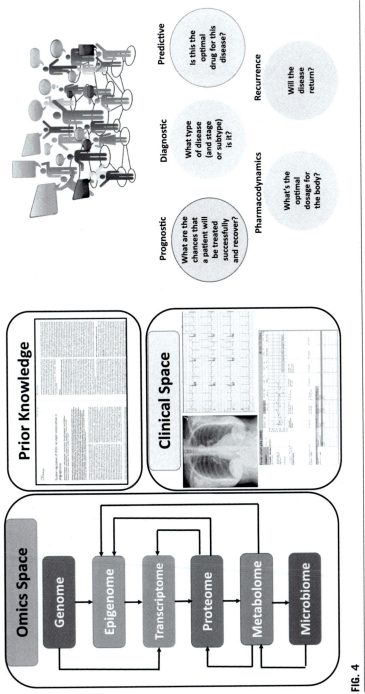

**FIG. 4**

Studying and analyzing the poly-omics data along with the clinical data and existing knowledge will help in better understanding of how a disease regulates in each patient. This would help in improvising the existing patient care and management facilities.

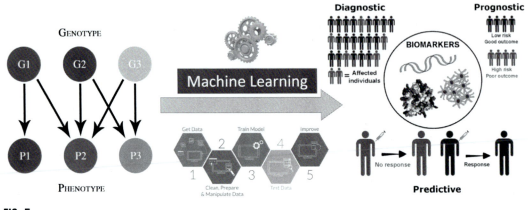

**FIG. 5**

Novel insights from the application of machine learning on poly-omics and clinical datasets may help bridging the genotype–phenotype relationships, like identification of novel biomarkers which can be used for either diagnostic, prognostic, or predictive purposes against a disease.

gastroenterology, ophthalmology, and other diseases. The genotype–phenotype associative analysis from this would help in translating the clinical management by early diagnosis and patient stratification, and thus, in the decision-making for selection among the available drug treatments, treatment alterations, and additionally in prognosis, providing personalized care to each patient.

In the past two decades, omics-based technologies have remarkably advanced, which is making a tremendous impact on a better understanding of complex diseases, like cancer. And with the growing data complexity, machine learning is helping to get insights, which help in the development of computational tools for early diagnosis for different cancer types. As in diseases like cancer, an early diagnosis ensures higher chances of survival for a patient. Leukemia, an hematological malignancy, has a high occurrence and prevalence rate, with its early diagnosis being a key challenge. To address this, diagnostic applications have been developed, which are based on CNN, SVM (support vector machines), hybrid hierarchical classifiers, and other pattern-based approaches (Salah et al., 2019). Similar studies have explored different supervised machine learning approaches being used for breast cancer diagnosis, primarily based on histopathological images and mammograms (Gardezi et al., 2019; Yassin et al., 2018). Also, there have been population-specific diagnostic predictors developed, considering the genetic and physiological differences amidst the human ethnicities. Like, models based on SVM, Least Squares Support Vector Machine (LS-SVM), Artificial Neural Network (ANN), and Random Forest (RF) to detect prostate cancer in Chinese populations using the prebiopsy data (Wang et al., 2018).

## 3.2 Prognosis of a disease

Disease prognosis can only be performed after a medical diagnosis had been made. And it primarily focuses on the prediction of susceptibility, i.e., risk assessment, recurrence, and survival of a patient against a particular disease. In terms of machine learning, susceptibility can be defined as the challenge for predicting the likelihood of developing a disease prior to its occurrence; while, recurrence is predicting the likelihood of regenerating the disease later to a treatment; and, survival is trying to predict an outcome postdiagnosis in terms of life expectancy, survivability, and disease progression. To address these challenges, prognostic prediction(s) need to consider factors besides the clinical diagnosis. For example, in cancer, a prognosis usually involves varied subsets of biomarkers along with the clinical factors, including the age and the general health of the patient, the location and type of cancer, as well as the grade and size of the tumor. Combining the genetic factors like somatic mutations in carcinoma genes, expression of specific tumor proteins, the environment of tumor cells with the clinical data, increases the robustness of cancer prognoses predictions (Cochran, 1997; Edge and Compton, 2010; Fielding et al., 1992; Gress et al., 2017). In 2016, the American Joint Committee on Cancer (AJCC) identified the need for personalized probabilistic predictions and therefore described the necessary characteristics and thus setting guidelines that shall help in developing prognostic applications (Kattan et al., 2016).

The majority of machine learning built prognostic applications use supervised learning, which is based on conditional probabilities. Cruz and Wishart have well investigated the different machine learning methods used in cancer prognosis (Cruz and Wishart, 2006). In general, artificial neural networks (Rumelhart et al., 1986), decision trees (Quinlan, 1986), genetic algorithms (Sastry et al., 2005), linear discriminant analysis (Duda et al., 2001), and nearest neighbor algorithms (Barber and Barber, 2012) have been the most frequently used algorithms for the aforesaid purpose. However, pertaining to a particular cancer type, the diagnostic accuracy of such models is important for its adoption under clinical settings. Like, a meta-analysis study performed to determine the diagnostic accuracy of machine learning algorithms for breast cancer risk prognosis showed an SVM-based model to be the best performing one (Nindrea et al., 2018).

In recent years, deep learning has demonstrated to be an effective method for illuminating novel findings from heterogeneous datasets. DeepSurv, a deep learning-based framework along with the state-of-the-art Cox survival method, designed for modeling interactions between a patient's covariates and treatment effectiveness, is been used for treatment recommendations (Katzman et al., 2018). Using a similar combination of an algorithm, GDP (Group lass regularized Deep learning for cancer Prognosis) was developed, which uses clinical and poly-omics data for survival prediction (Xie et al., 2019). One of the recent studies demonstrated the significance of genetic factors in prognosis (Ming et al., 2019). It showed a remarkable difference in the predictive accuracy for risk prognosis in breast cancer among geographically distinguishing populations. For the US-based population, a combination of adaptive boosting with random forest gave the best performance, in comparison to the Swiss-based population, for whom it was adaptive boosting with Markov chain Monte Carlo generalized linear mixed model.

## 3.3 Discovery of biomarkers and drug candidates

Definition of biomarker has evolved with time, and it may be best defined as "characteristic that is objectively measured and evaluated as an indicator of normal biological processes, pathogenic processes, or pharmacological responses to a therapeutic intervention" (Atkinson et al., 2001). Pertaining to healthcare, the development and use of biomarkers have primarily wedged varied aspects to diseases and corresponding patients. Therefore, the role of biomarkers in the development of precision medicine provides a strategic opportunity for technological developments to improve healthcare (Slikker, 2018).

Machine learning in these multidimensional data settings can accelerate the early stages of the bio-marker discovery process, inform the development of biomarker-driven therapeutic strategies, and give insights to enable better planning of patient treatment pathways. Translating candidate biomarkers into clinical applications is laborious with a high attrition rate and is very costly. A study by the pharmaceutical and diagnostic industry experts suggests an average of $100 M is being spent on developing and commercialization of new biomarker-based technology, with 55% of the amount being used in the initial phases associated with candidate identification, development, and validation (Graaf et al., 2018). Therefore, selecting the right candidate biomarker is of utmost importance, that has the best chance of successful adoption in the clinical setting.

In the last 5–10 years, many of the cancer clinical studies have tried exploring biomarkers discovery with the intra- and inter-tumor heterogeneity, as well as clonal and sub-clonal evolution in response to different treatments via tumor samples, to devise novel individualized and adaptive management strategies (Collins et al., 2017). Like, in lung cancer, attempts for identification of biomarkers by integrating different types of molecules into a biomarker panel along with the patient clinical data, to differentiate lung nodules into noncancer/cancer with poor survival probability and cancer with higher survival probability subtypes (Vargas and Harris, 2016). Besides, there also have been studies investigating tissue-specific biomarkers of human muscles with an age prediction task using Elastic-Net, Support Vector Machines, k-Nearest Neighbors, Random Forests, and feed-forward neural networks (Mamoshina et al., 2018).

This process may also support drug discovery, as it could help to identify endotypes, i.e., patients having the same underlying cause for a disease. The process benefits by leveraging the available vast-collection of patient-level data, gaining the knowledge from advanced poly-omics analysis and thus, reducing the need for wet-lab experiments. The key feature is capturing the patient heterogeneity along with the underlying biology leading to patient stratification. This provides an opportunity for early identification of responder patients, helping in the designing of effective clinical trials. Overall, this would help to reduce the patient attrition rate, especially in the stages of phase 2 and 3 trials. Companies like Deep Genomics (a Canada based start-up) has already begun developing platforms using machine learning to lessen the amount of costly trial and error in drug discovery (Home | Deep Genomics, n.d.).

## 4 Future opportunities

Application of machine learning in precision medicine presents the distinctive challenges of having clinical interpretability of a model for its adoption under clinical settings. Computationally, this provides a unique research challenge of forming a balance in-between the performance and interpretability of the model as well as the results. For example, a deep learning model may effectively be able to identify a diseased from a healthy person, but clinically it will be imperative to know, based on what features or parameters, these predictions are been made and why.

Also, based on what is known about precision medicine, it is clear that for tailoring patient care, the domain needs to explore varied data dimensionalities. This depends on multiple factors including clinical (patient history, observed features, diagnostic measures, etc.), genetic (genome, proteome, metabolome, etc.), and, less clear nevertheless to be studied in-depth, wellness (behavior, emotional problems, stress, social support, etc.) along with the lifestyle and environmental factors (smoking, alcohol, drugs, malnutrition, etc.). These additional factors may assist in understanding, why some

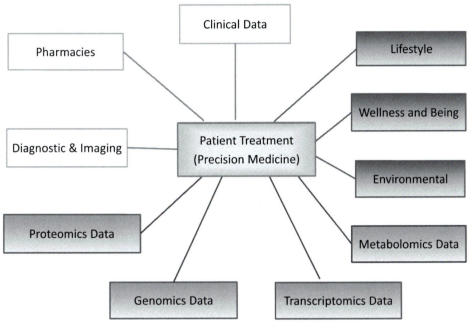

**FIG. 6**

Precision medicine targets to bring together different data types of an individual with the aim of providing better patient care facilities. The treatment can be thus planned based on a patient's detailed history which includes the clinical, genetic, as well as the information coming from his/her lifestyle, wellbeing, and environmental factors an individual is exposed to (pre- and postnatal).

people even with a disease genotype do not develop a disease or why a sub-group shows a healthier prognosis. The role of a few factors like smoking (active and passive) are well-established with triggering, expression, and progression of cancer, cardiovascular, or other diseases. Nevertheless can emotions like "happiness or hope" be also playing a role, which can be associated with the genetic or clinical expression of a disease? Only time and further research in this domain may probably answer such questions but for sure it gives an opportunity for an integrative approach to explore and analyze these data dimensionalities (Fig. 6).

# 5 Conclusions

By the advancements made in computational power, theoretical understanding, and an ever-increasing amount of data, the last decade has witnessed widespread applications of machine learning in every major field of human society, including medicine and healthcare. In the 21st century, heterogeneous and complex diseases like cancer, cardiovascular, and rare genetic disorders are some major and pressing medical problems. The holistic approach offered by precision medicine will likely become increasingly important in order to provide effective treatment and management strategies for such diseases. Machine learning is currently a vital tool in precision medicine and is almost certain to remain so in the future. It can effectively handle the massive poly-omics datasets and aid to solve a number of analytical problems within precision medicine and in numerous ways better than historically conventional statistical methods. As discussed in this chapter, the state-of-the-art algorithms and analytical techniques offered by machine learning have shown a wide range of applications in precision medicine. Machine learning thus presently offers a diverse and effective tool set for precision medicine research; a tool set that will grow and improve in the future.

# References

Akbani, R., Ng, P.K.S., Werner, H.M.J., Shahmoradgoli, M., Zhang, F., Ju, Z., Liu, W., Yang, J.Y., Yoshihara, K., Li, J., Ling, S., Seviour, E.G., Ram, P.T., Minna, J.D., Diao, L., Tong, P., Heymach, J.V., Hill, S.M., Dondelinger, F., Städler, N., Byers, L.A., Meric-Bernstam, F., Weinstein, J.N., Broom, B.M., Verhaak, R.G.W., Liang, H., Mukherjee, S., Lu, Y., Mills, G.B., 2014. A pan-cancer proteomic perspective on the cancer genome atlas. Nat. Commun. https://doi.org/10.1038/ncomms4887.

Ashley, E.A., 2015. The precision medicine initiative: a new national effort. JAMA 313, 2119–2120. https://doi.org/10.1001/jama.2015.3595.

Atkinson, A.J., Colburn, W.A., DeGruttola, V.G., DeMets, D.L., Downing, G.J., Hoth, D.F., Oates, J.A., Peck, C.C., Schooley, R.T., Spilker, B.A., Woodcock, J., Zeger, S.L., 2001. Biomarkers and surrogate endpoints: preferred definitions and conceptual framework. Clin. Pharmacol. Ther. https://doi.org/10.1067/mcp.2001.113989.

Ayodele, T.O., 2010. Types of machine learning algorithms. New Adv. Mach. Learn. https://doi.org/10.5772/56672.

Barber, D., Barber, D., 2012. Nearest neighbour classification. In: Bayesian Reasoning and Machine Learning., https://doi.org/10.1017/cbo9780511804779.019.

Brownlee, J., 2016. Supervised and Unsupervised Machine Learning Algorithms. Understand Mach. Learn. Algorithms.

Caruana, R., Niculescu-Mizil, A., 2006. An empirical comparison of supervised learning algorithms. In: ACM International Conference Proceeding Series., https://doi.org/10.1145/1143844.1143865.

Caruana, R., Karampatziakis, N., Yessenalina, A., 2008. An empirical evaluation of supervised learning in high dimensions. In: Proceedings of the 25th International Conference on Machine Learning., https://doi.org/10.1145/1390156.1390169.

Celebi, M.E., Aydin, K., 2016. Unsupervised learning algorithms. In: Unsupervised Learning Algorithms., https://doi.org/10.1007/978-3-319-24211-8.

Cochran, A.J., 1997. Prediction of outcome for patients with cutaneous melanoma. Pigment Cell Res. https://doi.org/10.1111/j.1600-0749.1997.tb00479.x.

Collins, F.S., 1999. Medical and societal consequences of the human genome project. N. Engl. J. Med. 341, 28–37. https://doi.org/10.1056/NEJM199907013410106.

Collins, F.S., Varmus, H., 2015. A new initiative on precision medicine. N. Engl. J. Med. 372, 793–795. https://doi.org/10.1056/NEJMp1500523.

Collins, D.C., Sundar, R., Lim, J.S.J., Yap, T.A., 2017. Towards precision medicine in the clinic: from biomarker discovery to novel therapeutics. Trends Pharmacol. Sci. 38, 25–40. https://doi.org/10.1016/j.tips.2016.10.012.

Cruz, J.A., Wishart, D.S., 2006. Applications of machine learning in cancer prediction and prognosis. Cancer Informat. 2. https://doi.org/10.1177/117693510600200030. 117693510600200.

Duda, R.O., Hart, P.E., Stork, D.G., 2001. Pattern Classification. John Wiley, Sect, New York.

Edge, S.B., Compton, C.C., 2010. The American joint committee on cancer: the 7th edition of the AJCC cancer staging manual and the future of TNM. Ann. Surg. Oncol. https://doi.org/10.1245/s10434-010-0985-4.

Esteva, A., Kuprel, B., Novoa, R.A., Ko, J., Swetter, S.M., Blau, H.M., Thrun, S., 2017. Dermatologist-level classification of skin cancer with deep neural networks. Nature 542, 115–118. https://doi.org/10.1038/nature21056.

Fielding, L.P., Fenoglio-Preiser, C.M., Freedman, L.S., 1992. The future of prognostic factors in outcome prediction for patients with cancer. Cancer. https://doi.org/10.1002/1097-0142(19921101)70:9<2367::AID-CNCR2820700927>3.0.CO;2-B.

Filipp, F.V., 2019. Opportunities for artificial intelligence in advancing precision medicine. Curr. Genet. Med. Rep. 7, 208–213. https://doi.org/10.1007/s40142-019-00177-4.

Gardezi, S.J.S., Elazab, A., Lei, B., Wang, T., 2019. Breast cancer detection and diagnosis using mammographic data: systematic review. J. Med. Internet Res. https://doi.org/10.2196/14464.

Ghahramani, Z., 2004. Unsupervised learning. Lect. Notes Comput. Sci. https://doi.org/10.1007/978-3-540-28650-9_5 (including Subser. Lect. Notes Artif. Intell. Lect. Notes bioinformatics).

Graaf, G., Postmus, D., Westerink, J., Buskens, E., 2018. The early economic evaluation of novel biomarkers to accelerate their translation into clinical applications. Cost Eff. Resour. Alloc. 16. https://doi.org/10.1186/s12962-018-0105-z.

Green, A.K., Reeder-Hayes, K.E., Corty, R.W., Basch, E., Milowsky, M.I., Dusetzina, S.B., Bennett, A.V., Wood, W.A., 2015. The project data sphere initiative: accelerating cancer research by sharing data. Oncologist. https://doi.org/10.1634/theoncologist.2014-0431.

Gress, D.M., Edge, S.B., Greene, F.L., Washington, M.K., Asare, E.A., Brierley, J.D., Byrd, D.R., Compton, C.C., Jessup, J.M., Winchester, D.P., Amin, M.B., Gershenwald, J.E., 2017. Principles of Cancer Staging., https://doi.org/10.1007/978-3-319-40618-3_1.

Handelman, G.S., Kok, H.K., Chandra, R.V., Razavi, A.H., Lee, M.J., Asadi, H., 2018. eDoctor: machine learning and the future of medicine. J. Intern. Med. 284, 603–619. https://doi.org/10.1111/joim.12822.

Hede, K., 2013. Project data sphere to make cancer clinical trial data publicly available. J. Natl. Cancer Inst. https://doi.org/10.1093/jnci/djt232.

Hodson, R., 2016. Precision medicine. Nature. https://doi.org/10.1038/537S49a.

Holzinger, A., 2014. Trends in interactive knowledge discovery for personalized medicine: cognitive science meets machine learning. IEEE Intell. Inf. Bull. 15, 6–14.

Home | Deep Genomics WWW Document, n.d. URL https://www.deepgenomics.com (Accessed 25 July 2020).

Kattan, M.W., Hess, K.R., Amin, M.B., Lu, Y., Moons, K.G.M., Gershenwald, J.E., Gimotty, P.A., Guinney, J.H., Halabi, S., Lazar, A.J., Mahar, A.L., Patel, T., Sargent, D.J., Weiser, M.R., Compton, C., 2016. American joint committee on Cancer acceptance criteria for inclusion of risk models for individualized prognosis in the practice of precision medicine. CA Cancer J. Clin. 66, 370–374. https://doi.org/10.3322/caac.21339.

Katzman, J.L., Shaham, U., Cloninger, A., Bates, J., Jiang, T., Kluger, Y., 2018. DeepSurv: Personalized treatment recommender system using a Cox proportional hazards deep neural network. BMC Med. Res. Methodol., 18. https://doi.org/10.1186/s12874-018-0482-1.

Kim, Y.A., Cho, D.Y., Przytycka, T.M., 2016. Understanding genotype-phenotype effects in Cancer via network approaches. PLoS Comput. Biol. 12. https://doi.org/10.1371/journal.pcbi.1004747.

König, I.R., Fuchs, O., Hansen, G., von Mutius, E., Kopp, M.V., 2017. What is precision medicine? Eur. Respir. J. https://doi.org/10.1183/13993003.00391-2017.

Li, J., Lu, Y., Akbani, R., Ju, Z., Roebuck, P.L., Liu, W., Yang, J.-Y., Broom, B.M., Verhaak, R.G.W., Kane, D.W., Wakefield, C., Weinstein, J.N., Mills, G.B., Liang, H., 2013. TCPA: a resource for cancer functional proteomics data. Nat. Methods. https://doi.org/10.1038/nmeth.2650.

Liu, J., et al., 2018. An integrated TCGA pan-Cancer clinical data resource to drive high-quality survival outcome analytics. Cell. https://doi.org/10.1016/j.cell.2018.02.052.

Love-Koh, J., Peel, A., Rejon-Parrilla, J.C., Ennis, K., Lovett, R., Manca, A., Chalkidou, A., Wood, H., Taylor, M., 2018. The future of precision medicine: potential impacts for health technology assessment. Pharmacoeconomics 36, 1439–1451. https://doi.org/10.1007/s40273-018-0686-6.

Maetschke, S.R., Madhamshettiwar, P.B., Davis, M.J., Ragan, M.A., 2014. Supervised, semi-supervised and unsupervised inference of gene regulatory networks. Brief. Bioinform. https://doi.org/10.1093/bib/bbt034.

Mamoshina, P., Volosnikova, M., Ozerov, I.V., Putin, E., Skibina, E., Cortese, F., Zhavoronkov, A., 2018. Machine learning on human muscle Transcriptomic data for biomarker discovery and tissue-specific drug target identification. Front. Genet. 9, 242. https://doi.org/10.3389/fgene.2018.00242.

Mardinoglu, A., Nielsen, J., 2012. Systems medicine and metabolic modelling, J. Intern. Med. John Wiley & Sons, Ltd, pp. 142–154. doi:https://doi.org/10.1111/j.1365-2796.2011.02493.x.

Ming, C., Viassolo, V., Probst-Hensch, N., Chappuis, P.O., Dinov, I.D., Katapodi, M.C., 2019. Machine learning techniques for personalized breast cancer risk prediction: Comparison with the BCRAT and BOADICEA models. Breast Cancer Res. 21. https://doi.org/10.1186/s13058-019-1158-4.

Mitchell, T.M., 1997. Machine Learning, McGraw-Hill Science/Engineering/Math. McGraw-Hill Science/Engineering/Math.

Nindrea, R.D., Aryandono, T., Lazuardi, L., Dwiprahasto, I., 2018. Diagnostic accuracy of different machine learning algorithms for breast cancer risk calculation: a meta-analysis. Asian Pac. J. Cancer Prev. https://doi.org/10.22034/APJCP.2018.19.7.1747.

Osler, W., 1903. On the educational value of the medical society. Boston Med. Surg. J. https://doi.org/10.1056/nejm190303121481101.

Pinho, J.R.R., 2017. Precision Medicine. 15 Einstein, Sao Paulo, pp. VII–X, https://doi.org/10.1590/S1679-45082017ED4016.

Quinlan, J.R., 1986. Induction of decision trees. Mach. Learn. 1, 81–106.

Rumelhart, D.E., Hinton, G.E., Williams, R.J., 1986. Learning representations by back-propagating errors. Nature 323, 533–536. https://doi.org/10.1038/323533a0.

Salah, H.T., Muhsen, I.N., Salama, M.E., Owaidah, T., Hashmi, S.K., 2019. Machine learning applications in the diagnosis of leukemia: current trends and future directions. Int. J. Lab. Hematol. 41, 717–725. https://doi.org/10.1111/ijlh.13089.

Samuel, A.L., 1959. Some studies in machine learning using the game of checkers. IBM J. Res. Dev. 3 (3), 210–229.

Sastry, K., Goldberg, D., Kendall, G., 2005. Genetic algorithms. In: Search Methodologies: Introductory Tutorials in Optimization and Decision Support Techniques. Springer, US, pp. 97–125, https://doi.org/10.1007/0-387-28356-0_4.

Sinha, K., 2014. Semi-supervised learning. In: Data Classification: Algorithms and Applications., https://doi.org/10.1201/b17320.

Slikker, W., 2018. Biomarkers and their impact on precision medicine. Exp. Biol. Med. 243, 211–212. https://doi.org/10.1177/1535370217733426.

Turing, A.M., 1950. Computing machinery and intelligence. Mind LIX, 433–460. https://doi.org/10.1093/MIND.

Uddin, M., Wang, Y., Woodbury-Smith, M., 2019. Artificial intelligence for precision medicine in neurodevelopmental disorders. NPJ Digital Med. 2, 1–10. https://doi.org/10.1038/s41746-019-0191-0.

Vargas, A.J., Harris, C.C., 2016. Biomarker development in the precision medicine era: lung cancer as a case study. Nat. Rev. Cancer 16, 525–537. https://doi.org/10.1038/nrc.2016.56.

Wade, N., 2010. A Decade Later, Human Genome Project Yields Few New Cures—The New York Times. The New York Times.

Wang, G., Teoh, J.Y.C., Choi, K.S., 2018. Diagnosis of prostate cancer in a Chinese population by using machine learning methods. In: Proceedings of the Annual International Conference of the IEEE Engineering in

Medicine and Biology Society, EMBS. Institute of Electrical and Electronics Engineers Inc, pp. 1–4, https://doi.org/10.1109/EMBC.2018.8513365.

Weil, A.R., 2018. Precision medicine. Health Aff. https://doi.org/10.1377/hlthaff.2018.0520.

Weinstein, J.N., et al., 2013. The cancer genome atlas pan-cancer analysis project. Nat. Genet. https://doi.org/10.1038/ng.2764.

Xie, G., Dong, C., Kong, Y., Zhong, J.F., Li, M., Wang, K., 2019. Group lasso regularized deep learning for cancer prognosis from multi-omics and clinical features. Genes (Basel) 10. https://doi.org/10.3390/genes10030240.

Xu, Z., Mo, M., King, I., 2012. Semi-Supervised learning. In: Computational Intelligence., https://doi.org/10.4018/978-1-60566-010-3.ch272.

Yassin, N.I.R., Omran, S., El Houby, E.M.F., Allam, H., 2018. Machine learning techniques for breast cancer computer aided diagnosis using different image modalities: a systematic review. Comput. Methods Programs Biomed. https://doi.org/10.1016/j.cmpb.2017.12.012.

Yu, K.H., Zhang, C., Berry, G.J., Altman, R.B., Ré, C., Rubin, D.L., Snyder, M., 2016. Predicting non-small cell lung cancer prognosis by fully automated microscopic pathology image features. Nat. Commun. 7, 1–10. https://doi.org/10.1038/ncomms12474.

# Index

Note: Page numbers followed by *f* indicate figures, *t* indicate tables, and *b* indicate boxes.